The ACP Handbook of
Women's Health

Rose S. Fife, MD, MPH
Sarina B. Schrager, MD, MS

ACP
PRESS.

AMERICAN COLLEGE OF PHYSICIANS   PHILADELPHIA

Associate Publisher and Manager, Books Publishing: Tom Hartman
Director, Editorial Production: Linda Drumheller
Editorial Coordinator: Angela Gabella
Cover Design: Lisa Torrieri
Index: Nelle Garrecht

Printed in the United States of America
Printing/binding by Versa Press
Composition by SPi

ISBN: 978-1-934465-10-3

09 10 11 12 13 / 10 9 8 7 6 5 4 3 2 1

The ACP Handbook of

Women's Health

Contributors

Sabina Agrawal, DO
Staff Physician
William S. Middleton Memorial
    VA Medical Center
Clinical Assistant Professor
University of Wisconsin
    School of Medicine and Public
    Health
Madison, Wisconsin

Rebecca Austin, MD, FAAP
Mercy Health System
Family Medicine Residency
    Program
Janesville, Wisconsin

Kimberly A. Bauer, MD
Clinical Research Fellow
Department of Dermatology
Northwestern University
    Feinberg School of Medicine
Chicago, Illinois

Jonathan Benson, MD
Indiana University School of
    Medicine
Indianapolis, Indiana

Kenneth Berman, MD
Fellow, Gastroenterology
Indiana University School
    of Medicine
Indianapolis, Indiana

Carolina Bruno, MD
Department of Medicine
Indiana University School of
    Medicine
Indianapolis, Indiana

E. Diana Burtea, MD
Program Director
Family Medicine Residency
Community Health Network
Indianapolis, Indiana

Anjali Butani, MD
Procedural Dermatology
    Fellow
Department of Dermatology
Northwestern University
    Feinberg School of Medicine
Chicago, Illinois

Melissa K. Cavaghan, MD
Assistant Professor of Clinical
    Medicine
Indiana University School of
    Medicine
Indianapolis, Indiana

Suparna M. Chhibber, MD
Faculty
San Jacinto Methodist Family
    Medicine Residency
Baytown, Texas

Shannon Connolly, BA
Medical Student
University of Southern
    California Keck School of
    Medicine

Robert V. Considine, PhD
Professor of Medicine
Indiana University School of
    Medicine
Indiana University
Indianapolis, Indiana

Lee T. Dresang, MD
Associate Professor of Family
  Medicine
University of Wisconsin
  School of Medicine and Public
  Health
Madison, Wisconsin

Deborah Dreyfus, MD
Department of Family Medicine
University of Wisconsin
  School of Medicine and Public
  Health
Madison, Wisconsin

James Edmondson
Professor of Medicine Emeritus
Indiana University School of
  Medicine
Indianapolis, Indiana

**Marguerite Elliott, DO, MS,
  FAAP**
Associate Professor
University of Wisconsin School of
  Medicine
Madison, Wisconsin

Ann Evensen, MD
Assistant Professor
Department of Family
  Medicine
University of Wisconsin
Madison, Wisconsin

Hala Fatima, MD
Assistant Professor of Medicine
Indiana University School of
  Medicine
Indianapolis, Indiana

Joanna R. Fields, MD
Indiana University School of
  Medicine
Indianapolis, Indiana

Rose S. Fife, MD, MPH
Associate Dean for Research
Barbara F. Kampen Professor of
  Women's Health
Professor of Medicine and
  Biochemistry and Molecular
  Biology
Adjunct Professor of Pediatrics
Indiana University School of
  Medicine
Indianapolis, Indiana

Charles C. Flippen II, MD
Associate Professor
David Geffen School of Medicine,
  UCLA
Sylmar, California

Sarah Fox, MD
Academic Fellow
Department of Family Medicine
University of Wisconsin
Madison, Wisconsin

Jennifer Frank, MD, FAAFP
Assistant Professor of Family
  Medicine
University of Wisconsin
  School of Medicine
  and Public Health
Appleton, Wisconsin

Howard K. Gershenfeld, MD, PhD
Associate Professor of Psychiatry,
  Integrative Biology and
  Psychology
University of Texas Medical
  Center Southwestern
Staff Psychiatrist
Zale-Lipshy University Hospital
Dallas, Texas

Andrew Goddard, MD
Professor of Psychiatry
Indiana University School of
  Medicine
Indianapolis, Indiana

Marji Gold, MD
Professor of Family and Social
    Medicine
Albert Einstein College of
    Medicine
Bronx, New York, New York

Rafael Grau, MD
Associate Professor of Clinical
    Medicine
Director, Division of Rheumatology
Indiana University School of
    Medicine
Indianapolis, Indiana

Judith A. Gravdal, MD
Professor and Chair Department of
    Family and Preventive Medicine
Rosalind Franklin University of
    Science and Medicine
The Chicago Medical School
Morris M. Goldberg Chair of
    Family Medicine
Advocate Lutheran General
    Hospital
Park Ridge, Illinois

Teri Greco, MD, MSc
Instructor in Medicine Brigham
    and Women's Hospital
Harvard Medical School
Fish Center for Women's Health
Chestnut Hill, Massachusetts

Amy Groff, DO
Academic Fellow
Department of Family Medicine
University of Wisconsin
Madison, Wisconsin

Rose M. Guilbe, MD
Assistant Professor of Family and
    Social Medicine
Albert Einstein College of
    Medicine Montefiore Medical
    Center
Bronx, New York

Joan E. Hamblin, MD
UW Health/Eau Claire Family
    Medicine
Associate Professor of Family
    Medicine
University of Wisconsin
    School of Medicine and Public
    Health
Madison, Wisconsin

Nasser Hanna, MD
Associate Professor of Medicine
Melvin and Bren Simon Cancer
    Center
Indiana University School of
    Medicine
Indianapolis, Indiana

Marissa Harris, MD
Clinical Instructor
Albert Einstein College of
    Medicine
Bronx, New York, New York

Debra Helper, MD
Associate Professor of Clinical
    Medicine
Indiana University School of
    Medicine
Indianapolis, Indiana

Julie Howard, MD
Faculty, Glendale Adventist
    Family Medicine
Glendale, California

Richard H. Huggins, MD
Clinical Research Fellow
Northwestern University
    Feinberg School of Medicine
Chicago, Illinois

Emily Jackson, MD
Clinical Instructor
Albert Einstein College of
    Medicine
Bronx, New York, New York

Shadia Jalal, MD
Hematology-Oncology Fellow
Indiana University School of
    Medicine
Indianapolis, Indiana

Jessica Johnston, MD
Resident Physician in Family
    Medicine
Fox Valley Family Medicine
    Residency Program
Appleton, Wisconsin

Rattan Juneja, MBBS, MD, MRCP
Associate Professor of Clinical
    Medicine
Indiana University School of
    Medicine
Medical Director
Clarian Diabetes Center—Indiana
    University
Indianapolis, Indiana

Anna Kaminski, MD, MS
Associate Medical Director
Planned Parenthood of Western
    Washington
Seattle, Washington

Mollie L. Kane, MD, MPH
Assistant Professor of Pediatrics
University of Wisconsin School of
    Medicine and Public Health
Department of Pediatrics
Madison, Wisconsin

Kari Kindschi, MD
Resident Physician in Family
    Medicine
University of Wisconsin
    Department of Family Medicine
Madison Residency Program

Kala Kluender
University of Wisconsin
Madison, Wisconsin

Raufu A. Lasisi, MD
Resident
Indiana University School of Medicine
Indianapolis, Indiana

Antoinette L. Laskey, MD, MPH
Assistant Professor of Pediatrics
Indiana University School of
    Medicine
Riley Hospital for Children
Indianapolis, Indiana

Tara D. Lathcop, MD
Community Preceptor
Alaska Family Medicine Residency
Anchorage, Alaska

Julia K. LeBlanc, MD
Assistant Professor of Medicine
Indiana University School of
    Medicine
Indianapolis, Indiana

Ruth Lesnewski, MS, MD
Assistant Professor of Family
    Medicine
Albert Einstein College of Medicine
Bronx, New York

Radha Lewis, MD
Family Planning Fellow
Women's & Children's Hospital
Los Angeles County and University
    of Southern California
Los Angeles, California

Jeffrey Lightfoot, MD
Psychiatry Department
Indiana University School of
    Medicine
Indianapolis, Indiana

Theodore Logan, MD
Associate Professor of Clinical
    Medicine
Indiana University School of
    Medicine
Indianapolis, Indiana

Anne-Marie Lozeau, MD, MS
Assistant Professor
University of Wisconsin School of
    Medicine and Public Health
Madison, Wisconsin

Helen Luce, DO
Department of Family Medicine
University of Wisconsin
Wausau, Wisconsin

Honor MacNaughton, MD
Attending Physician
Reproductive Health Advocacy
    Fellow
Institute for Urban Family Health
New York, New York

Katherine L. Margo, MD
Director of Student Programs
Department of Family Medicine
    and Community Health
University of Pennsylvania School
    of Medicine
Philadelphia, Pennsylvania

Lawrence A. Mark, MD, PhD
Indiana University School of
    Medicine
Indiana University Melvin and
    Bren Simon Cancer Center
Indianapolis, Indiana

David H. Mattson, MD, PhD
Professor of Neurology
Indiana University School of
    Medicine
Indianapolis, Indiana

Rosalilia Mendoza, BA
University of Wisconsin
Madison, Wisconsin

Laurel C. Milberg, PhD
Associate Professor of Family
    Medicine
Drexel University School of
    Medicine
Forbes Family Practice Residency
    Program
Western Pennsylvania Hospital
Forbes Regional Campus
Monroeville, Pennsylvania

Lida Mina, MD
Fellow, Hematology/Oncology
Indiana University School of
    Medicine
Indianapolis, Indiana

Ginat W. Mirowski, DMD, MD
Associate Professor of
    Dermatology
Northwestern University
    Feinberg School of Medicine
Chicago, IL
Adjunct Associate Professor
Indiana University School of
    Dentistry
Indianapolis, Indiana

Samina Naseer, MD
Resident
Family Practice
Forbes Campus
West Pennsylvania Hospital
Monroeville, Pennsylvania

Katherine Neely, MD
Assistant Professor of Family
    Medicine
Drexel University School of
    Medicine
Residency Program Director
Forbes Family Practice Residency
    Program
Western Pennsylvania Hospital
Forbes Campus
Monroeville, Pennsylvania

Rebecca O'Bryan, MD
Indiana University School of
    Medicine
Indianapolis, Indiana

Ann M. O'Connor, PA-C
Faculty Assistant and Associate
    Preceptor
Northeast Family Medical Center
University of Wisconsin-Madison
Physician Assistant Program
Madison, Wisconsin

Sean O'Connor, MD
Professor of Psychiatry and
    Biomedical Engineering
Indiana University School of
    Medicine
Indianapolis, Indiana

Kathy Oriel, MD, MS
Associate Professor of Family
    Medicine
University of Wisconsin School of
    Medicine and Public Health
Madison, Wisconsin

Heather L. Paladine, MD
Associate Residency Director
Visiting Assistant Professor of
    Clinical Family Medicine
University of Southern California
Los Angeles, California

Amy S. Paller, MD, PhD
Chair, Department of
    Dermatology
Professor of Pediatrics and
    Dermatology
Northwestern University
    Feinberg School of Medicine
Chicago, Illinois

Nancy Pandhi, MD, MPH
Clinical Instructor and Assistant
    Scientist
Department of Family Medicine
Health Innovation Program
University of Wisconsin
Madison, Wisconsin

Smitha Patibandla
Psychiatric Services
Reid Hospital
Indianapolis, Indiana

Iwona Podzelinski, MD
Indiana University School of
    Medicine
Indianapolis, Indiana

Emily Porter, MD
Family Medicine Resident
University of Wisconsin
Madison, Wisconsin

Linda W. Prine, MD
Associate Professor
Albert Einstein College of Medicine
Faculty
Beth Israel Residency in Urban
    Family Practice
Beth Israel, New York, New York

Tammy Quall, MSSW
Development Office
Access Community Health Centers
Madison, Wisconsin

Jo Marie R. Reilly, MD
Associate Clinical Professor of
    Family Medicine
University of Southern California
    Keck Medical School
Clinical Staff, Family Medicine
California Hospital
Los Angeles, California

Theresa Rohr-Kirchgraber, MD
Assistant Professor of Clinical
    Pediatrics
Indiana University School of
    Medicine
The Charis Center for Eating
    Disorders
Indianapolis, Indiana

Jeffrey M. Rothenberg, MD, MS
Associate Clinical Professor of
    Obstetrics and Gynecology
Indiana University School of
    Medicine
Indianapolis, Indiana

Mary Rouse, MD
Assistant Professor of Clinical
    Pediatrics
Indiana University School of Medicine
The Charis Center for Eating
    Disorders
Indianapolis, Indiana

Jeanne Marie Schilder, MD
Assistant Professor of Obstetrics and Gynecology
Indiana University School of Medicine
Indianapolis, Indiana

Bethanee Schlosser, MD, PhD
Assistant Professor of Dermatology
Director, Women's Skin Health Program
Northwestern University Feinberg School of Medicine
Department of Dermatology
Chicago, Illinois

Paul G. Schoon, MD
Assistant Professor of Clinical Obstetrics and Gynecology
Indiana University School of Medicine
Director, Urodynamics Lab
Wishard Memorial Hospital
Indianapolis, Indiana

Sarina B. Schrager, MD, MS
Associate Professor
University of Wisconsin
Department of Family Medicine
Madison, Wisconsin

Penina Segall-Gutierrez, MD, MS
Voluntary Clinical Instructor/ Contract Physician
University of Southern California
Planned Parenthood
Los Angeles and San Bernadino, California

Anantha Shekhar, MD, PhD
Associate Dean for Translational Research
Raymond E. Houk Professor of Psychiatry
Indiana University School of Medicine
Indianapolis, Indiana

Juliemarie M. Sicilia, MD
Clinical Assistant Professor of Family Medicine
University of Washington
Faculty Physician
Alaska Family Medicine Residency
Anchorage, Alaska

Tara B. Stein, MD
Clinical Instructor
Albert Einstein College of Medicine
Faculty Attending
Montefiore Medical Center
Bronx, New York, New York

Melissa M. Stiles, MD
Associate Professor of Family Medicine
University of Wisconsin School of Medicine and Public Health
Department of Family Medicine
Madison, Wisconsin

Anna Maria Storniolo, MD
Professor of Clinical Medicine
Division of Hematology/ Oncology
Indiana University School of Medicine
Indianapolis, Indiana

DaWana Stubbs, MD
Assistant Professor of Clinical Medicine
Indiana University School of Medicine
Indianapolis, Indiana

John W. Stutsman, MD
Assistant Professor of Clinical Obstetrics and Gynecology
Indiana University School of Medicine
Indianapolis, Indiana

Nighat Tahir, MD
Fellow, Rheumatology
Indiana University School of
    Medicine
Indianapolis, Indiana

Kiet A.T. Ton, MD
Family Medicine Residency
University of Wisconsin
Wausau, Wisconsin

Janet M. Townsend, MD
Associate Professor of Family
    and Social Medicine
Albert Einstein College of Medicine
    Montefiore Medical Center
Bronx, New York

Michael A. Umland, BS, MD
Family Practice Resident
Wausau, Wisconsin

Rakesh Vinayek, MD
Professor of Medicine
Indiana University School of
    Medicine
Indianapolis, Indiana

Elizabeth von der Lohe, MD
Professor of Clinical Cardiology
Indiana University School of
    Medicine
Indianapolis, Indiana

Beverly VonDer Pool, MD
Clinical Associate Professor
University of Alabama Birmingham
School of Medicine
Birmingham, Alabama

Michael J. Waddell, MD
Clinical Diabetes and Endocrine
    Fellow
Indiana University School of
    Medicine
Indianapolis, Indiana

Kathleen E. Walsh, DO, MS
Clinical Instructor
University of Wisconsin School of
    Medicine
Emergency Medicine/Internal
    Medicine
Monroe Clinic
Monroe, Wisconsin

Norma Jo Waxman, MD
Associate Clinical Professor of
    Family and Community Medicine
Family Medicine Residency
    Program
University of California,
    San Francisco
Attending Physician
San Francisco General Hospital
San Francisco, California

**Dennis P. West, PhD,
    FCCP, CIP**
Vincent W. Foglia Family Research
    Professor of Dermatology
Northwestern University
    Feinberg School of Medicine
Chicago, Illinois

Joanne E. Williams, MD, MPH
Assistant Professor
Emory University
Department of Family Medicine
Fairburn, Georgia

Linnea Williams, DO
Resident St. Luke's/ Central City
    Family Medicine Residency
Milwaukee, Wisconsin

**Joslyn N. Witherspoon, MD,
    MPH**
Clinical Research Fellow
Department of Dermatology
Northwestern University
    Feinberg School of Medicine
Chicago, Illinois

Contents

Part II   LIFE CYCLE STRUCTURE

Introduction

Rose S. Fife

Women's health has undergone a sea change in the last few decades. In addition to the transformations arising from ever-improving medical technologies, such as digital mammography and microsurgical procedures, which have greatly improved detection and treatment of a variety of diseases, many other features of medical practice have changed drastically to the benefit of women. Until 15–20 years ago, clinical trials were traditionally performed only on white males, and doses for everyone else, including all women, were adjusted accordingly based on the findings in the stereotypical 70-kg white male (1,2).

Additionally, it was not recognized that women could suffer from the same diseases as men, but present differently. For instance, women with chest pain or left arm numbness were often assumed to have musculoskeletal or psychogenic pain rather than a myocardial infarction. The effects of secondhand smoke, which often were principally endured by women and children, were unknown. The risks of the rise in tobacco consumption among women were not appreciated for a long time.

The National Institutes of Health and the Food and Drug Administration began to urge that women, and eventually children, be included in clinical trials, when appropriate. Thus, gradually, drugs emerged that had been tested on women and children, so the doses and frequency of administration were specifically identified for them (1,2).

In 1991, a meeting was held in Hunt Valley, Maryland, to "set the agenda for research on women's health" (3). A follow-up meeting was held in 1997 to "provide multidisciplinary interaction between women's health advocates and scientists to focus on a new era in women's health research," according to Vivian Pinn, MD, NIH Associate Director for Research on Health and Director of the Office of Research on Women's Health (3). The hope was that this meeting would "provide a springboard for women's health research into the 21st century" (3).

The Women's Health Initiative was undertaken as a 15-year study to assess the leading causes of death and morbidity (heart disease, cancer, and osteoporosis) in women and included over 161,000 participants (4). It included clinical trials to examine the effects of hormone treatment and other interventions in postmenopausal women. A significant component of the study, that of examining the effects of combined estrogen and progestin, was terminated early due to an excess of adverse outcomes, including breast cancer, cardiovascular disease, stroke, and pulmonary embolism (5). This was a critical event, demonstrating the overwhelming necessity of evidence-based studies, since these agents had long been thought to be beneficial for postmenopausal women.

During the last 10 years or so, the recognition that women get myocardial infarctions and other cardiac disorders that may present with symptoms different from their male counterparts, that women suffer from chronic obstructive lung disease and lung cancer as a result of smoking just like men do, and that many drugs are metabolized differently in women and thus must be given in doses not altered only by considerations of body size are but a few of the changes that have been wrought in our attitudes toward a better understanding of women's health.

Thus, this book was conceived with the goal of providing a concise yet comprehensive overview of the major issues in women's health that the primary care provider, in particular, is likely to encounter. Our aim was not to provide detailed therapeutic guidelines, since these change rapidly, but rather to enable the physician (or trainee) to find a quick summation of the key features, differential diagnoses, and overall approach to the care of the women he or she encounters, as well as to provide some of the social and behavioral contexts of women's health in today's world. References have been provided to help the practitioner who may want to explore a subject in greater depth. We have been very fortunate to have had the services of skilled and knowledgeable experts in their fields and are very grateful to them for their extraordinary contributions.

References

1. **Freedman, LS, et al.** Inclusion of women and minorities in clinical trials and the NIH Revitalization Act of 1993—The Perspective of NIH clinical trialists. Controlled Clin Trials. 1995;16:277–85.
2. **McCarthy, CR.** Historical background of clinical trials involving women and minorities. Acad Med. 1994;69:695–8.
3. NIH News Advisory (1997). NIH Office of Research on Women's Health sponsors national scientific workshop to set the agenda for research on women's health for the 21st century. (http://www.nih.gov/news/pr/nov97/od-13a.htm, accessed 4/28/08).
4. Women's Health Initiative (2008). (http://www.nhlbi.gov/whi/, accessed 4/28/08).
5. NIH New Release (2002). NHLBI stops trial of estrogen plus progestin due to increased breast cancer risk, lack of overall benefit. (http://www.nhlbi.nih.gov/new/press/02-07-09.htm, accessed 4/28/08).

Part I

Organ System Structure

1

Prevention and Screening in Women

A. Cancer Screening
Jennifer Frank, MD; Jessica Johnston, MD

B. Screening and Prevention
Sarina B. Schrager, MD, MS

A. Cancer Screening

Jennifer Frank and Jessica Johnston

KEY POINTS

- Breast cancer is the most common cause of cancer in women and the second leading cause of cancer death.
- Women of average risk should be offered screening for breast, cervical, and colorectal cancer based on their age.
- It is recommended that women who have certain known or suspected hereditary cancer syndromes be offered screening for endometrial and ovarian cancer.
- Breast magnetic resonance imaging (MRI) is recommended in addition to mammography for breast cancer screening in high-risk women.
- Cervical cancer screening may be performed using conventional Pap smear testing, liquid-based cytology (LBC), or human papilloma virus (HPV) DNA testing.
- Women at increased cancer risk may require more frequent screening, more extensive screening, or screening starting at younger ages.

Epidemiology of Disease

Breast cancer is the leading cancer diagnosis in women, accounting for 31% of diagnosed cancers and 15% of cancer deaths (1). Lung cancer, the second most commonly diagnosed cancer in women, is the most common cause of cancer deaths in women (1). Colorectal cancer is the third most common cancer diagnosis and cause of cancer death in women (1). Endometrial cancer accounts for about 6% of cancers in women and ovarian cancer accounts for approximately 3% of cancers. Cervical cancer is less common, affecting approximately 9710 women in the U.S. in 2006 (1). There is an increased incidence of breast, ovarian, colorectal, and endometrial cancers in women with certain familial cancer syndromes.

Evidence-Based Screening Recommendations

Breast Cancer

Screening for breast cancer may include self-breast exam (SBE), clinical breast exam (CBE), mammography, and/or MRI.

1. *Self-breast exam*. SBE is not associated with a decrease in mortality from breast cancer, but is associated with false-positive results

and an increased number of breast biopsies (7). For these reasons, neither the US Preventive Services Task Force (USPSTF) nor the American Cancer Society (ACS) recommend SBE to screen for breast cancer, although it is recommended that women are counseled about the benefits and risks of SBE (2,7). In high-risk women SBE may be encouraged (3).

2. *Clinical breast exam.* CBE has not demonstrated a benefit for detection of breast cancer either alone or in combination with mammography (7). The USPSTF does not recommend CBE for breast cancer screening, citing insufficient evidence. The ACS recommends CBE for breast cancer screening every 3 years in average-risk women aged 20–39 and annually for average-risk women 40 years and older (2). Women at increased risk may benefit from screening starting at younger ages and occurring more frequently (2,3).

3. *Mammography.* Screening with mammography demonstrates a reduction in mortality from breast cancer (7). For average-risk women, the USPSTF recommends mammography every 1–2 years starting at age 40 and the ACS recommends mammography annually starting at age 40 (2,7). Since screening with mammography also increases the number of false-positive results and breast biopsies, women should be counseled about the potential benefits and harms as well as the limitations of mammography (2). For women at increased risk of breast cancer due to family history, genetic predisposition, or history of receiving chest radiation therapy, mammography may be started before age 40 although data is limited regarding the optimal age to initiate screening (2). The ACS recommends annual mammography and breast MRI starting at age 30 for women at high risk (2). Sensitivity of mammography ranges from 56% to 95% with specificity of 94–97% (7). Age <50, dense breast tissue, and use of hormone replacement therapy all lower sensitivity (7). Specificity increases with a shorter interval between mammograms and the ability to review previous mammograms for comparison (7).

4. *Magnetic resonance imaging.* MRI of the breasts is not recommended for average-risk women although it may be used with mammography to screen certain populations of high-risk women (5). Sensitivity of MRI ranges from 80% to 100% and specificity ranges from 81% to 99% (5). Annual MRI plus mammography is recommended for women with a BRCA mutation, untested women who have a first-degree relative with a BRCA mutation, a lifetime risk of developing breast cancer of 20–25% based on a predictive model, history of radiation to chest between 10 and 30 years of age, and women affected with or first-degree relatives of people with certain hereditary syndromes (Li–Fraumeni syndrome, Cowden syndrome, Bannayan–Riley–Ruvalcaba syndrome) (5). MRI is usually done at the same time as mammography, although staggering MRI and mammography by 6 months is another option (5).

Cervical Cancer

Screening for precancerous and cancerous cervical lesions is performed using either conventional Pap smear testing or liquid based cytology (LBC).

Pap smear testing. Pap smears may be performed either with a conventional slide sent for cytology or LBC. The sensitivity of a single conventional Pap smear ranges from 30% to 80% with specificity 86–100% depending on clinician and cytologist expertise (8). Sensitivities for LBC are similar (6). Current evidence does not favor the use of one type of Pap smear testing over another (6). The ACS and USPSTF recommend screening for average-risk women beginning 3 years after the onset of sexual activity (vaginal intercourse) or by age 21, whichever occurs first (2,6), with either conventional cytology annually or LBC every 2 years (2). Starting at age 30, a woman who has had three consecutive normal results may be screened every 2–3 years with conventional or LBC or every 3 years with HPV DNA testing plus conventional cytology or LBC (2). A woman may elect to stop cervical cancer screening after age 65–70 if she has had three satisfactory, normal Pap smears and has had no abnormal cytology results in the preceding 10 years (2,6). Women with total hysterectomy for benign disease may also stop screening (2,6).

Human papillomavirus DNA testing. Testing for oncogenic (or high-risk) HPV is not recommended as the sole test for cervical cancer screening (6); however, it may be combined with Pap smear testing. The sensitivity of HPV testing for high-grade lesions is 82–91% with specificity of 73–79% (6). Screening recommendations are the same for women who have received vaccination against HPV (2).

High Risk Groups
1. Women exposed to diethylstilbestrol (DES) *in utero* should continue annual conventional cytology or biennial LBC after age 30 (2).
2. Immunocompromised women (HIV+, organ transplant recipients, chronic steroid use, or undergoing chemotherapy) should receive cervical cancer screening every 6 months in the year after initial diagnosis and annually after the first year (2).
3. Women with a history of cervical cancer, *in utero* DES exposure, or who are HIV+ should continue screening beyond age 70 if they would benefit from detection and treatment (2).

Colorectal Cancer

Screening for colorectal cancer (CRC) may include fecal occult blood testing (FOBT), fecal immunochemical testing (FIT), stool DNA testing (sDNA), colonoscopy, flexible sigmoidoscopy, double-contrast barium enema (DCBE), or computed tomographic colonography ("virtual colonoscopy") (9). The direct visualization tests (flexible sigmoidoscopy, DCBE, colonoscopy, and CT colonography) provide the ability to screen for adenomatous polyps as well, thereby offering CRC prevention (if adenomatous polyps are detected and removed) in addition to screening

(9). Screening should begin at age 50 for average-risk women. No age is defined for discontinuation of screening, although women with a limited life expectancy are unlikely to realize a benefit from screening (10).

1. *Fecal occult blood testing.* Use of guaiac-based test cards examining three consecutive stool samples collected by the patient demonstrate mortality reduction of between 15% and 33% when done periodically (annual or biennial) (10). If the stool samples are rehydrated, sensitivity increases from approximately 40% to 60% but is accompanied by a drop in specificity from over 96% to 90% (10). Annual FOBT testing is associated with decreased mortality from CRC compared to biennial screening, but is also associated with a higher false-positive rate, necessitating additional testing (10). Annual FOBT is recommended (9). A single FOBT obtained by the clinician during digital rectal examination is not recommended (2).

2. *Fecal immunochemical testing.* FIT presents advantages compared to FOBT. FIT does not require pretest dietary restriction, making patient compliance more likely. Additionally, FIT uses an automated analysis, thereby decreasing the chance of human error (11). FIT testing may have equal or greater sensitivity and specificity than FOBT for detecting distal CRC but has not been shown to be a superior test to FOBT (11). The impact of FIT testing on mortality from CRC has not been determined. Annual testing is recommended (9).

3. *sDNA testing* detects multiple DNA targets in the stool that may be shed from adenomatous or cancerous cells, using a single, entire stool sample (9). Sensitivity is reported to range from 52% to 91% and specificity from 93% to 97% (9). The optimal interval time between tests is undetermined (9).

4. *Colonoscopy.* Colonoscopy is a recommended option for CRC screening and provides the opportunity to biopsy any abnormal tissue or polyps detected on exam. For average risk women, the screening interval is 10 years (2,10). Women at increased risk of CRC may warrant earlier and/or more frequent testing. Colonoscopy is associated with rare but possible risks of perforation, bleeding, and death (12). The sensitivity of colonoscopy for detection of adenomas 1 cm or larger is 88–94% (12).

5. *Flexible sigmoidoscopy.* Screening for CRC with flexible sigmoidoscopy may be done with or without FOBT (2,10), although the ACS recommends the combination over either test alone (2). Flexible sigmoidoscopy screening is associated with decreased mortality from CRC (10). FOBT, when done, should be performed prior to flexible sigmoidoscopy (13). The combination of tests has not been shown to decrease mortality compared with either test alone (9). Flexible sigmoidoscopy should ideally be performed with an insertion depth of at least 40 cm and should be repeated every 5 years (9).

6. *CT colonography* uses CT technology to recreate a 3-dimensional image of the colon to screen for polyps and cancerous lesions. Sensitivity varies from as low as 70% for polyps measuring 6–9 mm up to 96% for

invasive CRC (9). Screening every 5 years is currently recommended, although this may change as more data is collected (9). CT colonography may be an option for patients either unwilling or unable to undergo colonoscopy (9).

Several groups of women are considered to be at increased risk of developing CRC. These include women with a first-degree relative or two second-degree relatives diagnosed with CRC or adenomatous polyps, women known or suspected of having familial adenomatous polyposis (FAP), hereditary nonpolyposis colorectal cancer (HNPCC), and women with inflammatory bowel disease (13).

1. Women who have a first-degree relative with either colon cancer or adenomatous polyps should start CRC screening with colonoscopy at age 40, or 10 years younger than the age at which the affected family member was diagnosed (whichever comes first) (13). If the affected family member was younger than age 60 at the time of diagnosis, colonoscopy should be repeated every 5 years (instead of every 10 years) (13).

2. Women who have 2 second-degree relatives with CRC should be screened with colonoscopy starting at age 40, or 10 years before the earliest diagnosis of an affected family member (whichever comes first). If the affected family members were younger than age 60 at the time of diagnosis, colonoscopy should be repeated every 5 years (13).

3. Screening with annual sigmoidoscopy is recommended for women with known or suspected FAP starting at age 10 to 12 years of age (13).

4. Women with known or suspected HNPCC should be screened with colonoscopy every 1–2 years starting at age 20–25 years of age or 10 years younger than the youngest age at which a family member was diagnosed with CRC (13).

Endometrial Cancer

Endometrial cancer screening for women of average and increased risk is not recommended. However, for women at very high risk (those with known or suspected HNPCC gene mutation carrier status or autosomal dominant predisposition to CRC), annual screening with endometrial biopsy is recommended starting at age 35 (2).

Ovarian Cancer

Screening for ovarian cancer in an average-risk woman is not recommended because of the lack of benefit versus risk in available screening tests and the rarity of ovarian cancer in the general population (4). However, ovarian cancer screening may be indicated in high-risk women, particularly those with a known BRCA gene mutation or whose family or personal history is associated with an increased risk (>10% lifetime risk) (4).

1. *Pelvic examination.* Screening for ovarian cancer with a pelvic examination is not recommended because of a low sensitivity and specificity (4).

2. *CA125 serum level*. CA125 is a tumor marker that may be elevated in ovarian cancer but also in benign conditions and other types of cancers. CA125 is usually combined with a transvaginal ultrasound (TVU) when used to screen for ovarian cancer. Using an absolute cutoff value of 30 U/mL may miss stage 1 ovarian cancer but may also be associated with mortality reductions in postmenopausal women (who are less likely to have benign gynecologic conditions causing a falsely elevated level) (4). An algorithm using the CA125 level compared with age and rate of rise demonstrated a sensitivity of 83% with a specificity of 99.7% reflecting that ovarian cancer often causes CA125 levels to both be elevated as well as to rise over time (4).

3. *Transvaginal ultrasound* has a reported sensitivity of 33.3% and a specificity of 84.5% in one study of high-risk women (14). Premenopausal women may have more physiologic or benign conditions of the ovary leading to an abnormal TVU result. Color-flow Doppler may increase specificity, and while not usually used as the first-line screening, can help further characterize abnormalities visualized on the ovaries with TVU (4).

4. *CA125 plus transvaginal ultrasound*. Screening high-risk women with CA125 and TVU twice yearly is currently recommended by the National Comprehensive Cancer Network (3,4). Screening is not recommended by the USPSTF (15) or the American College of Obstetricians and Gynecologists (ACOG) (16) because of a lack of proven mortality benefit with screening.

Screening in high-risk women may be recommended as young as age 30 if an affected family member was diagnosed at a younger age (4). However, screening before age 30 is unlikely to be beneficial given the rarity of ovarian cancer in women younger than 30, even in those who have a hereditary cancer syndrome (4).

As with other cancer screening recommendations, no set age has been determined at which screening should be discontinued, since consideration should be given to overall life expectancy and the woman's wishes regarding treatment if a cancer were detected.

References

1. American Cancer Society. Cancer Facts and Figures 2006. Atlanta: American Cancer Society, 2006.

2. **Smith RA, Cokkinides V, Eyre HJ.** Cancer screening in the United States, 2007: A review of current guidelines, practices, and prospects. CA Cancer J Clin. 2007;57:90–104.

3. National Comprehensive Cancer Network: Clinic Practice Guidelines in Oncology, version 1, 2007. http://www.nccn.org/physician_gls/f_guidelines.asp.

4. **Rosenthal A, Jacobs I.** Familial ovarian cancer screening. Best Pract Res Clin Obstet Gynaecol. 2006;20:321–38.

5. **Saslow D, Boetes C, Burke W, et al.** American Cancer Society guidelines for breast screening with MRI as an adjunct to mammography. CA Cancer J Clin. 2007;57:75–89.

6. US Preventive Services Task Force. Screening for cervical cancer. January 2003.

7. US Preventive Services Task Force. Screening for breast cancer. August 2002.

8. **Nanda K, McCrory DC, Myers ER, et al.** Accuracy of the Papanicolaou test in screening for and follow-up of cervical cytologic abnormalities: a systematic review. Ann Intern Med. 2000;132:810.

9. **Levin B, Lieberman DA, McFarland B, et al.** Screening and surveillance for the early detection of colorectal cancer and adenomatous polyps, 2008: a joint guideline from the American Cancer Society, the US Multi-Society Task Force on Colorectal Cancer, and the American College of Radiology. CA Cancer J Clin. epub March 5, 2008.

10. U.S. Preventive Services Task Force. Screening for Colorectal Cancer. July 2002.

11. **Allison JE, Sakoda LC, Levin TR, et al.** Screening for colorectal neoplasms with new fecal occult blood tests: update on performance characteristics. J Natl Cancer Inst. 2007;99:1462-70.

12. **Helken JP.** Screening for colon cancer. Cancer Imaging. 2006;6:S13-21.

13. **Ko C, Hyman NH.** Practice parameters for the detection of colorectal neoplasms: an interim report (revised). Dis Colon Rectum. 2006;49:299-301.

14. **Woodward ER, Sleightholme HV, Considine AM, et al.** Annual surveillance by CA125 and transvaginal ultrasound for ovarian cancer in both high-risk and population risk women is ineffective. BJOG. 2007;114:1500-9.

15. U.S. Preventive Services Task Force. Screening for ovarian cancer. May 2004.

16. American College of Obstetricians and Gynecologists. Committee Opinion: The role of the generalist obstetrician-gynecologist in the early detection of ovarian cancer. December 2002.

B. Screening and Prevention

Sarina B. Schrager

KEY POINTS

- ❖ Cardiovascular disease (CVD) is the leading cause of death among women in the U.S.
- ❖ Prevention of CVD begins with risk assessment and focuses on evidence-based screening tests.
- ❖ Women can modify their CVD risks by maintaining a healthy weight and performing regular exercise.
- ❖ All women should be screened routinely and repeatedly for intimate partner violence during primary care visits.

> ◆ Osteoporosis prevention begins in children with lifelong coun-
>   seling on adequate calcium intake.
> ◆ Normal-risk women should have a DEXA scan to assess their bone
>   density at age 65, and high-risk women should have one at age 60.

Prevention of diseases in women is an important part of overall primary care. Primary prevention is the most valuable because it prevents a condition from developing. An example of primary prevention is immunization of children. Secondary prevention interferes with the development of clinical outcomes from asymptomatic disease. An example of secondary prevention is routine screening for hypertension. Tertiary prevention focuses on interfering with clinical consequences of a disease already diagnosed. An example of tertiary prevention is aspirin to prevent cardiovascular events in someone with known coronary artery disease (1). This chapter will focus on secondary prevention and routine screening for common, non-cancer conditions in women (see Section A).

Many primary care providers include screening tests in annual physical exams and other health maintenance visits. A good screening test (1):

- Is acceptable to the patient (i.e., not particularly painful, easy to do, etc.)
- Confers minimal risk at a reasonable cost
- Is accurate (i.e., has a high sensitivity and specificity)
- Can detect the disease when it is asymptomatic

In addition, for a screening program to be effective there must be evidence that an early diagnosis of the condition affects the outcome (1). This chapter will review the evidence supporting common screening tests used in primary care. The top six leading causes of death among women are heart disease, malignancy, stroke, unintentional injuries, lower respiratory tract infections, and diabetes (2). As such, screening efforts should begin with a focus on these conditions.

Cardiovascular Disease

More women die each year from heart disease than from all types of cancers combined (2). It is estimated that the direct and indirect annual costs for treating heart disease (for both men and women) in the U.S. is over $400 billion (3). Prevention of heart disease focuses on establishing a woman's level of risk for CVD and then mediating the risk factors. Women are classified as high-risk, at-risk, and at optimal or low risk, based on their risk factors (4). Having a previous diagnosis of some type of vascular disease or diabetes puts a woman in the "high-risk" category (4). Lifestyle risk factors, including smoking, obesity, poor diet, or physical inactivity place a woman in the "at-risk" category. Having a family history of CVD also puts a woman in the "at-risk category" (4). Women in the low risk category have a healthy lifestyle with no other risk factors.

Table 1-1   Screening Tests for CVD Risk Factors in Women

Condition	Screening Test	USPSTF Level of Recommendation*	Comments
Hypertension	BP measurement	A	Starting at age 18, biannual measurement if BP <120/80 mm Hg, annual if BP 120–139/80–90 mm Hg
Hyperlipidemia	Serum total cholesterol and HDL	A—start at 45 B—between 20 and 45 if other risk factors	Not enough evidence to support adding triglycerides
Smoking	Clinical screen	A	Recommend screening and offer pharmacologic aid to people who want to quit
Diabetes	Serum fasting glucose	I—asymptomatic adults B—adults with hypertension or hyperlipidemia	Insufficient evidence to support screening in asymptomatic individuals In practice, consider screening women with a history of gestational diabetes and obese women with PCOS.
Carotid artery stenosis	Carotid artery ultrasonography	D	There is little evidence that screening asymptomatic adults prevents strokes, and may, in fact, cause harm via false-positive test results.

*For a description of level of recommendation, see Appendix A.
From US Preventive Services Task Force, Guidelines for Clinical Preventive Services, available at www.ahrq.gov; with permission.

There is good evidence to support screening for hypertension, smoking, and lipid disorders in women (Table 1-1) (5). Diabetes is another substantial risk factor for CVD and a leading cause of mortality in its own right. Though the US Preventive Services Task Force (USPSTF) does not recommend screening for diabetes in women who do not also have hypertension and hyperlipidemia, many other women are at high-risk of developing diabetes. For instance, women with a history of gestational diabetes and other abnormal glucose tolerance during pregnancy are at a very high risk of developing type 2 diabetes later in life (6). In addition, obese women with polycystic ovarian syndrome (PCOS) are at very high risk of developing diabetes (7). Women in both of these groups may benefit from regular fasting glucose measurements to screen for type 2 diabetes.

Maintaining a healthy lifestyle is the most important factor in heart disease and diabetes prevention in women. Women should exercise at least 30 minutes a day at least 3 days a week, but preferably every day. Women may need to exercise up to 60 or 90 minutes daily if they need to lose weight. Exercise can be defined as any activity that gets a person's heart rate up to a level of over 50–60% of their maximum heart rate. Women also should maintain a healthy weight and eat a diet high in fruits and vegetables. In addition, high-dose omega-3 fatty acids (fish oil or flax seed oil) may be considered as an adjunct to a healthy diet and exercise (4). There is not enough evidence to support the routine use of aspirin in healthy women under 65 to prevent a myocardial infarction (MI), and aspirin in these women may actually cause harm (4). Women at high-risk for CVD or women over 65 years should take aspirin therapy (4). There is not enough evidence to support routine screening ultrasounds to detect abdominal aortic aneurysms in women (8).

Unintentional Injuries and Violence

Unintentional injuries are another leading cause of death among women, especially in younger age groups. Several categories of injuries may be prevented. Motor vehicle accidents (MVA) are the leading cause of death among all adults under 35 years. The use of restraints (seat belts) can decrease the mortality rates from MVA by 45–70% (5). There have been many public health and community interventions aimed at increasing the use of seat belts, including legislating penalties for people who ride in cars without restraints in some states. The USPSTF states that there is insufficient evidence that primary care providers could increase the use of seat belts by counseling patients in the office (5).

Family violence is very common. It is estimated that at least 20–30% of women in the U.S. have been abused by a partner at some point in their lives (9). Many of these women sustain serious physical injuries from the abuse. Thus, many organizations recommend that all primary providers screen all women for violence as part of an overall prevention agenda. Routine and repeated screening of women can increase the detection rate of violence in the primary care setting (9). Clinicians can ask women questions about her safety or ask women to fill out a questionnaire at each office visit (10). One randomized trial in Canada of women attending family medicine clinics, women's health clinics, and emergency rooms found that women preferred to complete a questionnaire than to be asked about violence in person (11). It is unknown whether these results can be extrapolated in the U.S. Previous studies had found that women liked being asked directly by their provider (12). Either way, primary care offices should find a method that works and focus on screening all women for violence. Box 1-1 provides examples of specific questions that a clinician can use to screen for violence.

At present, there is no research supporting the link between increasing screening rates and decreased rates of abuse, likely due to the complex nature of this issue and the lack of studies (5,14) However, there are minimal negative outcomes of routine screening, and it is likely to increase a woman's access to community resources (15).

Box 1-1   Examples of Violence Screening Questions

- Violence has become so common in many women's lives that I now ask all my patients about violence in their homes. There are resources available for abused women.
- In the past year, have you been physically hurt by someone close to you?
- Are you physically threatened by anyone in your home?
- Do you feel safe in your current relationship?
- Are you afraid of any of your previous partners?

From The American College of Obstetrics and Gynecology, screening tools for domestic violence. Available at www.acog.org; with permission.

Osteoporosis

Osteoporosis is one of the most common conditions affecting women. Approximately 8 million women in the U.S. have osteoporosis, incurring annual direct and indirect costs of over $19 billion (16). Osteoporosis, itself, is asymptomatic. The most serious manifestation of osteoporosis is a fracture. Vertebral fractures can cause chronic pain and respiratory difficulties resulting from kyphosis. Hip fractures are associated with significant morbidity (inability to ambulate, nursing home placement, pneumonia, embolic phenomena) and mortality (16). Several different interventions, including organized exercise programs, home hazard assessments, vitamin D supplementation, and correction of visual deficiency, have all been effective in decreasing the rates of falling and risking fractures in the elderly (17) (Table 1-2).

Table 1-2   Osteoporosis and Fracture Prevention in Women

Age	Intervention	Comments
All ages	Counseling about adequate dietary calcium intake	Premenopausal women should eat 3 servings of dairy products a day, and postmenopausal women should eat 4 servings daily.
60	DEXA scan of hip and LS spine	High-risk women (family history of osteoporosis, early menopause, low calcium diet, weight under 127 lbs, thyroid disease, bone-affecting medications, such as chronic corticosteroid use)
65	DEXA scan of hip and LS spine	Normal risk
75 (USPSTF)	Screening for risk of falling	"Have you had any falls during the past year?"

Other Conditions

There is not enough evidence to support screening asymptomatic women for thyroid disease with a thyroid-stimulating hormone (TSH) level (5). However, in practice, some women in high-risk groups (elderly, post-partum, those with other autoimmune diseases, diabetics) may benefit from screening because of the higher prevalence of subclinical thyroid diseases in these women.

References

1. **Gordis L.** Epidemiology, 3rd Edition 2004, W.B Saunders, Philadelphia, PA.
2. The Office on Women's Health, quick data online, available at www.womenshealth.gov.
3. **Thom T, Haase N, Rosamond W, et al.** For the American Heart Association Statistics Committee and Stroke Statistics Committee. Heart disease and stroke statistics—2006 update: a report from the American Heart Association Statistics Committee and Stroke Statistics Subcommittee. Circulation. 2006;113:e85-151.
4. **Mosca L, et al.** Evidence-based guidelines for cardiovascular disease prevention in women: 2007 update. Journal of the American College of Cardiology. 2007;49:1230-50.
5. US Preventive Services Task Force, Guidelines for Clinical Preventive Services, available at www.ahrq.gov.
6. **Vambergue A, Dogninc C, Boulogne A et al.** Increasing incidence of abnormal glucose tolerance in women with prior abnormal glucose tolerance during pregnancy: DIAGEST 2 study. Diabetes Medicine. 2008;25:58-64.
7. American College of Obstetricians and Gynecologists. Clinical guidelines on diagnosis and treatment of polycystic ovarian syndrome. Obstetrics and Gynecology. 2002;100:1389-402.
8. **Cosford PA, Leng GC.** Screening for abdominal aortic aneurysm. Cochrane Database Systematic Review. 2007;2:CD002945.
9. The Family Violence Prevention Fund, Preventing domestic violence: clinical guidelines on routine screening. 1999, available at www.endabuse.org.
10. **Chen PH, Rovi S, Washington J, et al.** Randomized comparison of 3 methods to screen for domestic violence in family practice. Annals of Family Medicine. 2007;5:430-5.
11. **MacMillan HL, Wathen CN, Jamieson E, et al.** McMaster violence against women research group. Approaches to screening for intimate partner violence in health care settings: a randomized trial. JAMA. 2006;296:530-6.
12. **Fogarty CT, Burge S, McCord EC.** Communicating with patients about intimate partner violence: screening and interviewing approaches. Family Medicine. May 2002;34:369-75.
13. The American College of Obstetrics and Gynecology, screening tools for domestic violence. Available at www.acog.org.
14. **Gunter J.** Intimate partner violence. Obstetric and Gynecologic Clinics of North America. 2007;34:367-88.

15. **Houry D, et al.** Does screening in the emergency department hurt or help victims of intimate partner violence? Annals of Emergency Medicine. 2008;51:433–42.

16. National Osteoporosis Foundation, Fast facts about osteoporosis. Available at www.nof.org.

17. **Gillespie LD, Gillespie WJ, Robertson MC, et al.** Interventions for preventing falls in elderly people. Cochrane Database Systematic Review. 2003;4:CD000340.

2

Cancer in Women

A. Gynecologic Malignancies
   Jeanne M. Schilder, MD; Iwona Podzielinski, MD

B. Breast Cancer
   Anna Maria Storniolo, MD; Lida Mina, MD

C. Lung Cancer
   Shadia Jalal, MD; Nasser Hanna, MD

D. Colon Cancer
   Marguerite Elliott, DO, MS; Katri Kindschi, MD

E. Melanoma
   Theodore F. Logan, MD; Lawrence A. Mark, MD, PhD

F. Skin Cancer (Non-Melanoma Skin Cancer)
   Joslyn N. Witherspoon, DO, MPH; Bethanee J. Schlosser, MD, PhD;
   Dennis P. West, PhD; Anjali Butani, MD; and Ginat W. Mirowski, DMD, MD

A. Gynecologic Malignancies

Jeanne M. Schilder and Iwona Podzielinski

KEY POINTS

- Gynecologic malignancies represent approximately 8% of all malignancies in women and 10.7% of cancer deaths annually in the U.S.
- As with any malignancy, early identification of most gynecologic cancers leads to improved survival.
- Symptoms of ovarian cancer may present with vague constitutional symptoms and can mimic many other disease processes, including gastrointestinal disorders and benign gynecologic conditions. Accurate and timely diagnoses require a high index of suspicion and pelvic examination (including rectovaginal exam) in women with symptoms suggestive of ovarian cancer.
- Screening for cervical cancer leads to early detection and decreased incidence; screening guidelines should be followed by primary care physicians.
- Abnormal uterine bleeding in any post- or peri-menopausal woman requires evaluation to rule out endometrial cancer; younger women with risk factors should be evaluated as well.
- Vulvar and vaginal cancers are rare but can be diagnosed easily with biopsy of any abnormal lesion; risks are similar to those for cervical cancer.
- Gestational trophoblastic disease should be considered in any female of reproductive age presenting with symptoms suggestive of pregnancy complications or metastatic disease of unknown origin.

Epidemiology

Ovarian cancer incidence in the U.S. is approximately 23 000 cases per year, with 15 000 deaths, and is the most lethal gynecologic malignancy. The lifetime risk of developing ovarian cancer is 1.7%, or 1 in 70, and has remained stable over the last 3 decades, while the overall 5-year survival has improved from 37% in 1974 to 44% in 2006. Risk increases with age and with family history of ovarian and breast cancer. The median age of diagnosis is 63 years. Hereditary breast ovarian cancer (HBOC) syndromes are associated with BRCA-1 and -2 mutations and carry a risk of 28–40%. Ovarian cancer risk decreases with parity (women with any pregnancies have a 30–60% reduction in risk compared to nulliparous females), oral contraceptive use (up to 50% risk reduction), and other factors leading to decreased ovulation, such as breast-feeding (1,2).

Cervical cancer is the second most common malignancy worldwide following breast cancer. Pap smear screening in the U.S. has resulted in a dramatic reduction in incidence since implementation in the 1940s, and the incidence has declined by an additional one third during the past 2 decades. Human papillomavirus (HPV) testing has revolutionized cervical cancer screening, especially with the introduction of the HPV vaccine in 2006 (1,3). Unfortunately, despite effective screening measures, there are still approximately 10 000 new cases of cervical cancer annually in the U.S. (2008) and approximately 3700 deaths (4). Populations at highest risk include the elderly, economically disadvantaged, and other groups unable to participate in screening programs. Other risk factors include HPV infection, young age at first intercourse, multiple sexual partners, partners with multiple sexual partners, high parity, history of other sexually transmitted infections, cigarette smoking, immunodeficiency, poor diet (vitamin deficiency), and alcoholism (1).

Endometrial cancer is the fourth most common cancer in American women and the most common gynecologic malignancy, with 40 000 cases in 2007 and approximately 7000 deaths in the U.S. annually. The majority of patients have abnormal bleeding leading to early diagnosis (~75% are Stage I at presentation). The median age at diagnosis is 61 years. Peri- and post-menopausal presentation is typical, but 5% of women are diagnosed before age 40, and 20–25% are premenopausal. Incidence and survival are higher in white women compared with black women. Risk factors can be divided into 3 categories (Table 2-1).

Table 2-1   Risk Factors for Endometrial Cancer

Variants of normal anatomy or physiology
- Obesity, especially upper body obesity (2.5–4.5× RR)
- Nulliparity (2–3× RR)
- Early menarche, late menopause (2.4× RR)
- Older age
- White race

Frank abnormality or disease
- Diabetes mellitus (2.8× RR), hypertension (1.5× RR), gallbladder, or thyroid disease
- Hereditary non-polyposis colon cancer also known as Lynch II (40–60% lifetime risk)
- Stein-Leventhal or estrogen producing tumors
- History of infertility
- Menstrual irregularities

Exposure to external carcinogens
- Unopposed estrogen (9.5× RR)
- Tamoxifen (6.4× RR)

RR = relative risk
Adapted from Barakat RR, Grigsby PW, Sabbatini P, Zaino RJ. Corpus: Epithelial tumors.
In Hoskins WJ, Perez CA, Young RC (eds): Principles and Practice of Gynecologic Oncology.
Philadelphia: Lippincott Williams & Wilkins; 2000:919–59; with permission.

Mesenchymal tumors of the uterus, such as leiomyosarcoma, endometrial stromal sarcoma, and carcinosarcoma (or mixed Mullerian tumor), are much less common (1).

Clinical Presentation

Symptoms of ovarian cancer are often nonspecific and may include abdominal discomfort, fullness, early satiety, dyspepsia, fatigue, urinary frequency, dyspnea, changes in bowel habits, and abnormal uterine bleeding. Pelvic examination often reveals a solid or fixed pelvic mass, cul-de-sac nodularity, and ascites (5).

Early cervical cancer may be asymptomatic and can be diagnosed on Pap smear, with appropriate colposcopic evaluation with directed biopsies. Rarely a gross lesion is identified on routine pelvic examination, in which case Pap smear and colposcopy are not necessary; immediate biopsy should be performed. Advanced disease usually presents with symptoms including vaginal bleeding, discharge, postcoital bleeding, pelvic pain, or pain in the back, hip, or leg (6).

The most common presentation of endometrial cancer is postmenopausal bleeding. Any peri- or post-menopausal woman with abnormal uterine bleeding requires evaluation for endometrial cancer, including women with breakthrough bleeding on hormone replacement therapy. A high index of suspicion must be maintained if the diagnosis is to be made in young patients. Most young patients who develop endometrial cancer are obese, often with anovulatory menstrual cycles. In patients of reproductive age, bleeding associated with pregnancy must be ruled out prior to sampling the endometrium to evaluate for endometrial cancer.

Diagnosis

Women with persistent unexplained symptoms, such as abdominal pain, bloating, indigestion, early satiety, pelvic pain, change in bowel or bladder habits, abnormal uterine bleeding, and/or constitutional symptoms, should undergo a complete history and physical examination, including rectovaginal examination. If a gastrointestinal or other etiology is not determined, the index of suspicion for a gynecologic etiology must remain high. Transvaginal ultrasound is indicated to evaluate any abnormality detected on examination or if the patient's body habitus does not allow for an accurate assessment. If pelvic exam, ultrasound, and CA-125 are all normal, a gynecologic malignancy is highly unlikely. A patient with a suspicious mass, ascites, and elevated CA-125 requires further assessment, which may include laparoscopy or laparotomy, depending on the clinical scenario (5).

The Pap test is an effective screening test for cervical cancer. Abnormal Pap smear results, including atypical squamous cells of undetermined significance (ASCUS) with HPV-positive reflex testing, atypical glandular cells of undetermined significance (AGUS), low-grade squamous intraepithelial lesion (LSIL), or high-grade intraepithelial lesion (HSIL), require colposcopy for further evaluation; abnormal areas should be biopsied, and endocervical curettage should be performed. Once histologic confirmation of malignancy is obtained, clinical staging is performed to evaluate the extent of disease (6).

Historically, fractional dilatation and curettage (D&C) has been the preferred diagnostic procedure for evaluation of suspected endometrial cancer. The office endometrial biopsy (often obtained with a Pipelle curette) is an alternative for most patients, with an accuracy of approximately 90%. In the symptomatic patient, in whom inadequate tissue or no tissue is obtained for pathologic evaluation on Pipelle biopsy, a dilatation and curettage (D&C) must be considered. Differential diagnosis of abnormal uterine bleeding includes pregnancy (normal or abnormal), infection, atrophy, endometrial hyperplasia, and malignancy of the cervix, vagina, or vulva (7).

Clinical Care

Only 25% of patients with ovarian cancer will be diagnosed with localized or regional disease. Patients with Stages IA and IB have >90% 5-year survival rates. Comprehensive surgical staging is an important factor in determining appropriate adjuvant treatment and prognosis (8) (Table 2-2). Up to 30% of patients with apparent early-stage disease are found to have more severe disease based on nodal or distant intra-abdominal metastases. All peri- and post-menopausal patients with suspected ovarian cancer should have access to a gynecologic oncologist who can perform comprehensive staging, which includes total abdominal hysterectomy with bilateral oophorectomy, cytologic evaluation of ascites or washings, visualization and biopsy of the diaphragm, examination and biopsy of abdominal and pelvic peritoneum, pelvic and para-aortic lymph node sampling, and omentectomy. Adjuvant chemotherapy is recommended for patients with poor prognostic factors, including those with Stage IC or II disease, moderate- to high-grade tumor, and/or clear cell histology. Standard chemotherapy includes combination of platinum and taxane treatment.

Advanced epithelial ovarian cancer treatment includes comprehensive cytoreductive surgery followed by chemotherapy. Surgical debulking to a maximum residual tumor ≥1 cm in diameter offers a statistically significant survival benefit, even in advanced stages. Combination chemotherapy with platinum and a taxane results in response in 80% of patients, but up to 75% of these eventually relapse and die of disease. Intraperitoneal (IP) chemotherapy with cisplatin and paclitaxel has recently demonstrated improved overall survival for patients with optimal debulking (9).

Treatment for cervical cancer is stage-dependent (Table 2-3). Microscopic disease is first evaluated by cone biopsy. Patients with Stage IA1 disease can be managed with close surveillance (appropriate for

Table 2-2   Carcinoma of the Ovary—Staging FIGO TNM

	Primary tumor cannot be assessed	TX
0	No evidence of primary tumor	T0
I	Tumor confined to ovaries	T1
	IA Tumor limited to 1 ovary, capsule intact	T1a
	No tumor on ovarian surface	
	No malignant cells in the ascites or peritoneal washings	
	IB Tumor limited to both ovaries, capsules intact	T1b
	No tumor on ovarian surface	
	No malignant cells in the ascites or peritoneal washings	
	IC Tumor limited to 1 or both ovaries, with any of the following:	T1c
	Capsule ruptured, tumor on ovarian surface, positive malignant cells in the ascites, or positive peritoneal washings	
II	Tumor involves 1 or both ovaries with pelvic extension	T2
	IIA Extension and/or implants in uterus and/or tubes	T2a
	No malignant cells in the ascites or peritoneal washings	
	IIB Extension to other pelvic organ	T2b
	No malignant cells in the ascites or peritoneal washings	
	IIC IIA/B with positive malignant cells in the ascites or positive peritoneal washings	T2c
III	Tumor involves 1 or both ovaries with microscopically confirmed peritoneal metastasis outside the pelvis and/or regional lymph nodes metastasis N1	T3
	IIIA Microscopic peritoneal metastasis beyond the pelvis	T3a
	IIIB Macroscopic peritoneal metastasis beyond the pelvis 2 cm or less in greatest dimension	T3b
	IIIC Peritoneal metastasis beyond pelvis >2 cm in greatest dimension and/or regional lymph nodes and/or metastasis	T3c N1
IV	Distant metastasis beyond the peritoneal cavity	M1

Note: Liver capsule metastasis is Stage III, liver parenchymal metastasis is Stage IV. Pleural effusion must have positive cytology.
Reprinted from the International Federation of Gynecology and Obstetrics (FIGO): Benedict JL, Bender H, Jones H, Ngan HYS, Pecorelli S. Int J Gynecol Obstet 2000; 70:209–62; with permission.

patients desiring future child-bearing) or simple hysterectomy. Patients with Stage IA2 cervical cancer are treated with non-radical hysterectomy and pelvic lymph node assessment. For those with Stage IB1 disease, radical hysterectomy with pelvic lymph node dissection and pelvic radiation therapy (external beam followed by brachytherapy) are equally effective. Surgery offers the advantage of ovarian preservation and fewer detrimental effects to the vagina. Radiation therapy is usually recommended for patients who are not surgical candidates or those who wish to avoid surgical risks (6).

Advanced stage cervical cancer cannot be successfully managed surgically. Standard treatment for patients with Stages IB2–IVA includes concurrent weekly cisplatin chemotherapy and external beam radiation

Table 2-3 FIGO Staging Classification: Cervical Carcinoma

Stage 0	Carcinoma in situ
Stage IA1	Invasive carcinoma, confined to cervix, diagnosed only by microscopy Stromal invasion ≤3 mm in depth and ≤7 mm in horizontal spread
Stage IA2	Invasive carcinoma, confined to cervix, diagnosed only by microscopy Stromal invasion >3 mm and ≤5 mm in depth and ≤7 mm in horizontal spread
Stage IB1	Invasive carcinoma, confined to cervix, microscopic lesion >IA2 or clinically visible lesion ≤4 cm in greatest dimension
Stage IB2	Invasive carcinoma, confined to cervix, clinically visible lesion >4 cm in greatest dimension
Stage IIA	Tumor extension beyond cervix to vagina but not to lower third of vagina. No parametrial invasion
Stage IIB	Tumor extension beyond cervix. Parametrial invasion but not to pelvic sidewall and not to lower third of vagina
Stage IIIA	Tumor extension to lower third of vagina but not to pelvic sidewall
Stage IIIB	Tumor extension to pelvic sidewall or causing hydronephrosis or nonfunctioning kidney
Stage IVA	Tumor invasion into bladder or rectum
Stage IVB	Distant metastasis

FIGO, International Federation of Gynecology and Obstetrics.
Reprinted from the International Federation of Gynecology and Obstetrics
(FIGO): Benedict JL, Bender H, Jones H, Ngan HYS, Pecorelli S. Int J Gynecol Obstet 2000;
70:209–62; with permission.

therapy, followed by brachytherapy. Previously, these patients were managed with radiation alone, but recent clinical trials evaluating concurrent chemo-radiation demonstrated a reduction in the risk of death by 30–50% with the addition of platinum-based chemotherapy to radiation therapy. Patients with IVB cervical cancer are often treated with palliative chemotherapy and possibly radiation therapy to control bleeding or pain (6).

The standard initial management for endometrial cancer is surgical staging, which includes total abdominal hysterectomy, bilateral salpingo-oophorectomy, peritoneal cytology, bilateral pelvic and para-aortic lymph node sampling, and complete evaluation of the peritoneal cavity (Table 2-4). Patients undergoing complete surgical staging have significantly better survival (10). Even with Stage I cancer, as determined on endometrial biopsy, complete staging may impact therapy. Early stage disease is cured with surgical resection. Locally advanced disease is treated with radiation. Advanced disease (Stages III and IV) is treated with chemotherapy. Combination of cisplatin, doxorubicin, paclitaxel, and filgrastim is the accepted regimen (11).

Recurrences, especially those in the vaginal vault, can be treated with surgery, radiation therapy, or a combination of the two. Many recurrences

Table 2-4   Carcinoma of the Corpus Uteri—Staging FIGO TNM

Stages	Categories	
	Primary tumor cannot be assessed.	TX
	No evidence of primary tumor.	T0
0	Carcinoma in situ (pre-invasive carcinoma)	Tis
I	Tumor confined to the corpus uteri	T1
	IA Tumor limited to endometrium	T1a
	IB Tumor invades up to less than half of myometrium.	T1b
	IC Tumor invades to more than one half of myometrium.	T1c
II	Tumor invades cervix but does not extend beyond uterus.	T2
	IIA Endocervical glandular involvement only	T2a
	IIB Cervical stromal invasion	T2b
III	Local and/or regional spread as specified in IIIA, B, C T3 and/or N1	
	IIIA Tumor involves serosa and/or adnexae (direct extension or metastasis) and/or cancer cells in ascites or peritoneal washings.	T3a
	IIIB Vaginal involvement (direct extension or metastasis)	T3b
	IIIC Metastasis to pelvic and/or para-aortic lymph nodes	N1
	IVA Tumor invades bladder mucosa and/or bower mucosa.	T4
	IVB Distant metastasis (excluding metastasis to vagina, pelvic serosa, or adnexa, including metastasis to intra-abdominal lymph nodes other than para-aortic and/or inguinal nodes)	M1

Note: The presence of bullous edema is not sufficient evidence to classify a tumor as T4. Reprinted from the International Federation of Gynecology and Obstetrics (FIGO): Benedict JL, Bender H, Jones H, Ngan HYS, Pecorelli S. Int J Gynecol Obstet 2000; 70:209–62; with permission.

are distant, and radiation therapy may be of limited benefit. Hormone treatment or chemotherapy may be the treatment of choice (7).

Other Gynecologic Malignancies

Fallopian tube cancer and primary peritoneal cancer are similar to ovarian cancer. Histologically, these malignancies are identical to serous ovarian cancer. Epidemiology, risks factors, and treatment, including surgical staging or debulking and chemotherapy, are the same, although a recent publication notes that the etiology of primary peritoneal cancer may actually follow a separate pathway from ovarian and fallopian tube cancer (12). Nevertheless, all 3 entities are treated similarly and are considered the same for inclusion in clinical trials.

Vulvar and vaginal cancer are rare gynecologic malignancies, with less than a total of 5000 new cases and approximately 1500 deaths each year in the U.S. (4,13). Risk factors are similar to risks for cervical cancer, most importantly sexual behaviors leading to acquisition of human papillomavirus. Other risk factors include cigarette smoking, history of dysplasia or carcinoma of other genital organs (cervix, vulva, vagina, anus), sexually transmitted infections (gonorrhea, herpes simplex), and immunocompromised status. Vulvar and vaginal cancer are most prevalent after the age of 70 years, and the majority of the patients have squamous histology. A rare type of vaginal cancer, clear cell carcinoma, is associated with diethylstilbestrol (DES) exposure of a female fetus *in utero* (14).

Gestational trophoblastic disease (GTD) is a rare but important form of malignancy, which manifests as a complication of pregnancy (15). Worldwide the incidence varies significantly, with a 7–10-fold greater incidence in Asian countries versus North America and Europe. Socioeconomic and nutritional factors have been implicated as risk factors and possibly explain some of these regional differences. GTD is more common at the extremes of reproductive age (young and older gravidas); age >40 increases risk by 5–10-fold. Risk increases with history of prior pregnancy complicated by GTD, spontaneous abortion, or infertility. The incidence of complete or partial molar pregnancy in North America and Europe is 1/600 of therapeutic abortions or 1/1000–1200 of normal pregnancies. Fifteen percent of complete moles and 4% of partial moles will need treatment for malignant sequelae following evacuation. Gestational trophoblastic disease should be considered in any female of reproductive age presenting with symptoms suggestive of pregnancy complications, or metastatic disease of unknown origin (15).

References

1. **Brinton LA, Hoover RN.** Epidemiology of Gynecologic Cancers. In Hoskins WJ, Perez CA, Young RC (eds): Principles and Practice of Gynecologic Oncology. Philadelphia: Lippincott Williams & Wilkins; 2000:3–27.
2. **Lancaster JM, Powell CB, Kauff ND, et al.** Society of Gynecologic Oncologists Education Committee. Gynecol Oncol. 2007;107:159–62.
3. **Naucler P, Ryed W, Tornberg S, et al.** Human papillomavirus and papanicolau tests to screen for cervical cancer. N Engl J Med. 2007;357:1589–97.
4. **Jemal A, Siegel R, Ward E, et al.** Cancer statistics 2008. CA Cancer J Clin. 2008;58:71–96.
5. American College of Obstetricians & Gynecologists, ACOG Practice Bulletin Management of adnexal masses. Obstet Gynecol. 2007;110:201–14.
6. **Petignat P, Roy M.** Diagnosis and management of cervical cancer. BMJ. 2007;13:765–8.
7. **Irvin WP, Rice LW,** Berkowitz RS. Advances in the management of endometrial cancer. A review. J Repro Med. 2002;47:173–89.
8. **Earle CC, Schrag D, Neville BA, et al.** Effect of surgeon specialty on processes of care and outcomes for ovarian cancer patients. J Natl Cancer Inst. 2006;98:172–80.
9. **Armstrong DK, Bundy B, Wenzel L, et al.** Intraperitoneal cisplatin and paclitaxel in ovarian cancer. N Engl J Med. 2006;354:34–43.
10. **Roland PY, Kelly FJ, Kulwicki CY, et al.** The benefits of a gynecologic oncologist: a pattern of care study for endometrial cancer treatment. Gynecol Oncol. 2004;93:125–30.
11. **Fleming GF, Filiaci VL, Bentley RC, et al.** Phase III randomized trial of doxorubicin + cisplatin versus doxorubicin + 24 h paclitaxel + flitrastim in

endometrial cancer: a Gynecologic Oncology Group Study. Ann Oncol. 2004;15:1173–8.

12. **Jordan SJ, Green AD, Whiteman DC, et al.** Australia Cancer Study Group (ovarian cancer), Australian Ovarian Cancer Study Group. Serous ovarian, fallopian tube, and primary peritoneal cancers: a comparative epidemiologic analysis. Int J Cancer. 2008;122:1598–603.

13. **Canaran TP, Cohen D.** Vulvar cancer. Am Fam Physician. 2002;66: 1269–74.

14. **Herbst AL, Anderson D.** Clear cell adenocarcinoma of the vagina and cervix secondary to intrauterine exposure to diethylstilbesterol. Semin Surg Oncol. 1990;6:343–6.

15. **Soper JT.** Gestational trophoblastic disease. Obstet Gynecol. 2006;108: 176–87.

16. **Barakat RR, Grigsby PW, Sabbatini P, et al.** Corpus: Epithelial Tumors. In Hoskins WJ, Perez CA, Young RC (eds): Principles and Practice of Gynecologic Oncology. Philadelphia: Lippincott Williams & Wilkins; 2000:919–59.

B. Breast Cancer

Anna Maria Storniolo and Lida Mina

KEY POINTS

- Breast cancer is the second leading cause of cancer death in American women.
- Primary prevention through lifestyle modifications and the use of certain selective estrogen receptor modulators can have an impact on breast cancer incidence.
- Secondary prevention through risk assessment and adequate screening should be incorporated into general medical practice.
- The treatment of breast cancer consists of surgery, with or without radiation for local control, and systemic therapy, which can include anti-estrogens, chemotherapy, and some newer targeted biologic therapies, depending on the pathologic features of the cancer and extent of disease.

Epidemiology

Breast cancer is the most common malignancy in women in the U.S., accounting for nearly one third of all female cancers. Breast cancer is also responsible for 15% of cancer deaths in women, making it the second leading cause of cancer death following lung cancer. One in eight American women will be diagnosed with breast cancer during their lifetime, making the average lifetime risk 13.2%. It is estimated that 178 480 new cases of breast cancer will be diagnosed by the end of 2007, and 40 460 will die of this cancer (1).

After decades of increasing incidence, trends are finally shifting. There has been a decrease in breast cancer incidence from 1999 to 2003, and a steady plateau since that time (2).

Breast cancer rarely occurs in men and accounts for <1% of all cancers in men. The female:male ratio is approximately 100:1. The highest rates occur in Caucasian women, whereas the lowest occur in Native American women. Globally, breast cancer incidence rates are highest in North America and northern Europe and lowest in Asia and Africa. The higher a woman's socioeconomic status, the higher her risk of breast cancer. It has been suggested that these trends in breast cancer reflect lifestyle differences (such as age at first birth) as well as dietary influences. Age is the single most important risk factor associated with breast cancer. Incidence increases steadily until the eighth decade of life. Fifty percent of newly diagnosed cases of breast cancer occur in women over the age of 65 years.

Interestingly, breast cancer mortality is higher in African American women than in white American women despite a lower incidence of the disease. Socioeconomic disparities seem to account only partly for this difference; African American women are at higher risk of developing early-onset, more aggressive, ER (estrogen receptor)-negative breast cancer. It is still unclear whether breast tumor biology is different across different ethnicities (3).

Signs and Symptoms

The most common complaint, whenever symptoms are present, is a breast lump, which occurs in 65–76% of cases. Other symptoms include breast pain (5%), skin or nipple retraction (5%), nipple discharge (2%), breast enlargement (1%), and nipple erosions or crusting (<1%).

Diagnosis

Mammography is the first step toward diagnosing breast cancer. Mammography findings suggestive of malignancy include asymmetric lesions, micro-calcifications, and a mass or architectural distortion. Based upon a suspicious mammogram, the primary physician should order an adjunctive image, usually additional mammographic views and/or breast ultrasound. If suspicions persist, patients should be referred for breast biopsy. Most commonly, this is achieved through fine needle aspiration of a palpable lesion or ultrasound-guided core biopsy.

Prevention

Prevention is the key to reducing breast cancer incidence and mortality. Whereas secondary prevention involves early detection to find the cancer at an early, hopefully curable stage, primary prevention aims to alter the process of breast carcinogenesis, thus preventing the malignancy from occurring at all.

Risk Assessment

History

Adequately trained health care professionals are key to the successful integration of cancer risk assessment into clinical practice. A detailed history should be taken, including personal history (reproductive, hormonal, and prior cancers), as well as family history (including age of onset, type of cancer, and age at death) out to 3 generations, if possible. A family pedigree should be drawn in order to detect a cancer pattern.

Breast cancer risk factors other than age include: family history of breast cancer; personal history of certain benign breast conditions (atypical hyperplasia, lobular carcinoma *in situ*); early menarche; late menopause; nulliparity/late first birth; alcohol use; history of radiation; possibly high fat diet; and use of hormone replacement therapy (HRT). The Women's Health Initiative trial (WHI) assessed the risks and benefits of estrogen and progestin combination in healthy postmenopausal women and concluded that invasive breast cancer rates were significantly higher in the HRT group with hazard ratio of 1.26 (95% CI, 1–1.59) (4). It has been speculated that numerous other risk factors may increase the risk of breast cancer, but, despite all of the available data, 75% of women with breast cancer have no known risk factors.

The Gail Model

For women over the age of 35 years, several tools are available to identify those at increased risk. The Gail Model (5), the use of which was validated in the NSABP-P1 trial, is a computer-based mathematical model that incorporates several risk factors to arrive at an absolute risk of developing breast cancer in the next 5 years and also produces a lifetime risk. Those risk factors accounted for in the Gail model include age, age at menarche, age at first birth or nulliparity, number of first-degree relatives with breast cancer, number of previous benign breast biopsies, history of atypical hyperplasia, and race. Other risk models, most notably the Claus model (6), exist but have not been routinely incorporated into clinical practice. Recently, newer models combine previously identified risk factors and add several others, namely breast density, BMI, and hormone therapy use (7,8).

Genetics

Genetic-linkage studies in large families with multiple members who have breast cancer, ovarian cancer, or both, led to the discovery of two breast cancer susceptibility genes, BRCA1 and BRCA2, in 1994 and 1995, respectively. BRCA mutations are rare in the general population but are present in up to 2% in the Ashkenazi Jewish population. Five to ten percent of all breast cancers are attributable to deleterious BRCA mutations. Genetic testing should be done in a selected patient population per ASCO (American Society of Clinical Oncology) recommendations (9) (Box 2-1).

Box 2-1   ASCO Recommendations for Genetic Testing

1. High incidence of breast cancer in family, especially multiple people in multiple generations
2. Breast cancer occurring at an early age
3. Relatives with more than one breast cancer
4. Family history of ovarian cancer, especially in persons who have also had breast cancer
5. Related males with breast cancer
6. Ashkenazi Jewish descent

Screening

Secondary prevention consists of screening the general population. For women without strong family histories, discussions about breast cancer screening should start at the age of 40 years and end when life expectancy is less then 10 years. Although there has been some controversy regarding mammography screening (10), the data overwhelmingly support the conclusion that it results in a decrease in breast cancer mortality (11). Evidence supporting the usefulness of mammography screening is strongest for women between 50 and 69 years of age, and screening should be routinely recommended in this age group (11). The American Cancer Society guidelines currently recommend yearly mammograms starting at age 40 (12) (Table 2-5).

There are limited data supporting the use of ultrasound for breast cancer screening as an adjunct to mammogram in high-risk patients or patients with dense breasts. However, one study (DMIST) supported the benefit of digital mammography in young women and women with dense breasts (13).

Primary Prevention

Lifestyle modifications known to impact breast cancer include early age at first pregnancy, longer lactation, weight control, regular exercise, limited

Table 2-5   Mammography Screening Recommendations

	Women at Normal Risk	Women with Genetic Predisposition
Breast Self-Exam	Starting at age 20, women are instructed to do self-exams and report abnormalities.	Monthly starting at age 18
Clinical Breast Exam	• Every 3 y starting at age 20	Every 6 months starting at age 25
	• Annually starting at age 40	
Mammogram	Annually starting at age 40	Annually starting at age 25

alcohol intake, and avoidance of smoking. Breast-feeding was also found to play a pivotal role; a recent analysis showed that the relative risk of breast cancer is reduced by 4.3% (95% CI 2.5–5.8) for each year a woman breast-feeds (14). More recently, the WINS trial showed that reducing dietary fat intake also may improve relapse-free survival of breast cancer patients receiving conventional cancer management (15). One might extrapolate these data to conclude that reducing dietary fat intake may indeed result in primary prevention, but this has not yet been demonstrated in a clinical trial.

The selective estrogen receptor modulators (SERMs) tamoxifen and raloxifene have estrogen agonist or antagonist effects, depending on the target organ. In breast tissue, both have antagonistic effects, leading to their use as chemoprevention agents in breast cancer. Two large trials of tamoxifen for primary prevention (NSABP P-1 and IBIS-1) suggest a statistically significant decrease in the risk of ER-positive invasive breast cancer, but no influence on the incidence of ER-negative breast cancer (16,17). The National Comprehensive Cancer Network (NCCN) currently recommends tamoxifen as an option to reduce breast cancer risk in healthy pre- and postmenopausal women >35 years of age who have ≥1.7% 5-year risk of breast cancer (by Gail score) or who have lobular carcinoma *in situ* (LCIS). More recently the STAR trial suggested that raloxifene could be as effective as tamoxifen in reducing the incidence of invasive breast cancer in high-risk postmenopausal women, with a lower risk of thromboembolic events (9). The NCCN now offers raloxifene as an option for postmenopausal high-risk women (as defined above) or those who have LCIS.

Women at very high risk of breast cancer can go beyond chemoprevention and seek risk reduction surgery. Prophylactic mastectomy is, in fact, associated with a substantial decrease in the incidence of subsequent breast cancer in patients with a strong family history of breast cancer, ovarian cancer, or both, as well as in women with BRCA1/BRCA2 mutations (18). However, such surgery can negatively impact the body perception image of a woman and affect her relationships, and extensive psychosocial discussions are warranted before such a decision is made. An alternative to bilateral prophylactic mastectomies, especially in women with BRCA1/BRCA2 mutations, is bilateral salpingo-oopherectomy, which not only nearly eliminates the risk of ovarian cancer in these women at high risk for breast and ovarian cancer, but also reduces the risk of breast cancer by 75% (19,20).

Management of Breast Cancer

A central component of the management of breast cancer is full knowledge of the extent of the disease (staging) and its biologic features (hormone receptors and epidermal growth factor receptor-2 [HER-2] status). After breast tissue is obtained, it is of utmost importance to determine the status of the following biomarkers: ER (estrogen receptor), PR (progesterone receptor), and HER-2. Therapy is then tailored accordingly. Breast cancer can be divided into non-invasive carcinomas and invasive carcinomas and is staged based on the American Joint Committee on Cancer (AJCC), as illustrated in Table 2-6 (21).

Table 2-6   Breast Cancer Staging

Stage 0	Carcinoma in situ
Stage I	Tumor ≤2 cm, node negative
Stage II	• **IIA**: Tumor 2–5, node negative or tumor <2 cm, node positive
	• **IIB**: Tumor >5 cm, node negative or tumor 2–5 cm, node positive
Stage III	• **IIIA**: Tumor >5 cm, node positive or tumor <5 cm, node positive with lymph nodes attached to each other or other structures
	• **IIIB**: Tumor penetrated to skin of breast or chest wall, or spread to internal mammary nodes
Stage IV	Distant metastasis

For the operable local-regional carcinoma, the mainstay of initial treatment is local control. This is achieved either by mastectomy or by lumpectomy in addition to total breast irradiation. Sentinel lymph node dissection with either surgical option is warranted. In 2008, systemic adjuvant chemotherapy usually consists of an anthracycline with or without a taxane. New data suggest that one might avoid the potential cardiotoxicity of the anthracycline by using a combination of cyclophosphamide and docetaxel (22). Women with hormone receptor-positive breast cancer also should be treated with anti-estrogen therapy, which includes tamoxifen or an aromatase inhibitor, depending on menopausal status.

For locally advanced breast cancer, including inflammatory breast cancer, a multimodal approach is needed, based on the concept that breast cancer is already a systemic disease at presentation. Neoadjuvant chemotherapy (anthracycline-based combination with concurrent or sequential taxane) is generally recommended, followed by local therapy with surgery and, if feasible, radiation treatment. Breast conserving surgery is contraindicated in inflammatory breast cancer. For ER-positive breast cancer, adjuvant hormonal treatment also is recommended.

Ductal carcinoma *in situ* (DCIS) is also called Stage 0 breast cancer. It is considered a local disease, and, therefore, the treatment involves lumpectomy and radiation, or mastectomy. A retrospective analysis of data from the NSABP-24 trial has shown that women whose DCIS stains as ER-positive have approximately 50% lower risk for subsequent breast cancer compared to placebo when treated with 5 years of tamoxifen, in essence for secondary prevention (23,24).

Metastatic disease is unlikely to be cured; however, meaningful improvements in survival have been achieved in the last 2 decades. Because of its more favorable safety profile, endocrine therapy is usually initiated in ER-positive metastatic breast cancer. For non-responsive disease or for ER-negative disease, chemotherapy is an appropriate option. Fortunately, breast cancer is one of the most chemotherapy-sensitive solid tumors. Several classes of cytotoxic agents can be initiated as monotherapy or in combination regimens. In metastatic disease, attention to palliation of symptoms, such as pain, nausea, and weakness, is a critical aspect of patient care.

Targeted Therapy

Targeted therapy in breast cancer has transformed the landscape of this disease over the last generation. The most important advance in targeted therapy has been the ability to target the estrogen receptor. The success story continues with trastuzumab, a humanized monoclonal antibody that targets epidermal growth factor receptor-2 or HER-2. Trastuzumab is now indicated in the adjuvant as well as metastatic setting for all breast cancers that over-express HER-2 (25,26).

Finally, even the oldest chemotherapy can become targeted if we have the ability to select the patient population that will benefit the most and have the fewest side effects. The recent use of multigene reverse transcriptase polymerase chain reaction technology (Oncotype DX) in ER–positive, lymph node–negative breast cancer has revealed that even "older" chemotherapy regimens like cyclophosphamide, methotrexate, and fluorouracil (CMF) can be strikingly effective for a specific population of patients (27).

The future of all anti-cancer therapy will lie in the identification of new targets for anti-cancer drugs, using advanced tools, such as genomics and proteomics, and in better identifying the population subsets that would best benefit from these therapies.

References

1. **Jemal A, et al.** Cancer statistics, 2007. CA Cancer J Clin. 2007;57:43–66.
2. **Anderson WF, et al.** Shifting breast cancer trends in the United States. J Clin Oncol. 2007;25:3923–9.
3. **Newman LA, et al.** African-American ethnicity, socioeconomic status, and breast cancer survival: a meta-analysis of 14 studies involving over 10,000 African-American and 40,000 White American patients with carcinoma of the breast. Cancer. 2002;94:2844–54.
4. **Rossouw JE, et al.** Risks and benefits of estrogen plus progestin in healthy postmenopausal women: principal results from the Women's Health Initiative randomized controlled trial. JAMA. 2002;288:321–33.
5. **Gail MH, et al.** Projecting individualized probabilities of developing breast cancer for white females who are being examined annually. J Natl Cancer Inst. 1989;81:1879–86.
6. **Claus EB, Risch N, Thompson WD.** Autosomal dominant inheritance of early-onset breast cancer, Implications for risk prediction. Cancer. 1994;73:643–51.
7. **Chen J, et al.** Projecting absolute invasive breast cancer risk in white women with a model that includes mammographic density. J Natl Cancer Inst. 2006;98:1215–26.
8. **Barlow WE, et al.** Prospective breast cancer risk prediction model for women undergoing screening mammography. J Natl Cancer Inst. 2006;98:1204–14.
9. **Khatcheressian JL, et al.** American Society of Clinical Oncology 2006 update of the breast cancer follow-up and management guidelines in the adjuvant setting. J Clin Oncol. 2006;24:5091–7.

10. **Olsen O, Gotzsche PC.** Cochrane review on screening for breast cancer with mammography. Lancet. 2001;358:1340–2.

11. **Fletcher SW, Elmore JG.** Clinical practice. Mammographic screening for breast cancer. N Engl J Med. 2003;348:1672–80.

12. **Smith RA, Cokkinides V, Eyre, HJ.** American Cancer Society guidelines for the early detection of cancer, 2006. CA Cancer J Clin. 2006;56: 11–25;quiz 49–50.

13. **Pisano ED, et al.** Diagnostic performance of digital versus film mammography for breast-cancer screening. N Engl J Med. 2005;353:1773–83.

14. Breast cancer and breastfeeding: collaborative reanalysis of individual data from 47 epidemiological studies in 30 countries, including 50302 women with breast cancer and 96973 women without the disease. Lancet. 2002;360:187–95.

15. **Chlebowski RT, et al.** Dietary fat reduction and breast cancer outcome: interim efficacy results from the Women's Intervention Nutrition Study. J Natl Cancer Inst. 2006;98:1767–76.

16. **King MC, et al.** Tamoxifen and breast cancer incidence among women with inherited mutations in BRCA1 and BRCA2: National Surgical Adjuvant Breast and Bowel Project (NSABP-P1) Breast Cancer Prevention Trial. JAMA. 2001;286:2251–6.

17. **Cuzick J, et al.** First results from the International Breast Cancer Intervention Study (IBIS-I): a randomised prevention trial. Lancet. 2002;360:817–24.

18. **Hartmann LC, et al.** Efficacy of bilateral prophylactic mastectomy in BRCA1 and BRCA2 gene mutation carriers. J Natl Cancer Inst. 2001;93:1633–7.

19. **Kauff ND, et al.** Risk-reducing salpingo-oophorectomy in women with a BRCA1 or BRCA2 mutation. N Engl J Med. 2002;346:1609–15.

20. **Rebbeck TR, et al.** Prophylactic oophorectomy in carriers of BRCA1 or BRCA2 mutations. N Engl J Med. 2002;346:1616–22.

21. **Singletary SE, et al.** Revision of the American Joint Committee on Cancer staging system for breast cancer. J Clin Oncol. 2002;20:3628–36.

22. **Jones SE, et al.** Phase III trial comparing doxorubicin plus cyclophosphamide with docetaxel plus cyclophosphamide as adjuvant therapy for operable breast cancer. J Clin Oncol. 2006;24:5381–7.

23. **Fisher B, et al.** Tamoxifen in treatment of intraductal breast cancer: National Surgical Adjuvant Breast and Bowel Project B-24 randomised controlled trial. Lancet. 1999;353:1993–2000.

24. **Allred DC, B.J., Land S et al.** Estrogen receptor expression as a predictive marker of the effectiveness of Tamoxifen in the treatment of DCIS: findings from NSABP protocol B-24. Breast Cancer Research Treatment. 2002;76:36.

25. **Piccart-Gebhart MJ, et al.** Trastuzumab after adjuvant chemotherapy in HER2-positive breast cancer. N Engl J Med. 2005;353:1659–72.

26. **Marty M, et al.** Randomized phase II trial of the efficacy and safety of trastuzumab combined with docetaxel in patients with human epidermal growth factor receptor 2-positive metastatic breast cancer administered as first-line treatment: the M77001 study group. J Clin Oncol. 2005;23:4265–74.

27. **Paik S, et al.** A multigene assay to predict recurrence of tamoxifen-treated, node-negative breast cancer. N Engl J Med. 2004;351:2817–26.

C. Lung Cancer

Shadia Jalal and Nasser Hanna

KEY POINTS

- Lung cancer is the leading cause of cancer deaths in women.
- Death rate from lung cancer in women has increased dramatically over the last 50 years.
- Among nonsmokers, lung cancer is much more common in women than in men.
- Adenocarcinoma is the most common type of lung cancer in women, whereas squamous cell carcinoma is more common in men.
- Prevention or cessation of smoking is the most effective way to reduce lung cancer.
- Women have longer survival after a diagnosis of lung cancer but experience more toxicity from treatment than men.

Epidemiology

In 1999, cancer exceeded heart disease as the most common cause of death for people younger than 85 years of age (1). Of all cancers, lung cancer remains the leading cause of cancer-related death for both men and women in the U.S. Lung cancer accounts for 29% of all cancer-related deaths in women and claims more female lives every year than breast, uterine, and ovarian cancers combined (2). The death rate of lung cancer among U.S. women has become epidemic, increasing 600% from 1930 to 1997 (3).

The dramatic increase in cigarette consumption is primarily responsible for the lung cancer epidemic in women during the twentieth century. It is estimated that 22 million women in the U.S. currently smoke, including 500,000 teenage girls (2). Tobacco advertisements target young women by stressing images of independence, popularity, and beauty. The desire of some women to lose weight, and the belief that smoking helps with weight control, attracts some to start smoking. The addictive nature of nicotine results in the persistence of the habit even during pregnancy, where smoking rates range from 13% to 22% (2).

While cigarette consumption is by far the primary cause of lung cancer, nonsmokers may also be afflicted. Among non-smokers, lung cancer disproportionately occurs in women. It is estimated that 53% of all women with lung cancer worldwide are nonsmokers, compared to only 15% of men. In some Asian countries, never-smokers account for 70% of women diagnosed with lung cancer (4).

Clinical Features and Presentation

Like their male counterparts, the majority of women with lung cancer present with advanced-stage disease because early-stage disease is usually asymptomatic. Symptoms of lung cancer may be related to the primary tumor lesion or to metastatic disease. Common symptoms include cough, dyspnea (due to malignant pleural or pericardial effusions), hemoptysis, hoarse voice (due to recurrent laryngeal nerve injury), and chest pain. Symptoms of advanced disease include pain, fatigue, and weight loss. Less frequently, patients may present with Horner's syndrome (ptosis, miosis, and anhidrosis) due to superior sulcus tumors or superior vena cava (SVC) syndrome caused by compression of that vessel (5).

The most common sites of metastases are brain, liver, bone, and adrenals. Therefore, patients may experience headaches, visual or behavioral changes, bone pain, or persistent nausea and vomiting. Less commonly, paraneoplastic syndromes, including hyponatremia due to the syndrome of inappropriate ADH secretion, Cushing's syndrome due to elevated ACTH levels, or hypercalcemia due to the production of PTH-related peptide, can be seen at presentation (5).

Lung cancer histology is divided into small-cell and non-small-cell subtypes. Small-cell is primarily a disease of smokers in both men and women. Approximately 85% of all lung cancers are non-small-cell type. Adenocarcinoma is the more common histology in female smokers and never-smokers, compared to squamous cell carcinoma in male smokers (2). In one series, 73.9% of nonsmokers with lung cancer were women, and adenocarcinoma was present in 74.5% of them (6).

Sex-associated differences in presentation and survival also have been reported. In a study by Ferguson et al., women were younger at presentation (mean age 57.4 vs. 60.2) (7). Men were more likely to be current or ex-smokers and had higher overall tobacco consumption. Sex also was found to be an independent prognostic factor for survival, since women had better survival (independent of stage and histological subtype).

Diagnosis and Differential Diagnosis

The diagnosis of lung cancer is usually confirmed by biopsy of a suspicious mass or lymph node. Staging of non-small-cell lung cancer (NSCLC) utilizes the tumor, node, and metastasis (TNM) staging system developed by the American Joint Committee on Cancer (AJCC) (5). Staging of small-cell lung cancer (SCLC) follows the Veterans Administration Lung Group System, which divides the disease into limited and extensive stage. Limited-stage SCLC is defined as tumor confined to one hemithorax and regional lymph nodes (in the absence of a pleural effusion), while disease extending beyond this is defined as extensive-stage (8).

Patients diagnosed with lung cancer are usually staged with a computed tomography (CT) scan of the chest and abdomen, in addition to brain imaging (head CT scan or brain MRI). Bone scans and PET scans also are frequently utilized to define bone metastases or other

---

Box 2-2   Differential Diagnosis of Solitary Lung Mass

- Primary lung cancer
- Carcinoid tumor
- Metastatic cancer (melanoma, sarcoma, testicular cancer, colon cancer, breast cancer)
- Infectious granulomas (histoplasmosis, coccidioidomycosis, tuberculous or nontuberculous mycobacteria)
- Hamartomas

Box 2-3   Differential Diagnosis of Multiple Pulmonary Nodules

- Malignancy (solid organs, non-Hodgkin's lymphoma)
- Multiple abscesses
- Septic emboli
- Infectious granulomas (histoplasmosis, coccidioidomycosis, TB or nontuberculous mycobacteria)
- Wegener's granulomatosis
- Pulmonary arteriovenous malformation

---

unsuspected sites of disease, particularly when contemplating surgical resection for cure (8). Mediastinoscopy, mediastinotomy, endoscopic ultrasound of the esophagus, or bronchoscopy also are frequently utilized to more accurately stage the mediastinum.

The differential diagnosis of lung cancer is included in Boxes 2-2 and 2-3.

Prevention and Clinical Care

Since tobacco continues to be the primary risk factor for lung cancer in women, tobacco control remains the most effective preventative method against the development of lung cancer. Some studies have shown that females are less successful than males in quitting smoking when only pharmacologic interventions are used. Behavioral methods and treatment of problems that may have arisen during prior attempts at quitting, like weight gain or depression, should be addressed in women (2).

Chemoprevention (primary, secondary, and tertiary) has been studied in lung cancer. Retinoids and beta-carotene supplementation failed to demonstrate any benefit in reducing the incidence of lung cancer. The National Cancer Institute (NCI) is currently sponsoring a phase III trial evaluating selenium in preventing tumor recurrence in patients previously treated for stage I disease. Lastly, screening chest x-rays in high-risk patients have failed to reduce lung cancer mortality rates. Screening CT studies have demonstrated an ability to diagnose more stage I tumors, primarily adenocarcinoma, and lead to a high rate of surgical cure (9). However, ongoing trials are addressing whether screening CTs will ultimately reduce lung cancer mortality rates.

Etiologic Differences

As stated earlier, 53% of women with lung cancer worldwide have never smoked. Therefore, factors other than tobacco are thought to cause lung cancer in these individuals.

Environmental tobacco exposure or second-hand smoke is associated with an increased risk of lung cancer in never-smokers. A meta-analysis of 19 studies evaluating never-smoking women showed an increased risk of lung cancer by 20% due to environmental tobacco exposure (4).

Exposure to cooking fumes also is believed to be associated with increased risk of lung cancer in Chinese women. Type of cooking (especially frying), duration of cooking-years, and lack of proper ventilation play a role in the increased risk (4).

Women with prolonged exposure to radon (a uranium degradation product) were found to be at a higher risk for lung cancer in the Iowa Radon Lung Cancer Study. Asbestos also is a risk factor. Other heavy metals, including metal dust, nickel, cadmium, chromium, and arsenic, have been implicated in the pathogenesis of lung cancer (4).

Differences in Carcinogenesis of Tobacco

It is unclear whether women are more susceptible than men are to the carcinogenic effects of cigarette smoking. In a study by Henschke and Miettinen (10), 1200 female and male smokers were screened for lung cancer using CT scans. The risk of developing lung cancer was 2.7 times higher in women than in men. However, several other carefully conducted cohort studies, including the American Cancer Society (ACS) follow-up prevention trial, the Carotene and Retinol Efficacy trial (11), and an analysis of the Nurses' Health Study each reported no convincing evidence of an increased risk of lung cancer among women smokers compared to their male counterparts (12).

Biological Differences

Genetic differences involving enzymes that play a role in carcinogen metabolism are believed to exist between women and men. Examples include the increased expression of the CYP1A gene noted in the lungs of female smokers (13). CYP1A encodes for enzymes involved in the metabolism of carcinogenic polycyclic aromatic hydrocarbons (PAH). PAH leads to the formation of highly reactive substances that form DNA adducts. Lower DNA repair capacity also has been reported in women. A higher average of DNA adduct levels in lung tumors of women compared to men was reported by Kure *et al.*, even though females in that study had fewer pack-years of smoking (14).

Biological differences in lung cancers have been reported. For example, women with adenocarcinoma reportedly have a higher frequency of K-*ras* mutations. In addition, epidermal growth factor receptor (EGFR)-activating mutations occur at higher frequency in women (2).

Hormonal Differences

The estrogen receptors (ER) α and β have been reported in lung cancer tissue. However, the clinical significance of this expression is unclear. ERβ is the dominant estrogen in lung tissue and seems to regulate lung development, specifically alveolar formation and surfactant homeostasis. This expression might contribute to the greater lung maturity and higher surfactant levels noted in women. It has been observed that β-estradiol leads to proliferation of NSCLC cells, while estrogen blockade inhibits lung tumor growth. Crosstalk between EGFR and estrogen-ER signaling pathways has been reported in lung cancer. Furthermore, the metabolic products of estrogen (catechol estrogens) are believed to interact with DNA directly, forming DNA adducts, which result in critical mutations leading to carcinogenesis (15).

There is conflicting evidence regarding the effect of exogenous estrogens on the development and outcome of lung cancer in women. Ganti et al., (16) reported a longer overall survival in post-menopausal women who never used hormone replacement therapy (HRT), with median survival of 79 months versus 39 months in women who had used HRT (P = 0.02, HR [hazard ratio] = 1.77, 95% CI, 1.09 to 2.86).

In another study, postmenopausal women with breast cancer were randomized after 2–3 years of tamoxifen to receive either exemestane (steroidal aromatase inhibitor) or to continue on tamoxifen for the remainder of 5 years of total treatment. Women randomized to the tamoxifen group had an increased risk of second primary non-breast cancers, mainly lung cancer (12 women in tamoxifen group vs. 4 women in exemestane group) (17).

Outcome Differences

Sex differences in lung cancer survival have been observed for all stages and histological subtypes. Women have longer survival following surgical resection than their male counterparts. Female sex also is associated with a more favorable outcome in SCLC (18).

In a recently reported randomized trial, which evaluated adjuvant vinorelbine plus cisplatin versus observation in patients with resected NSCLC, factors associated with improved survival included female sex (19).

Treatment effects with individual agents also may differ depending on the sex of the patient. For example, EGFR inhibitors are more active in women than in men with NSCLC. In a study comparing erlotinib 150 mg po daily versus placebo in patients with stage III/ IV NSCLC (prior treatment with 1 or 2 chemotherapy regimens), the largest benefit in overall response rate was noted in women (14.4% compared to 6.0%, P = 0.006) (20). In addition, 2 recent phase III trials, STELLAR 3 and STELLAR 4, have reflected some of the effects gender can have on outcome. Both studies included chemo-naive patients with poor performance status (PS = 2) and advanced NSCLC. STELLAR 3 compared carboplatin/paclitaxel to paclitaxel poliglumex (PPX)/carboplatin. STELLAR 4 compared PPX to either gemcitabine or vinrelbine. Patients in both trials were stratified by age and gender. The primary endpoint of the trials was overall survival, which did not differ among the arms. However, an exploratory analysis revealed a trend towards improved survival in women in the PPX arms. Median survival advantage for

PPX-treated patients was greater in women <55 years old (10.0 vs. 5.2 months, P = 0.038) (21). A possible explanation for the improved survival in premenopausal women is that estrogen upregulates the activity of cathepsin B, a protease with increased expression in aggressive tumors that plays an important role in the efficient release of paclitaxel.

Toxicity differences related to lung cancer treatment also have been noted between men and women. Possible explanations for increased toxicity observed in women include a lower clearance rate of certain drugs like doxorubicin and 5-fluorouracil in women, and the higher baseline body-mass index in women due to increased body fat.

Conclusion

The epidemic of lung cancer in women must be aggressively confronted. Women who have the highest smoking prevalence have not reached the age at which they would be at greatest risk for lung cancer. Therefore, female mortality from lung cancer is expected to rise. Tobacco control measures are critical, and further study is needed to understand the unique biological differences and causes of lung cancer in women.

References

1. **Jemal A, Murray T, Ward E et al.** Cancer statistics. CA Cancer J Clin. 2005;55:10–30.
2. **Patel JD.** Lung cancer in women. J Clin Oncol. 2005;23:3212–8.
3. **Patel JD, Bach PB, Kris MG.** Lung cancer in women: a contemporary epidemic. JAMA. 2004;219:1763–8.
4. **Subramanian J, Govindan R.** Lung cancer in never smokers: a review. J Clin Oncol. 2007;25:561–70.
5. **Midthun DE, Jett JR.** Clinical presentation of lung cancer. In: Pass HI, et al. (eds), Lung Cancer: Principles and Practice. Philadelphia: Lippincott-Raven; 1996:421.
6. **Toh CK, et al.** The impact of smoking status on the behavior and survival outcome of patients with advanced non-small cell lung cancer: a retrospective analysis. Chest. 2004;126:1750–6.
7. **Ferguson MK, et al.** Sex-associated differences in presentation and survival in patients with lung cancer. J Clin Oncol. 1990;8:1402–7.
8. **Spira A, Ettinger DS.** Multidisciplinary management of lung cancer. N Engl J Med. 2004;350:379–92.
9. The International Early Lung Cancer Action Program Investigators. Survival of patients with Stage I lung cancer detected on CT screening. N Engl J Med. 2006;355:1763–71.
10. **Henschke CI, Miettinen OS.** Women's susceptibility to tobacco carcinogens and survival after diagnosis of lung cancer. JAMA. 2006;296:180–4.
11. **Bach PB, et al.** Variations in lung cancer risk among smokers. J Natl Cancer Inst. 2003;95:470–8.
12. **Bain C, et al.** Lung Cancer rates in men and women with comparable histories of smoking. J Natl Cancer Inst. 2004;96:826–34.
13. **Mollerup S, et al.** Sex differences in lung CYP1A1 expression and DNA adduct levels among lung cancer patients. Cancer Research. 1999;59:3317–20.

14. **Kure EH, Ryberg D, Hewer A, et al.** p53 mutations in lung tumors: Relationship to gender and lung DNA adduct levels. Carcinogenesis. 1996;17:2201–5.
15. **Dougherty S, et al.** Gender Difference in the activity but not expression of estrogen receptors α and β in human lung adenocarcinoma cells. Endocrine related Cancer. 2006;13:113–34.
16. **Ganti AK, et al.** Hormone replacement therapy is associated with decreased survival in women with lung cancer. J Clin Oncol. 2006;24:59–63.
17. **Coombes RC, et al.** A randomized trial of exemestane after two to three years of tamoxifen therapy in postmenopausal women with primary breast cancer. N Engl J Med. 2004;350:1081–92.
18. **Singh S, et al.** Influence of sex on toxicity and treatment outcome in small-cell lung cancer. J Clin Oncol. 2005;23:850–6.
19. **Winton T, et al.** Vinorelbine plus cisplatin vs. observation in resected non-small cell lung cancer. N Engl J Med. 2005;352:2589–97.
20. **Shepherd FA, et al.** Erlotinib in previously treated non-small-cell lung cancer. N Engl J Med. 2005;353:123–32.
21. **Ross H, et al.** Effect of gender on outcome in two randomized phase III trials of paclitaxel poliglumex (PPX) in chemo-naive patients with advanced NSCLC and poor performance status (PS2). J Clin Oncol. 2006 ASCO Annual Meeting Proceedings Part I. Vol 24, No. 18S (June 20 Supplement), 2006:7039.

D. Colon Cancer

Marguerite Elliott and Kari Kindschi

KEY POINTS

- Colon cancer is the third leading cause of all cancer deaths in females in the U.S.
- Lifetime incidence of colon cancer is approximately 6%.
- The stage of cancer at the time of presentation is an important determinant of long-term survival. In most cases, the initial diagnosis is established after the onset of symptoms. Unfortunately, about 20% of patients have metastatic disease at diagnosis.
- The prevalence of polyps increases with age, especially after age 50.
- Magnitude of risk is closely related to family history, specifically the number of family members affected, whether or not they are first-degree relatives, and the age of disease onset.
- Modifiable factors that potentially impact colon cancer risk include behaviors (alcohol use, obesity, physical activity, tobacco use), diet, and use of chemopreventive agents (supplements, aspirin, NSAIDs, hormone therapy).

> ◆ Psychosocial issues are both normal and expected with colon cancer.
> ◆ The primary care clinician may be the patient's main source of support and assistance with distress issues.
> ◆ Primary care clinicians need to be aware of potential "distressors" and be ready to help the patient to identify them and provide assistance in handling them.

Epidemiology

Colon cancer is responsible for 10% of all cancer deaths in the U.S., representing an estimated 52 180 deaths in 2007 (1). It is the second leading cause of cancer deaths in the U.S. among both sexes and the third leading cause of cancer death for women, behind lung and breast cancer, respectively (1). The mortality rate has been decreasing since the 1980s because of increased screening, earlier detection, and improved therapies (1).

In 2007, there were an estimated 112 340 new cases of colon cancer, with nearly equal numbers in men and women (1). The incidence of the disease increases with age, with 90% of cases diagnosed after the age of 50 years (1). The average lifetime risk is 6% (2) and is highest in developed countries (3). The majority of cancers are sporadic, but a family history of colon cancer can increase an individual's risk (4). There are also rare, autosomal dominant familial syndromes, specifically hereditary nonpolyposis colorectal cancer (HNPCC) and familial adenomatous polyposis (FAP), which account for approximately 5% of colon cancers (4).

Clinical Features

In the majority of cases, the initial diagnosis of colon cancer is established after the onset of symptoms (1). The most common symptoms include abdominal pain, a change in bowel habits, hematochezia, melena, weakness, anemia without GI symptoms, and weight loss (1). Many conditions can cause similar vague symptoms. The differential diagnosis includes malignancy, hemorrhoids, diverticulitis, infection, and inflammatory bowel disease. Presenting symptoms provide clues to the location of the tumor. Cancer in the right or proximal colon leads to occult bleeding and unexplained iron deficiency anemia. Left-sided or distal colon lesions cause bowel dysfunction, constipation, obstruction, or diarrhea (5). Imaging of left-sided tumors demonstrates characteristic annular or encircling lesions with an apple-core or napkin-ring appearance and a constricted bowel lumen (5).

At the time of diagnosis, about 20% of patients will have distant metastatic disease (2). Symptoms at diagnosis, especially bowel perforation or obstruction, are particularly ominous. An advanced disease process is suggested by the presence of right upper quadrant pain, distention, early satiety, or adenopathy. Hematologic or lymphatic dissemination usually causes liver involvement first, followed by spread to the lungs, bones, and skin (6).

The extent of the disease determines prognosis and therapeutic options. Staging is accomplished by a physical examination, endoscopic assessment, imaging modalities, laboratory testing, and findings during surgical resection/exploration. Clinically, physicians look for abdominal distention, masses, or signs of spread of the disease, especially focusing on the presence of hepatomegaly, ascites, or lymphadenopathy. CT scans are utilized to evaluate regional extension, regional lymphadenopathy, distant metastases, and complications of the tumor, such as obstruction, perforation, and fistula formation. PET scans may be valuable in localizing occult disease in cases with suspicious symptoms and a negative work-up for metastatic spread (6). Laboratory testing is also important. Carcinoembryonic antigen (CEA) and CA 19-9 are serum tumor markers for colon cancer that have prognostic significance but very low diagnostic value. CEA is the preferred marker. A level >5 ng/ml is considered abnormal (7). The higher the level at the time of diagnosis, the more likely advanced cancer is present (7) (Table 2-7).

Overall survival is highly-correlated by the stage at diagnosis (6). Five-year survival estimates are based on the staging system, as shown in Table 2-8.

Risk Factors

Most colon cancers are sporadic. One of the most important risk factors is age. The prevalence of polyps increases with age. Ninety percent of cases are found in people over the age of 50 years (1). A personal history of polyps is also significant. The risk of colon cancer increases with the number of polyps, the size of the lesions, and the presence of high-grade dysplasia or villous histology (6).

The magnitude of risk also is closely correlated with family history. Familial clustering is common in sporadic cases. The lifetime risk of colon cancer in the general population is 6% (2). The highest risk is seen in people who have 2 first-degree relatives with colon cancer or 1 first-degree relative with colon cancer who was diagnosed prior to age 50 (2). In these cases, the lifetime risk increases 3–4-fold (2). For people with 2 second-degree relatives with colon cancer or 1 first-degree relative with colon cancer, the risk is increased 2–3-fold (2). Colon cancer in a second- or third-degree relative increases the risk 1.5-fold (2). Simply having a first-degree relative with a polyp increases the risk 2-fold (2). Using these criteria, a substantial percentage of the population could be considered at increased risk for colon cancer.

Several hereditary conditions also predispose people to colon cancer. HNPCC is due to a mutation in a mismatch repair gene. It accounts for approximately 4% of all colon cancers (6). Generally, the lesions develop early in life (during the 30s or 40s) and are more likely to be found in the proximal colon (4). Polyps are not more prevalent but have a higher tendency to develop into cancer. There is also an association with extra-colonic cancers, including cancers of the endometrium, ovaries, stomach, small bowel, hepatobiliary system, renal pelvis, and ureter (2). The most common of these is endometrial cancer (4). FAP is due to

Table 2-7 Staging of Colon Cancer is Organized by a TNM-Based System with the Following Definitions

	0	1	2	3	4
T Tumor spread	Stromal invasion up to and including muscularis mucosa	Tumor invasion into submucosa	Tumor invasion into muscularis propria	Tumor invasion into subserosa	Direct tumor invasion into other organs or structures
N Node involvement	None	Invasion into 1–3 lymph nodes	Invasion into >3 lymph nodes		
M Metastatic spread	No metastatic spread	Metastasis present			

Detailed Guide: Colon and Rectum Cancer [Internet] [cited 2008]. Available from: http://www.cancer.org/docroot/CRI/CRI_2_3x.asp?dt=10. Adapted from the American Cancer Society, Inc.; with permission.

Table 2-8   Survival Based on Stage of Cancer

STAGE	I	IIA	IIB	IIIA	IIIB	IIIC	IV
T,N,M	T1,N0,M0 T2,N0,M0	T3,N0,M0	T4,N0,M0	T1,N0,M0 T2,N0,M0	T3,N1,M0 T4,N1,M0	Any T, N2,M0	Any T, any N,M1
Five-year survival rate (%)	93	85	72	83	64	44	8

a mutation in the APC gene on chromosome 5 (4). It accounts for about 1% of colon cancers (4). This inherited condition is associated with hundreds or thousands of polyps that are present throughout the colon (4). Tumors have usually formed by the age of 20 years, and nearly 100% of people with FAP will develop colon cancer by the age of 50 years in the absence of prophylactic colectomy (6).

Elevated risk is also seen in persons with certain chronic diseases. Inflammatory bowel disease, particularly ulcerative colitis, has been associated with an increased risk of colon cancer (5). The severity and duration of the disease are the primary determinants of risk. While the exact mechanism is unknown, it is thought that the inflammation predisposes the tissue to carcinogenesis (5). Established guidelines identify increased cancer risk after 10 years of pancolitis and after 15–20 years of colitis limited to the left side (6). Several studies have indicated a link between insulin resistance and a higher risk of colon cancer (3). One of the hypotheses is that in states of hyperinsulinemia insulin acts as a growth factor for the colonic mucosa and thus stimulates tumor cells in the colon (3).

Research focused on modification of behavioral risk factors is based on the premise that most colon cancer results from a complex interaction between genetic and environmental factors. High daily alcohol intake is consistently related to an increased risk of colon cancer and colonic adenomas (3). Physical activity is inversely associated with colon cancer risk (3). Individuals who are more physically active have a lower risk. In one study, a 50% reduction in colon cancer incidence was found in people with the highest activity levels (3). Many studies have demonstrated an association between smoking and colon cancer. Generally, there is a relatively long induction period, up to 30 years, from exposure to risk elevation (3).

Studies have evaluated the protective effects of a healthy diet and supplements. Unfortunately, in most instances, investigations have yielded conflicting results which makes the development of broad recommendations difficult. Several small studies have shown an association between a diet that is high in fruits and vegetables and a reduction in colon cancer rates (3). Many subsequent large studies have not identified a significant relationship (3). Several large epidemiologic studies demonstrated an increased risk in distal colon cancer with long-term consumption of red meats and processed meat (3). Others, however, failed to find any significant association (3). Some studies have shown a protective effect from high dietary fiber intake, but a systemic review and pooled analysis of 13 cohort studies did not show any definitive evidence that increased fiber intake decreased the incidence of cancer or the recurrence of polyps (3). Daily multivitamin use with 400 mcg of folic acid decreased the risk of colon cancer in the Nurses' Health Study (3). However, a large controlled trial did not show a decreased incidence of colon cancer in the folic acid group and, in fact, demonstrated an increased risk of adenomas and non-colorectal cancer in the group supplemented with folic acid (8). The Nurses' Health Study and Health Professionals Follow-Up Study indicated that calcium intake of 1250 mg daily was associated with a decrease in distal colon cancer (3). In addition to reduction of colon cancer risk, calcium supplementation may decrease the recurrence of adenomas (3).

Hormone replacement therapy may decrease the risk of colon cancer. The Women's Health Initiative reported a decreased risk of colon cancer in women who received estrogen and progesterone hormone replacement. Unfortunately, when women in this group did develop cancer, it was found at a more advanced stage (9).

Several investigations revealed a decrease in the incidence of adenomas with regular use of aspirin and other anti-inflammatory medications (3). Most, but not all, demonstrated a benefit (3). Conflicting results of studies have led to uncertainty about the dose and duration required to improve outcome. There is no general recommendation for the healthy population to use routine aspirin as a chemopreventive agent against colon cancer. Nonsteroidal anti-inflammatory drugs (NSAIDs) also have been shown to decrease both the risk of cancer and adenomas; however, side effects, such as bleeding, may preclude prophylactic use (3).

Psychosocial Issues

Anyone facing a diagnosis of cancer will have a multitude of emotions, fears, and concerns, and women dealing with colon cancer are no different. The National Comprehensive Cancer Network (NCCN) refers to these issues as "distress" (10). The NCCN definition of distress in cancer is "...a multifactorial unpleasant emotional experience of a psychological (cognitive, behavioral, emotional), social, and/or spiritual nature that may interfere with the ability to cope effectively with cancer, its physical symptoms, and its treatment. Distress extends along a continuum, ranging from common normal feelings of vulnerability, sadness, and fears to problems that can become disabling, such as depression, anxiety, panic disorder, social isolation, and existential and spiritual crisis" (10).

Primary care clinicians, as well as colon cancer patients, need to keep in mind that while undergoing treatment for cancer, likely overseen by an oncologist and utilizing a team of individuals who are involved in the cancer treatment itself, the other health needs of the patient continue to exist. Any preexisting chronic health conditions (diabetes, hypertension, thyroid disease, etc.) remain and need attention, as do routine health maintenance issues. In fact, many of the treatments involved in treating colon cancer may have a significant effect on a woman's chronic health conditions. Oncologists have neither the time nor resources to manage the total health of the patient. Thus, a partnership between involved physicians, clinical and ancillary support staff, and the patient needs to be forged in order to develop and deliver comprehensive healthcare to the patient.

A woman with cancer will place a great deal of her priorities and energies on what will happen to her family—children and partner. While going through treatments which may cause great fatigue and physical discomfort, she may feel that she needs to continue her pre-diagnosis level of activity, for example, cooking, providing transportation, keeping the house clean, working, leading the Girl Scout troop, shopping, and so on. After all, she was likely "living with her cancer" for many years prior to its diagnosis and doing all of these things. An encounter with her primary care clinician may be the key to her being able to acknowledge that she may need to adjust her priorities during this time. The primary care clinician's knowledge of the patient, her family situation, and other factors, such as local sources of help and support, may be what she needs to confront her situation.

Common psychosocial issues that face a woman with colon cancer include:

a   Practical problems (finances, insurance, job issues, discrimination).
b   Family problems (relationships)
c   Emotional problems (fears of recurrence and death, depression, anxiety, loss, and grief)
d   Spiritual/religious concerns
e   Physical problems (changes in body image due to surgical scars, radiation tattoos, etc.; significant changes in bowel habits or having a colostomy; loss of hair; neuropathy; cognitive changes; fatigue)

Primary care clinicians caring for patients undergoing treatment for colon cancer provide a great service to the patient by keeping in close touch and continuing the patient's normal routines for health maintenance exams as well as chronic care needs. These face-to-face encounters, as well as phone calls and other communication methods, provide opportunities to identify and discuss potential topics of distress with patients and to provide resources to help the patient with identified issues. Resources may include Internet resources, support groups, referrals to other professionals (traditional and nontraditional), assistance with information on the Family Medical Leave Act (FMLA), or conversations with the patient and/or her family, to name a few. While these may also be available from her oncologist and members of a multidisciplinary oncology care team, she may not feel comfortable in discussing these problems with that group or even be aware that there are sources of assistance available to her in that venue. The primary care clinician plays a valuable role for the cancer patient as she progresses through her cancer experience, maintaining her otherwise "normal health status" and discovering and adjusting to her new "normal."

Conclusion

Colon cancer is a prevalent and deadly disease that is largely preventable with regular screening. It is most often the primary care clinician who recommends and arranges for screening. While there are a number of screening options, a colonoscopy can be not only a screening tool but can treat and potentially cure an early-stage colon cancer. Ongoing research is helping to identify simpler screening tools, ways to modify risk factors, and to establish the protective effects of various chemopreventive strategies. The primary care clinician plays a very important role in the total health care of these patients.

References

1. Cancer Facts and Figures 2007 [Internet] [cited 2008. Available from: http://www.cancer.org/downloads/STT/CAFF2007PWSecured. pdf.
2. **Burt RW.** Colon cancer screening. Gastroenterology. 2000;119:837.
3. **Giovannucci E.** Modifiable risk factors for colon cancer. Gastroenterol Clin North Am. 2002 Dec;31:925-43.
4. **Burt RW, DiSario JA, Cannon-Albright L.** Genetics of colon cancer: Impact of inheritance on colon cancer risk. Annu Rev Med. 1995;46:371-9.
5. **Heuman D, Mills AS, McGuire Jr. H.** Gastrointestinal neoplasms. In: Gastroenterology. Philadelphia, Pennsylvania: W.B. Saunders; 1997.
6. Detailed Guide: Colon and Rectum Cancer [Internet] [cited 2008. Available from: http://www.cancer.org/docroot/CRI/CRI_2_3x.asp?dt=10.
7. Tumor Markers [Internet] [cited 2008. Available from: http://www.cancer.org/docroot/PED/content/PED_2_3X_Tumor_Markers.asp?sitearea=PED.
8. **Cole BF, Baron JA, Sandler RS, et al.** Polyp prevention study group. Folic acid for the prevention of colorectal adenomas: A randomized clinical trial. JAMA. 2007 Jun 6;297:2351-9.
9. **Chlebowski RT, Wactawski-Wende J, Ritenbaugh C, et al.** Women's health initiative investigators. Estrogen plus progestin and colorectal cancer in postmenopausal women. N Engl J Med. 2004 Mar 4;350:991-1004.
10. National Comprehensive Cancer Network. Distress Management V.1.2008. NCCN Clinical Practice Guidelines in Oncology. 11/06/07. Available at: http://www.nccn.org/professionals/physician_gls/PDF/distress.pdf. Accessed February 10, 2008.

E. Melanoma

Theodore F. Logan and Lawrence A. Mark

KEY POINTS

- Melanoma is the sixth most commonly diagnosed cancer in the U.S.
- The average age of onset of melanoma is 59 years.
- Those at greatest risk are fair-complected, may have a history of severe sunburns as children, and have family or personal histories of melanoma.
- Reducing exposure of the skin to ultraviolet light with protective covering and use of sunscreen is recommended and may decrease the incidence of melanoma.
- Melanoma is incurable, but the length of survival increases when it is identified early.

Cutaneous Melanoma

Introduction

Melanoma develops from the neural crest-derived melanocyte, or pigment-producing cell, which typically is found in the basal epidermis at the dermal-epidermal junction in the skin. Rests of melanocytes also may normally be found in the leptomeninges, choroid of the eye, cochlea of the ear, and capsule of lymph nodes.

Epidemiology

The incidence of melanoma is increasing. The National Cancer Institute's Surveillance, Epidemiology and End Results (SEER) database noted annual increases in incidence for all races of 1.2% and for non-Hispanic Whites of 2.3% (males 2.2%, females 2.5%) from 1995 to 2004 (1). In 2007, melanoma was estimated to be the sixth most commonly diagnosed cancer in the U.S., comprising 4% of all malignancies in men and women, with almost 60 000 new cases and over 8000 deaths. The gender ratio is approximately 1:1 (2). Over decades, the death rate from melanoma has risen less steeply than its incidence and may have leveled out (3). The mortality rate for males is greater (3.9/100 000) than for females (1.7/100 000) (1). The median age of onset is 59 years, approximately 10 years earlier than many other common malignancies, making it the second most common tumor responsible for the loss of many productive years of life (4). In women between the ages of 25 and 35 years, melanoma is the leading cause of cancer-related death (3). Caucasians in the U.S. have an estimated lifetime risk of developing melanoma of approximately 1 in 74, with 1 in 58 for men and 1 in 82 for women (3). These findings are similar for other Caucasian populations in Europe, Australia, and New Zealand. While they can occur at any site, melanomas are more common on the back in males and the lower leg in females (3).

The incidence of melanoma in non-White populations is much lower. In African Americans, Native Americans, and Latinos in the U.S., the incidence is 1.0, 2.9, and 4.5 per 100 000 persons, respectively, compared to 21.6/100 000. Whites (1). The pattern of skin distribution of melanoma is more commonly acral, such as foot or nailbed or mucosal surface, than other cutaneous malignancies (3).

Risk factors for the development of melanoma are numerous and include a history of intermittent high-dose ultraviolet (UV) light exposure (such as with blistering sunburns or tanning bed use), greater than 50 moles, greater than 5 dysplastic nevi, personal history of prior melanoma, organ transplantation, immunosuppression, older age, and psoralen with ultraviolet A light (PUVA) therapy. Genetic susceptibility is also important as a risk factor and includes those who burn easily, tan poorly, have fair complexions, easily freckle, have red or blond hair or blue eyes, and have a family history of first-degree relatives with melanoma or xeroderma pigmentosa. Pregnancy and estrogen usage do not appear to increase the frequency of melanoma (3).

Clinical Features and Presentation

Melanoma typically presents as a pigmented lesion that changes in size, shape, color, or elevation. The mnemonic ABCD (EF) has been used to summarize known melanoma characteristics (3): Asymmetry, Border irregularity, Color variation, Diameter >6 mm (E = elevation, evolution, enlargement, Funny-looking) (Figure 2-1). Other associated symptoms can include bleeding, itching, tenderness, and ulceration. However, none of these findings is specific, and the diagnosis can be difficult. Because of the limitations of this type of pattern recognition, some clinicians use the "ugly duckling" sign and teach this to their patients for surveillance. This is useful when the patient has many lesions, all of which have a fairly monomorphic appearance, in circumstances in which one can distinguish 1 or 2 lesions that are morphologic outliers from the general pattern of the other lesions.

Additionally, it is very important to distinguish melanoma from benign seborrheic keratoses, which are not melanocytic in origin and should be considered keratinocytic hyperplasia. These are typically brown in color, are seen on older individuals, and have a stuck-on or greasy appearance. Sharply demarcated edges and keratin pearls within the seborrheic keratosis may be seen with the aid of a hand lens or dermatoscope.

Distinction from atypical nevi, also termed dysplastic nevi or Clark's nevi, is also important. These have a "fried egg" appearance, consisting of a darker pigmented papule in the center of a lighter brown macule,

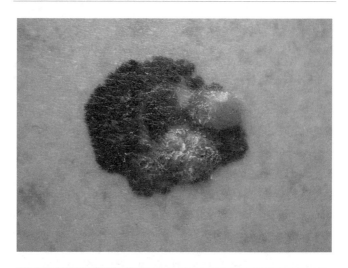

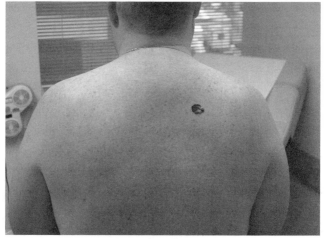

Figure 2-1   Primary melanoma.

>6 mm in diameter. Some asymmetry may be acceptable in these. Histologically, they are defined by architectural disorder, papillary dermal fibrosis, bridging of rete pegs, and some element of cytologic atypia. They are considered markers of elevated risk for melanoma when found in multiples but do not warrant excision unless they exhibit marked cytologic atypia. There is no evidence to support that removal of all atypical nevi reduces the risk of melanoma development.

Four main clinical types of melanoma are recognized. In superficial spreading melanoma (approximately 70%), the melanoma grows laterally (radial growth phase), often from a precursor lesion like a dysplastic nevus, and frequently displays ABCD characteristics before the appearance of a nodule (vertical growth phase). Nodular melanoma (approximately 15%) appears without a prior lateral growth phase and may not have a precursor lesion. Acral lentiginous melanoma (approximately 10%) develops on palms, soles, digits, subungually, or on mucosal surfaces. These occur in people of all ethnic/racial groups (Caucasian, African American, Latino, and Asian), may be distinct from other forms of melanoma, and are thought to be less related to ultraviolet irradiation exposure. Lentigo maligna melanoma (approximately 5%) generally develops in individuals >60 years, on chronically sun-exposed skin, such as the face. The radial growth phase is slow, typically evolving over many years before invasion occurs (3). A fifth type, desmoplastic melanoma, is recognized but is rare and usually presents as an amelanotic nodule on the head or neck.

Prevention

Metastatic melanoma is incurable at this time, but resection of localized disease is associated with prolonged survival depending upon stage at presentation (Table 2-9). Therefore, screening of persons at high risk has been recommended (4). While such approaches have identified a higher than expected proportion of early lesions, they have yet to demonstrate reduction in mortality. Persons at significantly increased risk for melanoma should, in general, have yearly full skin examinations, including mucous membranes. A full skin exam once every 2–3 years is probably sufficient for the general population. Monthly self-directed skin examination may be useful, but excision of atypical nevi with the goal of reducing risk is not, since melanoma often starts *de novo* (not in a preexisting mole) in patients with atypical moles (3). Efforts to reduce ultraviolet light exposure by covering up with clothing and brimmed hats, avoiding midday sun exposure, and using sunscreens, are recommended. While sunscreens are able to protect against sunburn and UV-induced damage (5), it is unclear whether they reduce the risk of melanoma (4).

Diagnosis

Suspicious lesions should be biopsied to establish the diagnosis. It is important that the pathologist reviewing the biopsy receives a history of the patient, a clinical description of the lesion, and a suspected differential diagnosis. Prognosis, surgical management, and therapeutic choices in melanoma are guided principally by tumor depth, degree of tumor invasion, and evidence of overlying epidermal erosion. Therefore, the optimal biopsy is performed either by using punch technique or by surgical excision for complete removal with narrow margins (1–3 mm). The pathologic evaluation for a melanoma should include careful measurement of the

Table 2-9   A. Melanoma TNM Classification

T	Thickness	N	Number of Nodes	M	Site	LDH
T1	≤1.0 mm	N1	1	M1a	Distant skin, subcutaneous, nodal	Normal
T2	1.01–2.00 mm	N2	2–3			
T3	2.01–4.00 mm		a. micrometastatic			
	a. without ulceration		b. macrometastatic (clinically palpable)	M1b	Lung	Normal
	b. ulceration T1a- without ulceration and Clark level II/III		c. in-transit/ satellite(s) without nodes	M1c	All other visceral	Normal
	T1b-with ulceration or Clark level IV/V	N3	≥4	Any distant mets	Elevated	
			Matted nodes or in-transit/satellite(s) with metastatic node(s)			

LDH- serum lactate dehydrogenase.
Adapted from Table 1 of Balch CM, Soong SJ, Atkins MB, et al. An evidence-based staging system for cutaneous melanoma. CA Cancer J Clin. 2004;54:131–49;.with permission.

B. AJCC Staging (Pathologic)

Stage	TMN			Approximate 5-year Survival (%)
0	T1s	N0	M0	
IA	T1a	N0	M0	95
IB	T1b, T2a	N0	M0	89–91
IIA	T2b, T3a	N0	M0	77–79
IIB	T3b, T4a	N0	M0	63–67
IIC	T4b	N0	M0	45
IIIA	T1-4a	N1a, N2a	M0	67
IIIB	T1-4b	N1a, N2a	M0	52–54
	T1-4a	N1b, N2b, N2c	M0	
	T1-4b	N2c	M0	
IIIC	T1-4b	N1b, N2b	M0	24–28
	Any T	N3	M0	
IV	Any T	Any N	Any M	1-year survival rate 41–59

Adapted from Tables 2 and 5 of Balch CM, Soong SJ, Atkins MB, et al. An evidence-based staging system for cutaneous melanoma. CA Cancer J Clin. 2004;54:131–49; with permission.

depth of the primary lesion, at the thickest point. This is usually reported as Breslow depth in millimeters and is the distance from epidermal basal layer to the tumor base (3). Additionally, melanomas <1 mm thick have altered staging based on level of tumor invasion, called Clark level. Therefore, all pathologic reports should include this level as defined by: I) tumor is confined to the epidermis; II) tumor invades the papillary dermis; III) tumor fills the papillary dermis to the reticular dermis; IV) tumor invades the reticular dermis; and V) tumor fills the reticular dermis and invades the fat. Shave biopsies are suboptimal since they often transect the tumor base, thereby losing these critical depth criteria (4). Subungual melanomas present with a new or growing pigmented linear streaking, most commonly under the nail of the great toe or thumb, and require biopsy obtained from under the nail plate, usually at the nail matrix (3).

AJCC Staging

This new staging system for melanoma (Table 2-9B) was developed by the Melanoma Staging Committee of the American Joint Committee on Cancer (AJCC) and was based on melanoma patient outcome data from 13 prospective databases, merging data from 30 450 patients to obtain a database containing 17 600 melanoma patients with complete information for all factors necessary for a tumor node metastasis (TNM) staging classification. The analysis forms the basis of the current AJCC staging system for melanoma and represents an impressive example of evidence-based medicine (6).

Multivariate analysis of 13 581 patients with primary-only melanoma from the AJCC data set allowed identification of factors associated with survival in patients with localized primaries. The two most powerful predictors of survival were tumor thickness (Breslow depth) and ulceration, defined as absence of intact epidermis overlying the primary tumor. Ulceration is determined microscopically by the pathologist. Other less powerful factors noted to confer worse prognosis were older age, primary site on head, neck, or trunk, higher Clark level, and male gender (3).

Complete data were available for 1201 patients with lymph node metastasis, and multivariate analysis showed that the number of involved nodes, tumor burden within the node (microscopic vs. macroscopic or clinically palpable nodes), and ulceration of the primary melanoma were the most powerful predictors for survival (3). Intralymphatic metastasis occurring between the primary site and the draining lymph nodes is called satellite or in-transit metastasis and confers poorer prognosis (3).

Data from 1158 patients with metastatic melanoma were similarly analyzed and showed that site of metastasis was an important prognostic predictor. Skin or lymph node metastases conferred better prognosis than lung metastases, which in turn was better than other visceral sites. Elevated LDH was added, based on other studies, and was found to be associated with a worse outcome (3).

Typically, melanoma progresses by growing laterally in the skin before growing vertically and spreading through the lymphatics to the draining lymph node group and subsequently metastasizing to other organs. As can be seen in Table 2-9, 5-year survival is critically depend-ent on the depth and ulceration status of the primary melanoma when resected. This underscores the rationale for dermatologic screening of patients at increased risk for melanoma, with removal of suspicious lesions in an attempt to remove any melanomas while still thin. Patients with thin melanomas (<1 mm) without other risk factors have a 95% 5-year survival, while patients with a deep, ulcerated, primary melanoma have a 45% 5-year survival. Involvement of regional draining nodes indicates stage III disease and significantly decreases expected 5-year survival, which ranges between 24–67%, depending upon node number, tumor burden (clinically palpable), and ulceration status of the primary. Metastatic disease, stage IV, has a dismal 41–59% 1-year survival (3,6).

Clinical Care

Wide Local Excision/Sentinel Lymph Node Biopsy

After diagnosis is made with excisional biopsy and pathological evalua-tion is performed to determine tumor depth and ulceration status, the patient will require a wide local excision (WLE) of the biopsy site. The local recurrence rate at the biopsy site goes up with increased depth of the primary melanoma. With local recurrence, survival is decreased. It has been suggested that for a T1 melanoma 1-cm margins around the original biopsy site are optimal, for T2 melanomas 1–2-cm margins, for T3 2-cm margins, and for T4 at least 2-cm margins.

If Breslow depth of the tumor is >1 mm, or the tumor either is ulcerated or invades to Clark level IV or V regardless of Breslow thick-ness, it is recommended that the WLE be performed simultaneously with sentinel node biopsy (SNBX) in order to obtain the most prog-nostic information. Sentinel node biopsy, first described in patients with melanoma, is performed to identify the proximal draining lymph node group for the primary melanoma and to assess the involvement of the proximal draining lymph node(s) by the melanoma (7). The pro-cedure is performed by injecting the biopsy site with both radiocolloid and vital blue dye, which travels via lymphatic drainage to the drain-ing lymph node group and allows identification of the initial draining lymph node(s). The node(s) are removed and examined pathologically. The yield of positive nodes increases with increasing depth of the primary (3). If the sentinel node(s) are negative, no further surgical intervention involving the draining lymph node group is required.

Lymph Node Dissection

Should lymph node metastasis be shown by biopsy of clinically palpa-ble adenopathy or should the sentinel node(s) be positive (stage III dis-ease), a formal lymph node dissection is recommended. If the sentinel node(s) is involved, additional nodes are involved in approximately 20% of cases (3). Patients with a positive sentinel node(s) should undergo an immediate lymphadenectomy (8).

Adjuvant Therapy/Surveillance

For patients with resected lymph node-positive melanoma, multiple adjuvant therapeutic strategies have been tested in clinical trials (4). High-dose interferon alpha-2b has shown to have benefit compared to no treatment (observation) or experimental vaccine in 3 randomized phase III studies performed by the Eastern Cooperative Oncology Group (ECOG) (9–11) High-dose interferon is given over a 1-year period and can have frequent and toxic side effects, which can result in dose delay, decrease, or discontinuation. Common toxicities include fever, flu-like symptoms, fatigue, decreased appetite, weight loss, cytopenias, hepatotoxicity, depression, and autoimmune reactions. Multiple low-dose interferon studies have failed to show benefit in the adjuvant setting, and, to date, high-dose interferon is the only FDA-approved adjuvant therapy for high-risk resected melanoma (12).

Nonetheless, high-dose interferon adjuvant therapy is somewhat controversial and not uniformly used in the U.S. or accepted internationally. Modest benefit, inconsistent overall survival benefit, and toxicity have been cited as reasons (4,13). Radiation therapy to the tumor bed is used sometimes in the adjuvant setting, even though there are no randomized trials proving its benefit. This is most common after resection of macroscopic parotid nodes, extracapsular spread, or metastases to multiple cervical nodes (3).

For nearly all patients, starting from the time of diagnosis, frequent follow-up is recommended: every 3 months for the first 2 years, followed by every 6 months for another 2–3 years, and by yearly visits thereafter. Follow-up visits should include history directed at any new or changing lesions, review of systems directed at any unexplained new findings, and physical exam targeting any "ugly ducklings," lymphadenopathy, or recurrence within the primary excision site. Liver function tests, LDH, and chest x-rays performed every 6–12 months may be offered to stage I patients but are recommended for stage II disease and greater. These recommendations are given because of the relative likelihood of local recurrence and distant metastasis, since many patients may be stratified into higher risk groups based on their AJCC stage (3). The patient also needs to be followed with full-body skin exams because of the increased risk of developing a second primary melanoma.

Local Recurrence Management

When arising after adequate surgical resection, local recurrence suggests that the melanoma is aggressive and portends in-transit, regional node, or distant metastases. Clinically negative regional nodes are involved with occult metastases in up to 50% of cases. Treatment is surgical (3). Regional relapse in skin lymphatics (in-transit metastases) is managed surgically, when possible, and, if confined to an extremity with metastases too numerous to be excised, with isolated limb perfusion (3). Regional node relapse also is managed surgically when possible. Radiation therapy may be considered if the melanoma is unresectable, partially resectable, or even in the adjuvant setting. Local or regional relapse worsens prognosis (3).

Metastatic Disease

The median survival time for patients with stage IV melanoma is 6–10 months, with fewer than 5% surviving for 5 years (4).

Solitary/Organ-Confined/Resection

For patients with solitary metastatic lesions or a limited number of localized lesions, surgery may provide both palliative and possible survival benefits (3).

Systemic Therapy

No treatment has demonstrated survival advantage in patients with metastatic melanoma in a randomized, controlled clinical trial. The FDA-approved treatments are dacarbazine and high-dose bolus Interleukin-2. Dacarbazine can be given to outpatients intravenously every 3–4 weeks, with an expected response rate of 15–20% and most responses being partial and of limited duration (4).

High-dose bolus Interleukin-2 was approved by the FDA in 1998, based on durable complete and partial responses demonstrated in phase II trials. The response rate is 15–17% with 5–6% complete responses (4). Due to its substantial toxicity, high-dose bolus Interleukin-2 is best given to selected patients by experienced physicians and staff in appropriate hospital settings (4).

Patients with metastatic melanoma in the central nervous system present a difficult challenge in that survival times tend to be short and therapeutic options few. The primary management is with external beam radiation therapy and/or focused radiation such as gamma knife radiosurgery.

Ocular Melanoma /Mucosal Melanoma

Both of these non-cutaneous melanomas are rare, with ocular melanoma more common among men (6.8 cases per million men vs. 5.3 per million women) and mucosal (especially genital tract) more common among women (2.8 cases per million women vs. 1.5 cases per million men) (14).

Conclusion

Melanoma is a common cause of cancer-related death in men and women. Primary care providers should be aware of the risk factors for and clinical presentations of melanoma.

References

1. SEER: Surveillance, Epidemiology and End Results Website. In: SEER Cancer Statistics Review 1975–2004. (Accessed March 19, 2008, at http://seer.cancer.gov/csr/1975_2004/results_single/sect_16_table.10.pdf).

2. **Jemal A, Siegel R, Ward E, et al.** Cancer statistics, 2007. CA Cancer J Clin. 2007;57:43–66.

3. **Balch CM, Atkins MB, Sober AJ.** Cutaneous Melanoma. In: Vincent T. DeVita, Jr., Samuel Hellman, Steven A. Rosenberg (eds) Cancer Principles & Practice of Oncology, 7th Edition, Philadelphia, Lippincott Williams & Wilkins, 2005:1754–1809.

4. **Tsao H, Atkins MB, Sober AJ.** Management of cutaneous melanoma. N Engl J Med. 2004;351:998–1012.

5. **Moyal DD, Fourtanier AM.** Broad-spectrum sunscreens provide better protection from solar ultraviolet-simulated radiation and natural sunlight-induced immunosuppression in human beings. J Am Acad Dermatol. 2008;58:S149–154.

6. **Balch CM, Soong SJ, Atkins MB, et al.** An evidence-based staging system for cutaneous melanoma. CA Cancer J Clin. 2004;54:131–49.

7. **Morton DL, Wen DR, Wong JH, et al.** Technical details of intra-operative lymphatic mapping for early stage melanoma. Arch Surg. 1992;127:392–9.

8. **Morton DL, Thompson JF, Cochran AJ, et al.** Sentinel-node or nodal observation in melanoma. N Engl J Med. 2006;355:1307–17.

9. **Kirkwood JM, Strawderman MH, Ernstoff MS, et al.** Interferon alfa-2b adjuvant therapy of high-risk resected cutaneous melanoma: The Eastern Cooperative Oncology Group Trial Est 1684. JCO. 1996;14:7–17.

10. **Kirkwood JM, Ibrahim JG, Sandak VK, et al.** High and low dose interferon Alfa-2b in high-risk melanoma: first analysis of intergroup Trial E1609/S9111/C9190. JCO. 2000;18:2444–58.

11. **Kirkwood JM, Ibrahim JG, Sosman JA, et al.** High-dose interferon Alfa-2b significantly prolongs relapse-free and overall survival compared with the gm2-klh/qs-21 vaccine in patients with resected stage iib-iii melanoma: results of intergroup trial e1694/s9512/c509801. JCO. 2001;19:2370–80.

12. **Kirkwood JM, Tarhini AA, Moschos SJ, et al.** Adjuvant therapy with high-dose interferon a2b in patients with high-risk stage iib/iii melanoma. Nat Clin Pract Oncol. 2008;5:2–3.

13. **Sabel MS, Sondak VK.** Pros and cons of adjuvant interferon in the treatment of melanoma. The Oncologist. 2003;8:451–8.

14. **McLaughlin CC, Wu XC, Jemal A, et al.** Incidence of noncutaneous melanomas in the U.S. Cancer. 2005;103:1000–7.

F. Skin Cancer (Non-Melanoma Skin Cancer)

Joslyn N. Witherspoon, Bethanee J. Schlosser,
Dennis P. West, Anjali Butani, and Ginat W. Mirowski

KEY POINTS

- Non-melanoma skin cancers (NMSC) are the most common cutaneous malignancies.
- Non-melanoma skin cancers have a >95% 5-year cure rate when diagnosed and treated early.
- Treatment includes surgical and nonsurgical modalities.
- Treatment depends on tumor type, location, size, and histological pattern, as well as the age and health status of the patient.
- Prevention of NMSC can be achieved through regular and consistent sun avoidance and protection.

Epidemiology

Non-melanoma skin cancer, consisting of basal cell carcinoma (BCC) and squamous cell carcinoma (SCC), is the most common malignancy in the U.S. (1). The incidence of NMSC is estimated to be greater than one million cases per year, of which 80% are BCCs and 20% are SCCs (2). The true incidence and prevalence are difficult to determine because these cancers are not routinely reported in tumor registries (1). Men and women are equally at risk for the development of these tumors, but increased rates of occupational and recreational ultraviolet (UV) exposure lead to a higher incidence in men. Mortality rates for NMSC are strongly age-related, with the highest mortality rate occurring in the individuals 85 years old and older. Mortality due to genital NMSC accounts for approximately half of all NMSC-related mortality in the U.S. Although men are 3 times as likely to die from non-genital NMSC compared to NMSC of the penis and scrotum, mortality rates among women are slightly higher for vulvar skin cancer than for non-genital NMSC (3).

Clinical Features (Presentations, Signs, Symptoms)

Basal Cell Carcinoma

BCCs, malignant tumors that arise from the epidermal basal cell layer, typically occur on the head, neck, trunk, arms, and legs of both men and women. Rates of BCC are highest in elderly men, but young women are increasingly at risk (4). Risk factors for the development of BCC include

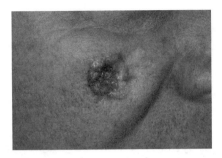

Figure 2-2   Nodular basal cell carcinoma on the cheek. Pearly papule with overlying telangiectases and a rolled border, with ulceration and crusting. (Courtesy of Bethanee Schlosser, MD.)

UV exposure, light hair and eye color, exposure to ionizing radiation, immunosuppression, tanning bed use, and smoking tobacco. A genetic predisposition is noted in certain genodermatoses (4).

BCCs have been classified on the basis of clinical and histopathologic features. Nodular BCC, the prototypic form, presents as a single pearly papule or nodule with overlying telangiectases and a rolled border, with or without ulceration and/or crusting (4) (Figure 2-2). Pigmented BCC appears as a hyperpigmented translucent papule, which may be eroded. Superficial BCC is clinically identified as a scaly erythematous patch or plaque that may resemble eczema (5). Morpheaform, or sclerosing, BCC is characterized by an ivory-white, scar-like appearance and demonstrates an aggressive growth pattern histologically (5).

If left untreated, BCCs may increase significantly in size (>5–10 cm in diameter) and can locally destroy cartilage and bone and can even invade soft tissues (Figure 2-3). The recurrence rate for primary BCCs treated by Mohs micrographic surgery (MMS) is 1%. The recurrence rate for standard excision is 10%, curettage and desiccation is 7.7%, radiation therapy is 8.7%, and cryotherapy is 7.5% (5). Nests of tumor cells may track along nerves (i.e., perineural invasion), resulting in involvement of skin distant and distinct from the primary lesion. Metastasis of BCC is extremely uncommon, with rates ranging from 0.0028 to 0.55% (4).

Actinic Keratosis

Actinic keratoses (AKs) are premalignant skin lesions that develop in response to prolonged exposure to UV radiation and may progress to become SCC (6). AKs present as ill-defined erythematous scaly papules, typically 2–6 mm in diameter, on sun-exposed areas, such as the face, scalp, posterior neck, and dorsal upper extremities (Figure 2-4). The dry

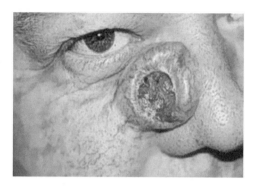

Figure 2-3   Nodular basal cell carcinoma approaching the orbit of the eye.
(Courtesy of Ginat Mirowski, DMD, MD.)

scale of AKs imparts a rough, gritty texture. Clinically, AKs may be more
easily detected by palpation than by visualization.

   Risk factors for the development of AKs include cumulative UV radiation exposure, older age, male gender, fair skin, blond or red hair, green
eyes, immunosuppression, prior history of AKs or other skin cancers, and
certain genetic syndromes (6).

   Actinic cheilitis, defined as severe solar damage of the vermilion border that may represent an AK, presents as a thickened and pale lower
lip with possible scale (Figure 2-5). Loss of the normal lip markings and
dissolution of the border between the cutaneous lip and the vermillion
border are other distinctive features. The presence of an induration,
erosion, or ulceration suggests progression to SCC and should prompt
immediate biopsy for histopathologic evaluation.

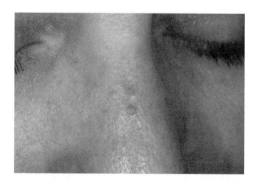

Figure 2-4   Erythematous scaly papules of actinic keratoses on the nose. (Courtesy
of Bethanee Schlosser, MD.)

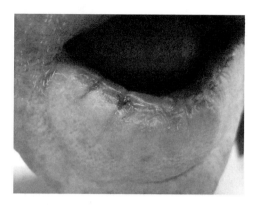

Figure 2-5   Actinic cheilitis of the lip. Due to chronic damage and loss of elasticity, patients may develop fissures as noted in this patient. (Courtesy of Bethanee Schlosser, MD.)

Squamous Cell Carcinoma

Most SCCs occur on sun-exposed skin of the head, neck, and trunk. They appear as firm, flesh-colored, or erythematous, hyperkeratotic papules and plaques with or without ulceration. SCCs also may be described by patients as itchy or painful non-healing wounds that bleed when traumatized (2) (Figure 2-6).

SCCs are twice as common in men as in women (7). Physical barriers, including longer hairstyles and use of lipstick, may account for

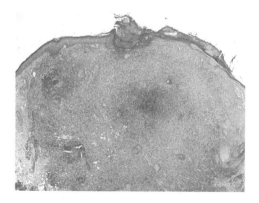

Figure 2-6   Histopathology of invasive squamous cell carcinoma showing extension of atypical keratinocytes beyond the epidermal basement membrane into the dermis. (Courtesy of Joan Guitart, MD.)

the lower frequency of SCC involving the ears and lips of women (7). Predisposing factors for the development of SCC include UV radiation exposure, ionizing radiation exposure, history of AKs, immunosuppression, scars, prior burns, and certain genodermatoses (7). A role for human papillomavirus (HPV) infection in some types of SCCs has been documented. HPV types 6 and 11 are frequently found in patients with tumors of the genitalia and type 16 in those with head, neck, and periungal tumors (2,7). Verrucous carcinoma also appears to be associated with several HPV types. HPV is most likely at least one etiologic factor in the higher prevalence of SCC in transplant patients (1).

Histologically, SCCs arise from keratinocytes in the epidermis. Loss of normal cytologic features, decreased organization, increased nuclear-to-cytoplasmic ratio, keratinocyte crowding, and mitotic figures are characteristic of malignant transformation. The histopathologic hallmark of invasive SCC is extension of atypical keratinocytes beyond the epidermal basement membrane into the dermis (7) (Figure 2-7). Primary invasive SCCs recur at a rate of 8% over 5 years. A 5-year metastasis rate of 5% has been documented (7).

Metastases, generally to regional lymph nodes, are detected 1–3 years after initial diagnosis (7). Perineural invasion is an ominous finding, with most patients dying of the disease within 5 years (2). Neurotropic spread results from contiguous movement of tumor cells along nerve fibers. Perineural spread occurs in only 5% of SCCs, but it confers a high risk of recurrence and metastasis (2). Metastasis is typically preceded by local recurrence at the site of the primary lesion. SCC of the ear has the

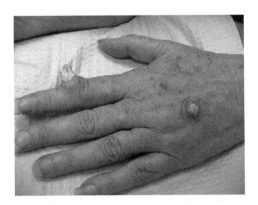

Figure 2-7   Squamous cell carcinoma on the hand of an immunocompromised patient. Notice the appearance of a cutaneous horn on the left index finger, as well as the keratotic papule with an erythematous base on the dorsal hand. (Courtesy of Ginat Mirowski, DMD, MD.)

highest rate of recurrence (18.7%), whereas lip SCC has the highest rate of metastasis (13.7%) (7). Palpation of regional lymph nodes for adenopathy is indicated prior to biopsy, and the presence of lymphadenopathy may greatly influence further evaluation of such patients.

Diagnosis and Differential Diagnosis

A diagnosis of NMSC relies on both clinical and pathological features (Table 2-10 Clinical differential diagnosis of actinic keratosis, BCC, and SCC). A biopsy should be performed on all suspicious, persistent, enlarging, or non-healing papules and plaques. Lesions with significant elevation and/or induration are most often biopsied using a shave technique, but areas of concern which are flat or depressed should be assessed by a punch biopsy.

Prevention

Primary prevention of skin cancer is based on increasing public awareness and providing patients with individualized guidance. Exposure to UV radiation (natural sunlight or tanning lamps) is the most important modifiable risk factor for the development of NMSC; avoidance of UV radiation exposure (sunlight or tanning lamps) is the most effective means by which to decrease this risk. The American Academy of Dermatology recommends the following sun avoidance and protection practices:

- Seek shade when appropriate, remembering that UV rays are most intense from 10:00 a.m. to 4:00 p.m.
- Wear light-colored, tightly-woven, protective clothing, like long sleeves and pants, a wide-brimmed hat, and sunglasses.
- Apply a broad-spectrum sunscreen that protects against both UVA and UVB rays, with a SPF (sun protection factor) of at least 15.
- Reapply sunscreen every 2 hours when in the sun and also on cloudy days, as well as after swimming or sweating.

UVA is responsible for tanning, while UVB exposure results in significant erythema and potential sunburn. Both UVA and UVB contribute to premature skin aging and the development of skin cancer. In late 2007, the Food and Drug Administration proposed revised labeling standards for sunscreen drug products with regard to levels of protection against both UVA and UVB. The level of UVB sunscreen protection is indicated by the numerical value reflecting the sun protective factor, or SPF. The SPF rating is calculated by comparing the amount of time needed to produce a sunburn on protected skin to the amount of time needed to cause a sunburn on unprotected skin. In a person who would experience a sunburn in 10 minutes without sun protection, a sunscreen with an SPF of 15 will delay onset of sunburn to 150 minutes. UVA protection is to be displayed using a four-star rating system that will be placed adjacent to the SPF rating for UVB protection on sunscreen labels.

Table 2-10   Clinical Differential Diagnosis of Actinic Keratosis and Non-Melanoma Skin Cancer

	Differential Diagnosis
Basal cell carcinoma	**Nodular BCC**
	Amelanotic melanoma
	Dermal nevus
	Dermatofibroma
	SCC
	Seborrheic keratosis
	Pigmented BCC
	Blue nevus
	Compound nevus
	Nodular melanoma
	Seborrheic keratosis
	Superficial BCC
	Eczematous dermatitis
	Inflamed seborrheic keratosis
	Psoriasis
	SCC *in situ*
	Morpheaform BCC
	Morphea
	Scar
	Trichoepithelioma
Actinic keratosis	Verruca vulgaris
	Cutaneous horn
	Porokeratosis
	SCC
	Seborrheic keratosis
	Psoriasis
	Seborrheic dermatitis
	Actinic cheilitis
	Discoid lupus erythematosus
	Lichen planus
Squamous cell carcinoma	AK
	Atypical fibroxanthoma
	BCC
	Deep fungal infection
	Eccrine poroma
	Melanocytic nevus
	Merkel cell carcinoma
	Pyogenic granuloma
	Seborrheic keratosis
	Trauma
	Verruca vulgaris

Clothing and accessories, such as hats, can provide significant protection from UV exposure. The UV protection factor (UPF) is a standardized, direct measure of how greatly UV radiation is reduced when it passes through a fabric; a UPF of 10 reduces penetration of UV radiation to the covered skin to 1/10 of that reaching bare skin. Only clothing with a UPF of at least 40 can be labeled as solar UV-protective. Clothing treatment products, such as *SunGuard*, increase the UPF of clothing by transferring an invisible shield of UV protectant, such as Tinosorb FD, to clothing fibers. This simple, at-home treatment can increase the UPF of a white cotton T-shirt from 5 to 30, thereby blocking >96% of UV rays.

Treatment and Follow-Up

Clinical evaluation of a patient for possible cutaneous malignancies includes a history and a complete physical examination. Specific attention should be given to the history of sun exposure during childhood, history of severe and/or blistering sunburns, occupational and recreational UV exposure (e.g., outdoor occupations, water sports, etc.), previous radiation treatment and potential causes of immunosuppression (e.g., post-transplantation, HIV/AIDS). Predisposition for the development of NMSC is well-described and significantly increased in some genetic syndromes, such as xeroderma pigmentosum and nevoid basal cell carcinoma syndrome. Screening for new or recurrent NMSC involves total body skin examination with subsequent biopsy of suspicious lesions.

Treatment of NMSC includes both surgical and nonsurgical modalities (Table 2-11: Treatment of Actinic Keratosis and Non-Melanoma Skin Cancer). Treatment aims to completely eradicate the malignancy while preserving and/or restoring normal anatomic function and providing optimal cosmesis (8). The choice of treatment modality is based on tumor type, location, size, histopathologic pattern, and risk of recurrence.

Surgery is most frequently employed in the treatment of NMSC and may include cryosurgery, electrodessication, and curettage, conventional excision, and Mohs micrographic surgery. Liquid nitrogen cryosurgery provides local destruction and is recommended for actinic keratoses and small, clinically well-defined, in situ or primary tumors. Liquid nitrogen is administered using either a spray device or cotton-tipped applicator. In electrodessication and curettage (ED&C), a curette is used to mechanically remove the tumor from surrounding normal skin, followed by electrocautery to destroy the lesion base and provide hemostasis. ED&C is most often employed in the treatment of small (<2 cm diameter), clinically well-defined, nodular BCCs located on the trunk or extremity. Five-year cure rates of 95% or more are possible with the use of either ED&C or cryosurgery for low-risk lesions (small, well-defined primary lesions on the trunk, arms, and legs). ED&C should not be employed in the treatment of recurrent, clinically ill-defined, or morpheaform tumors.

Surgical excision and MMS are treatments that offer a >99% 5-year cure rate. Simple excision of low-risk NMSC tumors is widely

Table 2-11   Treatment of Actinic Keratosis and Non-Melanoma Skin Cancer

	Treatment
Basal cell carcinoma	Cryosurgery with liquid nitrogen
	Electrodesiccation and curettage
	Standard surgical excision
	Mohs micrographic surgery
	5-fluorouracil cream, solution
	Imiquimod cream
	Photodynamic therapy
	Radiation therapy
Actinic keratosis	Cryosurgery with liquid nitrogen
	Currettage with or without electrocautery
	Shave excision
	5-fluorouracil cream, solution
	Diclofenac gel
	Imiquimod cream
	Chemical peel
	Cryopeeling
	Dermabrasion
	Laser resurfacing
	Photodynamic therapy
Squamous cell carcinoma	Cryosurgery with liquid nitrogen
	Electrodessication and curettage
	Standard surgical excision
	Mohs micrographic surgery
	Bleomycin (intralesional)
	Methotrexate (intralesional)
	5-fluorouracil (oral)
	Radiation therapy

utilized because it provides acceptable cure rates and is cost-effective (9). Unlike ED&C, the tumor status of the surgical margins can be assessed. MMS is the "gold standard" treatment of NMSC. MMS provides a complete histologic analysis of tumor margins, the highest cure rate, and maximal preservation of normal skin (9). Indications for MMS include recurrent tumors, tumors >2 cm diameter, tumors located in high-risk areas (i.e., lip, ear), tumors located in sites of previous radiation therapy and tumors with aggressive histopathologic features (i.e., micronodular, morpheaform, or infiltrating BCC) (9). The cost associated with MMS limits its utilization.

Nonsurgical treatment methods include topical chemotherapeutics, biological immune response modifiers, retinoids, and photodynamic therapy. Five-fluorouracil (5-FU), the topical chemotherapeutic agent most widely used for cutaneous tumors, interferes with DNA synthesis in rapidly dividing cells, resulting in tumor cell death. In contrast, imiquimod, a topical immune response modulator, promotes innate immune responses via activation of Th-1 cell-mediated immunity and local elevations in pro-inflammatory cytokines. Imiquimod is effective in the treatment of AKs, superficial BCCs, and SCCs in situ (9). Photodynamic therapy involves the topical administration of a tumor-localizing, photosensitizing agent and its subsequent activation with visible light to cause destruction of the tumor (4).

Oral retinoids, such as acitretin, are derivatives of vitamin A that can reduce the development of SCC and BCC. This chemopreventive effect is thought to occur by induction of apoptosis, cessation of tumor proliferation, and/or stimulation of normal keratinocyte differentiation (9). Oral retinoids are most often employed in post-solid organ transplant patients who, because of the required significant systemic immunosuppression, demonstrate significant increases in the incidence of NMSC as well as mortality from aggressive NMSC.

Following a diagnosis of NMSC, patients should be counseled regarding specific photoavoidance and photoprotection techniques. Patients with BCC or widespread AKs should be followed regularly with total body skin examinations every 6 months initially. According to the National Cancer Institute, patients with SCC should be re-examined every 3 months for the first several years and followed indefinitely at 6-month intervals due to the substantial risk of metastasis. Any suspicious lesion should be evaluated clinically and histologically.

References

1. **Ridky TW.** Nonmelanoma skin cancer. J Am Acad Dermatol. 2007; 57:484–501.
2. **Alam M, Ratner D.** Cutaneous squamous-cell carcinoma. N Eng J Med. 2001;344:975–83.
3. **Lewis KG, Weinstock, MA**. Trends in nonmelanoma skin cancer mortality rates in the United States, 1969 through 2000. Journal of Investigative Dermatology. 2007;127:2323–7.
4. **Rubin AI, Chen EH, Ratner D.** Basal cell carcinoma. N Eng J Med. 2005;353:2262–9.
5. **Carucci JA, Leffell DJ.** Basal cell carcinoma. In Wolff K, et al. (eds). Fitzpatrick's Dermatology in General Medicine, 2008; pp. 1036–42.
6. **Duncan KO, Geisse JK, Leffell DJ.** Epithelial precancerous lesions. In Wolff K, et al. (eds). Fitzpatrick's Dermatology in General Medicine, 2008; pp. 1007–15.
7. **Grossman D, Leffell DJ.** Squamous cell carcinoma. In Wolff K, et al. (eds). Fitzpatrick's Dermatology in General Medicine, 2008; pp. 1028–36.
8. **Martinez JC, Otley CC.** The management of melanoma and non-melanoma skin cancer: a review for the primary care physician. Mayo Clin Proc. 2001;76:1253–65.
9. **Neville J, Welch E, Leffell D.** Management of nonmelanoma skin cancer in 2007. Nature Clinical Practice Oncology. 2007;4:462–9.

3

Cardiovascular Disease in Women

A. Hypertension
Ann Evensen, MD

B. Hyperlipidemia
Amy Groff, DO; Sarina B. Schrager, MD, MS

C. Heart Disease
Elisabeth von der Lohe, MD

D. Overweight and Obesity
Carolina Bruno, MD; Robert V. Considine, PhD

E. Cigarette Smoking and Cessation in Women
Katherine Neely, MD; Samina Naseer, MD; Laurel C. Milberg, PhD

A. Hypertension

Ann Evensen

KEY POINTS

- Hypertension is extremely common, affecting 75% of women over the age of 70.
- Treating hypertension in women decreases the incidence of stroke and myocardial infarction.
- Diagnosis, treatment goals, and choice of antihypertensive agent are the same in men and non-pregnant women.
- Women who are pregnant or who may become pregnant should never receive angiotensin converting enzyme (ACE) inhibitors, angiotensin receptor blockers (ARB), or nitroprusside. The preferred agents for this group of women are methyldopa, hydralazine, labetolol, and nifedipine.
- Estrogen-containing contraceptives increase blood pressure.
- Women with hypertension who take hormonal contraception have a higher risk of stroke and myocardial infarction.
- Hypertension is twice as common in African American women as in Caucasian women.

Epidemiology

By age 70, about 75% of women will be diagnosed with hypertension (1). The prevalence of hypertension in African-American women is twice that of Caucasian women (23% vs. 12%) (2). Hypertension is the most important risk factor for the development of cardiovascular disease, which is the largest single cause of death among women worldwide (3). Risk of organ damage is directly proportional to the degree of blood pressure elevation (4). Treatment of hypertension in women successfully reduces risk of stroke and myocardial infarction (MI) (5).

Clinical Presentation

Hypertension is often asymptomatic and only diagnosed with routine screening. The US Preventive Services Task Force (USPSTF) strongly recommends that clinicians screen adults aged 18 and older for high blood pressure. Uncommon symptoms of hypertension are headache, dizziness, palpitations, fatigue, epistaxis, hematuria, blurred vision, dyspnea, and chest pain. If the hypertension is due to primary hyper-aldosteronism, the patient may experience polyuria, polydipsia, and muscle weakness. Cushing's syndrome can cause emotional lability and weight gain. A patient with pheochromocytoma may experience episodic symptoms (1,6).

Diagnosis and Differential Diagnosis

The diagnosis of hypertension should be made on the basis of the averaging of at least two blood pressures taken on two separate occasions. If hypertension is diagnosed, the patient should be examined for carotid, femoral, and abdominal bruits, heart murmurs and extra sounds, jugular venous distension, thyromegaly, rales, retinopathy, large kidneys, abnormal pulses, and Cushingoid features. The body mass index (BMI) should be calculated.

Essential hypertension is the diagnosis in >90% of all cases of hypertension. See Table 3-1 for the differential diagnosis of hypertension in women. Evaluation of a newly-diagnosed hypertensive

Table 3-1   Differential Diagnosis of Hypertension in Women

Essential hypertension (90% of all cases)
Kidney disease
• Renovascular
• Parenchymal
Arteriolar nephrosclerosis
Diabetic nephrosclerosis
Glomerulonephritis
Polycystic kidney disease
Cardiovascular disease
• Aortic regurgitation
• AV fistula
• Coarctation of the aorta
• Patent ductus arteriosis
Endocrine/Metabolic disease
• Cushing's syndrome
• Gestational hypertension
• Hyperaldosteronism
• Hypercalcemia
• Hyperthyroidism
• Pheochromocytoma
Neurologic disease
• Pain
• Increased intracranial pressure
• Sleep apnea
Drug effects
• Alcohol
• Appetite suppressants
• Decongestants
• Exogenous thyroid
• Hormonal contraception
• Complementary medications

From Dosh SA. The diagnosis of essential and secondary hypertension in adults. J Fam Pract. 2001;50:707–12. Fisher ND and Williams GH. Harrison's Principles of Internal Medicine. 16th edition. New York: McGraw Hill Companies; c2005. Chapter 230; Hypertensive Vascular Disease, p. 1463–81. Curtis KM, Mohllajee AP, Martins SL, et al. Combined oral contraceptive use in women with hypertension: a systematic review. Contraception. 2006;73:179–88; with permission.

woman should include: thyroid stimulating hormone, complete blood count, urinalysis, lipid panel, and comprehensive metabolic panel. Chest x-ray, electrocardiogram, and evaluation for rare causes of hypertension such as pheochromocytoma and renal artery stenosis also may be considered (7).

Clinical Care

Women have lower average systolic and diastolic blood pressure than men. Due to a loss of elastin and accumulation of collagen in the vascular tree at menopause, the blood pressure in the average woman after menopause increases disproportionately faster with age as compared to her male counterpart (8). Theoretically, these differences could result in different optimal medication choices for the treatment of hypertension in these two groups. No studies demonstrate such a difference, however. The ALLHAT study compared medications for hypertension in men and women over age 55 with at least one additional risk factor for heart disease. This study included a female subgroup analysis that found similar rates of cardiovascular events and all-cause mortality when different classes of medications were used (5). Currently the choice of medications and treatment goals for hypertension are the same in women as they are in men as outlined in the Seventh Report of the Joint National Committee on Prevention, Detection, Evaluation, and Treatment of High Blood Pressure (JNC VII) (9).

For all classes of hypertension, including pre-hypertension (SBP 120–139 mm Hg or DBP 80–89 mm Hg), clinicians should encourage weight reduction in overweight and obese individuals, implementation of the DASH (Dietary Approaches to Stop Hypertension) diet, dietary sodium reduction, increased physical activity, and moderate alcohol consumption (for women, this is <2 drinks per day).

For Stage 1 hypertension (SBP 140–159 mm Hg or DBP 90–99 mm Hg), treatment should start with a thiazide diuretic unless there is a compelling indication for an alternative medication (diabetes, chronic kidney disease, or established cardiovascular disease).

For Stage 2 hypertension (SBP ≥160 mm Hg or DBP ≥100 mm Hg), or for anyone who is >20/10 mm Hg above their goal blood pressure, clinicians should consider starting treatment with two medications. Typically, one medication would be a diuretic and the other an ACE inhibitor, ARB, beta blocker, or calcium channel blocker.

Most patients will require two or more medications to achieve their goal of ≤140/90 mm Hg (≤130/80 mm Hg for patients with diabetes, renal disease, or established cardiovascular disease). See Table 3-2 for a summary of antihypertensive medication choices (9).

Clinical Care of Special Populations

Hormone use—The average hormonal contraceptive user has a higher blood pressure than a non-user. Although low in all patients using

Table 3-2   Recommended Initial Drug Choices for Special Populations

Patient Characteristic:	ACE	Alpha Blocker	ARB	BB	CCB	Diuretic	Vasodilator
No compelling indication						X	
Black					X	X	
BP >20/10 mm Hg over goal (choose diuretic plus one other agent)	X		X	X	X	X	
Diabetes	X		X	X	X	X	
High risk cardiovascular disease	X			X	X	X	
Kidney disease			X	X			
Pregnant or may become pregnant*		X		X	X		X

*Preferred agents are methyldopa, labetolol, nifedipine, and hydralazine.
From Powrie RO. A 30-y-old woman with chronic hypertension trying to conceive. JAMA. 2007;298:1548–59. Safar ME, Smulyan H. Hypertension in women. Am J Hyperten. 2004;17:82–7; with permission.

oral contraception, rates of MI and stroke are 2–9 times higher in pill users, particularly if they have hypertension. Hypertensive oral contraceptive users have higher rates of cardiovascular events than hypertensive non-users. A WHO Expert Working Group on this subject stated that combined oral contraceptives are not recommended (unless other options are unacceptable or unavailable) for women with a history of hypertension who cannot have blood pressure checks, for those with Stage 1 hypertension (140–159 mm Hg systolic or 90–99 mm Hg diastolic), and for those with controlled hypertension. The working group also stated that oral contraceptives should not be used (without qualifier) in women with Stage 2 hypertension (over 160 mm Hg systolic or 100 mm Hg diastolic) or in those with known vascular disease (10). It is reasonable to consider the above risks and cautions applicable to the contraceptive patch and vaginal ring as well. Progesterone-only contraception is less likely to cause hypertension, but caution is still recommended in using this medication in women with hypertension, and it is contraindicated in those with vascular or thromboembolic disease. Hormone replacement therapy (HRT) does not increase blood pressure, but it has been found to increase the risk of MI and stroke.

African-American women—Due to an increased prevalence of cardiovascular disease, African-American women benefit more from treatment of their hypertension than do Caucasian women. For example, the number needed to treat to prevent one cardiovascular event for African-American women is 21, as compared to 78 in

Caucasian women (2). Male and female African-American hypertensive patients may respond better to diuretics and calcium channel blockers when used as monotherapy, but the response to drug combinations is similar regardless of race. Angioedema with use of ACE inhibitors is 2–4 times more common in African-American patients than in Caucasians (9).

Pregnant or who may become pregnant—Nitroprusside is contraindicated in pregnancy because of its potential for cyanide poisoning. Fetuses exposed to the ACE inhibitors and ARBs are at increased risk of early and late intrauterine death, cardiovascular and central nervous system defects, renal failure, oligohydramnios, preterm birth, low birth weight, and fetal distress. These agents have a "black box" contraindication for use in patients who are pregnant or who may become pregnant. Agents that are acceptable for use in pregnancy include methyldopa, hydralazine, and labetolol. Other beta blockers and sustained-release nifedipine are used less often. The management of preeclampsia, chronic hypertension in pregnancy, and gestational hypertension are beyond the scope of this review.

References

1. **Dosh SA.** The diagnosis of essential and secondary hypertension in adults. J Fam Pract. 2001;50:707–12.
2. **Quan A, Kerlikowske K, Gueyffler F, et al.** Efficacy of treating hypertension in women. J Gen Intern Med. 1999;14:718–29.
3. **Mosca L, Banka CL, Benjamin EJ, et al.** Evidence-based guidelines for cardiovascular disease prevention in women: 2007 update. Circulation. 2007;115:1481–501.
4. **Mason PJ, Manson JE, Sesso HD, et al.** Blood pressure and risk of secondary cardiovascular events in women: The Women's Antioxidant Cardiovascular Study (WACS). Circulation. 2004;109:1623–9.
5. Major outcomes in high-risk hypertensive patients randomized to angiotensin –converting enzyme inhibitor or calcium channel blocker vs diuretic: The Antihypertensive and Lipid-Lowering Treatment to Prevent Heart Attack Trial (ALLHAT). JAMA. 2002;288:2981–3196.
6. **Fisher ND and Williams GH.** Harrison's Principles of Internal Medicine. 16th edition. New York: McGraw Hill Companies; c2005. Chapter 230; Hypertensive Vascular Disease, p. 1463–81.
7. **Powrie RO.** A 30-year-old woman with chronic hypertension trying to conceive. JAMA. 2007;298:1548–59.
8. **Safar ME, Smulyan H.** Hypertension in women. Am J Hyperten. 2004;17:82–7.
9. **Chobanian AV, Bakris GL, Black HR et al.** The seventh report of the joint national committee on prevention, detection, evaluation, and treatment of high blood pressure. JAMA. 2003;289:2560–72.
10. **Curtis KM, Mohllajee AP, Martins SL, et al.** Combined oral contraceptive use in women with hypertension: a systematic review. Contraception. 2006;73:179–88.

B. Hyperlipidemia

Amy Groff and Sarina B. Schrager

KEY POINTS

- Cardiovascular disease (CVD) is the single leading cause of death among women.
- Elevated cholesterol is an important risk factor for CVD.
- Screening for lipids should occur every 5 years in average-risk women.
- Lifestyle changes are an essential first-line therapy in controlling hyperlipidemia in women and should be used in addition to any pharmaceutical therapy.
- LDL <100 mg/dL is the optimal level for all women.
- Recommendations for treating elevated lipids are the same for men and women.

Epidemiology

Worldwide, an average of >16 women per minute die of CVD, including both heart attack and stroke (1). Coronary heart disease (CHD) accounts for the majority of CVD-related deaths in women (2). Epidemiologic and clinical studies have established a causal relationship between elevated serum cholesterol levels and heart disease. There is also strong evidence showing that a reduction in cholesterol leads to a decrease in the rate of cardiovascular events (3). Data from the National Health and Nutrition Examination Survey (NHANES) in 2005–2006 showed that the prevalence of high serum total cholesterol was higher for women than for men (4). Data indicates that CHD may be preventable with management of cholesterol levels (5).

For the most part, there are no outward signs of hyperlipidemia. Box 3-1 lists some medical conditions that can be associated with hyperlipidemia.

Primary and secondary causes of hyperlipidemia are listed in Box 3-2. Most secondary causes can be reduced or eliminated by lifestyle modifications.

Screening Recommendations

The US Preventive Services Task Force (USPSTF) strongly recommends that clinicians routinely screen men ≥35 years of age and women ≥45 years of age for hyperlipidemia and treat abnormal lipids

---

Box 3-1   Possible Signs and Symptoms of Hyperlipidemia

- Xanthomas
- Claudication
- Bruits
- Angina
- Myocardial infarction
- Pancreatitis
- Cerebrovascular accident

Box 3-2   Primary and Secondary Causes of Hyperlipidemia

Primary:
- Genetics
- Family history (CVD at <65 years of age in a female relative and <55 y of age in a male relative)
- Age
- Sex

Secondary:
- Sedentary lifestyle
- Obesity
- Diet
- Tobacco use
- Liver disease
- Hypothyroidism
- Diabetes mellitus
- Kidney disease
- Medications including progestins, anabolic steroids, corticosteroids, some antihypertensive medications

From Executive Summary of the Third Report of the National Cholesterol Education Program (NCEP) Expert Panel on Detection, Evaluation, and Treatment of High Blood Cholesterol in Adults (Adult Treatment Panel III). JAMA. 2001;285:2486–97; with permission.

---

in people at increased risk for CHD. Routine screening of men 20–35 years of age and women 20–45 years of age for hyperlipidemia is recommended by the USPSTF if the patient has risk factors for CHD. In the absence of known risk factors for CHD, no recommendations for or against screening below the age of 20, for men or women, are given (6).

The USPSTF recommends screening using total cholesterol (TC) and high-density lipoprotein cholesterol (HDL-C). TC and HDL-C can be measured on non-fasting or fasting samples. There is insufficient evidence to recommend for or against routine triglyceride measurement (6).

Options for intervals of screening include: every 5 years for average-risk women, more frequently for people who have lipid levels close to those warranting therapy based on risk factors, and more than every 5 years for low-risk people who have had low or repeatedly normal lipid levels (6). Pharmacotherapy is warranted to lower LDL in very high risk women when their LDL level is >70 mg/dL. In high risk women with CHD or other risk factors, treatment is warranted to bring the LDL <100 mg/dL. For at risk women with multiple risk factors, the LDL level should be <130 mg/dL. LDL should be <160 mg/dL in at risk women and <190 mg/dL in all women, regardless of risk factors (8). Risk factors to help determine testing frequency include age, total cholesterol, smoking status, HDL level, and blood pressure using Framingham point scales (7). (To utilize a Framingham CHD risk scoring system based 10-year Risk Calculator, go to http://www.nhlbi.nih.gov/guidelines/cholesterol/index.htm.). The various risk levels are as follows: "At risk" includes women with greater than or equal to one risk factor for CVD (risk factors noted above), "high risk" includes women with CHD or a CHD equivalent, like diabetes, other atherosclerotic CVD, or 10 year Framingham global risk >20%, and "very high risk" includes women who have established CVD plus one of the following 3 items: multiple risk factors, poorly controlled risk factors, or CHD equivalent.

The National Cholesterol Education Program (NCEP) Expert Panel on Detection, Evaluation, and Treatment of High Blood Cholesterol in Adults (Adult Treatment Panel III) recommends that all adults 20 years or older receive a fasting lipoprotein profile once every 5 years (7). In women with elevated levels, more frequent screening may be appropriate. A fasting lipoprotein profile includes total cholesterol, LDL cholesterol, HDL cholesterol, and triglyceride levels. If unable to obtain fasting testing, then total cholesterol and HDL can be used. If total cholesterol is ≥200 mg/dL or HDL <40 mg/dL, then a follow-up fasting lipoprotein profile is needed to evaluate LDL (7).

General Recommendations for Lipid Management in Women

According to the *Evidence-Based Guidelines for Cardiovascular Disease Prevention in Women: 2007 Update* (8), all women >20 years of age should have LDL <100 mg/dL, HDL >50 mg/dL, triglycerides <150 mg/dL and non-HDL cholesterol <130 mg/dL (8).

Lifestyle changes are an essential first-line therapy in controlling hyperlipidemia in women. It is suggested that clinicians encourage women to quit tobacco use and recommend 30 minutes of moderate-intensity physical activity on most, and preferably all, days of the week. BMI should be maintained between 18.5 and 24.9 kg/m^2, and waist circumference should be ≤35 inches. Dietary recommendations include limiting saturated fat to <10% of caloric content (if possible to <7%), cholesterol to <300 mg/d, alcohol intake to no more than 1 drink per day, and sodium intake to <2.3 g/d (8).

Suggestions from the NCEP-ATP III report are similar, but not specific to women. They include reduced intake of saturated fats (<7% of total calories) and cholesterol (<200 mg/d), use of plant stanols/sterols (2 g/d) and increased viscous (soluble) fiber (10–25 g/d), weight reduction, and increased physical activity. They also recommend that at all stages of dietary therapy, clinicians refer patients to registered dietitians or other qualified nutritionists for medical nutrition therapy (7).

Pharmacotherapy Recommendations

The clinical recommendations regarding the use of pharmacotherapy to lower LDL in women have been discussed earlier (see Section on Screening Recommendations). Most of the recommendations do not differ from the recommendations for men. In addition to lifestyle modifications, very high risk women should be placed on an LDL-lowering medication if their LDL is >70 mg/dL, while high-risk women should begin treatment at an LDL >100 mg/dL. The treatment of at-risk women with multiple risk factors depends on their LDL and their Framingham risk score. Any woman with an LDL ≥190 mg/dL should be placed on an LDL-lowering medication.

High-risk women should be placed on niacin or fibrate therapy for low HDL or elevated non-HDL cholesterol. At-risk women with multiple risk factors and a Framingham global risk of 10–20% should also be started on niacin or fibrate therapy. These recommendations should be considered after a woman has already decreased her LDL to goal.

Table 3-3 lists various drug classes and non-pharmaceutical agents that can be used to correct hyperlipidemia and how each affects various types of cholesterol.

Gender Differences in Hyperlipidemia

In 2005, almost half of the 17.5 million victims of CVD, including heart disease and stroke, were women (10). According to NHANES reports in 2005–2006, among adults 20 years and older, 13.8% of men and 17.3% of women had serum total cholesterol levels that were ≥240 mg/dL, representing a statistically significant difference between the genders. The greatest difference between men and women was limited to those aged 60 years and older. More women than men have been screened for high cholesterol within the past 5 years, which is an improvement, but fewer women than men were told by their healthcare provider that they had hyperlipidemia (4). It is a clinician's responsibility to not only screen women for hyperlipidemia at various stages in life, but to inform and educate them about treatment and, most of all, prevention of CVD.

Table 3-3   Pharmaceuticals and Non-Pharmaceutical Therapy Used to Treat Dyslipidemia and Their Effects on Different Types of Cholesterol

Drug Class or Agent	Effect on LDL	Effect on Triglycerides	Effect on HDL
Nicotinic acid	Lowers	Lowers	Raises
Fibric acids	Lowers, but can have variable effects	Lowers	Raises
HMG-CoA reductase inhibitors (statins)	Lowers	Lowers	Raises
Bile acid sequestrants	Lowers	Raises, but can have variable effects	Raises
Fish Oil*		Lowers	
Plant stanols/sterols[†]	Lowers		
Fiber[‡]	Lowers		
Soy[§]	Lowers	Lowers	
Garlic, Nuts (walnuts), Artichoke extract[‖]	Lowers		

*Dosing fish oil: 3–4 g of EPA (Eicosapentaenoic acid) + DHA (Docosahexaenoic acid) = therapeutic dose for lowering triglycerides.
[†]Stanols/sterols: contained in spreads like *Take Control* or *Benecol* (2–3 g/d).
[‡]Pectin, Oat Bran, Ground flax seed (1–2 Tbsp/d), Psyllium and Guar gum (*Benefiber*) (1 Tbsp/d).
[§]20–50 g needed daily to lower cholesterol.
[‖]Garlic (1/2–1 clove/d), Nuts (1 oz/d), Artichoke extract (1800 mg divided twice a day or thrice a day.).
From Executive Summary of the Third Report of the National Cholesterol Education Program (NCEP) Expert Panel on Detection, Evaluation, and Treatment of High Blood Cholesterol in Adults (Adult Treatment Panel III). JAMA 2001;285:2486–97. Rakel D. Non-pharmaceutical therapy for lowering cholesterol: pearls for clinicians. Available at http://www.fammed.wisc.edu/integrative/modules/cholesterol. Accessed January 13, 2008; with permission.

References

1. Go Red for Women. World Heart Federation Website. Available at: http://www.worldheartfederation.org/whatwedo/goredforwomen/whygored. Accessed January 4, 2008.
2. American Heart Association. Heart Disease and Stroke Statistics-2007 Update. Dallas, TX: American Heart Association; 2006.
3. Levine GN, Keaney JF Jr., Vita JA. Cholesterol reduction in cardiovascular disease: clinical benefits and possible mechanisms. N Engl J Med. 1996;332:512–21.
4. Schober SE, Carroll MD, Lacher DA, et al. High serum total cholesterol—an indicator for monitoring cholesterol lowering efforts; U.S. adults, 2005–2006. NCHS data brief no 2, Hyattsville, MD: National Center for Health Statistics. 2007.
5. Mosca L, Grundy SM, Judelson D, et al. Guide to preventative cardiology for women. AHA/ACC scientific statement, consensus panel statement. Circulation. 1999;99:2480–84.

6. The Guide to Clinical Preventative Services 2006, Recommendations of the U.S. Preventative Services Task Force. Department of Health and Human Services, Agency for Healthcare Research and Quality; 2006.

7. Executive Summary of the Third Report of the National Cholesterol Education Program (NCEP) Expert Panel on Detection, Evaluation, and Treatment of High Blood Cholesterol in Adults (Adult Treatment Panel III). JAMA. 2001;285:2486–97.

8. **Mosca L, Banka CL, Benjamin EJ, et al.** Evidence-based guidelines for cardiovascular disease prevention in women: 2007 update. Circulation. 2007;115:1481–501.

9. **Rakel D.** Non-Pharmaceutical therapy for lowering cholesterol: pearls for clinicians. Available at http://www.fammed.wisc.edu/integrative/modules/cholesterol. Accessed January 13, 2008.

10. World Health Organization. Preventing chronic diseases: A vital investment. Geneva, 2005.

C. Heart Disease

Elisabeth von der Lohe

KEY POINTS

- Cardiovascular disease is **the** leading cause of death in women in the U.S.
- Deaths due to cardiovascular disease exceed the number of all cancer deaths combined.
- For decades, heart disease death rates have been falling rapidly for men but only slightly for women.
- More women under the age of 45 years are dying from heart disease than ever before.
- Diagnosis of coronary heart disease in women remains a challenge due to a high likelihood of atypical symptoms, such as dyspnea, extreme fatigue, and indigestion.
- Myocardial infarction and revascularization procedures (PCI and CABG) are associated with higher mortality and morbidity, primarily explained by age, risk factors, and body size.
- Primary angioplasty is the treatment of choice in patients with an acute myocardial infarction.
- Preventive care should be gender-specific and should avoid hormone replacement therapy.
- The most commonly encountered valvular abnormalities in women are aortic stenosis in the elderly and the mitral valve prolapse syndrome in young females.
- Peripartum cardiomyopathy is a serious illness that occurs in 1 in 3000 pregnant women.

Epidemiology

Cardiovascular disease is **the** leading cause of death in women in the U.S., accounting for nearly 500 000 deaths each year. Deaths due to cardiovascular disease in women exceed the number of deaths from all forms of cancers combined. About half of these deaths result from coronary heart disease (CHD) (1). In 2003, CHD claimed the lives of 233 886 women compared with 41 566 lives from breast cancer and 67 894 from lung cancer. Over the course of her lifetime, a woman faces a 32% probability of dying from CHD and resulting illnesses. For American women, the risk of developing breast cancer during their lifetimes is 13.2% (see Chapter 2b).

While it is true that the overall death rate caused by coronary artery disease is similar for both genders, the incidence pattern is strikingly different. Women develop CHD about 10 years later than men. Thus, CHD in women is a disease of the elderly. It is the leading cause of death among women aged 65 years and older. After age 75, cardiovascular mortality rates increase by a factor of 5 in men, compared to a factor of 9 in women. Taking into account that in the year 2025 about 390 million women in the U.S. will be >65 years of age, the epidemiologic and clinical impact of CHD is likely to markedly increase over the next 2 decades.

CHD also contributes significantly to hospitalizations and physical disabilities. Thirty-six percent of women between the ages of 55 and 64 and 55% of women over the age of 75 have significant limitations in their physical fitness due to CHD (1).

Clinical Presentation

Angina pectoris is the most common manifestation of CHD. However, up to 50% of women with angina have angiographically normal coronary arteries. Therefore, diagnosis of coronary heart disease in women remains a challenge. To complicate things further, many women with CHD have atypical symptoms as a manifestation of their atherosclerotic disease. This is particularly true for elderly women.

Typical angina is described as retrosternal heaviness, a pressure, or a squeezing sensation, with radiation across the precordium, up the neck or down the ulnar surface of the left arm. The right arm, the shoulders, and the lateral aspects of both arms may be involved as well. Some patients describe a "strangling" or "suffocating" sensation. Frequently the pain starts in the arm or neck and travels to the midsternal area.

Atypical symptoms, or "angina-equivalents," include dyspnea, sensation of epigastric fullness, retrosternal burning, and easy fatigability. The latter is seen in 70% of women who develop a myocardial infarction in the ensuing weeks (2).

Since there is a gradual transition from stable to unstable angina and, subsequently, to myocardial infarction, symptoms of a myocardial infarction are very similar to those of stable CHD. The only difference is the fact that at the time of a myocardial infarction these symptoms are persistent and frequently associated with diaphoresis, nausea, and shortness of breath. However, only 25% of women with an acute myocardial infarction present with typical symptoms. Twenty-five percent complain of indigestion or burning discomfort only. Another 25% of women present with arm, neck, jaw, or back pain as their only symptom, and a high percentage of female patients are truly asymptomatic and are unable to recall any symptoms at all. The most common symptoms seen in elderly women with an acute myocardial infarction are shortness of breath, marked weakness, or frank syncope (3).

Diagnosis and Differential Diagnosis

The following approach is helpful in determining the pretest likelihood of CHD in women: evaluation of the pain character (typical vs. atypical angina), followed by evaluation of risk factors (how many, how serious). Women with several risk factors (including menopause) and typical angina have a high likelihood of CHD (80–90%). On the other hand, the likelihood of CHD in pre-menopausal women with atypical symptoms and no cardiovascular risk factors is low (<4%). In other words, the more the risk factors and the more typical the chest pain, the higher the likelihood of disease. This approach should exclude diabetic women. Diabetic women have a high risk of CHD independent of age, symptoms (high likelihood of atypical or no symptoms), and menopausal status. Table 3-4 shows average pretest likelihoods of CHD in women with typical and atypical symptoms.

Differential diagnosis of angina-type symptoms includes vasospastic angina, syndrome X, hypertension, pulmonary hypertension, and depression. The next steps necessary in making or rejecting a diagnosis of CHD include physical examination, an EKG, and, frequently, an echocardiogram.

Table 3-4　Pretest Likelihood of Coronary Artery Disease in Symptomatic Patients According to Age and Sex (in Percentage)

Age	Typical Angina		Atypical Angina		Non-anginal Pain	
	Women	Men	Women	Men	Women	Men
30–39	26	70	4	22	1	5
40–49	55	87	13	46	3	14
50–59	79	92	32	59	8	22
60–69	90	94	54	67	19	28

Adapted from "Recommendations of the Task Force of the European Society of Cardiology: Management of stable angina pectoris." Eur Heart J. 1997;18:398 and Del Valle M, Frishman WH and Charney P in "Coronary Artery Disease in Women." American College of Physician. 1999;377; with permission.

Based on the pretest probability of CHD, these tests are either followed by no further cardiac testing (very low pretest probability), a stress test (intermediate or high pretest probability), or—as the definitive test—a coronary angiogram (high pretest probability). However, stress tests are contraindicated in patients with unstable angina and should not be performed earlier than 3 days after a myocardial infarction (4). Stress test selection depends upon the patient's ability to exercise to her target heart rate, presence of EKG changes, and/or comorbidities (e.g., bronchial asthma, obesity, and medication). An exercise stress test is preferable to a pharmacological stress test, because physical exertion most closely reflects physiological conditions and allows conclusions about functional capacities. However, the prerequisite is that the woman is able to achieve 85% of maximum predicted heart rate (220 minus the patient's age). A pharmacological stress test is indicated in all other cases.

The following stress tests are available:

1. Exercise electrocardiogram
2. Stress scintigram (thallium-201 or technetium-99)
3. Stress echocardiogram

The second and third tests above may be carried out in conjunction with exercise, as well as with pharmacological provocation with dobutamine, dipyridamole, or adenosine (4).

The choice of stress test (stress scintigram or stress echocardiogram) should depend on local expertise. The nuclear stress test is more sensitive than the stress echocardiogram but has a relatively high rate of false-positive results. In addition, the radiation exposure is substantive. A stress echocardiogram, on the other hand, is less sensitive and thus may miss the diagnosis. A stress electrocardiogram alone (without concomitant imaging) is not recommended, given its high rate of false-positive results in women.

Electron-beam-computed tomography (EBCT) is not very useful for the diagnosis of CHD, given its low specificity for significant lesions (varies from 41% to 76%). Positron emission tomography (PET) and magnetic resonance imaging (MRI) are not very practical and are very costly. A promising developing tool for the diagnosis of CHD—in particular, in young or middle-aged women—is a high-resolution (i.e., 64 slice- or dual source) cardiac CT. The main negative aspect of this test is the associated high level of radiation.

Clinical Care

Medical Treatment

All patients with CHD need medical treatment alone or in combination with revascularization procedures, such as percutaneous coronary intervention (PCI) or coronary artery bypass graft surgery (CABG).

Aspirin, beta-blockers, and nitrates are first-line medications for women with angina. Calcium channel blockers should only be used if beta blockers are contraindicated and should only be administered in long-acting form.

In women with an acute coronary syndrome, myocardial infarction, and/or PCI with stent placement, the dihydropyridine antagonist clopidrogel needs to be added to the regimen. Recommended duration of clopidrogel treatment is at least 1 month (but preferably 1 year) in patients who are treated medically and in patients who received a bare metal stent. All patients who received a drug-eluting stent should be placed on clopidrogel for 1 year to minimize the risk of acute and late in-stent thrombosis.

Percutaneous Coronary Intervention

Despite recent refinements in PCI techniques and improvements in adjunctive therapy, women continue to be at higher risk than men for complications from PCI and continue to have a higher in-hospital mortality, regardless of the device technology used. However, these gender differences are less pronounced in recent studies and should not discourage physicians from referring women for PCI, since long-term outcome is independent of gender.

Percutaneous Coronary Intervention in Patients with Acute Myocardial Infarction (Primary Angioplasty)

Primary angioplasty not only reduces in-hospital mortality but also cardiovascular complications, including early reinfarction and cerebral stroke. It, therefore, constitutes the treatment of choice in patients with acute myocardial infarction. However, primary angioplasty is only meaningful if the door-to-balloon time (i.e., time from presentation in the emergency department until inflation of the balloon) does not exceed 2 hours (ideally <90 minutes).

Coronary Artery Bypass Surgery

Although operative mortality is higher in women than in men, there is no gender difference in long-term survival. Seventy percent of women and 73% of men are still alive 18 years after CABG. The small difference in survival is most likely due to a higher operative mortality in women. However, despite similar long-term survival, more women than men remain symptomatic. One year after surgery, only 45% of women, but 69% of men are without angina.

Long-term outcomes for women who are candidates for either coronary angioplasty or bypass surgery are excellent and are independent of the choice of procedure. However, due to a higher likelihood of incomplete revascularization with PCI, patients who undergo coronary intervention experience more angina in the first 3 years thereafter than do CABG patients and more frequently require a second revascularization procedure.

Preventive Care

Prevention should be gender-specific and should avoid ineffective interventions such as antioxidants and hormone replacement therapy (5).

Valvular Heart Disease

Epidemiology

The most commonly encountered valvular abnormalities in women are:

1. Calcific or degenerative aortic stenosis (AS) in *elderly* women; and
2. Mitral valve prolapse (MVP) in *young* females (so-called mitral valve prolapse syndrome). The latter must be differentiated from MVP due to myxomatous changes or heritable disorders of the mitral valve, which occur more frequently in males.

All other valvular diseases either occur with similar frequency in both genders (i.e., severe mitral regurgitation [MR] secondary to left ventricular systolic dysfunction) or are less common (including, but not exclusively, aortic, pulmonic, and tricuspid regurgitation; pulmonic and tricuspid stenosis)

The prevalence of calcific aortic stenosis is approximately 5% in women over 75 years of age and close to 6% in those over 86 years of age. Moderate or severe aortic stenosis is more frequent in women (8.8% vs. 3.6% in men) (6). Calcification of the aortic valve with and without concomitant stenosis is associated with a 50% increased risk of cardiovascular death and myocardial infarction (6).

Mitral valve prolapse syndrome affects 2.4% of the population, with women (in particular, young women) affected twice as often as men. Unless it is associated with significant mitral regurgitation (MR), it generally has a benign long-term course (7).

Clinical Presentation

Calcific Aortic Stenosis: The most common symptoms are dyspnea on exertion, angina pectoris, syncope, and, eventually, heart failure. Angina in patients with aortic stenosis does not differ from that seen in CHD patients (6).

Mitral Valve Prolapse Syndrome: Symptoms are diverse and include stabbing chest pain, angina pectoris, palpitations, and syncope. In case of associated severe mitral regurgitation (MR), which is rare, patients can develop dyspnea on exertion, fatigue, and arrhythmias (7).

Diagnosis

Calcific Aortic Stenosis: All patients with aortic stenosis have a systolic murmur on physical examination. It is typically late-peaking and heard best at the base of the heart, with radiation along the carotid arteries. An echocardiography, including Doppler examination, typically confirms the clinical diagnosis and serves to determine the severity of the disease. It also allows measurements of the degree of left ventricular hypertrophy (LVH) and dysfunction (6). The EKG shows LVH in 85% of patients with severe aortic stenosis (AS); however, the absence of electrocardiographic signs of LVH does not exclude the diagnosis of AS. Cardiac catheterization is only indicated if noninvasive tests are inconclusive and/or surgical repair is necessary. In the latter case, the invasive diagnostic test is typically restricted to coronary angiography.

Mitral Valve Prolapse Syndrome: Physical examination of patients with MVP reveals a characteristic systolic click and a mid-to-late peaking systolic murmur along the left lower sternal border. Echocardiography, including Doppler examination, is necessary to confirm or reject the diagnosis and allows quantification of associated MR, if present.

Clinical Care

Calcific Aortic Stenosis: Since the prognosis for asymptomatic patients is excellent, they should be treated for cardiovascular risk factors only. However, these patients are advised to report new symptoms as early as possible. Sometimes an exercise test may be necessary to detect covert symptoms.

Symptomatic patients need aortic valve replacement, even if the severity of the stenosis (as determined by the transvalvular pressure gradient and/or the aortic valve area) is only moderate. An exercise stress test should absolutely be avoided in these patients. Balloon aortic valvotomy does not have a positive impact on long-term outcome but may be reasonable as a bridge to surgery in unstable patients or as a palliative procedure (6).

Mitral Valve Prolapse Syndrome: Many patients remain asymptomatic. In these patients, clinical follow-up with an occasional echocardiogram is sufficient. Patients with MVP syndrome and significant MR should be treated similarly to other patients with MR and may require MV repair (7).

Peripartum Cardiomyopathy

Epidemiology

Peripartum cardiomyopathy is defined as a dilated cardiomyopathy that occurs either in the last month of pregnancy or within 6 months of delivery. It is most likely an autoimmune disorder. The incidence is estimated to be 1 in 3000 pregnant women, with the highest risk in African-Americans, multiparous women, older women, and those with pre-eclampsia. Fifty percent of women will completely recover; in other words, their left ventricular function will normalize. The likelihood of recovery is highest in women with an initial ejection fraction exceeding 30%. Additional pregnancies should be avoided because of a great likelihood of disease recurrence associated with fatal outcome (8).

Clinical Presentation

Symptoms are the same as for other forms of congestive heart failure, particularly left-sided failure, and include fatigue, weakness, dyspnea, chest discomfort, pulmonary congestion, and peripheral edema.

Diagnosis

Physical examination typically reveals signs of heart failure with an S3 or S4 as well as a mitral regurgitation murmur. An echocardiogram is essential for establishing the diagnosis. The EKG may show nonspecific findings, such as sinus tachycardia, atrial and/or ventricular arrhythmias, intraventricular conduction defects, and nonspecific ST–T wave changes.

Clinical Care

Treatment does not differ from that of other forms of heart failure except that ACE (angiotensin-converting enzyme) inhibitors and angiotensin receptor blocking agents are contraindicated during pregnancy. In pregnant women, hydralazine and digoxin are safer alternatives. Anticoagulation with unfractionated heparin in pregnant women with an ejection fraction of <35% should be considered given the high risk of ventricular thrombus formation. Early induced delivery may be necessary in women with significant heart failure. In women with heart failure who are refractory to medical treatment, alternative treatment options should be considered, including implantation of a left ventricular assist device and heart transplantation (8).

References

1. **Thom T, Hasse N, Rosamond W. et al.** Heart disease and stroke statistics—2006 update: A report from the American Heart Association Statistics Committee and Stroke Statistics Subcommittee. Circulation. 2006;113:e85.
2. **Milner KA, Funk M, Richards S, et al.** Gender Differences in symptom presentation associated with coronary heart disease. Am J Cardiol. 1999;84:396.
3. **Vaccarino V, Parsons L, Every NR, et al.** Sex-based differences in early mortality after myocardial infarction. National Registry of Myocardial Infarction 2 Particip ants. N Engl J Med. 1999;341:217–25.
4. **Mieres JH, Shaw LJ, Arai A, et al.** Role of Noninvasive Testing in the Clinical Evaluation of Women With Suspected Coronary Artery Disease: Consensus Statement From the Cardiac Imaging Committee, Council on Clinical Cardiology, and the Cardiovascular Imaging and Intervention Committee, Council on Cardiovascular Radiology and Intervention, American Heart Association. Circulation. 2005;111:682–96.
5. **Mosca L, Banka CL, Benjamin EJ, et al.** Evidence-based guidelines for cardiovascular disease prevention in women: 2007 update. Circulation. 2007;115:1481–501.
6. **Freeman RV,** Otto CM. Spectrum of calcific aortic valve disease: pathogenesis, disease progression, and treatment strategies. Circulation. 2005;111:3316–26.
7. **Hayek E, Gring CN, Griffin BP.** Mitral valve prolapse. Lancet. 2005; 365:507–18.
8. **Pearson GD, Veille JC, Rahimtoola S, et al.** Peripartum cardiomyopathy: National Heart, Lung, and Blood Institute and Office of Rare Diseases (National Institutes of Health) workshop recommendations and review. JAMA. 2000;283:1183–8.

D. Overweight and Obesity

Carolina Bruno and Robert V. Considine

KEY POINTS

- Obesity is a chronic disease and a major health problem and is measured by the body mass index (BMI).
- Obesity is rapidly increasing in prevalence in developed countries worldwide.
- Obesity is associated with multiple comorbidities, including cardiovascular disease, type 2 diabetes, sleep apnea, gastrointestinal disease, osteoarthritis, and cancer.
- Goals of therapy are to prevent additional weight gain and enhance weight reduction.
- Treatments of obesity include diet, exercise, drugs, and/or surgery.

Epidemiology

It is estimated that there are now more than 1 billion overweight adults in the world, and at least 300 million of them are clinically obese. The U.S. has the highest rate of obesity in the developed world, with approximately 41.8% of adult women classified as obese (1). A significant proportion of the increase in body weight in the U.S. population has occurred since 1980. Data from the National Health and Nutrition Examination Surveys (NHANES) show that among adults aged 20–74 years the prevalence of obesity increased from 15.0% in the 1976–1980 survey to 32.9% in the 2003–2004 survey (2). In 2006, only 4 states had a prevalence of obesity <20%. Twenty-two states had a prevalence of obesity equal to or >25%; 2 of these states (Mississippi and West Virginia) had a prevalence of obesity ≥30% (3).

Clinical Characteristics

Body mass index (BMI) is a practical method for estimating adiposity that correlates reasonably well with body fat content. It is calculated by dividing the subject's weight by the square of her height: BMI = kg/m^2, or, using U.S./British units, BMI = $[pounds/inches^2] \times 703$. The World Health Organization and the National Center for Health Statistics define body weight status as follows:

BMI 18.5–24.9 kg/m^2	Normal range
BMI 25–29.9 kg/m^2	Overweight
BMI >30 kg/m^2	Obese

This classification is based on data obtained from large epidemiological studies conducted primarily in Caucasians that evaluated the relationship between BMI and mortality. In general, a higher BMI is associated with a greater risk of adiposity-related disease and premature mortality, until the age of 75. In elderly persons, BMI has less of an impact on mortality but possibly a greater effect on quality of life. Body fat distribution and ethnicity modify BMI-related risk. Overweight or obese subjects with excess upper body fat (central obesity or increased abdominal subcutaneous and visceral fat) are at greater risk for diabetes, hypertension, dyslipidemia, and ischemic heart disease. The absolute health risk for Chinese and South Asian people is higher at any level of BMI, and this should be taken into account during evaluation of women of these ethnicities (4).

The most common cause of overweight and obesity is sedentary lifestyle and increased caloric intake. Other etiologies include neuroendocrine disorders (Cushing's syndrome, hypothyroidism, polycystic ovary syndrome [PCOS]), medications (antipsychotics, antidepressants, antiepileptics, glucocorticoids), and cessation of smoking. Many overweight women gain excess weight after puberty. This weight gain may be precipitated by a number of events, including pregnancy, oral contraceptive therapy, and menopause (4).

The National Institutes of Health (NIH) guidelines suggest that all adult patients be screened for overweight and obesity by measuring BMI and waist circumference at the yearly health examination. Adiposity should be included in the evaluation of overall medical risk (5). The waist circumference is measured with a flexible tape placed on a horizontal plane at the level of the iliac crest as seen from the anterior view. In adults with a BMI of 25 to 34.9 kg/m², a waist circumference >88 cm (35 in) for women and 102 cm (40 in) for men is associated with a greater risk of hypertension, type 2 diabetes, dyslipidemia, and coronary heart disease.

Evaluation for comorbidities should include measurement of blood pressure, lipid profile, and fasting blood glucose.

Medical history should include age at onset of weight gain, previous weight loss attempts, change in dietary patterns, history of exercise, current and past medications, and history of smoking cessation.

Etiology

There are many factors that affect the balance between energy intake and energy expenditure, resulting in weight gain. The broad determinants of body weight can be classified as:

1. Biological influences: hormones and genetic factors
2. Behavioral influences: habits, emotions, beliefs, attitudes, and cognition
3. Environmental influences: physical, economic, and sociocultural factors

Perception of overweight as a desirable or undesirable trait is an important social determinant of obesity. Attitudes toward obesity vary greatly across social and ethnic groups and are related to the economic position of individuals. In many affluent countries, women experience social pressure to be thin. The social pressure toward thinness is greater for women than men and greater in women with higher levels of education (6).

Effect on Health

A number of large epidemiologic studies have evaluated the relationship between obesity and mortality. In general, a greater BMI is associated with increased rate of death from all causes and from cardiovascular disease. Obesity and increased central fat are associated with increased morbidity in addition to mortality, as discussed below (5). For a more detailed explanation of the following comorbidities and citation of original studies, see references 4 and 7.

Type 2 diabetes: There is strong association of type 2 diabetes with obesity in all ethnic groups. More than 80% of cases of type 2 diabetes can be attributed to obesity. A curvilinear relationship between BMI and the risk of type 2 diabetes was found in women in the Nurses' Health Study. Insulin resistance with hyperinsulinemia is characteristic of obesity and is present before the onset of hyperglycemia.

Hypertension: Blood pressure is positively correlated with BMI. The risk of hypertension is greatest in those subjects with upper body and abdominal obesity.

Dyslipidemia: Lipid abnormalities include high serum concentrations of cholesterol, low-density-lipoprotein (LDL) cholesterol, very-low-density-lipoprotein (VLDL) cholesterol, and triglycerides, and a reduction in serum high-density-lipoprotein (HDL) cholesterol of approximately 5%. Central fat distribution contributes to serum lipid abnormalities.

Coronary heart disease: Risk of coronary heart disease (CHD) and cardiovascular mortality is increased in obese subjects with excess abdominal fat distribution. After adjustment for other CHD risk factors, including hypertension, dyslipidemia, impaired glucose tolerance, and diabetes, overweight and obesity still increased the risk for CHD.

Stroke: Data from the Nurses' Health Study found that BMI $\geq 27 \, kg/m^2$, and weight gain after age 18, were associated with an increased risk of ischemic stroke.

Venous thrombosis: There is an increased risk of deep vein thrombosis and pulmonary embolus in the obese subject.

Hepatobiliary disease: Cholelithiasis is significantly increased in obese subjects. This is in part explained by increased cholesterol secretion, bile cholesterol supersaturation, and decreased gall bladder contractility. Non-alcoholic steatohepatitis (NASH) also is common. This spectrum of liver abnormalities includes hepatomegaly, abnormal liver biochemistry, steatosis, steatohepatitis, fibrosis, and cirrhosis. Steatosis affects approximately 75% of obese subjects and is associated with the presence of abdominal obesity.

Gastroesophageal reflux disease: A higher incidence of reflux symptoms is reported in most studies comparing lean and obese subjects.

Osteoarthritis: The incidence of osteoarthritis is increased in overweight and obese subjects, accounting for a major component of the cost of obesity. Although osteoarthritis is more common in the knees and ankles, it also develops in non-weight-bearing joints, suggesting that there are components of the obesity syndrome that alter cartilage and bone metabolism.

Malignancy: Cancer of the esophagus, colon and rectum, liver, gall bladder, pancreas, kidney, breast, uterus, cervix, and ovary is increased in overweight and obese subjects. Risks for non-Hodgkin's lymphoma and multiple myeloma also are increased. One explanation for the increased risk of endometrial and perhaps breast cancer in obese women is the increased production of estrogens by adipose tissue stromal cells. Obesity is also associated with consumption of a high-fat diet which is a risk factor for cancer development.

Endocrine dysfunction: Obesity is associated with Cushing's syndrome, hypothyroidism, and polycystic ovary syndrome (PCOS). Obese women are often affected by irregular menses, amenorrhea, and decreased fertility.

Kidney dysfunction: Multiple obesity-associated conditions, including hypertension, diabetes, and metabolic syndrome, compromise renal function. Glomerulosclerosis and obesity-related glomerulopathy-associated proteinuria also have been described in patients with severe obesity.

Skin changes: Acanthosis nigricans, striae, and hirsutism can be observed in obese subjects and often indicate the presence of concomitant disease including insulin resistance and PCOS.

Psychosocial changes: In the Nurses' Health Study, women who gained weight reported a deterioration in their quality of life. Depression is often associated with severe obesity, particularly in younger women.

Treatment

There are 2 goals to treatment of obesity: 1) prevention of further weight gain, and 2) weight loss.

Prevention of weight gain is an important strategy in overweight women, since it can delay onset of more serious comorbidities. Prevention of weight gain is also an important management strategy for obese women who are at high risk for weight-related comorbidities and are not psychologically ready to attempt weight loss. Effective prevention strategies need to focus on changes that are achievable, sustainable, simple, and relevant to the target population. The key behavioral modifications are to increase physical activity (decrease sedentary behavior) and maintain/decrease energy intake (8).

Effective treatment for weight loss must include a decrease in caloric intake. Guidelines issued by the NIH (5) recommend that individuals with BMI <34.9 kg/m^2 reduce their daily energy intake by 500 kcal/day, which would result in weight loss of approximately 1 pound per week and a 10% reduction of initial weight by 6 months. For women with more severe obesity (BMI ≥35 kg/m^2), a reduction of 500–1000 kcal/day is recommended. This reduction in caloric intake should result in weight loss of 1–2 pounds per week and 10% of initial body weight by 6 months. It is important for the health care provider to encourage the patient to accept a weight loss goal for initial therapy that is realistic, *e.g.*, no more than 10% of initial body weight. Most patients have an unrealistic view of the weight loss that they can achieve, and a loss of <15% is often viewed as a failure. However, a 10% weight loss is associated with significant improvement in comorbidities (8,9).

There are numerous dietary options for inducing weight loss. The choice of a diet may be left, in part, to patient preference, as well as to cost considerations. One of the keys to successful weight control is to identify a reduced-calorie eating plan that the woman finds acceptable, making long-term adherence more likely (8).

Dietary Intervention

Very-low calorie diet: This provides 400–800 kcal per day and large amounts of dietary protein. These diets usually are served in liquid form. They are safe when given under medical supervision. They are associated with an increased risk of symptomatic gallstones (8).

Low-carbohydrate, high-fat diets: Low-carbohydrate diets appear to facilitate dietary adherence and weight loss. Such diets simplify food choices by virtually eliminating carbohydrates, an entire class of macronutrients. In addition, the high protein content may increase satiation. A meta-analysis that examined 6 randomized controlled trials of low-carbohydrate versus low-fat diets, showed that low-carbohydrate diets induced significantly greater weight loss in the first 6 months of treatment, but that there was no difference in weight loss between the two diets at the end of a year. Low-carbohydrate diets also were associated with greater improvements in triglycerides and high-density lipoprotein cholesterol levels, whereas low-fat diets produced more favorable changes in low-density lipoprotein cholesterol and total cholesterol (10).

Low-glycemic index diets: The glycemic index of food is calculated by measuring the change in blood glucose following consumption of 50 g of target food. These diets encourage consumption of whole grains, legumes, fruits, and vegetables that have the potential to confer satiation while maintaining low insulin levels and not requiring marked restriction of the amount of food eaten (8).

Physical Activity

An increase in physical activity concomitant with dietary restriction is recommended for optimal weight loss. Several studies have documented that an increase in energy expenditure without caloric restriction will not result in significant weight loss; however, exercise is effective in promoting maintenance of reduced weight (5).

Regular bouts of aerobic activity also can reduce lipid levels, blood pressure, the risk of osteoporosis, and, in patients with type 2 diabetes, improve insulin sensitivity, reduce abdominal adiposity, and improve glycemic control. Studies suggest that patients are likely to engage in significantly more minutes of physical activity per week when instructed to exercise at home rather than exercising at a gym or medical facility. Exercising at home appears to reduce barriers to physical activity, such as travel time, cost, the need for child care, and public embarrassment about weight (8).

Weight regain is commonly observed following dietary and behavioral interventions. One way for patients to achieve long-term weight control is by participating in weight maintenance sessions after losing weight. Such sessions appear to provide the support and motivation needed for participants to continue to practice weight control behaviors that include regular monitoring of food intake, physical activity, and body weight (8).

Pharmacotherapy

Addition of pharmacotherapy to behavioral modification should be considered when weight loss goals are not met. Weight loss pharmacotherapy is approved for patients with no contraindications and a BMI >30 kg/m². Weight loss drugs can be used in overweight subjects (27> BMI >29.9 kg/m²) who have one obesity-related comorbidity. Treatment outcomes are significantly better when pharmacotherapy is administered as part of a weight loss program that includes diet, exercise, and behavioral modification (8,9).

Several anorexia-producing drugs derived from the amphetamine precursor beta-phenylethylamine are FDA-approved for short-term treatment of obesity. However, because weight regain occurs when drugs are discontinued, pharmacotherapy should be considered as a long-term treatment.

Two medications are approved for long-term use in the U.S.:

Orlistat: This is a lipase inhibitor that blocks digestion of dietary triglyceride and thus absorption of fatty acids. The compound itself is not absorbed by the GI tract and has little effect on systemic lipases. This drug is now available in over-the-counter formulations. Side effects include GI complaints due to fat malabsorption, which usually occur within the first 4 weeks of treatment. Treatment can decrease absorption of fat-soluble vitamins and some lipophilic medications. It is therefore recommended that patients receive a daily multivitamin and that orlistat not be taken 2 hours before or after ingestion of vitamins or lipophilic drugs. Orlistat administration has been associated with a reduction in serum cholesterol independent of weight loss. This may be due to reduced dietary cholesterol absorption (9).

Sibutramine: An inhibitor of the neuronal reuptake of serotonin, norepinephrine, and, to a lesser extent, dopamine, this compound reduces food intake and also stimulates a small increase in metabolic rate. Sibutramine stimulates a small increase in blood pressure (~2–4 mm Hg) and heart rate, but some patients experience much larger increases that require dose reduction or discontinuation of therapy. Other common side effects include dry mouth, headache, constipation, and insomnia (9).

Other drugs are under study but have not yet been approved for use in obesity.

Bariatric Surgery

Bariatric surgery is the most effective means of inducing significant weight loss in the extremely obese subject. Several studies have demonstrated that bariatric surgery-induced weight loss is effective in reducing obesity-related comorbidities. Benefits with respect to overall and cause-specific mortality have been demonstrated (11,12).

The NIH established guidelines for the surgical treatment of obesity in 1991. Eligible patients with a BMI ≥40 kg/m² should be well-informed and motivated. In addition, they should have demonstrated inability to lose weight with conventional therapy and have acceptable operative risks. Adults with a BMI ≥35 kg/m² who have a serious comorbidity, such as type 2 diabetes, hypertension, cardiomyopathy, sleep apnea, or severe joint disease, also may be surgical candidates. In-house mortality rates are <1% and are significantly affected by the experience of the surgeon and hospital staff (12). The National Institute of Diabetes, Digestive, and Kidney Diseases has established the Longitudinal Assessment of Bariatric Surgery (LABS) consortium to facilitate refinement of risk prediction for both patients and surgical programs (14). Bariatric surgery should be performed in conjunction with a comprehensive follow-up plan consisting of nutritional, behavioral, and medical monitoring (15).

Bariatric surgical procedures can be divided by mechanism of action into procedures that produce malabsorption (Roux-en-Y gastric bypass and biliopancreatic diversion) and procedures that cause gastric restriction (vertical banded gastroplasty and laparoscopic adjustable gastric banding). (For additional detail and anatomic representations of each procedure discussed below, consult Reference 13.)

Roux-en-Y gastric bypass: In this procedure, a small proximal gastric pouch is created, which empties into a segment of jejunum that is anastomosed to the pouch. The procedure is most often done laparoscopically. Complications associated with this procedure include marginal ulcers, stomal stenosis, dilatation of the bypassed stomach, staple line disruption, internal hernia, malabsorption of specific nutrients, and dumping syndrome.

Biliopancreatic diversion: This consists of a subtotal gastrectomy and enteroenterostomy much more distal than in the Roux-en-Y gastric bypass. The creation of a common channel of only 50–100 cm in length results in greater malabsorption.

Vertical banded gastroplasty: A small pouch is created from the gastroesophageal junction along the smaller curvature of the stomach. The pouch has a stoma restricted by a 1-cm polypropylene or silastic ring, which empties into the rest of the stomach. Complications associated with gastroplasty include staple line disruption, stomal stenosis, and gastroesophageal reflux.

Laparoscopic adjustable gastric banding: A silicone band is placed around the upper stomach, just below the gastroesophageal junction. The circumference of the band can be adjusted by inflating or deflating a balloon connected to a subcutaneously implanted port with percutaneous access. Complications include esophageal dilatation, erosion of the band into the stomach, band slippage, band or port infections, and leaks that result in inadequate weight loss.

Weight loss 10 years after surgery is greater with gastric bypass procedures than with gastric banding (12). This result is likely due to the combination of malabsorption and restriction of intake achieved with these procedures. Approximately 10–40% of patients do not achieve successful long-term weight loss after bariatric surgery. A major cause for lack of weight loss is ingestion of high-calorie soft foods and liquids. This finding reinforces the need for a comprehensive postsurgical plan for nutritional, behavioral, and medical monitoring.

References

1. **Ogden CL, Carroll MD, Curtin LR, et al.** Prevalence of overweight and obesity in the United States, 1999–2004. JAMA. 2006;295:1549–55.
2. World Health Organization website 2008. www.who.int/topics/obesity.
3. Centers for Disease Control and Prevention 2008 Website www.cdc.gov/nccdphp/dnpa/obesity.
4. **Klein S, Romijn JA.** Obesity. In: Williams Textbook of Endocrinology 10th Edition. Larsen PR, Kronenberg HM, Melmed S, and Polonsky KS eds. Saunders, Philadelphia, 2003:1619–41.
5. National Institutes of Health, National Heart, Lung and Blood Institute. Clinical Guidelines on the Identification, Evaluation, and Treatment of Overweight and Obesity in Adults – The Evidence Report. Obes Res. 6 Suppl 2:51S–209S; 1998. www.nhlbi.nih.gov.
6. **Seidell JC, Rissanen AM.** Prevalence of obesity in adults: The global epidemic. In: Handbook of Obesity Etiology and Pathophysiology 2nd Edition. Bray, GA, and Bouchard C, eds. Marcel Dekker, Inc, New York, 2004:93–107.
7. **Manson JE, Skerrett PJ, Willett WC.** Obesity as a risk factor for major health outcomes. In: Handbook of Obesity Etiology and Pathophysiology 2nd Edition. Bray, GA, and Bouchard C, eds. Marcel Dekker, Inc, New York, 2004:813–24.
8. **Wadden TA, Butryn ML, Wilson C.** Lifestyle modification for the management of obesity. Gastroenterol. 2007;132:2226–38.
9. **Bray GA, Greenway FL.** Pharmacological treatment of the overweight patient. Pharmacol Rev. 2007;59:151–84.
10. **Nordmann AJ, Nordmann A, Briel M et al.** Effects of low-carbohydrate vs low-fat diets on weight loss and cardiovascular risk factors: a meta-analysis of randomized controlled trials. Arch Intern Med. 2006;166;285–93.
11. **Buchwald H, Avidor Y, Braunwald E, et al.** Bariatric surgery: a systematic review and meta-analysis. JAMA. 2004;292:1724–37.
12. **Sjöström L, Narbro K, Sjöström CD, et al.** Swedish Obese Subjects Study. Effects of bariatric surgery on mortality in Swedish obese subjects. N Engl J Med. 2007;357:741–52.
13. **Elder KA, Wolfe BM.** Bariatric surgery: a review of procedures and outcomes. Gastroenterol. 2007;132:2253–71.

14. **Belle SH, Berk PD, Courcoulas AP, et al.** Longitudinal assessment of bariatric surgery consortium writing group. safety and efficacy of bariatric surgery: Longitudinal assessment of bariatric surgery. Surg Obes Relat Dis. 2007;3;116–26.

15. **McMahon MM, Sarr MG, Clark MM, et al.** Clinical management after bariatric surgery: value of a multidisciplinary approach. Mayo Clin Proc. 2006;81:S34–45.

E. Cigarette Smoking and Cessation in Women

Katherine Neely, Samina Naseer, and Laurel C. Milberg

KEY POINTS

- Smoking causes proportionately more morbidity and mortality among women than among men.
- Smoking cessation can reduce or eliminate extra health risks in 1–15 years.
- Nicotine addiction is a chronic, relapsing condition requiring ongoing attention.
- Women are more likely to quit with intervention than on their own.
- Most women require multiple attempts to successfully quit long-term smoking.
- Combined behavioral and pharmacologic interventions are most successful.
- Weight gain, stress relief and mental health issues, cervical cancer, and reproduction are areas of special concern for women smokers.
- Healthcare sites should have a comprehensive, system-based approach for smoking cessation.

Epidemiology

Cigarette smoking plays a major role in the mortality of U.S. women. Since 1980, when the Surgeon General's Report on Women and Smoking was released, about 3 million women have died, on average 14 years prematurely, of smoking-related diseases (1). Women smokers experience proportionately more morbidity/mortality than do men (the point estimate of the rate ratio for disease is 2.75 for women, 1.95 for men at 20+ cigarettes/day, a significant difference) (2). Tobacco cessation greatly reduces this risk. The relative benefits are greater when women stop smoking at younger ages, but smoking cessation is beneficial at all ages.

Tobacco smoking contributes to or causes the following (3):

Cancer

Cigarette smoking is the major cause of lung cancer among women. Since 1950, lung cancer mortality rates for U.S. women have increased to an estimated 600%. In 1987, lung cancer surpassed breast cancer to become the leading cause of cancer death among U.S. women (1). Currently, almost twice as many women die of lung cancer than of breast cancer each year (1). Smoking also contributes in varying degrees to an increased risk for cancer of the oropharynx, bladder, pancreas, kidney, liver, and colon and rectum (1). Smoking cessation is associated with decreasing risks, approaching never-smoker levels within 15 years (3).

Of particular importance to women, smoking is consistently associated with an increased risk of cervical cancer (1). The extent to which this association is independent of human papillomavirus (HPV) infection is uncertain. It is recommended that all women with cervical dysplasia and/or HPV infection be encouraged to quit smoking.

Cardiovascular Disease

Smoking is a major cause of atherosclerotic cardiovascular disease. For women <50 years, most coronary heart disease is attributable to smoking. Risks increase with the number of daily cigarettes smoked and the duration of smoking (4). This includes increased risks for coronary heart disease, ischemic stroke, subarachnoid hemorrhage, and peripheral atherosclerosis. Smoking cessation at any age substantially reduces the excess risk of coronary heart disease within 1 or 2 years. The increased risk of stroke associated with smoking reverses as well but takes 10–15 years to approach baseline. Cessation also appears to slow the progression of carotid atherosclerosis.

Lung Disease

Cigarette smoking is the primary cause of chronic obstructive pulmonary disease (COPD) in women, and the risk increases with the amount and duration of cigarette use. Adolescent girls who smoke have reduced rates of lung growth, and adult women who smoke experience a premature decline in lung function, which slows when women stop smoking (1).

Reproductive System

Cigarette smoking increases the risks for dysmenorrhea, secondary amenorrhea, and menstrual irregularity. Women smokers have natural menopause at a younger age than do nonsmokers, and experience more severe menopausal symptoms. Women who smoke have increased risk for primary and secondary infertility (1). Women who smoke during pregnancy risk premature birth, low-birth-weight infants, stillbirth, and infant mortality (1). Maternal smoking is associated with reduced lung function among infants and with increased risk of sudden infant death syndrome (SIDS) (1).

Other Smoking-Related Disease

Postmenopausal smokers have lower bone density and an increased risk of hip fracture. Women who smoke may have a modestly increased risk of rheumatoid arthritis, cataracts, and age-related macular degeneration (1).

Patterns of Tobacco Use among Women and Girls

While cigarette smoking was initially a male activity, its prevalence among women has increased as an unwelcome byproduct of increased equality and social freedom. The prevalence of current smoking among women in the U.S. increased from <6% in 1924 to 34% in 1965, and then declined to 22–23% in the late 1990s. In 1997–1998, smoking prevalence was highest among Native American women (34.5%), intermediate among Caucasian (23.5%) and African-American women (21.9%), and lowest among Latinas (13.8%) and Asian or Pacific Islander women (11.2%) (1). By educational level, smoking prevalence is nearly 3 times higher among women with 9–11 years of education (30.9%) than amongwomen with 16 or more years of education (10.6%) (1).

   Girls who start smoking are more likely to have parents or friends who smoke, weaker attachments to parents and family, and stronger attachments to peers and friends. They believe smoking is more common than it actually is, tend to favor risk-taking behaviors and rebelliousness, have less knowledge of the dangers and addictiveness of smoking, believe that smoking can control weight and negative moods, and have a positive image of smokers (5). Girls appear to be more affected than boys by the desire to smoke for weight control and by the perception that smoking controls negative moods; girls may also be more influenced than boys to smoke by rebelliousness or a rejection of conventional values (5).

   Women are heavily targeted in tobacco marketing, and tobacco companies have produced brands specifically aimed at women, both in the U.S. and overseas (5). Predominant themes are social desirability and independence: young, athletic, slim, beautiful women smoke cigarettes.

Clinical Care

Smoking cessation is associated with improvements in symptoms, prognosis, and survival, with reduction or elimination of extra health risks in 1–15 years. Will power, nicotine replacement therapy, group or individual multi-session psychological support and coaching, a variety of antidepressants, and nicotinic partial agonist agents have all been shown to contribute to successful smoking cessation (5). Unlike men, women are more likely to quit with intervention than on their own. The best chances for success can be obtained by combining behavioral and pharmacologic interventions (5).

   Using evidence from studies that vary in design, sample characteristics, and intensity of the interventions studied, researchers to date have not found consistent gender-specific differences in the effectiveness of intervention programs for tobacco use (5).

However, identification of factors that influence women's smoking and present barriers to quitting can help practitioners tailor their interventions with women smokers.

Biopsychosocial factors, such as pregnancy, depression, and the need for social support appear to be associated with smoking maintenance, cessation, or relapse for women (5). Among heavy smokers, women are more likely than men to report being dependent on cigarettes and have lower expectations about stopping smoking (5). Women who continue to smoke or fail quit attempts tend to have lower education and employment levels than do women who quit smoking (1).

Women and girls often have unstated roadblocks to quitting, such as fear of weight gain, increase in negative mood or anxiety, and girls, especially, may resist or rebel against advice to stop smoking (6). These factors may make motivational interviewing a particularly good intervention for women, because it emphasizes reflective listening and expression of empathy. The process of motivational interviewing also acknowledges many women's ambivalence toward quitting (7)

Motivational Interviewing

Motivational interviewing is a client-centered method of enhancing intrinsic motivation by exploring and resolving ambivalence about change (7). The principles of motivational interviewing are based on an understanding that the process of change involves a continuum of stages (Table 3-5) (8). The patient moves through these stages as the balance of forces supporting her behavior tip in the direction of forces that make the behavior less desirable. It is designed to elicit the patient's own motivation for change, a stark departure from the doctor's usual recommendations (7).

An overview of the steps in motivational interviewing follows:

1. Provide a brief medical recommendation to consider quitting smoking for specific reasons linked to the patient's health. Provide information, but leave the actual decision to quit up to the patient.

Table 3-5   Prochaska and DiClemente's Stages of Change

Stage of Change	Characteristics
Pre-Contemplation	Not currently considering change
Contemplation	Ambivalent about change; not considering change in the next month
Preparation	Some experience with change; trying to change; planning to act within one month
Action	Practicing new behavior
Maintenance	Continued commitment to sustaining new behavior
Relapse	Resumption of old behaviors

From Prochaska JO, DiClemente CC, Norcross JC. In search of how people change. American Psycholgist. 1992;47:1102–14; with permission.

Box 3-3   Resources for Patients

- U.S. Department of Health and Human Services: www.4woman.gov/QuitSmoking/
- HHS National Quitline Number: 1-800-QUITNOW
- You Can Quit Smoking Now: www.smokefree.gov
- Great Start (for pregnant smokers): www.americanlegacy.org/greatstart

2. Assess the patient's readiness for change by eliciting the full range of her thoughts and feelings about what was recommended; about what is good and not so good about smoking as opposed to quitting. Listen for "change talk" and focus on incongruities in what the patient says about how her current behavior differs from her ideal or desired behavior. In this process, the patient also becomes familiar with her own ambivalence and motivation for change.
3. Help the patient identify how important it is to her to quit smoking at this time and how confident she is in her ability to do so. Encourage the patient to consider even a small step toward change such as cutting down on the number of cigarettes she smokes a day, or not smoking in the car, and so forth.
4. If the patient is considering change, the clinician can provide printed information and resources (Box 3-3), support with return visits and phone calls, and help create a quit plan. If the patient is not considering change, the clinician can ask if it would be acceptable to check again at a subsequent visit (9).

Cessation Counseling (10)

Once a woman is ready to quit, counseling includes:

1. Helping her to recognize situations that increase the risk of smoking, such as negative affect, other smokers, drinking alcohol, time pressure, and urges.
2. Helping her to develop coping skills for dealing with dangerous situations, such as learning to anticipate and avoid temptation, learning cognitive strategies to reduce negative moods and counter urges to smoke, reducing stress, and increasing other sources of pleasure and relaxation.
3. Warning her about common nicotine withdrawal symptoms such as irritability, negative mood, anxiety, restlessness, difficulty concentrating, increased appetite, and constipation.
4. Encouraging her by communicating confidence, care, and concern, and a willingness to help, and by asking about her doubts and concerns as well as her reasons for quitting.

Special Considerations for Women

Special attention to fears about gaining weight and strategies for avoiding food as a substitute for the oral gratification and self-soothing that smoking provided is very important. Initiation of cigarette smoking is not associated with weight loss, but smoking does appear to attenuate weight gain over time, and smokers do have a moderately lower average weight. Smoking cessation among women typically is associated with a weight gain of about 6–12 pounds in the year after they quit (5). Women fear weight gain during smoking cessation more than do men. However, actual weight gain during cessation does not predict relapse to smoking.

An association between major depression and smoking is strong in women in general and, particularly, for subgroups of women such as the underserved, postpartum, and menopausal. A history of depression and negative mood has been associated with intervention failure, so special attention should be paid to assessing depression in women considering smoking cessation or as a source of resistance (11). Taking into account hormonal influences on mood, women are more likely to be successful if they time their quit date to avoid the premenstrual phase of their cycle (11).

The prevalence of smoking generally is higher among patients with anxiety disorders, bulimia, attention deficit disorder, and alcoholism (12). Some data indicate that women use cigarette smoking to regulate mood and cope with stress in the context of the pressures of our gendered society (12). Therefore, clinicians should routinely teach stress management techniques and consider treating any coexistent mental health issue prior to an attempt at smoking cessation.

Finally, pregnancy is an ideal time to encourage smoking cessation in women. A higher percentage of women stop smoking during pregnancy, both spontaneously and with assistance, than at other times in their lives (5). Only about one-third of women who stop smoking during pregnancy are still abstinent 1 year after the delivery (5).

Smoking is a chronic, relapsing condition requiring ongoing medical attention, and most women, like men, require multiple attempts to successfully quit long-term.

Pharmacologic Interventions

Nicotine replacement reduces the withdrawal syndrome and allows time to adjust to the habits of a nonsmoker while gradually tapering the nicotine dose. All forms of nicotine replacement have been shown to be effective, with an overall abstinence rate that is 1.5–2 times higher than control (10). Peak effectiveness is in those with moderate nicotine addiction, while those who smoke <10–15 cigarettes per day receive little benefit, and those with the highest addiction do better with combined therapy (13). Women should be encouraged to pick the route of administration that is best for them. A patch for long-acting effect, with a shorter acting form for rescue use, is currently common practice. It is crucial that the starting dose of nicotine is high enough to fully suppress withdrawal symptoms and then gradually taper over 6–12 weeks (13).

Antidepressants, particularly bupropion and nortriptyline, double the odds of abstinence at 6 months. Theoretical mechanisms of action include treating depressive symptoms of withdrawal, replacing antidepressant effects of nicotine, and direct action at the nicotine receptor. Treatment should be commenced 2 weeks prior to the planned quit date and continued for 6–12 weeks (13). Maintenance therapy has not been proven to decrease relapse.

Nicotine partial receptor agonists, of which only varenicline is currently available in the U.S., are another potent smoking cessation aid, with a 3-fold increase in successful abstinence at 1 year (14). Partial activation of the nicotine receptor may minimize withdrawal symptoms, while blocking the receptor blunts positive effects of smoking (15). The only comparison of varenicline with bupropion, using pharmaceutical industry-funded data, suggests that it is 1.7-fold more effective (14). Treatment should be instituted one week prior to quit date, with a gradually increasing dose, and cigarettes should be stopped once the full dose is reached. Therapy should be continued for 8–12 weeks. Studies on long-term maintenance are in progress (15). Post-marketing experience shows a possible risk of serious neuropsychiatric symptoms, both during treatment and after withdrawal (16). Patients should be warned to report any unusual mood or behavior changes. These symptoms are most marked in patients with chronic psychiatric illness, and varenicline should be avoided for now in that group.

Clonidine, a centrally acting antihypertensive, has limited and conflicting data, mostly in conjunction with behavioral therapy (13). It is somewhat more effective than placebo and is more effective in women than in men. Side effects and limited data would suggest that this be used only when other methods have failed or are contraindicated.

Strategies for Systematic Change

The most successful cessation programs are those that create a systematic approach to tobacco use among their staff and patients (17). Consider the following strategies:

Implement a tobacco-user identification system.

- Make smoking as a fifth vital sign, and assign someone to ask every patient at every visit.
- Provide education, resources, and feedback to promote provider interventions. Dedicate staff to provide tobacco dependence treatment and assess the delivery of this treatment in staff performance evaluations.
- Provide every woman who uses tobacco at least some treatment whether it be information about quitting, or medication to help remain tobacco free.
- Follow up by phone within a week after a woman commits to quitting.

References

1. Women and Smoking, US Surgeon General's Report, 2001.
2. **Mucha L, Stephenson J, Morandi N, et al.** Meta-analysis of disease risk associated with smoking, by gender and intensity of smoking. Gend Med. 2006 Dec;3:279–91.

3. **Brunnhuber K, Cummings KM, et al.** Putting evidence into practice: Smoking cessation. BMJ. Publishing Group, Summer 2007.

4. **Bolego C.** Smoking and gender. Cardiovasc Res, 2002 Feb 15;53:568–76.

5. **Sarna L.** Why tobacco is a women's health issue? Nurs Clin North Am. 2004 Mar;39:165–80.

6. **Greaves L.** Tobacco policies and vulnerable girls and women: toward a framework for gender sensitive policy development. J Epidemiol Community Health. 2006 Sep;60:57–65.

7. **Rollnick S, Mason P, Butler C.** Heath. Behavior Change: A Guide for Practitioners. Edinburgh: Churchill Livingstone. 1999.

8. **Prochaska JO, DiClemente CC, Norcross JC.** In search of how people change. American Psycholgist. 1992;47:1102–14.

9. **Miller WR, Rollnick S, Butler CC.** Motivational Interviewing in Health Care: Helping Patients Change Behavior. Guilford Publications, Inc. New York. 2007.

10. **Gritz ER.** Smoking cessation and gender: the influence of physiological, psychological, and behavioral factors. J Am Med Womens Assoc. 1996 Jan-Apr;51:35–42.

11. **Romans SE.** Cigarette smoking and psychiatric morbidity in women. The Australian and New Zealand Journal of Psychiatry [Aust N Z J Psychiatry], 1993 Sep;27:399–404.

12. **Talwar A, Jain M, Vijayan VK.** Pharmacotherapy of tobacco dependence. Med Clin North Am. 2004 Nov;88:1517–34.

13. **Talwar A, Jain M, Vijayan VK.** Pharmacotherapy of tobacco dependence. Med Clin North Am. 2004 Nov;88:1517–34.

14. **Cahill K, et al.** Nicotine receptor partial agonists for smoking cessation. Cochrane Database Syst Rev. 2007 Jan 24;(1):CD006103

15. **Hays JT, et al.** Efficacy and safety of varenicline for smoking cessation. Am J Med. 2008 Apr;121:S32–42.

16. FDA Public Health Advisory, 2/1/08, available at http://www.fda.gov/cder/drug/advisory/varenicline.htm

17. **Fiore MC, Bailey WC, Cohen SJ, et al.** Treating Tobacco Use and Dependence. Quick Reference Guide for Clinicians. Rockville, MD: U.S. Department of Health and Human Services. Public Health Service. October 2000.

4

Common Outpatient Reproductive
Health Issues

A. Abnormal Vaginal Bleeding in Reproductive Aged Women
Sarina B. Schrager, MD, MS

B. Abnormal Pap Smears
Diana Burtea, MD

C. Sexually Transmitted Infections
Suparna Chhibber, MD

D. Contraception
Norma Jo Waxman, MD; Anna Kaminski MS, MD;
Ruth Lesnewski, MS, MD; Shannon Connolly, BA;
Radha Lewis, MD; Penina Segall-Gutierrez, MD, MS

E. Female Sexual Dysfunction
Teri Greco, MD, MSc

F. Chronic Pelvic Pain
Sarina B. Schrager, MD, MS

G. Infertility
Juliemarie M Sicilia, MD; Tara D. Lathcop, MD

H. Uterine Fibroid Tumors
Sarina B. Schrager, MD, MS

I. Vaginitis
Suparna Chhibber, MD

J. HIV/AIDS Infection in Women
Jeffrey M. Rothenberg, MD, MS; Joanna R Fields, MD

K. Primary Care of Lesbian Women
Kathy Oriel, MD, MS

L. Primary Care of Women with Disabilities
Deborah Dreyfus, MD; Sarina B. Schrager, MD, MS

A. Abnormal Vaginal Bleeding in Reproductive Aged Women

Sarina B. Schrager

KEY POINTS

- The prevalence of abnormal vaginal bleeding is between 10–30% in women of childbearing age.
- Anovulation is the most common cause of abnormal vaginal bleeding in this age group.
- The 4 most common causes of secondary amenorrhea are pregnancy, hyperprolactinemia, thyroid disorders, and iatrogenic or medication-induced.
- Unstable women with acute heavy vaginal bleeding should be admitted to hospital for IV estrogen therapy or surgical intervention.
- Treatment of abnormal bleeding includes ovulation induction if a woman desires pregnancy and hormonal cycle control if she does not.
- Anovulatory women are at risk for endometrial hyperplasia or carcinoma due to unopposed estrogen and should have regular progesterone-induced withdrawal bleeds.

Normal menstrual bleeding is defined as regular vaginal bleeding that occurs at intervals from every 21 to 35 days. A woman's bleeding pattern usually remains stable throughout her life, with some variation after major reproductive events (i.e., pregnancy, miscarriage, etc.). A normal menstrual cycle is ovulatory, with two distinct phases: the follicular phase and the luteal phase. The follicular phase is the first half of the cycle, when the ovary is producing follicles. The luteal phase occurs after ovulation, when the corpus luteum develops in anticipation of a possible pregnancy. Box 4-1 defines vocabulary to describe different patterns of abnormal bleeding.

This chapter will discuss abnormal bleeding patterns in non-pregnant women of reproductive age. Please see related chapters on polycystic ovarian syndrome (PCOS) and hirsutism, menstrual irregularities in adolescent women, perimenopausal bleeding, and postmenopausal bleeding for more information about women of other ages.

Epidemiology

Abnormal vaginal bleeding is a common complaint in primary care. The prevalence of some type of abnormal bleeding is between 10–30%

Box 4-1 Abnormal Bleeding Patterns

Menorrhagia: prolonged or excessive bleeding at regular intervals
Metrorrhagia: irregular, frequent bleeding of varying amounts but not excessive
Menometrorrhagia: prolonged or excessive bleeding at irregular intervals
Polymenorrhea: regular bleeding at intervals of <21 d
Oligomenorrhea: bleeding at intervals greater than every 35 d
Amenorrhea: no bleeding for at least 6 mo
Intermenstrual bleeding: bleeding between menstrual cycles
Spotting: intermenstrual bleeding not requiring protection
Breakthrough bleeding: intermenstrual bleeding that requires protection
Dysfunctional uterine bleeding: all abnormal vaginal bleeding that is idiopathic and all anovulatory bleeding

---

among women of reproductive age (1). Women with abnormal bleeding have lower quality of life scores than women with normal bleeding. The estimated direct and indirect costs of abnormal bleeding are $1 billion and $12 billion annually, respectively (1). Indirect costs of abnormal bleeding include time off from work and cost of products to protect clothing from bleeding (e.g., tampons and pads). Abnormal bleeding is also a common reason for women to be referred to gynecologists and is an indication for up to 25% of all gynecologic surgery (2).

Diagnosis

The most common causes of abnormal bleeding in this age group are pregnancy complications, anovulatory disorders, and benign pelvic pathology. Thus, any woman who presents with a bleeding complaint should have a pregnancy test at the first stage in her evaluation. If the pregnancy test is negative, the next step is to determine whether her cycles are ovulatory or anovulatory. Characteristics of ovulatory cycles that are helpful in determining ovulatory status include regular cycle length, presence of premenstrual syndrome (PMS) symptoms, and changes in cervical mucus (Table 4-1). In contrast, anovulatory cycles tend to be unpredictable, with varying bleeding intervals and bleeding

Table 4-1 Signs and Symptoms of Ovulatory Cycles

Regular Cycle Length	Presence of PMS Symptoms
Dysmenorrhea	Mittleschmerz (pain at ovulation)
Changes in cervical mucus	Biphasic temperature curve
Premenstrual breast tenderness	Positive test result from luteinizing hormone (LH) predictor kit

Adapted from Oriel KA, Schrager S. Abnormal uterine bleeding. Am Fam Physician. 1999;60:1371–80; with permission.

amounts. Women do not notice a cyclic change in the cervical mucus and if a basal body temperature chart is kept, it is monophasic (i.e., no increase in temperature after ovulation).

Abnormal bleeding in ovulatory cycles includes menorrhagia, poly-menorrhea, oligomenorrhea, and intermenstrual bleeding. Menorrhagia, or heavy bleeding, can be associated with structural lesions (uter-ine leiomyomas, endometrial polyps, and endometrial hyperplasia). Bleeding abnormalities from a coagulation disorder (most commonly von Willebrand disease), liver failure, or chronic renal failure can also present as menorrhagia. Polymenorrhea (bleeding at short intervals) can be caused by a luteal phase disorder (not enough progesterone is pro-duced after ovulation to stabilize the endometrium) or a short follicular phase. Oligomenorrhea (infrequent bleeding) is commonly due to a pro-longed follicular phase. Intermenstrual bleeding can be caused by cervi-cal pathology (i.e., dysplasia or infection) or an IUD. It may be normal for some women to have bleeding at ovulation due to the dip in estrogen levels at that time (3).

Anovulation is the most common cause of abnormal vaginal bleeding. Box 4-2 describes the most common causes of anovulation. The major-ity of anovulation is related to hypothalamic abnormalities or PCOS. By definition, anovulatory cycles are unpredictable and cannot be classified by any one type of vaginal bleeding pattern. Their similarities lie in their unpredictability. A woman may experience 14 days of heavy bleeding 1 month, light spotting intermittently for the next month, and then go for 3 months without a cycle. The pathologic abnormality in these cycles is a lack of ovulation, which produces an unopposed estrogen state. The luteal phase of the menstrual cycle is dominated by progesterone, which is only produced after ovulation. This lack of progesterone contributes to irregular endometrial growth and non-uniform bleeding. In a nor-mal cycle, the entire endometrium sloughs off during menstruation. In

---

Box 4-2   Causes of Anovulatory Cycles

Hypothalamic
- Weight loss
- Eating disorders
- Female athlete triad
- Chronic illness
- Stress
- Excessive exercise

Polycystic ovarian syndrome
Thyroid disorders
Hyperprolactinemia
Idiopathic chronic anovulation
Medication-induced (i.e., after discontinuation of hormonal contraceptives)

Table 4-2   Clinical Evaluation of a Woman with Abnormal Bleeding

Ovulatory Abnormal Bleeding	Anovulatory Bleeding
History, physical exam, pregnancy test In menorrhagia: • Consideration of liver function tests, BUN/Cr, CBC, coagulation profile • Pelvic ultrasound to exclude uterine fibroids In intermenstrual bleeding: • Pap smear, cervical cultures Basal body temperature chart to determine length of follicular and luteal phase	History, physical exam, pregnancy test Laboratory studies: • TSH • Prolactin • CBC (if acute bleeding episode or frequent heavy bleeding) • Fasting glucose and insulin (see Chapter 11C) Screen for eating disorder, stress, female athlete triad

an anovulatory cycle, different sections of endometrium outgrow their blood supply at different times and bleed erratically. All women with abnormal bleeding should have a thorough history and physical examination and a pregnancy test. Table 4-2 describes the steps in evaluation of a woman with abnormal bleeding.

Another common presentation of abnormal bleeding is an acute bleeding episode. In this situation, a woman may be ovulatory but is more likely to be anovulatory. Evaluation in an acute bleeding episode should include a hemoglobin and hematocrit if the bleeding is heavy, assessment of volume status, and an endometrial biopsy.

Lastly, a woman may present with amenorrhea. Again, pregnancy should be the first item on any differential diagnosis of a woman with amenorrhea. The 4 most common causes of secondary amenorrhea (when a woman who previously had normal menses stops having menses for at least 6 months) are pregnancy, hyperprolactinemia, thyroid disorders, and medication-induced (e.g., hormonal contraceptives). Causes of hyperprolactinemia are discussed in Chapter 12D. Other reasons for amenorrhea include outflow obstruction (i.e., Asherman's syndrome, a condition caused by scarring of the uterus from instrumentation) or cervical stenosis and primary ovarian failure.

Evaluation of a woman with amenorrhea begins with a history and physical examination. Laboratory studies should include a pregnancy test, a thyroid-stimulating hormone (TSH) level, and prolactin level. The next step is an induced withdrawal bleed after administering progesterone for 10–14 days. If a woman has a menstrual bleed after the progesterone, outflow obstruction and low estrogen state (as in primary ovarian failure) are excluded as the causes of amenorrhea. If a woman does not have a withdrawal bleed after progesterone administration, a trial of estrogen supplementation for 3 weeks should be given before another course of progesterone is attempted. In this situation, if a woman has a withdrawal bleed, the diagnosis of primary ovarian failure is considered and levels of gonadatropins (FSH, and LH) should be obtained. If a woman does not have a withdrawal bleed after estrogen and progesterone administration, a hysterosalpingogram (special x-ray of uterus and ovaries after dye is injected into the endometrium) should be obtained to evaluate for outflow obstruction.

Abnormal bleeding is also quite common in women who use hormonal contraception. Women who take combination estrogen/progestin oral contraceptive pills, patches, or rings often have intermenstrual bleeding for the first 3 months of treatment. This is a common cause of discontinuation of pills. Abnormal bleeding is more common in women who smoke and can be associated with chronic endometritis (4). In addition, missed pills are a very frequent cause of abnormal bleeding. Abnormal bleeding is also very common in women who are using progestin-only methods of contraception (e.g., depot medroxyprogesterone acetate, progestin-only contraceptive pills, or implantable progestin rods). In these women, the abnormal bleeding usually is caused by the progestin-induced endometrial atrophy. As the endometrium becomes atrophic, various sections slough off individually (a mechanism similar to anovulatory bleeding).

Treatment

If a woman presents with heavy bleeding and exhibits any signs or symptoms of hypovolemia, she should be admitted to hospital and either treated with IV estrogen to stop the bleeding or have a surgical procedure (such as dilatation and curettage or D & C). If the bleeding is heavy, but the woman is stable and her hemoglobin level and hematocrit are close to normal, outpatient treatment with high-dose oral contraceptive pills (OCPs), estrogen, or progesterone is indicated (5).

Treatment of women with either ovulatory or anovulatory bleeding is not necessary unless the woman wishes to become pregnant or is bothered by her bleeding pattern. However, anovulation is an unopposed estrogen state, and treatment with some type of progesterone is necessary to reduce the risk of endometrial hyperplasia or carcinoma. Unopposed estrogen is a risk factor for endometrial cancer, along with obesity, diabetes, nulliparity, and age >35 years. To protect against the development of endometrial hyperplasia, a precursor to endometrial cancer, all women with chronic anovulation should have a progesterone-induced withdrawal bleed (6). In general, once the type of bleeding has been established and any secondary causes elucidated and treated, treatment of abnormal bleeding consists of ovulation induction if pregnancy is desired or cycle control with hormonal contraceptives if it is not. In women who are not candidates for estrogen-containing contraceptives, a monthly cycling of progesterone or continuous administration of progestin contraception (e.g., depot medroxyprogesterone acetate or levonorgestrel IUD) is an effective treatment as well. Continuous administration of progestin contraceptives

---

---

has the benefit of inducing amenorrhea in many women. For women who do not want to take any hormonal medications, some nonsteroidal anti-inflammatory drugs (NSAIDs) can decrease the amount of bleeding (5) (Box 4-3).

Treatment of women with abnormal bleeding on OCPs involves education and support to try to get them through the first 3 months on the pills. After that, consideration of supplemental estrogen, changing to a higher dose of an estrogen pill, changing to a pill with a different class of progestin, use of supplemental NSAID to decrease the amount of bleeding or changing to a non-hormonal type of contraception are all potential treatments (5). Treatment of bleeding in women on progestin contraception only can be more of a clinical challenge. A recent Cochrane review on this topic concluded that, although some women benefit from treatment with supplemental estrogen, estrogen/progestin contraceptive pills, mifepristone, and NSAIDs, there is not enough evidence to recommend any of these treatments (7).

References

1. **Liu Z, Doan QV, Blumenthal P, et al.** A systematic review evaluating health-related quality of life, work impairment, and health-care costs and utilization in abnormal uterine bleeding. Value Health. 2007;10:183–94.
2. **Goodman A.** Abnormal genital tract bleeding. Clin Cornerstone. 2000; 3:25–35.

3. **Oriel KA, Schrager S.** Abnormal uterine bleeding. Am Fam Physician. 1999;60:1371–80.
4. **Schrager S.** Abnormal bleeding associated with hormonal contraception. Am Fam Physician. 2002;65:2073–80, 2083.
5. **Ely JW, Kennedy CM, Clark EC, et al.** Abnormal uterine bleeding: a management algorithm. J Am Board Fam Med. 2006;19:590–602.
6. **Albers JR, Hull SK, Wesley MA.** Abnormal uterine bleeding. Am Fam Physician. 2004;69:1915–26.
7. **Abdel-Aleem H, d'Arcangues C, Vogelsong KM, et al.** Treatment of vaginal bleeding irregularities induced by progestin only contraceptives. Cochrane Database Syst Rev. 2007(4):CD003449.

B. Abnormal Pap Smears

Diana Burtea

KEY POINTS

- The Bethesda system of Pap smear nomenclature was developed to provide a uniform system of terminology to guide clinical management.
- Human papillomavirus (HPV) DNA testing for the presence of high-risk types of HPV is a useful adjunct tool to cervical cytology.
- Eighty percent of women under 20 years of age will clear an infection with the HPV within 2 years of infection.
- Colposcopy and endocervical sampling are the main diagnostic modalities used to evaluate abnormal Pap smears.
- Low-grade cervical lesions are evaluated with conservative management protocols based on a woman's age, as well as both severity and persistence of the lesion.
- High-grade cervical lesions are managed with aggressive treatment protocols using electrosurgical excision techniques.
- Primary prevention of cervical disease can now be achieved through HPV immunization programs.

Epidemiology of Cervical Cancer

It is estimated that in 2008 there will be over 11 000 new cases of cervical cancer and 3870 deaths (1). The Pap smear was developed to screen for cervical cancer, and since its inception in the 1940s, the incidence of cervical cancer has decreased by almost 80%. The annual expenditure on the evaluation and management of abnormal cervical cytology in the U.S. in 2006 was $3.6 billion (1). Worldwide, cervical cancer is the second leading cause of cancer in women.

The 2001 Bethesda Nomenclature

The Bethesda system for reporting the results of cervical cytology was developed as a uniform system of terminology to provide clear guidance for clinical management. The most important contribution of this was the creation of a standardized framework for laboratory reports that included a descriptive diagnosis and evaluation of specimen adequacy. A detailed description of the general components, as well as the significance of each component, is provided in Table 4-3 (2).

It is important to note that the Bethesda system applies only to cytological results (Pap smears) and is not interchangeable with histological results (biopsy results from colposcopy or excisional procedures). More detail can be obtained from histologic samples, such as the extent or invasiveness of disease. Cervical histologic lesions are reported as cervical intraepithelial neoplasia or CIN. CIN I refers to a low-grade lesion and commonly follows a Pap smear result of LGSIL (low-grade squamous intraepithelial lesion). CIN 2 or 3 lesions are considered high-grade and are associated with a Pap smear result of HSIL (high-grade squamous intraepithelial lesion). The management of CIN can be viewed at www.asccp.org. This chapter will focus on the management of abnormal cytology.

Human Papillomavirus

The evidence of correlation between HPV and cervical cancer is now overwhelming. More than 100 types of HPV have been identified, 40 of which infect the genital tract. The anogenital types of HPV are generally divided into 2 categories: "low-risk" and "high-risk," based on the chance of developing cervical cancer if infected. The best characterized low-risk types include HPV 6 and 11 and are most commonly associated with external genital warts. The best characterized high-risk types include HPV 16 and 18 and are most commonly associated with cervical cancer (3).

Most women are infected with HPV after their first sexual relationship, with the highest prevalence seen in women <25 years of age. HPV infection can be identified by cytology as a premalignant or low-grade lesion on a Pap smear. In most women, these HPV infections are transient and spontaneously clear within 2 years (4). In some women, however, HPV infections persist and can result in high-grade precancerous or cancerous lesions on the cervix.

With the greater understanding of the epidemiology of HPV and its role in cervical cancer, the primary focus of screening has changed from one of frequent testing with the hope of identifying any and all premalignant lesions to a more targeted approach that takes a comprehensive

Table 4-3

General Component	Detailed Description	Discussion
Specimen adequacy	Satisfactory for evaluation (note presence/absence of endocervical/transformation zone component) Unsatisfactory for evaluation (specify reason) Specimen rejected/not processed (specify reason) Specimen processed and examined but unsatisfactory for evaluation of epithelial abnormality because of (specify reason)	This component is important from a quality assurance perspective to insure the presence of the transformation zone in the specimen.
General categorization (Optional)	Negative for intraepithelial cell or malignancy Epithelial cell abnormality Other	This optional component is designed to allow a nurse or physician to triage reports quickly.
Interpretation/result	Negative for intraepithelial cell or malignancy Organisms: • *Trichomonas vaginalis* • fungal organisms morphologically consistent with *Candida* species • shift in flora suggestive of bacterial vaginosis • bacteria morphologically consistent with *Actinomyces* species • cellular changes consistent with herpes simplex virus Other non-neoplastic findings: • reactive cellular changes associated with inflammation • radiation • intrauterine contraceptive device • glandular cells status posthysterectomy • atrophy	While the purpose of the Pap smear is to identify cervical abnormalities, other abnormalities can be identified via microscope in the otherwise normal Pap smear. These abnormalities are placed as comments following a negative result and can include specific organisms that are identified or other non-neoplastic findings.

Epithelial cell abnormality	Squamous cell	Atypical squamous cells of undetermined significance (ASCUS)	The ASC category represents an equivocal category, as reactive changes at times do not allow for a clear cytologic designation. However, 10–20% of these equivocal readings are actually high-grade, which led to the necessity of creating the ASC-H category.
		Atypical squamous cells cannot exclude HSIL (ASC-H)	
		Low-grade squamous intraepithelial lesion (LSIL)	This category is considered the transient HPV infection.
		High-grade squamous intraepithelial lesion (HSIL)	This category is considered the persistent HPV infection and higher risk for progression to cervical cancer. Finding HSIL is the primary reason for Pap smear screening.
		Squamous cell carcinoma	
	Glandular cell	Atypical glandular cells, NOS	The presence of atypical glandular cells in general has a higher incidence of underlying high-grade disease than atypical squamous cells.
		Atypical glandular cells, favor neoplasia	
		Endocervical adenocarcinoma in situ (AIS)	
		Adenocarcinoma	
	Other	Endometrial cells in a woman ≥ 40 years of age	May be associated with risk of endometrial abnormalities.
Automated review and ancillary testing	HPV DNA testing noted if appropriate		
Educational notes and suggestions	Used to direct clinician to appropriate consensus guidelines		

view of a woman's individual risk for cervical cancer. Furthermore, over the past decade, new testing modalities, such as HPV DNA and liquid-based cytology, have become available, providing the clinician with better results. Thus, current screening guidelines aim to identify high-grade lesions in order to prevent progression to cervical cancer. At the same time, providers try not to be overly aggressive in evaluation of probable low-grade lesions, thereby avoiding unnecessary testing or treatment (5,6).

Management Protocols

Current management protocols have been developed through consensus meetings using the best available evidence, or, when evidence is not available, expert opinion. The most recent consensus guidelines were established in September 2006, by a group of 146 experts representing 29 organizations and professional societies, led by the American Society for Colposcopy and Cervical Pathology (7). Treatment algorithms are available at www.asccp.org and are discussed based on the Bethesda classification of the Pap smear result. Table 4-4 also summarizes the initial and subsequent work-up.

Atypical Squamous Cells of Undetermined Significance (ASC-US). This represents an equivocal result. Up to 20% of results in this category can actually correlate with high-grade lesion on biopsy. The advent of HPV DNA testing has made the management of this category better defined. The preferred approach to evaluation is to check for presence of HPV. If liquid-based cytology was used for the initial Pap smear, HPV DNA testing may be performed on the same sample. If liquid-based cytology was not used, the patient may return for HPV DNA testing. If DNA testing is negative for the presence of high-risk HPV, cytology can be repeated in 12 months. If DNA testing is positive for the presence of high-risk HPV, these women should be treated as if they have LSIL and undergo colposcopy (7,8).

Alternate acceptable approaches to the management of ASC-US include: 1) immediate colposcopy; or 2) repeat cytology at 6 and 12 months. For those who choose immediate colposcopy, it is important to remember that the routine use of diagnostic excisional procedures, such as the loop electrosurgical excision procedure (LEEP), is unacceptable for women with an initial ASC-US in the absence of histologically confirmed CIN 2 or 3 (high-grade) lesions. The potential for over-treatment is too high with this "see and treat" method (7). If colposcopy reveals CIN, it should be managed as per ASCCP Guidelines for Cervical Intraepithelial Lesions (7). If colposcopy does not reveal CIN, and the patient is known to be HPV-positive, then cytology can be repeated at 6 and 12 months or HPV DNA testing can be repeated at 12 months. If HPV status is unknown, cytology can be repeated at 12 months. For those choosing the repeat cytology approach, if both tests are negative, the woman may return to routine screening. However, if either result shows ASC or greater, then colposcopy is recommended (8).

Table 4-4

Bethesda Category	Initial Management	Subsequent Management	Comments
ASCUS	HPV DNA testing (*preferred approach*)	If HPV negative, repeat cytology at 12 mo. If HPV positive, do a colposcopy.	• "See and treat" method unacceptable • **Adolescent women with ASCUS**—repeat cytology at 12 mo, if the result shows HSIL or greater proceed to colposcopy. If the result is less than HSIL, then repeat cytology once again 12 mo later. If negative, return to routine screening. If ASC or greater results persist at 2 y, then proceed to colposcopy.
	Repeat cytology at 6 and 12 mo	If both results are negative, return to routine screening. If repeat cytology shows either ASC or greater, proceed with colposcopy.	
	Colposcopy	If CIN is found on biopsy, manage per appropriate guidelines. If no CIN is found but patient is HPV positive, may repeat cytology at 6 and 12 mo or do HPV DNA testing at 12 mo. If HPV is unknown, repeat cytology at 12 mo.	
ASC-H	Colposcopy	If CIN 2, 3 are found on biopsy, manage per appropriate guidelines. If no CIN2, 3 are found, proceed with repeat cytology at 6 and 12 mo or HPV DNA testing at 12 mo. If all are negative, may return to routine screening. If either cytology shows ASC or greater or the HPV testing is positive repeat colposcopy.	
LSIL	Colposcopy with endocervical sampling	If CIN 2 or 3 found, manage per appropriate guidelines. If no CIN2 or 3, cytology at 6 and 12 mo or HPV DNA testing at 12 mo. If negative, may return to routine screening. If either cytology shows ASC or greater or the HPV testing is positive repeat colposcopy.	• **Adolescent women with LSIL**—same as ASCUS above • **Pregnant women with LSIL**—colposcopy without endocervical sampling (preferred management) in non-adolescent pregnant women, repeat cytology at 12 mo for adolescent women as above, or defer colposcopy until 6 wk post-partum.

cont'd

Table 4-4   (cont'd)

Bethesda Category	Initial Management	Subsequent Management	Comments
HSIL	Colposcopy with endocervical sampling "see and treat"—LEEP	If colposcopy is chosen and CIN 2 or 3 is found, it is managed per applicable guidelines. If no CIN 2 or 3 is found, and the colposcopy was deemed unsatisfactory, proceed to diagnostic LEEP. If colposcopy was satisfactory, but biopsies are normal, review material to confirm diagnosis, and proceed to diagnostic LEEP or close follow-up with colposcopy and cytology every 6 mo for 1 y. If either repeat results reveal HSIL, proceed to LEEP. If both are negative, return to routine screening. Any other results should be managed per applicable guidelines.	• **Pregnant women with HSIL** Colposcopy should be performed by an experienced clinician. Endocervical sampling is contraindicated. Diagnostic excisional biopsy is also contraindicated unless invasive cancer is suspected. • **Adolescent women with HSIL**—"see and treat" is unacceptable. See text for complete management
AGC	Colposcopy, HPV DNA testing, and endometrial sampling if >35 y or at risk for endometrial neoplasia If initial abnormality was atypical endometrial cells, perform endometrial and endocervical sampling first if both negative then proceed to colposcopy.	*Initial Pap: AGC—favor neoplasia or AIS* If no invasive disease is evident, then proceed to a diagnostic excisional procedure. *Initial Pap: AGC-NOS* If results show CIN with or without glandular neoplasia, manage per appropriate CIN guidelines. If no CIN or neoplasia are seen, repeat cytology and HPV testing at 6 mo if HPV positive and 12 mo if HPV negative. If all results are negative, then routine testing may be resumed. If results show either ASC or greater or HPV positive, repeat colposcopy.	Note that subsequent management depends on the initial Pap and whether the initial work-up revealed neoplasia.

Atypical Squamous Cells: Cannot Exclude High-grade SIL (ASC-H). The results in this category are more concerning for high-grade lesions. Therefore, ASC-H should be considered to represent equivocal HSIL and, thus, be managed as if it is HSIL with immediate colposcopic examination (7,8). If the biopsy reveals CIN 2 or 3, management is as per the ASCCP Guidelines. If the biopsy does not reveal CIN 2 or 3, then cytology can be repeated at 6 and 12 months or HPV DNA testing can be done at 12 months. If both cytology results are negative, or if DNA testing is negative, then routine screening may be resumed. However, if either DNA testing was positive, or one or more of the cytologies revealed ASC or greater, then the colposcopy should be repeated (8).

Low-grade Squamous Intraepithelial Lesion. A cytology result of LSIL is a strong indicator of HPV infection, with a prevalence as high as 76.6% (7). Because of this high prevalence of positive HPV DNA testing, using HPV as a triage in women who have a Pap smear result of LSIL is not recommended. While conservative treatment of LSIL is appropriate in some special populations, in general LSIL is associated with a 12–16% prevalence of CIN 2 or greater on initial colposcopy (7). Thus, the preferred management of LSIL is colposcopic examination with endocervical sampling. If CIN 2 or 3 is present, this should be managed per ASCCP Guidelines. If there is no CIN 2 or 3 found on the biopsy, then repeat cytology can be performed at 6 and 12 months or HPV DNA testing can be done at 12 months. If both cytology results are negative, or if DNA testing is negative, then routine screening may be resumed. However, if either DNA testing was positive or 1 or more of the cytologic results revealed ASC or greater, then colposcopy should be repeated (8).

Special Populations—Adolescent Women with ASC-US or LSIL. The risk of developing invasive cervical cancer in women 20 years old and younger is very low. Furthermore, the chance of HPV clearance is up to 80% within 2 years (2) and 91% at 36 months in this population (8). Therefore, in the adolescent population, the management of these cytological abnormalities is less aggressive. Treatment with LEEP or other excisional procedures can cause complications, such as stenosis of the cervix with subsequent infertility, pre-term birth, low birthweight, and neonatal intensive care unit admissions, and should be avoided unless necessary to prevent invasive disease (9). The recommended follow-up of a result of ASC-US or LSIL in an adolescent is repeat cytology at 12 months. If the repeat cytology shows HSIL or greater, then colposcopy is recommended. Otherwise, repeat cytology should be performed in another year. If the repeat cytology is negative, then routine screening should resume. However, if at this time, 2 years after the initial abnormal Pap, the result is still ASC or greater, a colposcopy should be performed (8).

Special Populations—Pregnant Women with LSIL. The purpose of cytology screening in pregnancy is to detect high-grade lesions. Thus, low-grade lesions in pregnancy do not require urgent evaluation or treatment.

Acceptable options for management of LSIL in pregnancy include: 1) colposcopy for non-adolescent women; 2) deferral of colposcopy until 6 weeks postpartum; and 3) repeat cytology at 12 months in adolescent women. Colposcopy is the preferred method of follow-up. If no visible signs of CIN 2 or 3 are evident on colposcopy, then follow-up with colposcopy and biopsies can be performed postpartum. Repeat colposcopies during pregnancy are not necessary. If CIN 2 or 3 appears to be present at colposcopy, then biopsy should be performed by an experienced clinician, due to the risk of excess bleeding with cervical biopsy in this population (8). Endocervical sampling is contraindicated in pregnancy.

High-grade Squamous Intraepithelial Lesions (HSIL). The finding of HSIL carries a high risk for significant cervical disease. On colposcopic examination, 53–66% of women with a Pap smear result of HSIL will have CIN 2 or greater on biopsy. On diagnostic excision, 84–97% of women will have CIN 2 or greater (7). As a result of these statistics, failure to detect CIN 2 or greater by colposcopy is not necessarily reassuring and usually requires further diagnostic procedures. Consequently, many advocate a more aggressive "see and treat" approach as first-line management of HSIL (i.e., perform an excisional diagnostic procedure at the initial colposcopic examination).

The standard management algorithm for HSIL is: 1) immediate loop electrosurgical excision; or 2) colposcopic examination with endocervical assessment. If the colposcopic examination reveals CIN 2 or 3 the patient is managed per ASCCP guidelines. If no CIN 2 or 3 is found, and the colposcopy was technically unsatisfactory (i.e., the entire transformation zone was not visualized), one should proceed to a diagnostic excisional procedure. If the colposcopy was satisfactory and CIN 2 or 3 was not found, then there are 3 acceptable approaches: 1) review all results with the cytopathologist to ensure that the diagnosis is correct; 2) proceed to diagnostic excisional procedure; or 3) observation with *both* colposcopy and cytology at 6-month intervals for 1 year. If HSIL persists on cytology at either visit, a diagnostic excisional procedure is recommended. If the cytology is negative at both visits (6 and 12 months), then the woman may return to routine screening. Any other results should be managed per the appropriate ASCCP guidelines (8).

Special Populations—Adolescent Women with HSIL. Many CIN 2 or 3 lesions spontaneously regress in adolescent women within 2 years (7). Therefore, an aggressive approach may lead to over-treatment and long-term complications. The recommended management for women 20 years and younger with HSIL on Pap smear is colposcopic examination. If CIN 2 or 3 is present, patients should be managed per ASCCP guidelines. If no CIN 2 or 3 is found, close observation with *both* colposcopy and cytology at 6-month intervals for up to 2 years is recommended. If CIN 2 or 3 is found on biopsy, it should be managed per ASCCP guidelines. If no CIN 2 or 3 is found on biopsy, observation should continue for another year. If HSIL persists for 24 months with no CIN 2 or 3 identified, then a diagnostic excisional procedure should be performed. If the woman has 2 consecutive negative Pap smears *and* no high-grade colposcopic abnormality, then she may return to routine screening.

Special populations—Pregnant Women with HSIL. Colposcopy by a specialist is recommended for pregnant women with HSIL. Biopsy of lesions suspicious for CIN 2 or 3 or greater is preferred. Endocervical sampling is contraindicated in pregnancy. Diagnostic excisional biopsy is contraindicated unless invasive cancer is suspected based on prior cytology, biopsy, and colposcopic appearance. If CIN 2 or 3 is not suspected on colposcopic examination, repeat evaluation with cytology and colposcopy should be performed no sooner than 6 weeks post-partum (7).

Atypical Glandular Cells (AGC). While AGC are an uncommon finding on Pap smear, this result carries a significant risk for an underlying neoplastic condition. Adenocarcinoma has been reported in 9–38% of women with AGC (7). Therefore, the initial evaluation for AGC is comprehensive and includes: 1) colposcopy with endocervical sampling; 2) HPV DNA testing; and 3) endometrial sampling in women over 35 years or in those who have clinical risk factors for endometrial neoplasia, such as unexplained vaginal bleeding or chronic anovulation. If the atypical cells are endometrial cells only, the initial work-up can include endometrial and endocervical sampling only. In this situation, if no endometrial pathology is found, a colposcopy should be performed (8).

Subsequent follow-up of AGC depends on the initial Pap smear result. If the cytology showed AGC that is suggestive of neoplasia, or demonstrated AIS (adenocarcinoma in situ), and the initial evaluation did not reveal any invasive disease, a diagnostic excisional procedure is recommended because of the high risk for neoplasia. If the initial Pap smear showed AGC-NOS, and the initial work-up revealed any type of CIN or glandular neoplasia, the patient should be managed per the appropriate ASCCP guidelines. If the initial Pap smear showed AGC-NOS and no CIN or glandular neoplasia was found on initial evaluation, further management depends on the HPV status. If HPV status is positive for high-risk HPV, repeat cytology and HPV DNA testing should be performed at 6 months. If both are negative, routine screening may be resumed. If either result is abnormal, colposcopy should be performed. If HPV status is negative for high-risk HPV, repeat cytology and HPV DNA testing should be done at 12 months. If both are negative, routine screening may resume. If either result is abnormal, colposcopy should be performed (8).

Primary Prevention

Cervical cancer prevention entered a new era on June 8, 2006, with the approval by the U.S. Food and Drug Administration (FDA) of the first vaccine against HPV. This quadrivalent vaccine, marketed under the name of Gardasil®, has been heralded as a major breakthrough in the primary prevention of cervical cancer. The HPV vaccine contains highly purified recombinant virus-like particles of HPV types 6, 11, 16, and 18. These 4 types are responsible for approximately 70% of cervical cancers, 90% of genital wart cases, and 35–50% of precancerous lesions (9). The vaccine does not eradicate HPV infection that is already present, but it may still provide some benefit to women who were already infected with HPV because it prevents infection with other subtypes. Based on current trials, the efficacy of the vaccine is 96% for preventing persistent HPV infections and 100% for preventing CIN 2 or 3 lesions (10). The vaccine is administered in a 3-dose series, with the second dose given 2 months after the first dose, and the third dose 6 months after the first. The ACIP (Advisory Committee on Immunization Practices) recommends administration to girls beginning at the age of 11–12 years (11).

References

1. Cervical cancer epidemiology. www.cancer.gov/cancertopics. Accessed 2/28/08.
2. **Solomon D, Davey D, Kurman R, et al.** The 2001 Bethesda System. JAMA. 2002;287:2114-9.
3. **Ferris DG, Cox JT, O'Connor DM, et al.** Modern Colposcopy, Textbook and Atlas, 2nd ed. Dubuque: Kendall Hunt; 2004.
4. **Moscicki AB, Schiffman M, Kjaer S, et al.** Updating the natural history of HPV and anogenital cancer. Chapter 5. Vaccine. 2006;24:S42–S51.
5. ACOG Practice Bulletin: Clinical management guidelines for obstetrician-gynecologists. Obstet Gynecol. 2003;102:417–27.
6. **Wright TC, Schiffman M, Solomon D, et al.** Interim guidance for the use of Human Papillomavirus DNA testing as an adjunct to cervical cytology for screening. Obstetrics & Gynecology. February 2004;103:304-9.
7. **Wright TC, Massad S, Dunton CJ, et al.** 2006 consensus guidelines for the management of women with abnormal cervical cancer screening tests. American Journal of Obstetrics and Gynecology. October, 2007;197:346-55.
8. **Wright TC, Massad S, Dunton CJ, et al.** 2006 consensus guidelines for the management of women with abnormal cervical cancer screening tests. Journal of Lower Genital Tract Disease. October 2007;11:201–22.
9. **Suh-Burgmann B, Kinney W.** On maintaining the balance. Journal of Lower Genital Tract Disease. 2006;10:109–10.
10. **Villa LL, Costa RLR, Petta CA, et al.** Prophylactic quadrivalent human papillomavirus (types 6,11,16,and 18) L1 virus-like particle vaccine in young women: a randomized double-blind placebo-controlled multicentre phase II efficacy trial, http://oncology.thelancet.com Published online April 7, 2005.
11. Centers for Disease Control and Prevention, Quadrivalent Human Papillomavirus Vaccine. MMWR 2007;56:1–23.

C. Sexually Transmitted Infections
Suparna Chhibber

KEY POINTS

- Sexually transmitted infections (STIs) are some of the most common infectious diseases in the U.S.
- Often asymptomatic, STIs affect both sexes, but consequences can be more severe in women, resulting in pelvic inflammatory disease, infertility, and ectopic pregnancy.
- Rates of STIs are highest among adolescents and among African-American women.
- All pregnant women should be screened for STIs because of their potential for severe perinatal consequences.
- Gonorrhea, chlamydia, syphilis, chancroid, and HIV/AIDS are reportable in every state.

There are approximately 25 or more infections that can be transmitted through sexual intercourse. STIs are a major public health problem in the U.S. Nineteen million new cases of STIs occur every year, half of them in men and women between 15 and 24 years old (1). This leads to physical, psychological, and economic consequences. The direct medical cost associated with STIs in 2006 was about $14.7 billion dollars (2). This chapter will discuss the common STIs; however, discussion of HIV/AIDS is covered elsewhere (refer to Section J).

Epidemiology

Infection by *Chlamydia trachomatis* is the most commonly reported notifiable disease in the U.S. (2). The Centers for Disease Control and Prevention (CDC) estimates that there are approximately 2.8 million new cases of chlamydia every year, most commonly in young women (2). Chlamydia is common among all races and ethnicities. However, reported cases show a disproportionately high prevalence in African American women. African American women are affected twice as often as Latino women and 7 times more often than Caucasian women (2).

The second most commonly reported STI in the U.S. is gonorrhea (2). Gonorrhea is under-diagnosed and under-reported, and it is estimated that there are actually more than twice as many cases as those reported every year (2). Diagnosis rates of gonorrhea are 18 times greater in African-Americans than in Whites (2). An increasing concern in prevention and treatment of gonorrhea is the emergence of drug resistance (2). Infections with gonorrhea and chlamydia can lead to serious health consequences in women, including pelvic inflammatory disease, infertility, and ectopic pregnancy.

Syphilis has also increased in incidence over the past 6 years (3). In 2006, there were almost 37 000 cases of syphilis in the U.S. (4). The infection rate in African-Americans is 6 times higher than in Causasians (3). Syphilis is spread most commonly by sexual intercourse, but it also may be contracted by vertical transmission via the placenta (congenital syphilis) (3). Patients are most infectious early in the disease, and become less so as the disease progresses. An immunocompetent person does not transmit syphilis through sexual contact after 4 years of becoming infected (3). Other STIs, like genital herpes caused by *Herpes simplex* virus appear to be increasing, although case reports are not required for HSV, so the information is limited (4).

Trichomoniasis is another common STI, causing over 7 million new cases in 2006 (4). However, the most common STI of all is HPV. In a 2003 prevalence survey, 40% of all sexually active women between 14 and 19, and 50% of those between 20 and 24 were infected with HPV (4).

Twenty-six percent of the female adolescent population between the ages of 14 and 19 years in the U.S. has at least one of the common STIs: human papillomavirus (HPV), chlamydia, HSV, or trichomoniasis (2). Sexually active adolescents are at very high risk for these infections, since they frequently engage in unprotected sex and often have sexual partners for short durations (2). They also may face difficulty in accessing healthcare and may not acknowledge high-risk behavior (5).

Clinical Features

Chlamydia

Chlamydia trachomatis is a gram-negative bacterium that is an obligate intracellular parasite, and can live asymptomatically in the human genital tract. Active infection with chlamydia may cause cervicitis, endometritis, and pelvic inflammatory disease in females (6). It may cause conjunctivitis and reactive arthritis in both sexes. Infected infants may have conjunctivitis or pneumonitis. Immunity to the disease is relatively short-lived and immunotype-specific, so reinfections are common (6). Women infected with chlamydia may complain of mucopurulent vaginal discharge, dysuria, dyspareunia, or may be asymptomatic. Chlamydia may be the cause of a culture-negative cystitis in women. The most important complication of this infection is pelvic inflammatory disease (PID), which can damage the Fallopian tubes resulting in infertility and ectopic pregnancies (6). Chronic infection can also lead to puerperal fever, infections, and death *in utero* and in newborns (6). Diagnostic testing can be performed using swab or urine specimens. Culture, direct immunofluorescence, enzyme linked immunosorbant assay (EIA), nucleic acid hybridization, and nucleic acid amplification tests are available for detection of chlamydia. Patients who test positive should be tested for other STIs. Table 4-5 describes treatment recommendations for Chlamydia.

Table 4-5   Treatment of Chlamydia

Recommended Regimens	Alternative Regimens
1. Azithromycin 1 g orally in a single dose **or** 2. Doxycycline 100 mg orally twice a day for 7 d	1. Erythromycin base 500 mg orally 4 times a day for 7 d **or** 2. Erythromycin ethylsuccinate 800 mg orally 4 times a day for 7 d **or** 3. Ofloxacin 300 mg orally twice a day for 7 d **or** 4. Levofloxacin 500 mg orally once daily for 7 d
Recommended Regimens in Pregnancy	**Alternative Regimens in Pregnancy**
Azithromycin 1 g orally in a single dose **or** Amoxicillin 500 mg orally 3 times a day for 7 d	Erythromycin base 500 mg orally 4 times a day for 7 d **or** Erythromycin base 250 mg orally 4 times a day for 14 d **or** Erythromycin ethylsuccinate 800 mg orally 4 times a day for 7 d **or** Erythromycin ethylsuccinate 400 mg orally 4 times a day for 14 d

From Workowski K, Berman S. Centers for Disease Control and Prevention. Sexually Transmitted Diseases Treatment Guidelines. MMWR. 2006;55:51–7. Updated recommended treatment regimens for gonococcal infections and associated conditions—United States, April 2007; with permission.

Treatment of infected individuals prevents spread of the infection to sexual partners and, in the case of pregnant women, to infants. Treatment of sexual partners is required to prevent reinfection. A test of cure in 3–4 weeks is not warranted, except in pregnant women (6).

Gonorrhea

Neisseria gonorrhoeae, a gram-negative diplococcus, is responsible for gonorrhea. The risk of transfer of the infection from the female to the male partner is about 20% per episode of unprotected intercourse, and from male to female it is approximately 50–70% (7). The primary site of infection in women is the endocervix. Vaginal discharge, dysuria, abdominal pain, and intermenstrual bleeding, especially after intercourse, are common complaints of women affected by gonorrhea (7). Gonorrhea is rarely asymptomatic. Physical examination shows mucopurulent cervical discharge, erythema, and a friable

Table 4-6   Treatment of Uncomplicated Gonococcal Infection

Recommended Regimens	Alternative Regimens
Ceftriaxone 125 mg IM in a single dose **or** Cefixime* 400 mg orally in a single dose **plus** Treatment for Chlamydia if Chlamydial infection is not ruled out * not available in the U.S.	Spectinomycin* 2 g in a single IM dose **or** Single-dose cephalosporin regimens *not available in the U.S.

Single-dose Cephalosporin Regimens
Ceftizoxime 500 mg IM; **or** Cefoxitin 2 g IM, administered with Probenecid 1 g orally; **or** Cefotaxime 500 mg IM
Oral alternatives: Cefpodoxime 400 mg and Cefuroxime axetil 1 g

From Workowski K, Berman S. Centers for Disease Control and Prevention. Sexually Transmitted Diseases Treatment Guidelines. MMWR. 2006;55:51–7. Updated recommended treatment regimens for gonococcal infections and associated conditions—United States, April 2007; with permission.

cervix. Concomitant infection with chlamydia is very common. PID may occur in 10–20% of infected women and may be associated with endometritis, salpingitis, tubo-ovarian abscess, and pelvic peritonitis (7). Disseminated gonococcal infection is rare but may lead to septic arthritis and dermatitis.

Diagnosis is made by isolation of *N. gonorrhoeae*. Culture in Thayer-Martin agar medium, nucleic acid hybridization tests, and nucleic acid amplification tests are available for the detection of *N. gonorrhoeae* (5). Treatment recommendations for gonorrhea from the 2007 CDC updates are summarized in Table 4-6. Women with gonorrhea also should be treated for Chlamydia; the reverse is not true (2).

Fluroquinolone-resistant gonorrhea is widespread in the U.S., so treatment with this group of antibiotics is no longer recommended (8). PID may be treated with oral antibiotic therapy in mild to moderately severe cases. Clinical outcomes of both oral and parental therapy are similar. Table 4-7 summarizes the CDC recommendations for treatment of PID.

Syphilis

Syphilis is caused by the spirochete *Treponema pallidum*. Syphilis is a complex multisystem disease that has been called "the great imitator" (3). The clinical manifestations include early infective primary and secondary stages, followed by a latent period that ultimately progresses to tertiary syphilis (3). The average incubation period is 21 days, with a spirochetemia that leads to spread of the organism throughout the body. Primary syphilis is characterized by the primary chancre, which appears at the site of inoculation, most commonly the external genitalia. It begins as a painless papule that later becomes ulcerated and indurated, with a cartilaginous consistency. The ulcer has a raised border with a smooth base from which treponemes

Table 4-7   Treatment of Pelvic Inflammatory Disease

Parenteral Treatment of PID:	
Recommended Parenteral Regimen A	**Recommended Parenteral Regimen B**
Cefotetan 2 g IV every 12 h **or** Cefoxitin 2 g IV every 6 h **plus** Doxycycline 100 mg orally or IV every 12 h	Clindamycin 900 mg IV every 8 h **plus** Gentamicin loading dose IV or IM (2 mg/ kg), followed by a maintenance dose (1.5 mg/kg) every 8 h. Single daily dosing may be substituted.

Alternative Parenteral Regimens
Ampicillin/Sulbactam 3 g IV every 6 h **plus** Doxycycline 100 mg orally or IV every 12 h

Recommended Oral Regimen
Ceftriaxone 250 mg IM in a single dose **or** Cefoxitin 2 g IM single dose and Probenecid, 1 g orally in a single dose **or** other parenteral third-generation cephalosporin (e.g., ceftizoxime or cefotaxime)

plus
Doxycycline 100 mg orally twice a day for 14 d
With or without
Metronidazole 500 mg orally twice a day for 14 d

From Workowski K, Berman S. Centers for Disease Control and Prev1ention. Sexually Transmitted Diseases Treatment Guidelines. MMWR. 2006;55:51–7. Updated recommended treatment regimens for gonococcal infections and associated conditions—United States, April 2007; with permission.

can be easily identified (3). This must be differentiated from other STIs that are associated with ulcerative lesions, that is genital herpes and chancroid. The initial lesion usually heals within 2–8 weeks but may persist longer, especially in HIV-infected persons.

In the secondary stage of syphilis spirochetes invade other organs. The classic lesions of secondary syphilis involve the skin. The rash starts with development of macules, papules, and occasionally pustules over the trunk and extremities (3). Vesicular lesions are absent, except in congenital syphilis. All of the different types of lesions may persist concomitantly and may involve the entire body, including the palms and soles. The rash coalesces in intertriginous areas to form broad, painless, highly infectious plaques known as condyloma lata. Similar lesions can develop on mucus membranes and are called mucous patches (3). Constitutional symptoms, such as low-grade fever, anorexia, malaise, pharyngitis, and painless lymphadenopathy, especially in the epitrochlear region, are common. Other organ involvement can include cranial nerve damage, syphilitic hepatitis, glomerulonephritis, synovitis, osteitis, and infiltration of the gastrointestinal tract (3).

The latent stage of syphilis is the period during which there are no outward manifestations of the disease, but the specific treponemal antibody test (fluorescent treponemal antibody absorption, or FTA-abs) is positive (3). Late or tertiary syphilis is a slowly progressing disease associated with cardiovascular and central nervous system manifestations and a granulomatous lesion called a gumma that can develop on skin, bones, and internal organs (e.g., liver and spleen) (3). The classic pathologic change suggestive of syphilis is obliterative endarteritis.

Laboratory diagnosis can be established in primary, secondary, and congenital syphilis by direct visualization of *T. pallidum* through dark-field examination or immunofluorescent staining. Serologic tests include nonspecific non-treponemal reaginic antibody tests, such as VDRL and RPR, and specific antitreponemal antibody tests (e.g., FTA-abs). The 2 types of serologic tests are used together for definitive diagnosis, since the non-treponemal reaginic test may be falsely positive in certain unrelated medical conditions (3).

Penicillin G administered parenterally is the treatment of choice for all stages of syphilis (5). It is also the only therapy recommended in pregnant women (5). The CDC recommends skin testing of all pregnant patients reporting penicillin allergy and desensitization of all who test positive (5). Table 4-8 summarizes the treatments of syphilis. A re-evaluation with clinical and serological testing should be performed 6 months and 1 year after completion of treatment (5). All patients who have syphilis should be tested for HIV.

Table 4-8   Treatment of Syphilis

Primary and Secondary Syphilis
- Benzathine penicillin G, 2.4 million units IM in a single dose

Early Latent Syphilis
- Benzathine penicillin G, 2.4 million units IM in a single dose

Late Latent Syphilis or Latent Syphilis of Unknown Duration
- Benzathine penicillin G, 3 doses of 2.4 million units IM each at 1-wk intervals

Tertiary Syphilis
- Benzathine penicillin G, 3 doses of 2.4 million units IM each at 1-wk intervals

Neurosyphilis
- Recommended Regimen: Aqueous crystalline penicillin G, 3–4 million units IV every 4 h or continuous infusion, for 10–14 d
- Alternative Regimen: Procaine penicillin 2.4 million units IM once daily PLUS Probenecid 500 mg orally 4 times a day, both for 10–14 d

Syphilis in Pregnancy
- Penicillin regimen appropriate for the stage of disease.

Primary and Secondary Syphilis in HIV positive
- Benzathine penicillin G, 2.4 million units IM in a single dose, some recommend additional weekly doses for 3 wk

Latent Syphilis in HIV positive
- Benzathine penicillin G, at weekly doses of 2.4 million units for 3 wk

---

From Workowski K, Berman S. Centers for Disease Control and Prevention. Sexually Transmitted Diseases Treatment Guidelines. MMWR. 2006;55:51–7; with permission.

The Jarisch–Herxheimer reaction is a systemic response resembling gram-negative sepsis that is seen within 1–2 hours of initiation of treatment with penicillin. It is characterized by fever, chills, headache, myalgia, tachycardia, and hyperventilation, and it is due to release of pyrogens from spirochetes (3). The symptoms are usually self-limited, and can be managed with anti-inflammatory medications such as ibuprofen.

All sex partners of infected patients need to be evaluated. People exposed >90 days after the diagnosis of a sex partner should be treated empirically if serology is unavailable or uncertain.

Chancroid

Chancroid is an STI caused by the gram-negative coccobacillus, *Haemophillus ducrei*. It is characterized by painful genital ulcers and lymphadenopathy. Along with syphilis and genital herpes, it is a cofactor for HIV transmission (4). Diagnosis can be made if the patient has one or more painful genital ulcers, regional lymphadenopathy, no evidence of infection with syphilis after at least 7 days of onset of ulcers, and ulcers are negative for genital herpes (6). Definitive diagnosis can be made by culturing *H. ducreyi* on special media not commonly available.

Chancroid can be treated with a single oral dose of azithromycin 1 gram (5). A single IM dose of 250 mg of ceftriaxone may also be used. Alternatively, ciprofloxacin 500 mg orally twice a day for 3 days or erythromycin base 500 mg orally 3 times a day for 7 days are recommended (5). Patients should be re-evaluated after 3–7 days of treatment. Sex partners who had sexual contact with the infected patient need to be treated (5).

Lymphogranuloma Venereum

Lymphogranuloma venerum is caused by serovars L1, L2, and L3 of *C. trachomatis*. It is more common in men than women, and is characterized by unilateral tender inguinal and/or femoral lymphadenopathy (5). A genital ulcer may form in the area of inoculation, and subsequently heals. The lymph nodes may coalesce to form a stellate abscess, and heal with scarring. Doxycycline 100 mg orally twice a day for 21 days is the CDC-recommended treatment. Sexual contacts need to be treated. Pregnant and lactating women may be treated with erythromycin (5).

Genital Herpes

Herpes simplex type 1 (HSV1) and *Herpes simplex type 2* (HSV2) have been identified as causes of genital herpes infection. HSV2 is the most common cause of genital herpes, though. The first episode is often characterized by systemic symptoms like fever, malaise, headaches, and myalgias, and local symptoms such as itching, pain, vaginal discharge, and dysuria. Vesicular lesions, pustules, and painful ulcerated lesions can be present. In 80% of cases, the cervix or the urethra is involved (5). The clinical course of both HSV1 and HSV2 is similar, except that the recurrence rates are higher in HSV2 infections. At least 50 million people in the U.S. have genital herpes infection (5). The majority of whom are unaware, asymptomatic, undiagnosed, and shed the virus intermittently. Clinical diagnosis should be confirmed by laboratory testing. Viral culture is still the gold standard; however, PCR testing (not FDA-approved for genital specimens) and type-specific serology are more sensitive and specific. Patient education and counseling about the natural history of the disease and its transmission and complications are vital in preventing transmission (5). Acyclovir 400 mg orally 3 times daily or 200 mg five times daily for 7–10 days or longer if necessary is used to treat the first episode of genital herpes (5). Suppressive therapy may be required in patients who have >6 recurrences in a year. Daily therapy with acyclovir, famciclovir, or valacyclovir can be used. All three have similar efficacy, but acyclovir is much less expensive (5). If episodic therapy is required, then medications need to be started within one day of onset of symptoms. Genital herpes acquired during late pregnancy often results in a high risk of transmission to the infant. Most women with infants affected with neonatal herpes do not have a clinical history of genital herpes. Most specialists recommend that women with active herpetic lesions deliver by Caesarean section to prevent neonatal herpes (5). However, this does not completely eliminate the risk of transmission. Acyclovir may be used to treat pregnant women with genital herpes to decrease asymptomatic viral shedding, transmission, and frequency of recurrence (5).

Human Papillomavirus

Genital infection with the human papillomavirus (HPV) is the most common STI in the U.S. About 100 HPV subtypes have been identified so far, of which about 40 infect the genital area (6). There are 6.5 million new cases every year (9). Usually self-limited and asymptomatic, persistent HPV can cause cervical cancer in women and anogenital cancers and warts in both men and women infected with subtypes HPV 16 and 18, in particular. Over 50% of sexually active females have been infected with one or more of subtypes at some time of their lives. The most clearly established risk factor for acquiring HPV is increased number of lifetime sexual partners. In immunocompetent individuals, most HPV infections are cleared by the body's defenses.

About 20 anogenital types of HPV are associated with malignancy. Over 70% of anogenital cancers have been related to HPV 16 or HPV 18 (9). High-risk HPV subtypes, including 16, 18, 31, 33, 35, 39, 45, etc., are associated with malignancy, and low-risk HPV (e.g., 6 and 11) are associated with external genital warts, or condyloma (10). Condyloma acuminata is the most common clinical presentation of HPV infection. It is also the most prevalent STI in the world (9). The vast majority of condylomas are attributable to HPV 6 and 11 (11). The warts may range in size and appearance from small verrucous papules to large cauliflower-like growths, which may be flesh-, pink-, or brown-colored, and are often found in areas of highest friction during sexual activity. These are often asymptomatic but may cause some burning and pruritus.

Though condylomas are benign, many people opt for treatment due to the appearance or discomfort of the lesions, especially when large. The common treatment options for condylomas include antiproliferative agents such as podophyllotoxin creams or solutions, destructive methods like application of trichloroacetic acid, cryotherapy, and electrocautery, and excision by laser. Imiquimod, a topical immunomodulator, may also be used for treatment (11) (refer to Section B).

Differential Diagnosis

STIs can be divided into infections that cause ulcerative lesions and those that cause non-ulcerative lesions. In women, non-ulcerative lesions usually present as vaginitis, cervicitis, or PID. Mucopurulent cervicitis in women is caused by *N. gonorrhoeae* and *C. trachomatis*. Other organisms may produce vaginal discharge, and may be clinically distinguished by the nature of the discharge and wet mount exam (refer to Section I). Vulvar itching and burning, edema, and erythema are symptoms of vulvitis, which may be caused by Candida, HSV, or HPV (7). Pubic lice and scabies also can cause severe pruritus and inflammation and excoriation of the genital area (10).

Genital ulcerations may be caused by HSV, syphilis, or chancroid. Differential diagnosis of genital ulcers should also include scabies, Behcet's disease, Reiter's syndrome, trauma, and malignancy (10). When STIs are diagnosed in children, evaluation for sexual abuse is mandatory (refer to Chapter 5F).

Prevention

STIs are treatable and preventable. It is important for healthcare providers to elicit a sexual history from women during an office encounter in order to be better able to identify risky behaviors and provide education and counseling. Discussions concerning a woman's sexual practices, any methods used to prevent pregnancy or STIs, and previous history of STIs can identify individuals at risk. Patients seeking diagnosis and treatment for a particular STI should be evaluated for all other common STIs as well. Abstinence or a mutually monogamous relationship are obviously the best way to avoid STIs, though they are not always realistic options. Patients should be counseled to abstain from sex if they are being treated for an STI. Correct use of male latex condoms has been shown to decrease the transmission of HIV, chlamydia, gonorrhea, syphilis, and trichomoniasis (10). Condoms may also decrease risk of transmission of HSV and HPV conditions.

Adolescents are a group that deserve special mention, since they have a very high prevalence of STIs. In most states, adolescents can be medically treated for STIs without parental consent (5). All sexually active women under the age of 24 years should be screened annually for chlamydia (4). Women at high risk because of sexual behaviors (i.e., multiple sexual partners) also should be screened for gonorrhea, syphilis, and HIV (12). Many states require STI screening of all pregnant women.

Vaccination can be a useful way to prevent specific STIs. In 2006, the quadrivalent HPV vaccine was approved by FDA for use in females aged 9-26 years. The vaccine protects uninfected individuals from the diseases associated with HPV types 6, 11, 16, and 18, especially cervical cancer. The recommended age for vaccination of females is 11-12 years (9). It is a 3 vaccine series and costs about $300.

References

1. **Weinstock H, et al.** Sexually transmitted diseases among American youth: incidence and prevalence estimates, 2000. Perspectives on Sexual and Reproductive Health 2004;36:6-10.
2. CDC, Trends in Reportable Sexually Transmitted Diseases in the United States, 2006.
3. **Tramont EC.** Chapter 235—Treponema pallidum (Syphilis), Mandell, Bennett, & Dolin: Principles and Practice of Infectious Diseases, 6th ed.
4. CDC, 2006 STD Surveillance Report, http://www.cdc.gov/std/stats/other.htm accessed on February 27, 2008.
5. **Workowski K, Berman S.** Centers for Disease Control and Prevention. Sexually Transmitted Diseases Treatment Guidelines. MMWR. 2006; 55:51-7.
6. **Pekka Al Saikku.** Chapter 236—Chlamydia, Cohen & Powderly: Infectious Diseases, 2nd ed.
7. **Handsfield H, Sparling P.** Chapter 209—Neisseria gonorrhoeae, Mandell, Bennett, & Dolin: Principles and Practice of Infectious Diseases, 6th ed.
8. **Workowski K, Berman S.** Centers for Disease Control and Prevention. Sexually Transmitted Diseases Treatment Guidelines. MMWR. 2006;55:51-7. Updated recommended treatment regimens for gonococcal infections and associated conditions—United States, April 2007.
9. **Markowitz LE, Dunne EF, Saraiya M, et al.** Quadrivalent human papillomavirus vaccine: Recommendations of the Advisory Committee on Immunization Practices (ACIP). MMWR Recommendations and reports 2007;56:1-24.
10. **Ahmed AM.** Human papillomaviruses and genital disease, Dermatology Clinics—01-APR-2006;24:157-65, vi From NIH/NLM MEDLINE.
11. **Markowitz LE, Dunne EF, Saraiya M, et al.** Quadrivalent human papillomavirus vaccine: Recommendations of the Advisory Committee on Immunization Practices (ACIP). MMWR Recommendations and Reports. 2007;56:1-24.
12. **Tyndall MW.** Chapter 148—Sexually transmitted diseases, Cohen & Powderly: Infectious Diseases, 2nd ed.

13. **Melville J, Sniffen S, Crosby R.** Psychosocial impact of serological diagnosis of herpes simplex virus type 2: as qualitative assessment; Sex Transm Infect. 2003;79:280–85.
14. **Duncan B, Hart G, Scoular A.** Qualitative analysis of psychosocial impact of diagnosis of Chlamydia trachomatis: implications for screening, BMJ. 2001 Jan 27;322:195–99.

D. Contraception

Norma Jo Waxman, Anna Kaminski, Ruth Lesnewski, Shannon Connolly, Radha Lewis, and Penina Segall-Gutierrez

---

KEY POINTS

- The ideal form of birth control is well-tolerated and highly effective.
- Every office visit is an opportunity to assess the risk of unintended pregnancy, provide contraceptive counseling, and initiate contraception.
- Long-acting reversible contraceptives have the lowest failure and highest continuation rates. Wider use of these methods could lower unintended pregnancy rates.
- Pelvic exams are not required prior to starting any form of contraception except intrauterine devices (IUDs).
- All forms of contraception can be initiated at any point in the menstrual cycle. When pregnancy can be reasonably excluded, women may begin a new method on the day of their office visit.
- Extended use of birth control pills or ring offers non-contraceptive benefits and may improve efficacy.
- The WHO *Medical Eligibility Criteria for Initiating Contraceptive Methods* helps clinicians determine which method of contraception can be safely used by women with medical problems.

Epidemiology

Unintended pregnancy rates in the U.S. are much higher than in other developed nations. Approximately 50% of the 6.4 million U.S. pregnancies each year are unintended, and almost half of those end with abortion (1). Forty-eight percent of unintended pregnancies occur during a month when some form of birth control was used (1). Poor and non-white women are at highest risk of unintended pregnancy. Unintended pregnancy is associated with many medical and social problems, including higher infant and maternal morbidity and mortality, delayed onset of prenatal care, increased use of tobacco and other toxic substances during pregnancy, inadequate folic acid intake, higher rates of domestic violence, and lower rates of breast-feeding (2).

Over the past decade, contraceptive options have expanded and improved. Weekly contraceptive patches, a monthly vaginal ring, continuous use of combined hormonal contraception, and hormone-containing intrauterine contraception represent advances that can improve adherence and offer non-contraceptive benefits. Declining abortion rates during the past decade speak to improved use of contraception (3), but myths, barriers to access, politicization of abortion, and providers' knowledge deficits remain widespread and must be overcome. Educating patients and providers can help to reduce unintended pregnancy in the U.S.

Barriers to Access

Low-income and minority women and teens are disproportionately vulnerable to unintended pregnancy because they often have limited access to basic medical care. Uninsured women cannot obtain prescription or procedure-based contraceptives without paying for an office visit. Even insured women may confront obstacles to timely access to contraception. Many physicians prescribe a limited supply of contraceptives at the initial visit, requiring patients to return for a follow-up visit in order to obtain the next prescription. Since job pressures, problems getting child care, lack of provider availability, and myriad other life events may all lead to difficulty making the next appointment, gaps in treatment frequently occur. Insurance coverage and formulary changes also impact access. Dispensing contraceptives in the office, prescribing a 3–12 month supply (4), and allowing office staff to call in contraceptives—even for new patients—can lead to improved access. Office systems should facilitate contraceptive adherence.

Providers can further improve access by eliminating some of the unnecessary screening that has traditionally been required prior to the provision of contraception. Although Pap tests, breast exams, pelvic exams, and testing for sexually transmitted infections (STIs) are often needed for non-contraceptive purposes, they are not necessary prior to the initiation of most birth control methods. Simplified guidelines for prescribing contraception mandate only screening for hypertension and contraindications to estrogen. Eliminating any additional requirements improves access for women who may not have time for an extended appointment or who do not wish to have a pelvic exam (5).

Choosing a New Contraceptive Method

Successful use of contraception depends on a thorough history, review of eligibility criteria, and comprehensive patient education. Successful contraceptive selection requires thorough knowledge of available options and individual patients' preferences and circumstances. The best method for a 17-year-old may not be ideal at age 27, 37, or 47. The most effective methods are independent of users' actions. Once women undergo sterilization, implant, or IUD insertion, they need do nothing to assure the method's success. The lowest efficacy methods, such as withdrawal, require that users perform consistent actions before or during intercourse, a time when many couples are unable or unwilling to focus on preventing pregnancy. Many user-dependent methods such as "the pill" demonstrate a large gap between perfect use and average use because users must remember to take regular action in order for it to be effective. Table 4-9 describes the effectiveness of commonly available methods.

Table 4-9   Contraceptive Efficacy

Method	% of Women Experiencing an Unintended Pregnancy within the First Year of Use	
	Typical Use	Perfect Use
No method	85	85
Spermicides	29	18
Withdrawal	27	4
Fertility awareness-based methods	25	
Standard Days method (avoids intercourse on cycle days 8 through 19)		5
Ovulation method (measures cervical mucus)		3
Sponge		
Parous women	32	20
Nulliparous women	16	9
Diaphragm	16	6
Condom		
Female (Reality)	21	5
Male	15	2
Combined pill and progestin-only pill	8	0.3
Evra patch	8	0.3
No method	85	85
Spermicides	29	18
NuvaRing	8	0.3
Depo-Provera	3	0.3
IUD		
ParaGard (copper T)	0.8	0.6
Mirena (progestin-releasing)	0.2	0.2
Implanon	0.05	0.05
Female sterilization	0.5	0.5
Male sterilization	0.15	0.10

Adapted from Hatcher RA, Trussell J, Nelson AL, Cates W, Stewart FH, Kowal D. Contraceptive Technology: Nineteenth Revised Edition. New York: Ardent Media, 2007; with permission.

Some women consider mechanism of action when selecting a contraceptive. No contraceptive method works by aborting an implanted pregnancy. The copper IUD inhibits sperm motility and makes the endometrium less hospitable to implantation. All hormonal contraceptives, including the progestin IUD, cause thickening of cervical mucus and/or prevent ovulation. Unfortunately, hormonal contraceptives do not protect users against STIs. Women at risk for both STIs and unintended pregnancy should use condoms in addition to a high efficacy method.

Choosing an appropriate contraceptive method requires a thorough medical history. Some medical conditions, like migraine with aura, are contraindications for estrogen-containing contraceptives. Other medical problems, such as acne, are indications for combined hormonal contraceptives. Social factors also influence contraceptive selection. For teenagers who may be hiding their sexual activity from parents, injections, IUDs, and implants provide a discreet yet highly effective user-independent method. Women who are homeless, travel often, or live in multiple locations may have trouble remembering to take a pill at the same time every day. Successful contraception requires consideration of multiple medical and social factors.

Patient-centered contraceptive counseling enhances adherence. Clinicians should listen to patients' concerns and preferences, taking advantage of those that may bolster patient satisfaction. For example, women who request a particular brand of birth control pill should receive that pill unless it is contraindicated. On the other hand, many women are unaware of the full range of contraceptive options or have unfounded concerns about health risks. Whenever a patient requests a low-efficacy method, the clinician should inform her about the safety and benefits of higher efficacy, user-independent alternatives. Clinicians must address patients' concerns directly and respectfully, even concerns that seem trivial or unscientific. Widespread myths influence patients' attitudes toward and utilization of contraception. Women who expect hormones to harm them are more likely to experience side effects from hormonal methods, while those who expect a benefit from a particular method are more likely to use it without difficulty. Counseling women about expected side effects, such as change in bleeding patterns, has been shown to significantly improve continuation (6).

Women's child-bearing goals affect the appropriate choice of contraceptive as well. Women who plan to delay child-bearing by 2 years or more may consider implants or an IUD. Long-acting, fully reversible, and cost-effective, implants and IUDs do not depend on their user for efficacy. Recently expanded eligibility criteria allow IUD use by teenagers, nulliparous women, and those with a past history of pelvic inflammatory disease (PID), STIs, or ectopic pregnancy (7). Despite these new guidelines, many providers fail to inform their patients about the option of intrauterine contraception.

Non-contraceptive benefits may also influence choice of method (Table 4-10). Women with premenstrual syndrome, irregular periods, dysmenorrhea, and other menstrual disorders may benefit from continuous use of combined oral contraceptives or the contraceptive ring; such women may

Table 4-10   Non-Contraceptive Benefits of Hormonal Contraceptives

Medical Conditions Caused or Exacerbated by Menses	<ul><li>Menorrhagia</li><li>Dysmenorrhea</li><li>Irregular menses</li><li>Premenstrual syndrome</li><li>Endometriosis</li><li>Fibroids</li><li>Adenomyosis</li><li>Menstrual migraines</li><li>Iron-deficiency anemia</li><li>Some seizure disorders</li><li>Menstrual flares of chronic illness (e.g., rheumatoid arthritis)</li><li>Coagulopathies (e.g., menstrual porphyria)</li></ul>
Conditions in the group above often improve with any hormonal contraceptive product. Extended cycling can lead to enhanced benefits.	
Other Conditions Alleviated by Hormonal Contraceptives	<ul><li>Vasomotor symptoms of perimenopause</li><li>Acne</li><li>Hirsutism</li><li>Polycystic ovary syndrome</li></ul>
Risk Reduction through Use of Hormonal Contraceptives	<ul><li>Ovarian cancer</li><li>Endometrial cancer</li><li>Colorectal cancer</li><li>Osteoporosis</li></ul>

Adapted from Selected Practice Recommendations for Contraceptive Use, 2nd ed. Geneva, World Health Organization, 2004 and Edelman AB, Gallo MF, Jensen JT, Nichols MD, Schulz KF, Grimes DA. Continuous or extended cycle versus cyclic use of combined oral contraceptives for contraception. Cochrane Database Syst. Rev 2005;3:CD004695; with permission.

benefit equally from progestin injections or the progestin IUD. Although some women feel uncomfortable with methods that induce amenorrhea, others appreciate the convenience of having fewer menstrual periods. Clinicians can confidently assure patients of the safety and efficacy of continuous hormone use and can inform women that there are no health risks associated with giving up withdrawal bleeding.

Medical Eligibility

The WHO's *Medical Eligibility Criteria for Contraceptive Use 2004* (3) offers recommendations based on systematic review of clinical and epidemiological research. Table 4-11 guides clinicians in determining the safety of contraceptive methods for women with medical problems.

Initiating a Birth Control Method

Any contraceptive method may be initiated once pregnancy can be reasonably excluded. When contraceptive use begins during the first five days of the menstrual cycle, immediately postpartum, or immediately after an abortion, no back-up method is needed. Women who initiate contraception at any other time should use a back-up method for the first week (8).

Many women become pregnant while waiting for their next menses before initiating a new contraceptive method (8). Because hormonal contraceptives do not cause birth defects, most women can begin a new method on the day of their office visit. This is known as Quick Start. Those who have had unprotected intercourse in the past five days may take levonorgestrel emergency contraception before beginning their new method (8). Figure 4-1 provides an algorithm for determining appropriate initiation of a new contraceptive method.

Table 4-11   World Health Organization Medical Eligibility for Initiating Contraceptive Methods

Risk Level		
1	Method can be used without restriction	These contraceptive methods do not protect against sexually transmitted infections (STIs). Condoms should be used to protect against STIs.
2	Advantages generally outweigh theoretical or proven risks	For more information, see www.who.int/reproductive-health/publications/mec/mec.pdf
3	Method not usually recommended unless other, more appropriate methods are not available or not acceptable	
4	Method not to be used	

Condition	Qualifier for condition	Estrogen/ progestin: pill, patch, ring	Progestin-only: pill	Progestin-only: injection	Progestin-only: implant	Progestin IUD	Copper IUD
Anemia	Thalassemia	1	1	1	1	1	2
	Sickle cell disease	2	1	1	1	1	2
	Iron-deficiency anemia	1	1	1	1	1	2
Breast cancer	Family history of cancer	1	1	1	1	1	1
	Current	4	4	4	4	4	1
	In past, no evidence of disease for >5 y	3	3	3	3	3	1
Breast problems, benign	Undiagnosed mass	2	2	2	2	2	1
	Benign breast disease	1	1	1	1	1	1
Cervical cancer	Cervical intraepithelial neoplasia	2	1	2	2	2	1
	Awaiting treatment	2	1	2	2	4	4
Cervical ectropion		1	1	1	1	1	1
Depression		1	1	1	1	1	1
Diabetes mellitus (DM)	History of gestational DM only	1	1	1	1	1	1
	DM without vascular disease	2	2	2	2	2	1
	DM with end-organ damage or >20 y duration	3	2	3	2	2	1
Drug interactions	Antiretrovirals	2	2	2	2	2	2
	Certain anticonvulsants	3	3	2	3	1	1
	Griseofulvin	2	2	1	2	1	1
	Rifampin	3	3	2	3	1	1
	ALL OTHER ANTIBIOTICS	1	1	1	1	1	1
Endometrial cancer		1	1	1	1	4	4
Endometriosis		1	1	1	1	1	2
Gallbladder disease	Asymptomatic gallstones	2	2	2	2	2	1
	Symptomatic gallstones, without cholecystectomy	3	2	2	2	2	1
	Gallstones treated with cholecystectomy	2	2	2	2	2	1
	Pregnancy-related cholestasis in past	2	1	1	1	1	1
	Hormone-related cholestasis in past	3	2	2	2	2	1
Headaches	Non-migranous	1	1	1	1	1	1
Headaches: migraines	Without aura, age <35	2	1	2	2	2	1
	Without aura, age >35	3	1	2	2	2	1
	With aura, any age	4	2	2	2	2	1
HIV infection	High risk	1	1	1	1	2	2
	HIV infected	1	1	1	1	2	2
	AIDS (without drug interactions)	1	1	1	1	3	3

cont'd

Table 4-11   World Health Organization Medical Eligibility for Initiating Contraceptive Methods (cont'd)

Condition	Qualifier for condition	Estrogen/progestin: pill, patch, ring	Progestin-only: pill	Progestin-only: injection	Progestin-only: implant	Progestin IUD	Copper IUD
Hypertension	During prior pregnancy only – now resolved	2	1	1	1	1	1
	Well controlled	3	1	2	1	1	1
	Systolic 140–159 or diastolic 90–99	3	1	2	1	1	1
	Systolic >160 or diastolic >100	4	2	3	2	2	1
	With vascular disease	4	2	3	2	2	1
Ischemic heart disease	Past or current	4	2	3	2	2	1
Liver disease	Cirrhosis–mild	3	2	2	2	2	1
	Cirrhosis–severe	4	3	3	3	3	1
	Tumors–benign	4	3	3	3	3	1
	Tumors–malignant	4	3	3	3	3	1
	Viral hepatitis–carrier	1	1	1	1	1	1
	Viral hepatitis–active	4	3	3	3	3	1
Obesity	BMI >30 kg/m²	2	1	1	1	1	1
Ovarian cancer		1	1	1	1	3	3
Ovarian cysts	& benign tumors	1	1	1	1	1	1
Pelvic inflammatory disease	Past, with subsequent pregnancy	1	1	1	1	1	1
	Past, without subsequent pregnancy	1	1	1	1	2	2
	Current	1	1	1	1	4	4
Postpartum, not breastfeeding	<48 h	3	1	1	1	3	2
	2–21 d	3	1	1	1	3	3
	3–4 wk	1	1	1	1	3	3
	>4 wk	1	1	1	1	1	1
Postpartum, & breastfeeding	<6 wk postpartum	4	3	3	3	See above	See above
	6 wk–6 mo postpartum	3	1	1	1	1	1
	>6 mo postpartum	2	1	1	1	1	1
Post-abortion	First trimester	1	1	1	1	1	1
	Second trimester	1	1	1	1	2	2
	Immediately after septic abortion	1	1	1	1	4	4
Sexually transmitted infections	Vaginitis	1	1	1	1	2	2
	High risk	1	1	1	1	3	3
	Current GC/Chlamydia/ Purulent cervicitis	1	1	1	1	4	4
Smoking	Age <35	2	1	1	1	1	1
	Age >35, <15 cigarettes/d	3	1	1	1	1	1
	Age >35, >15 cigarettes/d	4	1	1	1	1	1
Seizure disorder	Without drug interactions	1	1	1	1	1	1
Stroke		4	2	3	2	2	1
Surgery	Minor, without prolonged immobilization	1	1	1	1	1	1
	Major, without prolonged immobilization	2	1	1	1	1	1
	Major, with prolonged immobilization	4	2	2	2	2	1
Thyroid disorders	Simple goiter, hyperthyroidism, hypothyroidism	1	1	1	1	1	1
Uterine fibroids	Without distortion of uterine cavity	1	1	1	1	1	1
	With distortion of uterine cavity	1	1	1	1	4	4
Valvular heart disease	Uncomplicated	2	1	1	1	1	1
	Complicated	4	1	1	1	2	2
Varicose veins		1	1	1	1	1	1
Venous thrombosis	Family history (1st-degree relatives)	2	1	1	1	1	1
	Superficial thrombophlebitis	2	1	1	1	1	1
	Past DVT	4	2	2	2	2	1
	Current DVT	4	3	3	3	3	1

WHO Medical Eligibility Criteria for Contraceptive Use Third edition 2004; This adaptation courtesy of RHEDI (Center for Reproductive Health Education In Family Medicine), Department of Family and Social Medicine at Montefiore Medical Center in the Bronx, New York.
Copies of this chart may be reproduced and distributed using http://www.reproductiveaccess. org/contraception/downloads/WHO_Chart.pdf

Contraceptive Methods

Only the male and female condoms offer STI protection. Clinicians should counsel all sexually active patients regarding STI prevention.

Sterilization is available for both men and women. These methods are permanent. Reversals are variably effective and not covered by insurance.

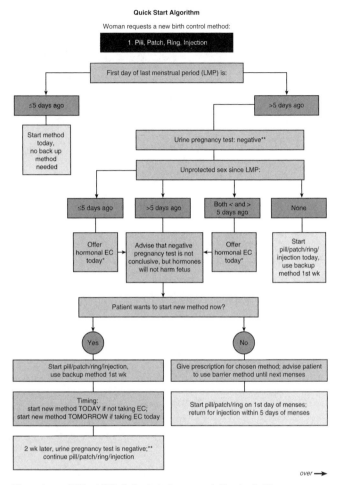

Quick Start Algorithm

Woman requests a new birth control method:

1. Pill, Patch, Ring, Injection

First day of last menstrual period (LMP) is:

≤5 days ago

>5 days ago

Start method today, no back up method needed

Urine pregnancy test: negative**

Unprotected sex since LMP:

≤5 days ago

>5 days ago

Both < and > 5 days ago

None

Offer hormonal EC today*

Advise that negative pregnancy test is not conclusive, but hormones will not harm fetus

Offer hormonal EC today*

Start pill/patch/ring/injection today, use backup method 1st wk

Patient wants to start new method now?

Yes

No

Start pill/patch/ring/injection, use backup method 1st wk

Give prescription for chosen method; advise patient to use barrier method until next menses

Timing: start new method TODAY if not taking EC; start new method TOMORROW if taking EC today

Start pill/patch/ring on 1st day of menses; return for injection within 5 days of menses

2 wk later, urine pregnancy test is negative;** continue pill/patch/ring/injection

over →

* Because hormonal EC is not 100% effective, check urine pregnancy test 2 weeks after EC use.
** If pregnancy test is positive, provide options counseling.

Figure 4-1   Quick start algorithm. (Adapted from the Reproductive Health Access Project website; with permission.)

Consider sterilization when pregnancy/childbearing is no longer desired or would seriously threaten the woman's health.

Vasectomy: The minimally invasive no-scalpel technique is the most commonly performed vasectomy procedure. Mild post-procedure bruising, swelling, and tenderness occur often and improve with support, NSAID, and rest. Less common side effects include transient sperm granulomas, proximal testicular infection, and thrombus. Semen analysis 6–8 weeks

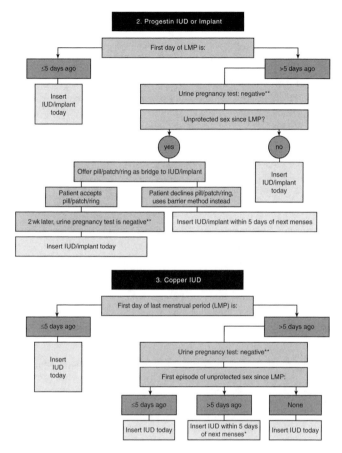

* Pill/patch/ring may be started as a bridge to copper IUD.
** If pregnancy test is positive, provide options counseling.

Note: These algorithms are based on the algorithm for injected progestin that appears in the 2005 *Pocket Guide to Managing Contraception* by Hatcher RA, Zieman M et al, page 135.

Figure 4-1   Continued.

after the procedure ensures absence of motile sperm. Couples should use back-up contraception until sperm is absent (9).

Tubal sterilization may be done by Fallopian tube separation (laparoscopic or laparatomy) or occlusion (transvaginal, hysteroscopic Essure). Essure induces tubal closure over 6–12 weeks in most cases (9). Couples should use a back-up method until a hysterosalpingogram demonstrates occlusion. Tubal ligation by laparoscope has a 1–2 day recovery period. Vessel or bowel injury occurs rarely.

Intrauterine contraceptives (IUDs) are long-acting and reversible methods available with and without progestin. Current evidence and FDA labeling support IUD use for most women. Contraindications include current cervicitis, PID, and active endometrial or cervical cancer (see Table 4-11). Women who cannot tolerate irregular bleeding or who want to avoid hormones may prefer the copper IUD. Fertility returns rapidly when the IUD is removed, allowing the woman control over child spacing. Uterine perforation is rare (1/1000); it occurs most often at the time of insertion and with extreme uterine flexion (9). Infection risk is slightly increased in the first 20 days after insertion but is the same as in non-users thereafter (7).

Copper IUD (Paragard) is effective for 10–12 years. It may be used as emergency contraception up to 5–8 days following unprotected intercourse. Abnormal uterine bleeding (meno- and metrorrhagia) or dysmenorrhea can occur in the first few months. *Dysmenorrhea may persist*; in some women, it may warrant switching to another method (9).

Progestin (levonorgestrel) IUD (Mirena) is effective for 5–7 years. Endometrial thinning from progestin reduces total menstrual blood loss by 70–80% in some users; amenorrhea occurs in 20% of users at 1 year and in 60% of users at 5 years (9). Many women develop irregular menstrual bleeding and amenorrhea with this method (9).

Progestin-based methods can be associated with unpredictable spotting or bleeding, decreased bleeding, and amenorrhea. These hormonal contraceptives are safe during lactation and are good choices for women unable to tolerate estrogens. *Adherence improves with counseling and discussion of typical side effects* (6).

Progestin (levonorgestrel) single rod implant (Implanon) is inserted subdermally by a trained clinician and is effective for 3 years. Amenorrhea is common, but unpredictable bleeding may persist in some women. Fertility returns promptly after removal of Implanon (9). Some premenstrual symptoms, including mood variability and headaches, lessen with use.

Depo-medroxyprogesterone acetate (Depo-Provera, DMPA) is administered IM by a clinician or SQ by the client. It is effective for 12 weeks but is often repeated at 10–12 week intervals to offer flexible appointment access. With a long history of use and an excellent safety record, DMPA has the longest list of known benefits and side effects. It is known to decrease seizure potential, sickle cell crisis, PID risk, and symptoms of endometriosis and fibroids (9). Of all hormonal methods, it causes the slowest return of fertility and the slowest resolution of side effects. Disadvantages include weight gain/loss, hair and skin changes, depression, irregular bleeding patterns, and lower libido, all of which resolve after discontinuation. Although depot progestin carries a black box warning regarding decreased bone density, recent studies demonstrate that bone density loss plateaus after 2 years and recovers completely when depot progestin is discontinued (10). Lifestyle factors (including diet, exercise, and pregnancy) have a greater effect on bone density than does depot progestin (10).

Progestin-only oral contraceptives are less effective than other progestin-only methods but remain a good choice for some women who cannot tolerate estrogens (9). Progestin-only pills need to be taken at *the same time each day*. Like other progestin-only methods, they may cause irregular bleeding, which can persist for months (9).

Combined hormonal contraceptives are the most commonly used method in the U.S. There are many non-contraceptive benefits and multiple formulations available to ameliorate side effects. All may be started on the same day as the office visit (QuickStart) and offer predictable menses once established (in 1–2 months) (8). The oral and ring forms may be used for extended cycles or with shorter hormone-free intervals, allowing the user to determine the timing of menses or induction of amenorrhea (11). All allow rapid return to fertility and reversal of side effects on cessation. Clinicians should educate patients regarding strategies to maximize adherence: for example, using cell phone alarms as a reminder to take the pill daily. Extended or continuous cycling may improve efficacy, as well as decrease PMDD symptoms, dysmenorrhea, or menorrhagia (11).

Vaginal ring (Nuvaring) has unique advantages in being the "most hidden" method. In some women, vaginal discharge, infection, or irritation may increase. Options for use include shorter ring-free (hormone-free) time of 2–3 days or extended cycle with replacement every 21–30 days for continuous cycles. The ring cannot be used with other intravaginal barrier methods but can be used with male condoms (9).

Transdermal patch (Ortho-Evra) delivers combined hormones using 3 consecutive patches for a week each followed by a hormone-free interval of one week. Skin irritation can occur at the patch site. The patch delivers higher estrogen levels than pills containing 30 mcg of estrogen, leading some women to have estrogen-mediated side effects such as nausea and breast tenderness. Venous thromboembolism (VTE) risk with the patch may be higher than with low-dose pills, but data on this issue are conflicting and incomplete (12). The patch may be less effective for women over 198 pounds (9).

Combined oral contraceptives are very commonly used and requested in all age groups. New options include pills packaged for extended use and those with shorter hormone-free intervals. (However, women can choose to have extended cycles using any birth control pill; they simply skip placebo pills and go straight to the next pack.) Rare adverse health risks include VTE, myocardial infarction, and stroke. Smokers over age 35 years have the highest risk of serious cardiovascular events (9) (see Table 4-11).

Visible barrier methods are less effective for pregnancy prevention, but offer STI protection. They are easy to buy and use but require planning or interruption of sexual activity to be effective. Allergy to latex can limit use and non-latex products may be less accessible. Educating on correct usage is recommended.

Male condoms require male partner participation and cooperation. Diminished penile sensation can be a deterrent or help relieve early ejaculation. Condoms can break or slip off. Polyurethane condoms may be less effective than latex condoms.

Female condoms (Reality) can also relieve early ejaculation. They can produce a "crackly" sound and some users may find them difficult to insert or irritating to the skin. They can slip out of place, or the penis can move to the outside of the condom.

Invisible barrier methods include the diaphragm and cervical cap. They cost very little and can last for several years but have relatively low efficacy (see Table 4-9) and must be remembered and used with each sexual encounter. A clinician must fit and evaluate the device for placement. The patient must be able to insert the diaphragm or cervical cap each time she has intercourse. These devices can be left in place for 24 hours. Spermicide must be used and reapplied each time. Allergies or sensitivity to nonoxynol-9 may occur. Diaphragms have been associated with increased risk of bladder infection (9). Cervical caps (Leah's Shield, Femcap) are available in limited sizes and may not fit all women. Efficacy decreases significantly in parous users (9).

Other family planning methods are variably reliable, and "perfect use" may increase success. The practitioner should educate and assist in the selection of more reliable methods as needed.

Emergency contraception (Plan B) is a progestin method that reduces the risk of mistimed pregnancy when taken within 5 days of unprotected intercourse or contraceptive error. It is more effective when taken sooner after exposure (9). It is available for purchase by women or men over the age of 18 years and is covered by several states' insurance programs. Prescribing Plan B is standard-of-care following sexual assault. The patient may take 2 doses at once or 2 tablets 12 hours apart (9).

Continuous breast-feeding lactational amenorrhea is effective if the mother breast-feeds continuously. Return to fertility (ovulation) is unpredictable. The woman should start a more effective method when menstruation returns *or* when frequency of breast-feeding is >3 hours *or* at 6 months (9).

Spermicide (nonoxynol-9) is available as cream, gel foam, or film; it is easy to buy and use. Some forms are messy. Spermicide can cause skin irritation in either partner. *Spermicide may increase the risk of HIV infection and should never be used for anal sex* (9).

Period abstinence eliminates pregnancy risk through avoidance of sexual intercourse. Many people fail to resume an effective method once they choose to initiate sexual activity again. There are no side effects.

Withdrawal can be used with condom use for almost 100% effectiveness and can be used if no other method is available or desirable. It requires a trusted male partner with significant self-control and awareness. *Withdrawal is not recommended for teens and offers no protection from STIs.*

Internet resources are given in Box 4-4.

Box 4-4   Internet Resources for Further Reading

- The complete book, *Managing Contraception*
  www.managingcontraception.org
- WHO Medical Eligibility Criteria for Contraceptive Use 2004
  www.who.int/reproductive-health/publications/mec/mec.pdf
- Association of Reproductive Health Professionals (ARHP)
  www.arhp.org
- Alan Guttmacher Institute
  www.agi-usa.org
- Contraception Online: A resource for clinicians, researchers, and educators
  www.contraceptiononline.org
- Planned Parenthood Federation of America
  www.plannedparenthood.org
- The Center for Reproductive Health Education in Family Medicine
  www.rhedi.org
- The Reproductive Health Access Project
  www.reproductiveaccess.org

References

1. **Finer LB, Henshaw SK.** Disparities in rates of unintended pregnancy in the United States, 1994 and 2001. Perspect Sex Reprod Health. 2006;38:90-6.
2. **Kost K, Landry DJ, Darroch JE.** The effects of pregnancy planning status on birth outcomes and infant care. Fam Plann Perspect. 1998;50:223-30.
3. Medical Eligibility Criteria for Initiating Contraceptive Methods, 3rd ed. Geneva, World Health Organization, 2004.
4. **Foster DG, Parvataneni R, DeBocanegra HT, et al.** Number of oral contraceptive pill packages dispensed, method continuation, and costs. Obstet Gynecol. 2006 Nov;108:1107-4.
5. **Stewart FH, Harper CC, Ellerston CE, et al.** Clinical breast and pelvic examination requirements for hormonal contraception: current practice vs evidence. JAMA. 2001;285:2232-9.
6. **Canto-DeCetina TEC, Canto P, Luna MO.** Effect of counseling to improve compliance in Mexican women receiving depot-medroxyprogesterone acetate. Contraception. 2001;63:143-6.
7. **Nelson A.** Contraindications to IUD and IUS use. Contraception. 2007;75:576-81.
8. Selected Practice Recommendations for Contraceptive Use, 2nd ed. Geneva, World Health Organization, 2004.
9. **Hatcher RA, Trussell J, Nelson AL, et al.** Contraceptive Technology: Nineteenth Revised Edition. New York NY: Ardent Media, 2007.
10. **Kaunitz AM, Arias R, McClung M.** Bone density recovery after depot medroxyprogesterone acetate injectable contraception use. Contraception. 2008;77:67-76.

11. **Edelman AB, Gallo MF, Jensen JT, et al.** Continuous or extended cycle versus cyclic use of combined oral contraceptives for contraception. Cochrane Database Syst Rev. 2005;3:CD004695.
12. **Jick S, Kaye JA, Li L, et al.** Further results on the risk of nonfatal venous thromboembolism in users of the contraceptive transdermal patch compared to users of oral contraceptives containing norgestimate and 35 microg of ethinyl estradiol. Contraception. 2007;76:4–7.

E. Female Sexual Dysfunction

Teri Greco

KEY POINTS

- Female sexual dysfunction (FSD) is defined as a disorder of sexual desire, orgasm, arousal, and sexual pain that results in significant personal distress.
- It is a multifactorial and multidimensional condition, combining several biological, psychological, medical, interpersonal, and social components.
- Approximately 43% of women experience sexual problems, with low libido being the most common complaint (51%), followed by problems with arousal (33%) and pain disorders (16%).
- After identification of a problem, a comprehensive evaluation should be performed, which includes a medical, psychosocial, and sexual history; physical examination; and potential laboratory testing.
- Most, if not all, treatments for female sexual dysfunction are not evidence-based; therefore, more well-designed clinical trials are needed to define which medical or psychological treatment components are most effective.
- Other than estrogen therapy for dyspareunia related to genitourinary atrophy, no medications are currently approved by the Food and Drug Administration (FDA) for the treatment of FSD.

Epidemiology

Female sexual dysfunction (FSD) is a prevalent and often underestimated problem in the general community. FSD is defined as a disorder of sexual desire, orgasm, arousal, and sexual pain that results in significant personal distress. It is multifactorial and multidimensional and includes biological, psychological, medical, interpersonal, and social components (1).

Although it is recognized as a widespread problem, some controversy exists about its prevalence, because of variation in assessment techniques and use of non-standardized definitions of sexual dysfunction. The U.S. National Health and Social Life Survey, which evaluated 1749 women aged 18–59 years, showed that 43% reported a sexual problem. Low libido was the most common complaint (51%), followed by problems with arousal (33%) and pain disorders (16%). FSD was shown to be associated with various psychosocial characteristics, such as less education, poor physical and emotional health, and negative experiences in sexual relationships. The survey also showed that African American women were more likely to suffer from decreased libido than Caucasian or Latina women (2).

In the recent study of 1550 American women aged 57–85 years, the National Social Life, Health, and Aging Project, showed that about half of the women surveyed reported at least 1 bothersome sexual problem. The most prevalent sexual problems among women were low desire (43%), difficulty with lubrication (39%), and inability to climax (34%). Women who rated their health as being poor were less likely to be sexually active, and, of those respondents who were sexually active, they were more likely to report sexual problems (3).

Definition and Classification

Initial definitions of FSD, as outlined in the Diagnostic and Statistical Manual of Mental Disorders, 4th edition (DSM-IV), were based on the Kaplan model of desire, arousal, and orgasm. A new 5-phase model for female sexuality proposed by Basson, *et al.* (4), suggested that intimacy and desire are essential for women to participate in sexual activity. Once intimacy and sexual stimuli lead women to arouse emotionally, sexual arousal and desire occur and culminate in emotional and physical satisfaction. Rather than the traditional view of a sexual response progressing through discrete phases in sequence (desire, arousal, orgasm, and resolution), it is now recognized that these phases overlap and that the sequence can vary (4).

The Sexual Functional Health Council of the American Foundation for Urologic Disease convened an interdisciplinary consensus panel in 1999 that expanded the DSM-IV classification system. Sexual dysfunction in women is now classified into sexual desire disorders, subdivided into hypoactive sexual desire disorder (HSDD) and sexual aversion disorder, female sexual arousal disorder (FASD), sexual orgasmic disorder, and sexual pain disorders, which may be further subdivided into dyspareunia and vaginismus (Table 4-12). An essential element of this new diagnostic system is the personal distress criterion, which means that a condition is considered a disorder only if it creates distress for the female experiencing the condition (1).

Evaluation

Although there is insufficient evidence for or against screening women for sexual dysfunction, physicians should consider questioning women

Table 4-12   Definitions of Sexual Dysfunction

Disorder	Definition
Sexual Desire Disorders*	
Hypoactive sexual desire disorder (HSDD)	Absent or diminished feelings of sexual desire and/or sexual thoughts or fantasies; Lack of responsive desire
Sexual aversion disorder	Persistent or recurring phobic aversion leading to avoidance of sexual contact
Sexual Arousal Disorders*	
Subjective arousal disorder	Absent or markedly reduced feelings of sexual arousal from any type of stimulation; Vaginal lubrication and other signs of physical response still occurs
Genital arousal disorder	Absent or impaired genital sexual arousal (minimal vulvar swelling, vaginal lubrication, and genital sensations with stimulation); Subjective sexual excitement still occurs
Combined arousal disorder	Absent or markedly reduced feelings of sexual arousal from any type of stimulation; Absent or impaired genital sexual arousal
Orgasmic Disorder*	
Female orgasmic disorder	Lack of orgasm or markedly diminished intensity of orgasmic sensations, or marked delay of orgasm from any kind of stimulation; Self-reported high sexual desire and arousal
Pain Disorders*	
Dyspareunia	Recurrent or persistent genital pain associated with sexual intercourse; May be further classified as superficial (associated with the vulva and/or vaginal entrance) or deep (perceived in the abdomen or internal organs and often associated with penile thrusting)
Vaginismus	Persistent difficulties to allow vaginal entry of a penis, finger, and/or object, despite the woman's expressed wish to do so; There may be a component of involuntary pelvic muscle contractions and avoidance and anticipation/fear of pain

* In order to diagnosis female sexual dysfunction, in addition to symptoms, all disorders must cause personal distress.

about their sexual activity and function at annual exams or after a change in health status, such as pregnancy, menopause, pelvic surgery, or a newly diagnosed medical problem. Attempts should be made to incorporate questions about sexual function into current and past medical history, review of systems, and social history by using open-ended, direct questions. Screening acknowledges the importance of sexual health to a woman's quality of life and general health and well-being.

After identification of a problem, a comprehensive evaluation should be performed, which includes a medical, psychosocial, and sexual history, physical examination, and potential laboratory testing. The medical history should focus on medical and psychiatric disorders, previous surgeries, medication use (Table 4-13), and substance abuse history. Patients with a history of sexual abuse, relationship problems, and concurrent psychiatric diagnoses should undergo assessment by a therapist to determine if they would benefit from psychotherapy in conjunction with medical treatment. Although several self-reported questionnaires are available to assess sexual dysfunction, their use may not be practical in a clinical setting since they are time-intensive and may not assess all the domains of sexual dysfunction (Table 4-14).

Physical examination should focus on detecting signs of endocrine, vascular, neurologic, infectious, or gynecologic abnormalities that may contribute to sexual dysfunction. A careful and systematic examination of the external genitalia, pelvic floor musculature, and internal genitalia, including a manual and speculum exam should be performed on all patients (Table 4-15). Patients with complaints of pain may not tolerate an internal exam, but, if tolerated, the location of their pain should be determined.

Laboratory Testing
Basic laboratory tests, including a serum chemistry, liver function tests, complete blood count, and lipid profile, may be indicated to assess for underlying diseases, such as diabetes, hyperlipidemia, and renal or liver disease. Specific hormonal tests, including thyroid-stimulating hormone (TSH), prolactin, and dehydroepiandrosterone-sulfate (DHEA-S), may be performed if endocrine abnormalities, such as thyroid dysfunction, hyperprolactinemia, or adrenal insufficiency, are suspected. If menopausal status is uncertain, estradiol, follicle-stimulating hormone, and luteinizing hormone may be obtained. Serum androgens may not be useful diagnostically because there are no precise definitions of androgen deficiency, the "normal" ranges for serum androgens in women of different ages are poorly characterized, the accuracy of available testosterone assays in women is questionable, and two large population studies failed to show a correlation between low serum testosterone level and low sexual desire. If measured, androgen levels ideally should be obtained in the morning and in the mid-third of the menstrual cycle using equilibrium dialysis or liquid chromatography mass spectrometry (5,6).

Differential Diagnosis

Many common medical disorders have negative effects on desire, arousal, orgasm, and freedom from pain during intercourse. Diseases and medical interventions can directly interfere with central and peripheral sexual physiology, so a thorough evaluation should be performed in every patient to uncover any potentially correctable medical illness, medication usage, or chronic condition leading to sexual dysfunction (Table 4-16).

Table 4-13   Medications Associated with Female Sexual Dysfunction

Medication	Mechanism of Action	Sexual Side Effects	Comments
Antidepressants			
SSRIs	Stimulation of serotonin receptors	Decreased desire; delayed or absence of orgasm	Bupropion may have fewer sexual side effects
Antipsychotics	Reduced dopamine; increased prolactin; α-blockade and muscarinic blockade	Delayed or absence of orgasm	Second generation antipsychotics that do not raise prolactin may have fewer sexual side effects
Antihypertensives	Effects on sympatholytic and vascular system	Decreased desire	ACE inhibitors, ARBs, and CCB may have fewer sexual side effects in women
Beta-blockers			
Anti-androgens	Suppression of GnRH or LH; antagonism of androgen receptor	Delayed or absence of orgasm	
GnRH agonists			
Cyproterone acetate			
Spironolactone (high dose)			
Cimetidine			
Testosterone-binding meds	Suppression of total and free testosterone	Decreased desire; vaginal dryness	No studies evaluating if the patch or vaginal ring have fewer sexual side effects than OCPs
Tamoxifen			
OCPs			
Statins			
Narcotics	Suppression of GnRH	Decreased desire	
Anti-epileptics	Induction of P450 hepatic enzymes; increased SHBG and decreased FT	Decreased desire	Oxcarbazapine and lamotrigine may have fewer sexual side effects
Phenytoin			
Phenobarbitone			
Primidone			
Carbamazepine			
Corticosteroids	Suppression of hypothalamic pituitary axis; decreased DHEA and DHEA-S	Decreased desire	

SSRI = selective serotonin reuptake inhibitors; GnRH = gonadotrophin releasing hormone; LH = luteinizing hormone; ACE inhibitors = angiotensin-converting enzyme inhibitor; ARBs = angiotensin receptor blockers; CCB = calcium channel blocker; OCPs = oral contraceptive pills; SHBG = sex-hormone binding globulin; FT = free testosterone; DHEA(S) = dehydroepiandrosterone (sulfate).

Table 4-14   General Assessment and History

History	Assessment
Presenting Problem	
	• Have you experienced a change in your interest in sex?
	• Do you have difficulty becoming aroused, achieving orgasm, or with sufficient vaginal lubrication?
	• Do you have superficial or deep pain with intercourse?
	• Quantify severity (global vs. situational), chronicity (primary vs. secondary), and context.
Psychosocial History*	
Sexual history	• First sexual experience
	• History of physical or sexual abuse, or female circumcision
Relationship history	• Quality of relationship
	• Partner sexual dysfunction
Psychosocial history	• Family or religious attitudes toward sex
	• Issues of self-esteem
	• Increased life stressors
Past Medical History	
Medication	• Review prescription medications, alcohol and tobacco use, and recreational drug use (see Table 4-13)
Psychiatric history*	• Mood and anxiety disorders
	• Eating disorders and body image disturbance
	• Substance abuse
Medical history	• Sexually transmitted diseases
	• Cancer (especially breast and gynecological cancers), chemotherapy, and radiation treatment
	• Neurologic disorders (multiple sclerosis, seizures, spinal cord or traumatic brain injury)
	• Endocrine disorders (diabetes, hyperthyroidism, hyperprolactinemia)
Surgical history	• Hysterectomy, incontinence repairs
Gynecologic History	
Obstetrical history	• Type of delivery
	• Episiotomy or vaginal tear
Gynecologic history	• Recurrent vaginal infections
	• Endometriosis
	• Uterine fibroids

*Patients with a history of sexual abuse, relationship problems, and concurrent psychiatric diagnoses should undergo assessment by a therapist to determine if they would benefit from psychotherapy.

Table 4-15   Physical Examination

Component of Exam	Assessment	Diagnosis
Nongenital Examination		
Thyroid	Thyroid enlargement, masses, or tenderness	Hypothyroidism, hyperthyroidism
Breasts	Nipple discharge	Hyperprolactinemia
Musculoskeletal	Limited mobility	Osteoarthritis
Neurological	Neurologic impairment	Multiple sclerosis, Parkinson's disease
	Abnormal genital/perineal sensation or abnormal bulbocavernosus reflex	Pudendal neuropathy
External Genitalia		
Mons pubis	Sparse pubic hair	Suggests low adrenal androgens
Vulvar skin inspection	Lesions	Herpes
	Cracks or fissures in the intralabial folds	Candidiasis
	Dermatitis	Eczema, lichen planus, lichen sclerosus
Labia majora and minora	Allodynia of the crease between the outer edge of the hymen and inner edge of labia minora; variable erythema of vestibule	Vulvar vestibulitis
Posterior forchette/ hymen	Scar tissue	Episiotomy scars
Clitoris	Adhesions, scar tissue	Female circumcision
Internal Genitalia		
Bladder and urethra	Protrusion of tissue or tenderness	Prolapse, infection, interstitial cystitis
Pelvic floor muscles	Inability to tighten and relax perivaginal muscles	Dyspareunia
	Increased tone or tenderness on palpation of levator ani muscle	Vaginismus
Vagina	Atrophy, decreased lubrication, erythema, tenderness	Postmenopausal atrophic vaginitis; scleroderma or Sjogren's syndrome
Cervix	Erythema, tenderness, discharge	Infection, dysplasia, cancer
Uterus	Tenderness, boggy, mass	Fibroids, endometriosis
Valsalva maneuver	Protrusion of tissue, leakage of urine	Cystocele, rectocele, uterine prolapse, incontinence

Table 4-16   Differential Diagnosis of Female Sexual Dysfunction

Disease	Pathophysiology of FSD
Endocrine Disorders	
Hypopituitarism	Compromised adrenal and ovarian function; low plasma concentrations of androgens
Adrenal insufficiency	Lack of precursor hormones
Diabetes mellitus	Patients report low desire with hyperglycemia; possible vascular and neurologic damage causing diminished genital sensation and decreased lubrication
Hyperprolactinemia	Overproduction of prolactin by adenoma, hypothyroidism, or medications resulting in decreased desire and arousal
Thyroid disorders	Over or underproduction of thyroid hormone leading to decreased desire
Psychiatric Disorders	
Depression	Neurotransmitters of frontal limbic system thought to be affected; side effects of antidepressants
Schizophrenia	Treatment with antipsychotics lead to low desire
Atherosclerotic disease	Low motivation or desire because of fear of another MI; no proven correlation between vascular disease and sexual dysfunction in women
Renal failure	Anovulation (no LH surge) and high prolactin secretion lead to low desire
Pelvic trauma/surgery	
Urinary incontinence	Leakage of urine with penetration or with orgasm reduces sexual motivation
Bilateral oophorectomy	Loss of ovarian androgen and androgen precursor production leading to decreased desire and vaginal lubrication
Neurologic Disorders	
Head injury	Direct damage to regions involved in processing sexual stimuli; hypothalamic or pituitary damage
Parkinson's disease	Neurologic symptoms secondary to a decrease in dopamine-producing cells leading to decreased desire
Multiple sclerosis	Demyelination of CNS; nerves of the reproductive organs may be impaired leading to decreased sensation, arousal, and orgasm
Cachexia	
Low-weight HIV	Decreased gonadotrophins and/or ovarian dysfunction
Anorexia nervosa	Decreased gonadotrophins

LH = luteinizing hormone; CNS = central nervous system; HIV = human immunodeficiency virus.

Treatment

Most treatment of FSD by clinicians is not evidence-based, since long-term outcome studies are lacking (Table 4-17). Other than estrogen therapy for dyspareunia related to genitourinary atrophy, no medications are currently approved by the FDA for the treatment of FSD. Several

Table 4-17   Treatment for Female Sexual Dysfunction

Disorder	Pharmacologic Treatment	Nonpharmacologic Treatment
Sexual Desire Disorders		
Hypoactive sexual desire disorder	Transdermal testosterone patch (300 μg) in surgically induced menopausal women (not FDA approved) Bupropion for SSRI-induced desire disorders	Cognitive behavioral therapy
Sexual Arousal Disorders		
Subjective arousal disorder Genital arousal disorder Combined arousal disorder	Transdermal testosterone patch (300 μg) in surgically induced menopausal women (not FDA approved) Bupropion for SSRI-induced arousal disorders Phosphodiesterase inhibitors for SCI and SSRI-induced arousal disorders Topical alprostadil (900 μg) Zestra (herbal oil applied to clitoris prior to intercourse)	EROS clitoral device (FDA approved) Cognitive behavioral therapy Individual or couples sex therapy
Orgasmic Disorder		
Female orgasmic disorder	Bupropion for SSRI-induced orgasmic disorders	EROS clitoral device (FDA approved) Directed masturbation Anxiety reduction techniques Kegel exercises
Pain Disorders		
Dyspareunia	Topical anesthetic applied to vestibule 10–15 min prior to intercourse Low dose TCAs or anticonvulsants Oral fluconazole in women with positive candida cultures	Vaginal muscle EMG biofeedback and pelvic floor PT Surgical excision of painful vestibular tissue

cont'd

Table 4-17   Treatment for Female Sexual Dysfunction (cont'd)

Disorder	Pharmacologic Treatment	Nonpharmacologic Treatment
Vaginismus	Local injection of botulism toxin	Graduated vaginal dilators 10–15 min 5×/wk
All Sexual Disorders		Weight reduction, exercise, smoking cessation, and treatment for substance abuse problems

FDA = federal drug administration; SSRI = selective serotonin reuptake inhibitor; SCI = spinal cord injury; TCAs = tricyclic antidepressants.

off-label uses of drugs, including testosterone, often are used for treatment, although data about effectiveness are sparse.

Sexual Desire Disorders

Epidemiological studies have shown little correlation between symptoms of sexual dysfunction and androgen levels. However, women undergoing surgical menopause do experience a significant decline in androgen levels. Treatment with vaginal estrogen should be initiated first because many symptoms related to sexual dysfunction, especially vaginal atrophy and dyspareunia, may improve and result in overall improvement in quality of life. All forms of vaginal estrogen preparations, including cream, tablet, and ring are effective. Long-term intravaginal use of estrogen cream should be avoided because it results in systemic absorption, while both tablets and ring relieve atrophy with minimal absorption. The addition of progestin to prevent endometrial hyperplasia is generally not advocated; however, evidence for endometrial safety beyond 1 year is lacking (6).

The results of 4 recent placebo-controlled, randomized trials involving 1619 women who had undergone surgically-induced menopause and were treated with estrogen replacement therapy and a 300-μg testosterone patch reported increased sexual desire, as measured by validated questionnaires, and an increased number of sexually satisfying events per month. Despite positive efficacy data, the patch was not approved by the FDA due to lack of long-term safety data regarding cardiovascular disease and breast cancer risk (4,7). The U.S. Endocrine Society has recommended that clinicians should not diagnose androgen deficiency in women, until it is a well-defined clinical syndrome and normative data on total and free testosterone levels across the lifespan have been established (5).

Sexual Arousal and Orgasmic Disorders

There are no approved pharmacological treatments for female arousal or orgasmic disorder, but the FDA has approved the ErosClitoral Therapy Device, which is a handheld battery-powered vacuum pump that can be used to increase blood flow to and around the clitoris. In large multi-center trials involving pre- and postmenopausal women, no benefit from sildenafil was reported, but a substantial (30–40%) placebo response was noted (4). Several smaller studies in women with spinal cord injury or selective serotonin reuptake inhibitor (SSRI)-associated arousal disorder showed an improvement in sexual function with sildenafil (8). Additionally, in a small study, women with FSD treated with 900 µg of topical alprostadil, a prostaglandin E1 agonist, did show an improvement in arousal scores, but further studies are needed to clarify the role of alprostadil in the treatment of arousal disorders (6). There is a high incidence of adverse sexual side effects, including inhibited or delayed orgasm, noted with antidepressant treatment, especially with SSRIs. Drug holidays, decreased dosages, addition of bupropion, or changing antidepressant therapy to a medication that has a lower incidence of sexual side effects, such as nefazodone, mirtazapine, bupropion, or duloxetine, may be effective, though data are limited (9). Although there is a lack of well-designed clinical trials proving efficacy, sex therapy, directed masturbation, cognitive behavioral therapy, pelvic floor exercises are routinely recommended for treatment of arousal and orgasmic disorders.

Pain Disorders

In regard to treatment of sexual pain disorders, a distinction is made between women with vulvar vestibulitis (the most common subtype of chronic dyspareunia that is characterized by pain confined to the vulvar vestibule that occurs upon attempted introital entry), women with dyspareunia not identified as vulvar vestibulitis, and women with vaginismus, although these disorders frequently overlap in clinical presentation (10). Ideally, a multidimensional and multidisciplinary approach for sexual pain should be implemented, but, unfortunately, there are a paucity of trials examining treatment efficacy. If possible, treatment should be individualized for each woman and her partner, and psychological and interpersonal issues should be addressed early on through psychotherapy. Evaluation and therapy also should address issues common to all of the sexual pain disorders, including the overall experience of pain, emotional and psychological issues, any past context of genital mutilation or sexual abuse, the genital mucus membrane, the pelvic floor, and sex and partner therapy.

Interventions, such as vaginal muscle EMG biofeedback, pelvic floor physical therapy with cognitive behavioral therapy, avoidance of scented soaps and panty liners, application of topical cromolyn or xylocaine to sites of allodynia, and use of fluconazole for associated recurrent candidiasis, have been used individually and in combination with reported clinical benefit but without scientific evidence. On the not-yet-proven assumption that neuropathic pain is at least in part responsible for sexual pain disorders, tricyclic antidepressants, venlafaxine, and anticonvulsants, usually carbamazepine or gabapentin are often used as part of the treatment and may offer some pain relief, although total pain resolution is infrequent. Most treatment plans for vaginismus include use of vaginal dilators that attempt to gradually reduce involuntary muscle tightening. Although this intervention is generally acknowledged to be highly effective and necessary for treating vaginismus, there has never been a randomized controlled treatment study examining it or any other therapy protocol.

References

1. **Basson R, Berman J, Burnett A, et al.** Report of the international consensus development conference on female sexual dysfunction: definitions and classifications. J Urol. 2000;163:888-93.
2. **Laumann EO, Paik A, Rosen RC.** Sexual dysfunction in the United States: prevalence and predictors. JAMA. 1999;281:537-44.
3. **Lindau ST, Schumm LP, Laumann EO, et al.** A study of sexuality and health among older adults in the United States. N Engl J Med. 2007;357:762-74.
4. **Basson R.** Clinical practice. Sexual desire and arousal disorders in women. N Engl J Med. 2006;354:1497-506.
5. **Bhasin S, Enzlin P, Coviello A, et al.** Sexual dysfunction in men and women with endocrine disorders. Lancet. 2007;369:597-611.
6. **Potter JE.** A 60-year-old woman with sexual difficulties. JAMA. 2007;297:620-33.
7. **Shifren JL, Braunstein GD, Simon JA, et al.** Transdermal testosterone treatment in women with impaired sexual function after oophorectomy. N Engl J Med. 2000;343:682-8.
8. **Raina R, Pahlajani G, Khan S, et al.** Female sexual dysfunction: classification, pathophysiology, and management. Fertil Steril. 2007;88: 1273-84.
9. **Taylor MJ, Rudkin L, Hawton K.** Strategies for managing antidepressant-induced sexual dysfunction: systematic review of randomised controlled trials. J Affect Disord. 2005;88:241-54.
10. **Meston CM, Bradford A.** Sexual dysfunctions in women. Annu Rev Clin Psychol. 2007;3:233-56.

F. Chronic Pelvic Pain

Sarina B. Schrager

KEY POINTS

- Chronic pelvic pain is an indication for 40% of the laparoscopies performed in the U.S.
- The rate of major depression among women with chronic pelvic pain is between 30% and 50%.
- The 4 most common causes of chronic pelvic pain are endometriosis, pelvic adhesions, interstitial cystitis, and irritable bowel syndrome.
- Up to 70% of women with chronic pelvic pain have more than one cause for their pain.
- Laparoscopy is controversial for the evaluation of chronic pelvic pain because 35–40% of the exams are normal and do not determine the cause of pain.
- Treatment of chronic pelvic pain is multidisciplinary and may include a physical therapist, a mental health professional, and a clinician.

Epidemiology

Chronic pelvic pain is defined as non-cyclical pain that lasts for over 6 months. It is very common, affecting about 15% of all women in their reproductive years. Chronic pelvic pain is a diagnosis associated with up to 10% of all outpatient gynecologic consultations, 40% of all laparoscopies, and 18% of all hysterectomies performed each year in the U.S. (1). In 1990, the estimated cost of services related to chronic pelvic pain was $2 billion (2).

Women with chronic pelvic pain have a much higher incidence of past sexual abuse than women in the general population, and they frequently have psychiatric comorbidities that accompany their chronic pain. Up to 50% of women diagnosed with chronic pelvic pain have major depression (2). Drug and alcohol abuse are associated with an increased likelihood of pain (3). There is no difference in prevalence based on race, ethnicity, education, or socioeconomic status (4).

The etiology of chronic pelvic pain is frequently multifactorial and comes from multiple organ systems. Up to 70% of women have more than one cause of their pain (5). The most common gynecologic causes of chronic pelvic pain are endometriosis and pelvic adhesions. The most common gastrointestinal cause is irritable bowel syndrome, and the most common urologic cause is interstitial cystitis (6). In addition, many women who have chronic pelvic pain also have some myofascial pain from the pelvic floor muscles (Table 4-18).

Table 4-18   Common Causes of Chronic Pelvic Pain

Gynecologic	Gastrointestinal	Urologic	Musculoskeletal
Endometriosis	Irritable bowel syndrome	Interstitial cystitis	Myofascial pain (abdominal wall or pelvic floor muscles)
Pelvic adhesions	Inflammatory bowel disease	Chronic urinary tract infections	Fibromyalgia
Pelvic congestion	Chronic constipation	Urethral syndrome	Coccygeal or low back pain
Pelvic inflammatory disease	Colitis	Radiation cystitis	Nerve pain
Adenomyosis Vulvodynia Uterine myomas	Diverticulitis	Urinary calculi	

Adapted from Reiter RC. Chronic pelvic pain. Clinical Obstetrics and Gynecology. 1990;33: 117–18 and Bordman R, Jackson B. Below the belt: approach to chronic pelvic pain. Canadian Family Physician. 2006;52:1556–62; with permission.

Pelvic congestion syndrome is an emerging cause of pelvic pain and has been described as pelvic aching that worsens with prolonged standing. Interstitial cystitis is a well-recognized contributor to chronic pelvic pain and is very common in women with established endometriosis (7).

Newer understanding of the chronic pain model has helped to clarify a multifactorial basis for chronic pelvic pain. The transition from an acute pain to a chronic pain state involves neuroplastic changes in the dorsal horn of the spinal cord (5). These changes cause allodynia, which is defined as a lower pain threshold resulting from a loss of inhibition of dorsal horn neurons. The neuropathic up-regulation of pain fibers results in multiple abnormal pain pathways that also connect different pelvic organs through common spinal cord innervation. Pain in one pelvic organ can therefore cause pain in a neighboring organ, which underlies the multifactorial cause of most pelvic pain syndromes.

Clinical Features

Initial evaluation of a woman with chronic pelvic pain includes a careful history to determine any pattern of the pain that would lead to a possible diagnosis. A complete medical, surgical, family, sexual, and psychological history should also be completed. It is important to get a sense of how the pain is affecting a woman's daily life. There are several screening questionnaires that have been validated to identify women with irritable bowel syndrome, interstitial cystitis, and domestic violence (6). Physical exam should include a general exam in addition to a thorough pelvic exam. Every effort should be made to replicate the pain through a bimanual or rectovaginal exam.

Laboratory evaluation is geared toward the likely diagnosis. Many women have a pelvic ultrasound to further evaluate her pelvic anatomy. Ultimately, many women undergo a diagnostic laparoscopy to evaluate the etiology of the pain. Laparoscopy is normal in 35–40% of these women. Endometriosis is diagnosed in about 30% of women at laparoscopy, and adhesions are diagnosed in about 25% (8). Many women also undergo a cystoscopy or a potassium sensitivity test to evaluate for interstitial cystitis. A potassium sensitivity test is an office-based test that involves inserting a catheter and filling the bladder with saline, then a potassium solution. Women with interstitial cystitis have more pain from the potassium solution than other women.

Treatment of a woman with chronic pelvic pain should be multi-modal to address the multifactorial nature of her pain. A strong relationship between the patient and the clinician is imperative as a basis for treatment to be successful. The first line of treatment includes pain control with non-narcotic medication. Hormonal manipulation with medroxyprogesterone acetate, oral contraceptive pills, or GnRH (gonatropin releasing hormone) analogues can be effective treatments for endometriosis-related pain. GnRH analogues can only be used for up to 6 months because of side effects, such as menopausal symptoms and osteoporosis. Medical treatment specific to the presumed cause of the pain is an important next step.

Laparoscopic treatment of endometriosis and lysis of dense adhesions (lysis of adhesions that are not severe is not proven to consistently decrease pain) are helpful in a subset of women. Hysterectomy is performed in women with untreatable pain and is most effective if accompanied by bilateral oopherectomy. This is a major surgical procedure that may include a myriad of complications, but can cure some pain related to endometriosis and pelvic congestion syndrome. Embolization of pelvic veins is an emerging treatment for pelvic congestion syndrome and shows promise in managing pain (9).

None of the above treatment modalities addresses the physiology of chronic pain. Several newer anticonvulsants (gabapentin, topiramate, valproic acid, pregabalin) and antidepressants, such as tricyclic antidepressants (TCAs) and selective serotonin reuptake inhibitors (SSRIs), have been successful in treating neuropathic pain from other sources. However, limited data are available in women with pelvic pain. Trigger point injections and botox injections in pelvic floor muscles show promise for treating myofascial pain (10). Multidisciplinary treatment teams should include mental health professionals, physical therapists, as well as physicians. Good quality evidence supports the treatment options in Box 4-5.

Box 4-5   Treatment Strategies for Chronic Pelvic Pain Supported by Consistent, High Quality Scientific Studies

- Combined oral contraceptive pills are an effective treatment for chronic pelvic pain, especially in women with dysmenorrhea.
- GnRH analogues are effective in decreasing symptoms caused by endometriosis and irritable bowel syndrome. Empiric treatment with these medications is an acceptable treatment strategy even without a laparoscopic diagnosis of endometriosis.
- NSAIDs are good for moderate pelvic pain, especially dysmenorrhea.
- Daily high dose progesterone is an effective treatment for pelvic pain associated with endometriosis and pelvic congestion syndrome.
- Laparoscopic destruction of endometriosis lesions is an effective treatment.
- Medical treatment plus counseling is more effective than medical treatment alone in decreasing pain.

Adapted from ACOG Practice Bulletin no. 51. Chronic pelvic pain. Obstetrics and Gynecology 2004;103:589–605; with permission.

References

1. **Zondervan K, Barlow DH.** Epidemiology of chronic pelvic pain. Bailliere's Best Practice and Research in Clinical Obstetrics and Gynecology. 2000;14:403–14.
2. **Reiter RC.** Chronic pelvic pain. Clinical Obstetrics and Gynecology. 1990;33:117–8.
3. **Latthe P, Mignini L, Gray R, et al.** Factors predisposing women to chronic pelvic pain: systematic review. BMJ. 2006;332:749–55.
4. ACOG Practice Bulletin no. 51. Chronic pelvic pain. Obstetrics and Gynecology. 2004;103(3):589–605.
5. **Butrick DW.** Chronic pelvic pain: how many surgeries are enough? Clinical Obstetrics and Gynecology. 2007;50(2):412–24.
6. **Bordman R, Jackson B.** Below the belt: approach to chronic pelvic pain. Canadian Family Physician. 2006;52:1556–62.
7. **Stanford EJ, Dell JR, Parsons CL.** The emerging presence of interstitial cystitis in gynecologic patients with chronic pelvic pain. Urology. 2007;69:53–9.
8. **Howard RM.** The role of laparoscopy as a diagnostic tool in chronic pelvic pain. Best Practices and Research in Clinical Obstetrics and Gynecology. 2000;14:467–94.
9. **Kim HS, Malhotra AD, Rowe PC, et al.** Embolotherapy for pelvic congestion syndrome: long term results. Journal of Vascular Interventional Radiology. 2006;17:289–97.
10. **Gomel V.** Clinical Opinion: chronic pelvic pain: a challenge. Journal of Minimally Invasive Gynecology. 2007;14:521–6.

G. Infertility

Juliemarie M. Sicilia and Tara D. Lathcop

KEY POINTS

- Infertility is becoming a more common diagnosis as women increasingly delay child-bearing until later years.
- An optimal work-up of female and male infertility can be conducted by primary care physicians.
- In women over 35 years of age, an infertility work-up should be considered with a 6-month duration of infertility rather than a 1-year duration.
- Infertility work-ups should be specific, cost-effective, and targeted to the individual couple/patient.
- There are several resources available to patients and physicians, including some alternative therapies, that have been shown to be helpful.
- Patients need the support of a primary care physician, since the diagnosis of infertility has the potential to be life-altering in many ways.

Epidemiology

Infertility is a disease that affects up to 15% of the population in the U.S. (1). The etiology of infertility in women includes ovulatory dysfunction (40%), tubal and pelvic pathology (40%), unexplained infertility and unusual problems (20%). In couples, the causes of infertility include male factor (35%), tubal and pelvic pathology (35%), ovulatory dysfunction (15%), and unexplained infertility and unusual problems (15%) (1).

Clinical Presentation

Women present for care, complaining that they are unable to become pregnant. This condition has physical, cultural, financial, and psychosocial implications that differ widely among different individuals. Some women may seek medical care after an "infertile" duration of a month, while some patients will not seek care until after many years of infertility.

The formal definition of primary infertility is failure to conceive after 1 year of attempting pregnancy with regular, unprotected intercourse. Secondary infertility is defined as the situation in which couples have achieved 1 pregnancy but have been unable to conceive a second time.

Practically, in women over the age of 35 years, a physician may consider an infertility diagnostic work-up after only 6 months of attempting pregnancy, rather than waiting the full year, because of the decrease in fecundity in women as they age (2).

Our emphasis in this chapter is on women, but male factor infertility requires at least brief discussion, since it is the cause of about a third of all infertility cases. The initial evaluation for male factor infertility includes a detailed history and physical examination and semen analysis. It is an easier, less invasive work-up than what female patients frequently have to undergo.

Differential Diagnosis

The most cost-effective, accurate way to begin an infertility work-up is with a detailed, meticulous medical history and physical examination. Medical history questions and physical examination details that should be investigated in women are included in Table 4-19.

Table 4-19   Evaluation of Infertility

Medical History Details	Physical Exam Details
Menarche	Bimanual exam and uterine size
Duration/regularity of periods	Any pelvic masses
Amount of clotting and bleeding of periods	
Gravity/parity within each relationship	Thyromegaly
Genetic disorders (i.e., Turner's syndrome)	Signs of androgen excess (hirsuitism, clitoromegaly, acne)
Endocrine disorders (i.e., thyroid, DM, PCOS)	Secondary sex characteristics (breast development, pubic and axillary hair distribution)
STD exposure/PID history	Any galactorrhea
Psychological stressors	Vaginal discharge
Uterine, cervical abdominal surgery (i.e., D and C, LEEP)	Cervical discharge
Duration of infertility	Vaginal patency and structure
Frequency of coitus	Cervical patency and structure
Lubricants, douches used during intercourse	Acanthosis nigrans
Substance abuse (tobacco and caffeine)	Weight loss/gain
Toxin exposure	
Radiation exposure	
Medications taken (i.e., anticholinergics and hormones)	
Type of cervical mucous	
Premenstrual symptoms	
Breast tenderness	
Mittelschmurtz	
Age	
Eating disorder history	

Ovulatory dysfunction is the most common cause of female infertility. A cycle day 21 serum progesterone level >3 ng/ml is indicative that ovulation has occurred. A level >10 ng/ml is suggestive of normal corpus luteum function and a normally functioning endometrium. A luteal phase defect is due to the inadequate secretion of progesterone post-ovulation and can potentially contribute to infertility. An endometrial biopsy performed on cycle day 25–28 also has been used to determine if a luteal phase defect exists. The laboratory is able to determine whether the endometrium is developed adequately for the cycle day when the specimen was obtained. The prevalence and clinical relevance of luteal phase defect diagnosed by endometrial biopsy as a cause of infertility have been questioned (2).

Clinically, breast tenderness, mittelschmurtz (mid-cycle pelvic pain from ovulation), a menstrual cycle length of 25–35 days, a biphasic basal body temperature curve, pre-menstrual symptoms (breast tenderness, mood swings, etc.) and the change from E type (estrogen-predominant, thin watery, stretchy) to P type (progesterone-predominant and thicker) mucous suggests normal ovulatory cycles. Ovulation dysfunction is the most common reason for infertility in women over the age of 35 years. The differential diagnosis of ovulatory dysfunction includes PCOS (polycystic ovarian syndrome), premature ovarian failure, hypothalamic amenorrhea, congenital adrenal hyperplasia, and pituitary- or androgen-secreting tumors. Low FSH levels may be indicative of PCOS or hypothalamic amenorrhea. Galactorrhea may be a sign of a pituitary tumor, which can cause anovulation. Serum TSH (thyroid stimulating hormone) and prolactin levels are used to exclude hypothyroidism and pituitary tumors, respectively.

Structural abnormalities of the uterus and fallopian tubes are the second most common cause of female infertility. Uterine factor infertility includes uterine fibroids, uterine polyps, uterine structural anomalies such as bicornuate uterus and uterine synechiae (Asherman's syndrome). Clinically, menorrhagia, or dysfunctional uterine bleeding, as well as an enlarged uterus on bimanual examination, may be found with uterine factor infertility. Hysterosalpingogram (HSG) or sonohystogram (SHG) assists in the diagnosis of uterine structural abnormalities by providing a clear view of the anatomy of the uterus. Hysteroscopy also may be necessary to evaluate the endometrial cavity. Not all uterine abnormalities will require surgical correction, but surgical consultation is recommended. Tubal factor infertility may result from an assortment of pelvic pathology, including endometriosis, adnexal adhesions from previous abdominal or pelvic surgery, STDs, or previous ectopic pregnancy. Diagnostic testing options to rule out the diagnosis of tubal obstruction include HSG and laparoscopy. A 2005 Cochrane review suggests that HSG with tubal flushing can be used as treatment to increase pregnancy rates (3).

Cervical factor infertility is less common and can be overcome with IUI (intrauterine insemination) and IVF (in vitro fertilization). Differential diagnosis includes cervical infection, anti-sperm antibodies, and cervical stenosis. The postcoital test (PCT) is usually performed at mid-cycle

(cycle day 12–15). The couple is advised to have intercourse and present for examination 6 hours afterward. Cervical mucus and sperm motility are measured to assess for an abnormal immune response by the woman to the man's sperm. The PCT is no longer a required test in the diagnostic work-up for every couple. It can be useful in couples hoping to be able to have timed intercourse, and it may be helpful with decision-making to pursue aggressive treatment versus continued watchful waiting (2).

Oocyte production and quality worsen as women age. A cycle day 3 serum FSH (follicle stimulating hormone) and estradiol levels are an estimate of egg quality and ovarian reserve or failure. A serum FSH level above 10 IU/L and a serum estradiol level >80 pg/ml may indicate ovarian failure and/or low ovarian reserve and poor egg quality. Inhibin levels show promise as another method of assessing ovarian reserve but are currently not a recommended part of the initial diagnostic evaluation (2).

A clomiphene challenge test may be useful in determining ovarian reserve. To perform this test, serum FSH is measured serially on cycle days 3 and 10. Clomiphene citrate (Clomid) 100 mg is taken orally by the patient daily on cycle days 5–9. In women with poor ovarian reserve, an FSH level >2 standard deviations above the mean (this will vary from laboratory to laboratory) correlates with a poor response to ovulation induction (1,2).

Polycystic ovarian syndrome (PCOS) is a common cause of ovulatory dysfunction, with an increasing incidence in the general population. It is estimated that over 3 million women of reproductive age in the U.S. have PCOS (1). PCOS can be diagnosed clinically by irregular menses with central obesity (waist >35'') and diagnostically with a 2-hour 75 g glucose tolerance test measuring both the glucose and the insulin levels. Measurement of a single fasting glucose: fasting insulin ratio has fallen out of favor as the preferred diagnostic test (1). Sonographically, women with PCOS can have normal-appearing ovaries, so this is not the best diagnostic test. If hyperandrogenic signs are present, a total testosterone as well as a morning fasting 17-hydroxyprogesterone should be measured to look for androgen-secreting tumors (see chapter on PCOS).

Hypercoagulable disorders, such as antiphospholipid antibody syndrome, will usually manifest as repeated spontaneous abortion. In women who have 2–3 repeat spontaneous pregnancy losses, testing for anti-phospholipid antibodies is warranted. Literature review of prospective trials shows that the presence of anti-phospholipid antibodies does not affect success with IVF (2). A summary of diagnostic laboratory testing is found in Table 4-20.

Clinical Care and Prevention

There are some preventable factors in female infertility. These include cessation of smoking tobacco, maintaining a healthy body weight (BMI 20–27), and limiting caffeine and alcohol consumption. Data from the Nurse's Health Study suggest that diets rich in dairy products and vegetable protein, yet low in trans-fats, may help women avoid ovulatory dysfunction and be more likely to conceive (4).

Table 4-20   Diagnosis of Infertility

Differential Diagnosis	Diagnostic Labs Used
Uterine factor	Hysterosalpingogram
	Sonohysterography
	Hysteroscopy
Cervical factor	Postcoital test
	Cervical cultures for chlamydia
Male factor	Semen analysis
Ovulatory dysfunction	Day 21 progesterone level
	Endometrial biopsy
Ovarian reserve	Day 3 FSH and estradiol levels
	Clomiphene Challenge test
Tubal factor/endometriosis	HSG
	Laparoscopy + /− biopsy,
Endocrine factors	TSH
	Antithyroid antibodies
	Prolactin
Hypercoagulable states	Anti-phospholipid antibodies
PCOS	2 h, 75 g GTT
	LH:FSH > / = 2:1 ratio
Androgen excess	17-hydroxyprogesterone
	Testosterone

Basal body temperature (BBT) measurement to predict ovulation is based on the thermogenic effect of progesterone on the body. BBT measurement is performed by the patient and measured at the same time daily upon awakening. Any thermometer with degree separation can be used. BBT is inexpensive and can be tracked by women to determine ovulation. Normal BBT is 97–98°F. A rise in temperature of 0.4–0.8°F above this baseline is seen within 48 hours after an LH (lutenizing hormone) surge, with return to baseline temperature with menses if no pregnancy occurs. BBT also can be used to identify short or long follicular and luteal phases in a woman's cycle.

Physicians can counsel patients on natural family planning techniques for assessment of ovulation as well. A urinary LH detection kit can be used by women to determine ovulatory cycles with greater ease and accuracy than BBT alone. The Clear-Blue Easy ovulation predictor kit can be used daily by women to sample their urine to assess for the LH surge. A change in the test strip occurs when the LH level rises. It is reported out as low, moderate, or high fertility. It is recommended that couples have intercourse on the days of high fertility to maximize success. The monitor kit costs approximately $225.00, and a month's refill of test strips is about $35.00. Women can buy simple test strips at the pharmacy that determine the level of LH in their urine.

Some women may be interested in alternative modalities for treating infertility. Data on acupuncture for improving pregnancy and birth rates after embryo transfer have been somewhat controversial, although a recent meta-analysis indicates support for acupuncture (5). The most scientific mind–body medicine research has been published by Alice Domar, PhD (7). Dr. Domar's program consists of mindful meditation, guided imagery, and yoga, which may help relieve depressive symptoms and ameliorate psychological stress in women undergoing infertility treatment (Box 4-6).

Treatments of infertility will vary, depending on the etiology of infertility (Table 4-21). Every woman has different factors contributing to her infertility, so every treatment plan must be individualized for maximum success and cost-effectiveness. Timed intercourse is a viable inexpensive option for some couples who have no tubal, cervical, uterine patency, or male infertility problems. Timed intercourse can be practiced with or without combined ovulation induction.

Clomid (clomiphene citrate) is an oral medication for ovulation induction. There are many reasons for infertility patients to be treated with Clomid, so pregnancy rates will vary depending on the age and etiology of infertility, but approximately 50% of women who respond to Clomid and ovulate conceive within 6 cycles of Clomid therapy (2). Clomiphene's mechanism of action involves binding to estrogen receptors for long durations thereby preventing endogenous estrogen from binding to the receptors. Clomid is usually begun at an initial dose of 50 mg/day initiated on cycle days 2–5 and is continued for a total of

Table 4-21   Infertility Treatment Problems

Infertility Problem	Treatment Options
Ovulatory dysfunction	Ovulation induction +/− IVF or IUI
Tubal pathology	HSG with tubal flushing or IVF
Cervical factor	IUI or IVF
PCOS	Metformin +/− ovulation induction
Uterine factor	Consultation for possible surgical correction
Hupercoagulation disorder	Heparin, aspirin
Unexplained infertility	IVF, IUI, ovulation induction
Ovarian failure	Donor oocytes or embryos
Male factor	IVF with ICSI

5 days of dosing. If the first trial of 50 mg/day is unsuccessful, Clomid can be increased to 100 mg/day for the same 5-day cycle (100 mg is the maximal allowed dose by the FDA). In women with PCOS, Clomid is often combined with metformin in doses of 1000–2000 mg/day total dosage. For some women with PCOS, weight loss and metformin may be successful without resorting to clomiphene ovulation induction (2).

The content and description of every possible gonadotropin ovulation induction protocol is well beyond the scope of this chapter. Basically, most ovulation induction protocols utilize a low-dose GnRH agonist (such as leuprolide) for suppression of endogenous LH surges. Pregnancy rates are increased by combining suppression with exogenous gonadotropins. Gonadotropins (either human menopausal gonadotropin, such as Repronex, or recombinant FSH, such as Follistim) are used for follicle stimulation and development of multiple oocytes which can be harvested and used for assisted reproductive procedures. Next, hCG (human chorionic gonadotropin) administration is used to complete oocyte maturation and is followed by either ovulation (for IUI) or by trans-vaginal oocyte retrieval and harvest (for IVF and ICSI cycles) (1,2).

IUI can be used in women who have patent fallopian tubes but have cervical factor infertility. IUI bypasses the cervix by placing a washed sperm sample inside the uterine cavity. Fertilization and embryo implantation are then allowed to naturally occur within the uterus. IUI can be used in a natural cycle (no ovulation induction) or in combination with clomiphene or exogenous gonadotropins in women who have ovulatory dysfunction but tubal patency.

IVF is the treatment of choice for most women with tubal obstruction or idiopathic infertility. There are 2 ways by which IVF can be performed. Natural-cycle IVF allows follicles to develop naturally without gonadotropins. The oocytes are then surgically harvested for IVF. Ovulation-induction IVF uses gonadotropins to stimulate follicle recruitment and development prior to oocyte retrieval. Once the oocytes are retrieved, they are combined with the sperm sample in the laboratory. Fertilization then takes place via cell culture, and embryos develop. Embryos can be transferred back into a woman's uterus for implantation on day 3 (cleavage stage) of development or on days 5–6 of development (blastocyst stage) (1,2). The pregnancy rates are similar for cleavage transfers and blastocyst transfers in most patients. Blastocyst transfers are thought to produce better implantation than cleavage transfers (2). Some fertility centers cite over 50% pregnancy rates in couples with infertility (8).

Patients undergoing ovulation induction with gonadotropins or Clomid require frequent measurement of follicle size via trans-vaginal ultrasound and frequent monitoring of serum estradiol levels prior to oocyte harvest or IUI. Gonadotropins, Clomid, IUI, and IVF carry risks of multiple gestations, ectopic pregnancy, possible allergic reaction to medications, possible infection, and the ovarian hyperstimulation syndrome. In addition, IVF also carries the risk for increased preterm births and preterm labor (9).

ICSI (intracytoplasmic sperm injection) is the treatment of choice for male factor infertility problems of low sperm motility. ISCI has been shown to be safe and effective without any difference in development as compared with children born as the result of standard IVF therapy (10). ICSI is performed once oocytes are retrieved, and an individual sperm is injected into an individual oocyte with microscopic surgical technique (2).

Treatment for unexplained infertility is controversial. A 2005 Cochrane review concluded that the advantage of IVF for unexplained infertility could not be proved over IUI or expectant management because the studies were just too small to have adequate power to prove clear benefit (11). However, another source reports utility of short-term (<6 cycles) of IUI and IVF (2).

In women with ovarian failure or poor ovarian reserve, donor oocytes or donor embryos are the most successful option for achieving pregnancy. The success rates for donor embryos or oocytes are directly related to the age of the donor, not the age of the recipient (3).

The cost of IVF and ISCI is prohibitive for many patients. The average cost of an IVF cycle is around $10 000–$15 000 with no guarantee of success. These financial stressors also contribute to a patient's psychological stress level. Eleven states, including New York, Massachusetts, and California, have legislatively mandated health insurance coverage for assisted reproductive technology; however, in most states, insurance companies are not required to cover assisted reproductive procedures.

Some women will opt for the adoption option after many failed attempts at infertility treatment. Information about types of adoption and support of the patient's decision to stop infertility treatment is crucial to these patients. This diagnosis is extremely stressful, both physically, from the gonadotropins and hormone supplementation, as well as psychologically, while waiting for treatment to produce a pregnancy, or making decisions about treatment. Offering patients a referral for counseling is prudent and frequently necessary. A physician who is available to act as a source of information and support to women can be invaluable to infertility patients.

References

1. **Speroff L.** Clinical Gynecologic Endocrinology and Infertility, 7th ed. Philadelphia, Lippincott, 2005
2. American society of reproductive medicine: compendium of practice committee reports, vol 86, sup 4. Birmingham, AL, Nov 2006.
3. **Johnson N, et al.** Tubal flushing for subfertility. Cochrane Database of Systemic Reviews. 2005;(2):CD003718.
4. **Chavarro J.** Diet and lifestyle in the prevention of ovulatory disorder infertility. Obstet Gynecol. 2007;110:1050–58.
5. **Manheimer E, et al.** Effects of acupuncture on rates of pregnancy and live birth among women undergoing in vitro fertilization: systematic review and meta-analysis. BMJ. 2008; Feb 7 [Epub ahead of print].
6. **Pandian Z, et al.** Invitro fertilization for unexplained subfertility. Cochrane Database of Systemic Reviews. 2005;(2):CD003357.
7. **Domar A.** Conquering Infertility. NYC, New York, Penguin Books, 2002.

8. 2004 Assisted Reproductive Technology Report, available at www.cdc. gov/ART, accessed 4/7/08.

9. **Van Voorhis BJ.** Outcomes from assisted reproductive technology. Obstet Gynecol. 2006;107:183–200.

10. **Place I, Englert Y.** A perspective longitudinal study of the physical, psychomotor and intellectual development of singleton children up to 5 years who were conceived by ISCI compared with children conceived spontaneously and by IVF. Fertil Steril. 2003;80:1388–97.

11. **Pandian Z, et al.** In vitro fertilization for unexplained subfertility. Cochrane Database of Systemic Reviews. 2005;(2):CD003357.

H. Uterine Fibroid Tumors

Sarina B. Schrager

KEY POINTS

- Uterine fibroid tumors occur in up to 30% of reproductive aged women.
- African American women have a higher risk of fibroids than Caucasian women.
- Family history is an important risk factor for developing fibroids.
- Gonadotropin releasing hormone (GnRH) analogues are an effective treatment before surgical intervention to shrink the size of the fibroids.
- Submucous fibroids that distort the uterine cavity significantly decrease fertility
- Fibroids are the leading indication for hysterectomy in the U.S.
- Uterine artery embolization and hysteroscopic myomectomy are 2 less invasive procedures that provide treatment options for women with fibroids who do not want a hysterectomy.

Epidemiology

Uterine leiomyomas (fibroid tumors) are very common, occurring in up to 30% of all reproductive aged women. One prevalence study looked at ultrasounds of over 1300 Caucasian and African American women between the ages of 35 and 49. This study found that over 80% of the African American women and 70% of the Caucasian women had ultrasound evidence of fibroids (1).

Fibroid tumors are benign growths of uterine smooth muscle cells and are estrogen-dependent. The incidence of fibroids increases with age. Women are most likely to be diagnosed with fibroids when they are in their 40s. African-American women and women with a family history of fibroid tumors are more commonly affected. African American women have a 2.9 times higher incidence of uterine fibroids, and women who have a first degree relative with fibroids have a 2.5 times higher incidence (2). Smoking, grand multiparity (>5 pregnancies), prolonged use of hormonal contraception (both progestin only and estrogen- and progestin-containing contraceptives), and postmenopausal status all decrease the risk of uterine fibroids.

Clinical Features

Many fibroid tumors are asymptomatic. The most common symptoms of fibroid tumors are menorrhagia and pelvic pain. Uterine fibroids also have been implicated in recurrent pregnancy loss and infertility. Extremely large fibroid tumors can cause obstructive symptoms, such as constipation and urinary obstruction. Menorrhagia from fibroids can cause anemia. However, due to a paucity of controlled studies, it is difficult to determine whether the fibroids were the cause of each of the symptoms (3).

Diagnosis of fibroid tumors begins with the palpation of uterine abnormalities on bimanual exam. Subsequently, pelvic ultrasounds are an excellent first step in confirming the diagnosis. In some situations, if the ultrasound is not confirmatory, a pelvic MRI may be helpful. Sonohysterography and hysteroscopy also can help evaluate the characteristics of submucosal fibroid tumors. Differential diagnosis of a palpated uterine mass should include a uterine leiomyosarcoma, ovarian pathology (both benign and malignant), or another type of pelvic malignancy arising from the bladder or colon. Distinguishing between a uterine myoma (fibroid) and a leiomyosarcoma may be accomplished with a pelvic MRI and a total serum LDH and LDH isoenzyme-3 (2).

Treatment of Uterine Fibroids

In cases when the fibroid is asymptomatic and a woman is not anemic, no treatment is necessary. Choosing appropriate therapeutic options depends on many factors, including the woman's age, her desire for future fertility, the type and size of the fibroid, and the specific symptoms experienced. If a woman is in her late 40s and close to anticipated menopause, often a watchful waiting approach is considered, since the symptoms will resolve with involution of the fibroid after menopause. Medication treatment with GnRH analogues effectively reduces the size of the fibroids and is a useful adjunct before surgery, making the surgical procedure easier. Side effects of menopausal symptoms and osteoporosis limit the long-term use of these medications (4). There is not enough evidence to support the use of nonsteroidal anti-inflammatory drugs (NSAIDs), hormonal therapy, raloxifene or tamoxifen, or mifepristone, although some of these therapies show promise in decreasing the size and symptoms associated with fibroids (Table 4-22).

Surgical options to treat fibroids range from hysterectomy to uterine artery embolization. If a woman wants to maintain fertility, specific

Table 4-22   Medical Treatments for Uterine Fibroids

Medication	Benefits	Disadvantages
GnRH analogues	Induce "medical menopause," thereby causing a hypoestrogenic state and shrinking the fibroid tumor.	Expensive. Many side effects (menopausal symptoms and osteoporosis) that limit use for much >6 months. Usually used prior to hysterectomy to shrink the fibroids. Fibroids regrow rapidly when discontinued (4).
Selective estrogen reuptake modulators (tamoxifen or raloxifene)	Act as estrogen antagonists in the uterus to decrease the size of the uterus.	No evidence yet to support the routine use of these medications (8).
Mifepristone	Acts as a progesterone antagonist and may decrease size of fibroid.	Small studies only. Needs larger trial before recommendation in practice (9).
Hormone therapy	Combined estrogen/ progestin may decrease endogenous estrogen levels.	No evidence to show effectiveness in limiting fibroid growth or improving symptoms.
NSAIDs	Decrease prostaglandin levels.	No evidence to show effectiveness in limiting fibroid growth or improving symptoms.
Depot medroxyprogesterone acetate	Induce endometrial atrophy and possibly decrease serum estrogen levels.	Small, uncontrolled study showed decreased menorrhagia in women with fibroids (10).
Levonorgestrel intrauterine system (Mirena IUD)	May induce endometrial atrophy and decrease menstrual bleeding.	Research shows that the Mirena IUD may decrease menstrual blood loss in women with menorrhagia secondary to fibroids but does not affect fibroid size (11).

Table 4-23   Surgical Treatment for Uterine Fibroids

Procedure	Description	Benefits	Disadvantages
Hysterectomy	Surgical removal of the entire uterus either abdominally or vaginally (easier recovery).	Definitive therapy.	Invasive procedure, several-day hospital stay, no future fertility.
Myomectomy	Removal of fibroid tumor surgically or via hysteroscopy.	Preserves fertility, less invasive than hysterectomy.	Recurrence rate of 15–30% at 5 years.
Myolysis	Destruction of fibroid tumors with heat, laser, or cryotherapy.	Minimally invasive, fewer complications than other surgical interventions.	Unknown recurrence rate. May cause uterine adhesions.
Uterine artery embolization	Interventional radiologists insert a catheter through the femoral artery to the uterine artery and inject particles that block the blood flow to the fibroid, causing it to infarct.	Less invasive than other surgical options, so has fewer side effects and faster recovery times. May preserve fertility.	Post-procedure pain necessitates at least one night in the hospital. Future fertility unknown. Long-term data unknown.

From Evans P, Brunsell S. Uterine fibroid tumors: diagnosis and treatment. American Family Physician. 2007;75:1503–8 and Smith SJ. Uterine fibroid embolization. American Family Physician. 2000;61:3601–7, 3611–12; with permission.

surgical interventions should be avoided. Half of all hysterectomies performed in the U.S. include uterine myomas as an indication (5). Uterine artery embolization is a less invasive procedure that is effective in decreasing the size of the fibroids. Other surgical options include myomectomy, myolysis, and hysteroscopic resection of a submucous fibroid (Table 4-23).

Infertile Women

Controversy exists regarding whether fibroids actually cause infertility. A meta-analysis found that submucous fibroids that distort the uterine cavity significantly decrease fertility. However, intramural and subserosal fibroids did not affect fertility rates (6). In women with large fibroids and either recurrent pregnancy loss or infertility, myomectomy should be considered to improve chances for future fertility.

Pregnant Women

Most fibroids in pregnant women do not significantly change in size during the pregnancy. When fibroids do grow during pregnancy, the majority of the growth occurs in the first trimester. Large submucosal fibroids cause the most pregnancy complications, such as pain from degeneration, vaginal bleeding, placental abruption (when the fibroid is sub-placental), intrauterine growth retardation, and preterm labor (7). Large fibroids can degenerate and cause severe pain in pregnant women. This phenomenon usually happens during the late first trimester or early second trimester and can necessitate inpatient pain control.

References

1. **Day Baird D, Dunson DB, Hill MC, et al.** High cumulative incidence of uterine leiomyoma in black and white women: ultrasound evidence. American Journal of Obstetrics and Gynecology. 2003;188:100–107.
2. **Parker WH.** Etiology, symptomatology, and diagnosis of uterine myomas. Fertility and Sterilit. 2007;87:725–36.
3. **Evans P, Brunsell S.** Uterine fibroid tumors: diagnosis and treatment. American Family Physician. 2007;75:1503–8.
4. **Lethaby A, Vollenhoven B, Sowter M.** Pre-operative GnRH analogue therapy before hysterectomy or myomectomy for uterine fibroids. Cochrane Database Systematic Review. 2001;(2):CD000547.
5. **Olive DL, Lindheim SR, Pritts EA.** Conservative surgical management of uterine myomas. Obstetrics and Gynecology Clinics of North America. 2006;33:115–24.
6. **Pritts EA.** Fibroids and infertility: a systematic review of the evidence. Obstetrical and Gynecologic Survey. 2001;56:483–91.
7. **Ouyang DW, Economy KE, Norwitz ER.** Obstetric complications of fibroids. Obstetric and Gynecologic Clinics of North America. 2006;33:153–69.
8. **Lingxia X, Taixiang W, Xiaoyan C.** Selective estrogen receptor modulators (SERMs) for uterine leiomyomas. Cochrane Database Systematic Review. 2007;(2):CD005287.
9. **Fiscella K, Eisinger SH, Meldrum S, et al.** Effect of mifepristone for symptomatic leiomyomata on quality of life and uterine size: a randomized controlled trial. Obstetrics and Gynecology. 2006;108:1381–7.
10. **Venkatachalam S, Bagratee JS, Moodley J.** Medical management of uterine fibroids with medroxyprosterone acetate (Depo Provera): a pilot study. Journal of Obstetrics and Gynaecology. 2004;24:798–800.
11. **Kaunitz AM.** Progestin-releasing intrauterine systems and leiomyoma. Contraception. 2007;75:S130–3.
12. **Smith SJ.** Uterine fibroid embolization. American Family Physician. 2000;61:3601–7, 3611–12.

I. Vaginitis
Suparna Chhibber

KEY POINTS

- Bacterial vaginosis (BV) is the most common cause of vaginitis in the U.S., followed by yeast and trichomonas.
- BV results from a disturbance of normal vaginal flora and loss of hydrogen peroxide production by lactobacilli, leading to an overgrowth of predominantly anaerobic bacteria, such as *Gardnerella vaginalis*, *Mobilincus*, *Bacteriodes*, *Peptostreptococcus*, and genital *Mycoplasmas*.
- Metronidazole is the drug of choice for the treatment of BV.
- BV during pregnancy is associated with an approximately two-fold risk of preterm labor, premature rupture of the membranes, and low birth-weight.
- *Candida albicans* is the most common yeast associated with vulvovaginal candidiasis. Non-*albicans* species are rare but are responsible for more resistant infections.
- Yeast vaginitis presents with vulvar pruritus and a "cottage cheese"-like vaginal discharge.
- Treatment of yeast vaginitis with topical antifungal preparations leads to resolution of infection in most cases.
- Trichomonal vaginitis is associated with copious, frothy malodorous vaginal discharge.
- The sexual partner of a woman with trichomonal infections should be treated.
- Patients should be offered screening, since vaginitis may be associated with other sexually transmitted infections (STIs).

One of the most frequent gynecological diagnoses encountered by physicians providing healthcare to women is vaginitis (1). Normal vaginal secretions arise from vulvar and vaginal glands and contain exfoliated cells, cervical mucus, and microorganisms. The normal flora in the vagina is composed of an average of 6 aerobic bacteria, the most common of which is hydrogen peroxide-producing lactobacillus. Vaginal cells stimulated by estrogen synthesize glycogen, which is broken down to lactic acid by the cells themselves and by lactobacilli. The production of lactic acid maintains the normal vaginal pH below 4.5 (2). Vaginitis develops as a result of a change in the vaginal flora by introduction of a pathogen or change in the environment that permits proliferation of pathogens (1). It is most often associated with infection or atrophic changes. Vulvovaginal candidiasis, BV, and trichomoniasis are the 3 most common forms of infectious vaginitis (3). Evaluation of these conditions includes a thorough history and physical examination, speculum examination of the vagina, pH testing, and wet mount and potassium hydroxide (KOH) preparations of the vaginal discharge.

Bacterial Vaginosis

Epidemiology

BV is the most common form of vaginitis in U.S. (2). It is more prevalent in African American women (30–50%) compared to non-Hispanic white women (10–20%) (2). Risk factors associated with BV include number of sexual partners in the last year, douching, smoking, and low socio-economic status (4,5).

Clinical Features

Women with BV usually complain of a thin, off-white discharge with a "fishy odor" that is accentuated after sexual intercourse. Clinical examination reveals the characteristic-smelling discharge adhering to normal-appearing vaginal walls (1).

Diagnosis and Differential Diagnosis

In clinical practice, BV is diagnosed primarily using the Amsel's criteria (1) which include: 1) thin homogenous discharge, 2) vaginal pH >4.5, 3) positive whiff test, and 4) clue cells (vaginal epithelial cells coated with bacteria) present on microscopic examination of the discharge. Three out of the 4 criteria are required for making the diagnosis (1). Ninety percent of women can be diagnosed correctly using these criteria. Another method of diagnosis is using Gram-stained vaginal smears. Since *Gardnerella vaginalis* can be found in asymptomatic women, a vaginal culture is not helpful in diagnosing BV. The differential diagnosis includes other common causes of vaginitis, such as vulvovaginal candidiasis, trichomoniasis, atrophic vaginitis, chemical irritation, and allergies (1).

Treatment of BV

The CDC recommends treatment of BV with metronidazole 500 mg orally twice a day for 7 days (6). Other treatment options and alternative regimens may also be used (Table 4-24). Because BV is associated with adverse pregnancy outcomes, all pregnant women with symptomatic infection require treatment. Metronidazole 500 mg orally twice a day for 7 days is the recommended regimen. Alternatively, metronidazole 250 mg orally 3 times a day for 7 days or clindamycin 300 mg orally twice a day for 7 days can be used. One month after the completion of treatment, a follow-up evaluation should be done to assess the effectiveness of therapy (6).

Table 4-24   Treatment of Bacterial Vaginosis

Treatment of choice		
Metronidazole	500 mg orally	One tablet twice a day for 7 days
Other treatment options		
Metronidazole	0.75% gel	5 g intravaginally for 5 days
Clindamycin	2% cream	5 g intravaginally for 7 days
Alternative regimen		
Clindamycin	300 mg orally	One tablet twice a day for 7 days
Clindamycin	100 mg ovules	One ovule intravaginally for 3 days

From Workowski K, Berman S. Centers for Disease Control and Prevention. Sexually Transmitted Diseases Treatment Guidelines, MMWR 2006;55:51–57; with permission.

Vulvovaginal Candidiasis

Epidemiology

Vulvovaginal candidiasis is the second most common cause of vaginitis in the U.S. (1). Seventy-five percent of women have an episode of vaginal candidiasis at some time during their lives, and about 5% will have recurrent infections (1). *Candida albicans* is the causative agent responsible for most cases. It is commonly found in vaginal flora and may be found in asymptomatic women. Less common species like *C. glabrata* may contribute to more resistant infections (7). The organism is commensal and becomes pathogenic when the host environment changes. Predisposing factors leading to vulvovaginal candidiasis include uncontrolled diabetes, antibiotic use, oral contraceptives, immunosuppression, HIV/AIDS, douching and use of similar feminine products, and orogenital intercourse (8).

Clinical Features

Patients with symptomatic vulvovaginal candidiasis usually present with acute pruritus and a thick, white, and "cottage cheese"-like discharge. Vaginal soreness, irritation, and vulvar burning are other associated symptoms. Dysuria and dyspareunia also are common during symptomatic episodes (9).

Diagnosis

A thorough evaluation is necessary since most of the symptoms and signs are nonspecific. Examinations should include a thorough inspection of the vulva and vagina, speculum examination of vagina and cervix, vaginal pH measurement, and microscopic examination of saline wet mount and KOH preparation of the discharge. Vaginal pH usually remains normal (<4.5) and may help to exclude some of the other causes of vulvovaginitis, like BV and trichomonal vaginitis. Microscopic examination of a saline preparation of the discharge usually reveals yeast or pseudohyphae. A 10% KOH preparation of the discharge makes it easier to visualize the fungal elements because it dissolves the vaginal epithelial cells (8). Routine culture is not necessary if microscopy is positive, but may be indicated if negative and the pH is normal. A positive culture by itself cannot be used to definitely diagnose vaginal candidiasis since 10–15% of asymptomatic women are colonized by *Candida*. Ideally, correlations of clinical findings, microscopic examination of the discharge, and culture are required for the diagnosis (9). Differential diagnosis includes other common causes of vaginitis, like BV and trichomonial vaginitis.

Prevention and Clinical Care

Vulvovaginal candidiasis is a common disease for which there are no specific prevention strategies. Therapy with probiotic lactobacilli has not proven to be beneficial in preventing recurrence after antibiotic therapy (9). Over-the-counter availability of topical antifungals leads to self-diagnosis and treatment with the possibility of emerging resistance (9). Care should be taken by the physician not to treat on the basis of such self-diagnosis.

Vulvovaginal candidiasis can be classified as uncomplicated and complicated. Uncomplicated infection is a mild to moderate infection, likely to be *Candida albicans* occurring sporadically in non-immunocompromised women. Recurrent (4 or more infections in 1 year) or severe infection with *Candida sp.* other than *C. albicans* in women with uncontrolled diabetes, immunosuppression, or debilitation, or in pregnant women is considered as complicated vulvovaginosis. The Centers for Disease Control and Prevention (CDC) recommends treatment of uncomplicated vulvovaginosis with a short course of topical azoles (6). These are more effective in treating vulvovaginal candidiasis than nystatin. Relief of symptoms and negative culture is obtained in 80–90% of patients who complete the therapy (6) (Table 4-25).

Patients with recurrent vulvovaginitis need to be evaluated for diabetes or immunodeficiency. If there are no identified factors for recurrence,

Table 4-25   Treatments of Uncomplicated Vulvovaginitis

Miconazole (OTC)	100 mg vaginal suppository	One suppository for 7 d
Miconazole (OTC)	200 mg vaginal suppository	One suppository for 3 d
Miconazole (OTC)	1200 mg vaginal suppository	One suppository for 1 d
Nystatin	100 000 unit vaginal tablet	One tablet for 14 d
Ticonazole	6.5% ointment	5 g intravaginally in a single application
Terconazole	0.4% cream	5 g intravaginally for 7 d
Terconazole	0.8% cream	5 g intravaginally for 3 d
Terconazole	80 mg vaginal suppository	One suppository for 3 d
Fluconazole	150 mg oral tablet	One tablet in a single dose

From Workowski K, Berman S. Centers for Disease Control and Prevention. Sexually Transmitted Diseases Treatment Guidelines, MMWR 2006;55:51–57; with permission.

Table 4-26 Treatment of Recurrent Vulvovaginitis

Initial therapy
- Topical therapy for 7–10 days.
- 100 mg, 150 mg, or 200 mg of oral fluconazole every third day for a total of 3 doses (day 1 h, 4, and 7).

Maintenance therapy
- Oral fluconazole (100 mg, 150 mg, or 200 mg) weekly for 6 months (first line of treatment).
- Topical clotrimazole 200 mg twice a week.
- Topical clotrimazole 500-mg vaginal suppositories once a week.

From Workowski K, Berman S. Centers for Disease Control and Prevention. Sexually Transmitted Diseases Treatment Guidelines, MMWR 2006;55:51–57; with permission.

vaginal cultures should be obtained to confirm the diagnosis and rule out infection with non-*albicans* species, which are more resistant to traditional antimycotic therapies. After the initial therapy is completed, maintenance therapy may be indicated for remission. Also, a longer duration (7-10 days) of initial therapy may be required. Treatment of sex partners is not necessary (6) (Table 4-26).

Trichomonal Vaginitis

Epidemiology

Trichomonal vaginitis is caused by the flagellated parasite *Trichomonas vaginalis*. Trichomonas is sexually transmitted and can be found in 30–80% of male sexual partners of infected women (1). Trichomonal vaginitis is the most common STI in U.S., with 3–5 million new cases reported annually (10). The prevalence of this infection is 3.5% and is disproportionately higher in non-Hispanic black women than in other groups. Risk factors include multiple sexual partners, smoking, certain feminine hygiene practices like douching, and IUD use (10).

Clinical Features

Trichomoniasis is associated with profuse, frothy, malodorous discharge, and vaginal irritation and dysuria. Up to 50% of infected women may be asymptomatic. Physical exam reveals vaginal edema, erythema, and an elevated pH (>4.5). An inflamed (or "strawberry") cervix may be present in 25% of cases. Microscopic examination of the wet mount shows motile trichomonads and increased numbers of polymorphonuclear leukocytes (1,2).

Diagnosis

Clinical symptoms and signs are unreliable in diagnosing trichomonal vaginitis. Identification of motile trichomonads by microscopic exam of wet mount preparations is essential for diagnosis; however, the exam lacks sensitivity (4). Culture on specialized media like Diamond's or Hollander has high sensitivity, and can be done if the wet mount is negative and clinical suspicion is high (11). PCR testing and tests using DNA probes have high sensitivity and specificity (4).

Treatment

Trichomonas is highly transmissible and is often associated with other STIs. The incidence of PID and tubal infertility is significantly higher among women infected with *T. vaginalis*. It is also associated with increased risk of acquiring HIV; thus, symptomatic and asymptomatic infections should be treated (3,4,12). The treatment recommended by the CDC is metronidazole 2 g orally in a single dose or tinidazole 2 g orally in a single dose. An alternative regimen includes metronidazole 500 mg orally twice a day for 7 days. The sexual partner also should be treated (6).

Psychosocial Issues

Vaginal infections are seen in the medical community as a disease process caused by microbes that are treatable with antibiotics or antifungals. However, these symptoms may lead to anxiety and sometimes severe emotional distress in patients. Many women associate these symptoms with serious diseases, like cancer and HIV. Infections during pregnancy may lead to worries about fetal heath and well-being. Concerns about STIs and sexual morality also may occur in some cases. Some women consider these conditions as concrete evidence of their partner's infidelity (13). Recurrent infections also may seriously interfere with a woman's sexual and emotional relationships (14). Future research is needed to explore psychosocial issues related to vaginitis in order to improve outcomes.

References

1. **Egan ME, Lipsky MS.** Diagnosis of vaginitis. American Family Physician. 2000;62:1095–104.
2. **Soper DE.** Genitourinary infections and sexually transmitted diseases. In Berek and Novak's Gynecology. Philadelphia: Lippincott Williams Wilkins; 2006.
3. **Owen MK, Clenney TL.** Management of vaginitis. American Family Physician. 2004;70:2125–32.
4. **Sobel JD.** What's new in bacterial vaginosis and trichomoniasis? Infectious Disease Clinics of North America. 2005;19:387–402.
5. **Eschenbach DA.** History and review of bacterial vaginosis. Am J Obstet Gynecol. 1993;169:441–45.
6. Workowski K, Berman S. Centers for Disease Control and Prevention. Sexually Transmitted Diseases Treatment Guidelines, MMWR 2006;55:51–57.
7. **Clenney TL, Jorgensen S, Owen M.** Vaginitis Clinics in Family Practice, March 2005 (Vol. 7/No. 1, pp. 57–66, DOI: 10.1016/j.cfp.2004.11.004)

8. **Nyirjesy P, Sobel JD.** Vulvovaginal candidiasis. Obstetric Gynecol. Clinic North America. 2003;30:671–84.

9. **Sobel JD.** Vulvovaginal candidosis. The Lancet. 9 June 2007–15 June 2007;369:1961–71.

10. **Sutton M. Sternberg M.** The Prevalence of Trichomonas vaginalis Infection among Reproductive-Age Women in the United States, 2001–2004. Clinical Infectious Diseases 2007;45:1319–26.

11. **Patel SR. Wiese W.** Systematic review of diagnostic tests for vaginal trichomoniasis. Infect Dis Obstet Gynecol. 2000;8:248–57.

12. **McClelland RS, Sangare L.** Infection with Trichomonas vaginalis increases the risk of HIV-1 acquisition. J Infect Dis. 2007 Mar 1;195:698–702.

13. **Karasz A, Anderson M.** The vaginitis monologues: women's experiences of vaginal complaints in a primary care setting. Social Science & Medicine. March 2003;56:1013–21.

14. **G Irving, D Miller.** Psychological factors associated with recurrent vaginal candidiasis: a preliminary study. Sexually Transmitted Infections. 1998;74:334–8. Copyright © 1998 by Sexually Transmitted Infections.

J. HIV/AIDS Infection in Women

Jeffrey M. Rothenberg and Joanna R. Fields

KEY POINTS

- HIV/AIDS in women is a global epidemic.
- HIV/AIDS disproportionately affects racial and ethnic minorities in the U.S., especially females.
- Social burdens add to the complexity of caring for and treating the disease in women.
- Understanding the mode of transmission to women as well as maternal-to-child transmission is important.
- Several gender-specific gynecologic diseases are associated with HIV/AIDS in women.

Epidemiology

Globally, the number of women with HIV/AIDS continues to rise. The World Health Organization (WHO) estimated that in 2005 there were at least 17.5 million infected women worldwide (1). The rate of rise in the U.S. is greater for women than men. Between 2000 and 2004, the Centers for Disease Control and Prevention (CDC) estimated that the increase was 10% for females and only 7% for males (2). Unfortunately, the disease disproportionately affects racial/ethnic minorities in the U.S. African American and Latino women represent about 25% of the U.S. female population but account for 79% of the HIV/AIDS cases in women (3). In 2005, of the 126 964 women with HIV/AIDS in the U.S., 64% were African American, 19% were White, and 15% were Latino, with the remainder representing 1% or less of the population (3). HIV/AIDS is the leading cause of death for Black women between the ages of 25 and 34 years and is the fifth leading cause of death in all women aged 35–44 years (4). For women of all races and ethnicities, the youngest cohort has the highest incidence.

Social Issues

Socially, women bear more of the burden of caring for their families, who may also suffer from the disease. Women with HIV/AIDS face more barriers to care because of the responsibilities that they may have as sole income earner in the household, being a single mother, and/or caring for other sick family members (5). Many other barriers to care exist for women, including lack of transportation, lack of insurance, and psychological and social barriers (fear of disclosure, stigmatization, denial, and cultural mistrust of the health care system). Women traditionally lack access to the same level of health care that is available to men in many parts of the world. It is this lack of access and social support that interferes with the ability of many women to obtain and adhere to treatment regimens (5). The NIAID (National Institute of Allergy and Infections Diseases) and other organizations have approached some of these challenges through support of ongoing research projects and clinical trials in an effort to combat the disease and its social implications in women (6).

Transmission

Worldwide, the main mode of transmission of HIV is through heterosexual encounters (7). Due to the fragility of the vaginal mucosa, coupled with the large surface area of mucosal exposure, women are at increased risk of infection when compared to males (8). High-risk factors, such as sex without condoms, non-consensual sex, and sex with high-risk male partners increases their overall risks. Other factors associated with an increased risk include alcohol and drug abuse, a history of childhood sexual abuse, and current domestic violence. In the U.S., the CDC estimates that 70% of HIV transmission to women is heterosexual and 28% is due to parenteral drug use (3). In the U.S., the risk of male-to-female transmission is greater than female-to-male (8). This phenomenon may not be true worldwide, however, but its biological basis is unclear. It has been postulated that it may be due to lack of circumcision in men, which increases their mucosal exposure to the virus (9). What is clear is that any disease that results in mucosal or epithelial ulcerations, such as syphilis, *Herpes simplex* virus (HSV), and chancroid increases a woman's chance of acquiring the infection (7).

It is also evident that the diligent and correct use of male condoms can lessen the risk of transmission. Unfortunately, however, it has been reported that the concomitant use of the most widely used spermicide, nonoxynol-9, may actually increase the risk of transmission. Current research is focused on determining the overall decrease in transmission when discordant couples are given anti-retroviral drugs along with prevention education (10).

Gender-Specific Manifestations

Men and women experience the same medical complications of HIV/AIDS, but there are obvious gender-specific manifestations that are encountered clinically. For instance, Kaposi's sarcoma is 8 times more common in men, while women seem to have higher rates of HSV infections (11). Perhaps some of the reasons that certain infections, such as pneumonia, are more commonly seen in women are not a result of the biology of the disease but rather arise from delay in seeking care or, simply, less access to care. Treatments for HIV/AIDS and associated conditions appear to be similarly efficacious in men and women (6).

Depression is more common in women and may be a contributory factor that worsens outcomes. In one prospective cohort study in the U.S., women with chronic depressive symptoms were twice as likely to die as were those with mild or no depressive symptoms, using multivariate analysis controlling for clinical features and treatment (12). For women with chronic, intermittent, or limited depressive symptoms who had CD4 counts below $200/mm^3$, the mortality rates were 54%, 48%, and 21%, respectively, higher than in non-depressed patients (12).

Mother-to-Child Transmission

A unique situation for women is mother-to-child transmission (MTCT) (often referred to as vertical transmission) of HIV. Data from the U.S. have demonstrated that 25% of infected women transmit the virus to their child in the absence of any intervention. The first sentinel study in the U.S. (PACTG 076) demonstrated a two-thirds decrease when using zidovudine (AZT) alone (13). The effect was so pronounced that the study was halted before it was completed, during the interim analysis, because it was deemed unethical to continue with the placebo arm. When utilizing full therapeutic anti-retroviral regimens, the risk of transmission decreases to <2% (14). Only 57 infants were reported to be infected vertically in 2005, which is in obvious contrast to what is seen in the rest of the world. Many factors contribute to MTCT, but foremost among them is the status of the mother. Parturients with more advanced disease, high viral loads, or low CD4 counts are most likely to transmit the virus (14). Chorioamniotis, prolonged rupture of fetal membranes, operative vaginal delivery, and drug use also increase transmission risk. An affordable and practical algorithm was developed and proven effective in a major NIAID study from Uganda (HIVNET 012) (15). This study demonstrated that a single oral dose of nevirapine given intra-partum to HIV+ women, followed by a second dose given to the newborn within 3 days after birth, reduced the transmission risk by almost half and improved survival at 18 months of life. The regimen was found to be not only effective but safe as well. This has implications for women, even in the U.S., who present in labor with no prior treatment to help minimize MTCT.

HIV+ mothers also can transmit the virus during nursing, which increases the risk by about 14% (16). Many studies have documented this risk, and UNAIDS recommends that HIV+ women in developing countries be educated and counseled about the transmission risks so that they can decide best on how to feed their newborns (17). Many studies are underway to examine strategies, both pharmacologic and temporal (early weaning), that might reduce this risk. Women in developed countries who have access to safe infant formula should not breast feed.

Pregnant women should be routinely tested for HIV. However, mandatory testing may keep at-risk women from seeking prenatal care, at least in the U.S. When considering testing, most agree that mandatory testing simply keeps at-risk women from seeking care, at least in the U.S. A better solution is the so-called opt-out strategy, which encourages testing all pregnant women, unless they refuse. This currently is the recommendation of the American College of Obstetrics and Gynecology (18).

Gynecologic Conditions and HIV/AIDS

There are many specific gynecologic conditions that increase in severity and frequency in HIV+ women. *Candida* vaginitis, which is a common and easily treated clinical entity in non-immunocompromised women, is often more frequent and persistent in HIV+ women (19). It occurs in 24–71% of HIV+ women. Recurrent vaginal yeast infections are the most common initial manifestations of HIV/AIDS infection in women. As with most opportunistic infections, as CD4 counts decline the incidence of *Candida* infections increase, and they become more refractory to treatment. Weekly doses of fluconazole can be helpful in preventing oropharyngeal and vaginal *Candida* infections without initiating drug resistance (19).

Vaginitis due to other etiologies, such as bacterial vaginosis, and sexually transmitted infections (STIs), like gonorrhea, *Chlamydia*, and trichomoniasis, also occur more frequently and with greater severity in HIV+ women (20). Of particular importance is the occurrence of severe ulcerative HSV infections of the perineum, which significantly affect quality of life and are sometimes difficult to treat with antiviral medications (21). Idiopathic genital ulcers also occur and can mimic HSV infections (22).

Human papillomavirus (HPV) infections are common and can lead to cervical dysplasia and cervical cancer in addition to genital warts. HIV+ women should be screened with Pap smears, with colposcopy, and with biopsy as needed. Invasive cervical cancer is the most common cancer seen in HIV+ women world-wide and is an AIDS-defining illness. Vulvar and vaginal dysplasia due to HPV are seen with an increased frequency in this population (23).

Pelvic inflammatory disease (PID) is common and often aggressive in HIV+ women. In certain instances, chronic recalcitrant PID occurs and can severely affect a woman's quality of life. HIV-infected women with PID present with more severe signs and symptoms and have a more prolonged clinical course, with longer duration of fever and hospitalization (24). HIV-infected women also are more likely to require a change in antibiotic therapy but are not more likely to require surgery. However, in HIV+ women with more complications, such as tubo-ovarian abscesses, surgery is more likely to be performed. Approximately 25% of HIV-infected women undergo surgical intervention, compared with 12% of those without HIV. Generally, HIV-infected women suffer higher rates of nausea, dysuria, lymphadenopathy, fever, genital ulcers, and cervical friability, as well as higher erythrocyte sedimentation rates and less leukocytosis than do non-infected women with PID (24).

Menstrual irregularities do not seem to be more prevalent in HIV+ women, but some contradictory results have been reported (25). Many of these occurred early in the course of the epidemic. Infected women do, however, suffer from an increase in postcoital bleeding (25). All abnormal bleeding in HIV+ women should be evaluated and managed in the same manner as for those without HIV.

Conclusion

The HIV/AIDS epidemic has affected women disproportionately (26). In the U.S., various racial/ethnic minorities, especially African Americans, represent a much higher proportion of those living with this disease than would be expected from the size of the these groups in the population (3). Apart from risky sexual behavior and drug use, other societal factors, such as poverty and the lack of education, have impacted these groups greatly. What has become clear is that, as in men, early diagnosis and access to care are of the utmost importance in bringing this devastating disease under control (27).

References

1. http://www.who.int/globalatlas/default.asp
2. http://www.cdc.gov/hiv/topics/surveillance/basic.htm
3. Centers for Disease Control & Prevention. HIV/AIDS Surveillance Report 2002; 13(2):1–44. http://www.cdc.gov/hiv/topics/women/resources/factsheets/women.htm
4. WISQARS Leading causes of death reports, 199–2004. http://webappa.cdc.gov/sasweb/cipc/leadcaus10.html
6. http://www3.niaid.nih.gov/healthscience/healthtopics/WomensHealth/PDF/womenshealth.pdf
5. **Piot P, Bartos M, Ghys, PD, et al.** The global impact of HIV/AIDS. Nature. 2001;410:968–73.
7. **Cohen OJ, Fauci AS.** Host factors that affect sexual transmission of HIV. International Journal of Infectious Diseases. 1998;2:182–5.
8. **Fleming DT, Wasserheit JN.** From epidemiological synergy to public health policy and practice: the contribution of other sexually transmitted

diseases to sexual transmission of HIV infection. Sexually Transmitted Infections. 1999;75:3–17.

9. **Weiss HA, Quigley MA, Hayes RJ.** Male circumcision and risk of HIV infection in sub-Saharan Africa: a systematic review and meta-analysis. AIDS. 2000;14:2361–70.

10. **Stephenson JJ.** Widely used spermicide may increase, not decrease, risk of HIV transmission. JAMA. 2000;284:949.

11. **Kaplan JE, Hanson D, et al.** Epidemiology of human immunodeficiency virus-associated opportunistic infections in the United States in the era of highly active antiretroviral therapy. Clin Infect Dis. 2000;Apr 30: S5–14.

12. **Dwight L Evans, Thomas R Ten Have, et al.** Association of depression with viral load, CD8 T lymphocytes, and natural killer cells in women with hiv infection. Am J Psychiatry. 2002;159:1752–59.

13. **Sperling RS, Shapiro DE.** Maternal viral load, zidovudine treatment, and the risk of transmission of human immunodeficiency virus type 1 from mother to infant. Pediatric AIDS Clinical Trials Group Protocol 076 Study Group, NEJM. 1996;335:1621–9.

14. **Goetghebuer T, Haelterman E, et al.** Vertical transmission of HIV in Belgium: A 1986–2002 retrospective analysis. Eur J Pediatr. 2009; 168:79–85.

15. **Guay LA, Musoke P, et al.** Intrapartum and neonatal single-dose nevirapine compared with zidovudine for prevention of mother-to-child transmission of HIV-1 in Kampala, Uganda: HIVNET 012 randomised trial. Lancet. 1999;354:795–802.

16. **Coutsoudis A, Pillay K, Kuhn L, et al.** Method of feeding and transmission of HIV-1 from mothers to children by 15 months of age: prospective cohort study from Durban, South Africa. AIDS. 2001;15:379–87.

17. http://www.cdc.gov/hiv/topics/perinatal/resources/meetings/2007/ pdf/Fogler_MTCT.pdf, April 2007.

18. http://www.acog.org/from_home/publications/ethics/co389.pdf

19. **Williams A, Yu C, Tashima K, et al.** Weekly treatment for prophylaxis of candida vaginitis.7th Conf Retrovir Oppor Infect Jan 30 Feb 2 2000 Conf Retrovir Oppor Infect 7th 2000 San Franc Calif 2000 Jan30–Feb 2;7:202 (abstract no. 677).

20. **Sobel, JD.** Vaginitis. N Engl J Med. 1997;337:1896–903.

21. **Wald A, Link K.** Risk of human immunodeficiency virus infection in herpes simplex virus type 2-seropositive persons: a meta-analysis. J Infect Dis. 2002;185:45–52.

22. **LaGuardia KD, White MH, Saigo, PE, et al.** Genital ulcer disease in women infected with human immunodeficiency virus. Am J Obstet Gynecol. 1995;172;553–62.

23. **Keller JM, Sewell C, Anderson J.** Incidence of recurrent cervical dysplasia in HIV positive women after cervical excisional treatment. Int Conf AIDS. 2000Jul9–14;13:abstract no. MoOrB237.

24. **Korn AP, Landers DV, Green JR, et al.** Pelvic inflammatory disease in human immunodeficiency virus-infected women. Obstet Gynecol. 1993;82:765–8.

25. **Harlow SD, Schuman P, Cohen M, et al.** Effect of HIV infection on menstrual cycle length. J Acquir Immune Defic Syndr Hum Retrovirol. 2000;24:68–75.

26. **Espinoza I, Hall HI, Hardnett F, et al.** Characteristics of persons with heterosexually acquired HIV infection, United States, 1999–2004. American Journal of Public Health. 2007;97:144–9.

27. **Valdiserri RO, Holtgrave DR, West, GR.** Promoting early HIV diagnosis and entry into care. AIDS. 1999;13(17):2317–30.

K. Primary Care of Lesbian Women

Kathy Oriel

KEY POINTS

- The primary care of lesbian women is the same as that of heterosexual women with a few important distinctions.
- Lesbian women may fear judgment or discrimination from healthcare providers, so physicians must make a special effort to communicate inclusivity and acceptance.
- Sexual behavior and sexual identity are 2 distinct concepts that may change throughout a woman's lifespan.

The designation "lesbian" defines women who are sexually attracted to women, sexually active with women, and may be used for individuals who identify as lesbian irrespective of sexual behavior. Sexual behavior—sexual partners past and present—can differ from sexual orientation, or identity. For example, a woman who is married and identifies herself as heterosexual may become sexually active with another woman while still identifying as heterosexual or "straight." Similarly, a woman who identifies as lesbian may be celibate but still carries a lesbian identity because of her social structure and connections.

Identifying a woman's sexual *behavior* is important for understanding the patient's risk of sexually transmitted infections (STIs), as well as her needs regarding contraception, and may help reduce discomfort during exams. Understanding a women's sexual *identity* is important in appreciating her support system, utilizing appropriate community resources, and gaining trust during joint medical decision-making.

Population-based studies in the U.S. and elsewhere indicate that approximately 8.6% of women identify some degree of same-gender sexuality. Eighty-eight percent of those women (7.6% of the population) report same-gender sexual attraction, 41% (3.5% of the population) report same-gender sexual behavior, and 16% of those (1.4% of the population) report a lesbian identity (1).

Establishing Patient Rapport

Sexual orientation is one of many demographic variables that may impact health, health behaviors, and access to health care. Unlike age, gender, race, ethnicity, and sometimes socioeconomic status, patients routinely do not disclose sexual orientation to healthcare providers. Despite a slowly improving societal acceptance of lesbians and gay men, past surveys of lesbian women consistently demonstrate fear of discrimination or disapproval in the medical setting if they disclose their orientation to healthcare providers (2).

Physicians and other providers can create a welcoming environment for lesbian women through the following actions:

- Intake forms that include "partnered" as a relationship status in addition to married, single, or divorced. Similarly, forms for minors should indicate "parent and parent" rather than "mother and father."
- Questions regarding family structure should not assume heterosexual relationships: "Who is important in your life?" "Do you have a partner?" "Who serves as your key source of support?" instead of "Are you married?" or "Do you have a husband?" Patients will be more comfortable if these social questions are asked prior to inquiring about sexual behavior.
- Questions about sexual behavior for all patients should be matter-of-fact and gender-neutral: "Are you sexually active?" "In the past have your sexual partners been men, women, or both?" "Tell me about your recent sexual partners."
- Office displays, even small or subtle ones, go a long way in increasing comfort for lesbian women. These may include non-discrimination policies, or posters and brochures that include and acknowledge same-sex families. Some practitioners display signs or buttons with a pink triangle or rainbows to designate "safe space." Both are symbols that the lesbian, gay, bisexual, and transgender community has used for years to demonstrate inclusivity.

One of the most ubiquitous challenges for gays and lesbians is the assumption of heterosexuality. When physicians and other healthcare providers assume women need contraception, routinely ask about husbands, or utilize forms that include only "single, married, divorced, or widowed," but not "partnered," lesbian women feel their existence was not considered and worry that clinic personnel will be insensitive or unsupportive of their needs.

By routinely utilizing lines of questioning that do not presume heterosexual status, physicians may provide benefit to heterosexual patients as well. This type of questioning demonstrates non-judgmental attitudes about gays and lesbians, reinforces the fact that one cannot make assumptions regarding sexual orientation by a person's physical appearance, and shows that the provider is an open, non-judgmental person. Demonstrating non-judgmental attitudes may help heterosexual patients broach other sensitive topics such as intimate partner violence, substance use issues, or sexual dysfunction.

Common Misperceptions Regarding Health Risks in Lesbian Women

Cervical Cancer Screening

Lesbian women and their physicians commonly believe they do not need papanicolaou (Pap) smears. Seventy to ninety percent (4) of lesbian women have had sexual intercourse in the past with male partners, and the human papillomavirus (HPV) can be transmitted between female partners. Lesbian women are less likely to receive routine Pap smears, perhaps because of discomfort with the medical profession, the lack of need for contraception, or because of the mistaken belief these tests are unnecessary in lesbians. In any event, lesbian women should receive Pap smears based on their individual risks, as outlined by the United States Preventative Services Task Force or the Association of Obstetricians and Gynecologists.

Sexually Transmitted Infection Screening

STI screening should be based on individual risk factors. There are reports of syphilis, HIV, and trichomonas transmission between women. Though little is known about chlamydia, gonorrhea, or syphilis transmission between women, usual screening guidelines based on number of sexual partners should be followed. It is important to address HIV prevention with lesbian women. Lesbian women who are also sexually active with men may have higher risk sexual activity with those men, including sex with bisexual men and anal intercourse (5).

Safe Sex Counseling

Lesbian women should understand that STIs can be transmitted between women. Transmission is more likely with the use of shared insertive sex objects, and HIV transmission is more likely to occur during the menstrual cycle. Women may use gloves for digital sexual contact, especially when there is broken skin. Dental dams are rectangular pieces of latex that can be used during genital-oral contact. Latex gloves are more available, and they can be opened with scissors to create an appropriate latex barrier for oral-genital or oral-anal contact.

Intimate Partner Violence

Intimate partner violence exists in lesbian relationships with lower prevalence than in heterosexual ones (6). Still, lesbian women should be screened for partner violence in a similar manner to heterosexual woman. Emotional and physical abuse in lesbian relationships is complicated by perpetrators threatening to "out" victims (tell others about her sexual orientation) if the victim leaves. Lesbian women in abusive relationships face the same barriers to leaving as do heterosexual women, but may also feel additional shame that such victimization was caused by another woman.

Vaginitis/Vaginosis

There are no infections that are unique to lesbians. Studies have identified that bacterial vaginosis may be more common in lesbian women, and that female partners are usually bacterial vaginosis-concordant, either both having bacterial vaginosis or both being symptom-free. Treatment of female partners of lesbians with bacterial vaginosis is a sound approach, especially when symptoms are recurrent (5).

Parenting and Pregnancy

More than 1 in 3 adult lesbians have given birth, and 41% of all lesbian women express a desire to have children (7). Lesbian couples choose to parent through adoption, foster-parenting, anonymous donor insemination, known donor insemination, and by parenting children from one partner's previous heterosexual relationship. Children raised by lesbian parents do not differ in intelligence, sexual identity, gender role preference, or family and peer relations (8). Lesbian women considering pregnancy should undergo preconception counseling and appropriate testing. Those considering pregnancy through a known donor via fresh (rather than frozen, quarantined semen through a certified sperm bank) should be counseled regarding risk of STIs, including HIV, and should be encouraged to meet with a knowledgeable attorney regarding donor parental rights. Myriad published and Internet resources exist for women considering parenthood through pregnancy, adoption, or foster parenting that patients can easily locate through the Internet or their local lesbian/gay advocacy organization.

Health Risk Screening

Tobacco and Substance Use

Studies consistently demonstrate that lesbians have higher smoking rates than those of heterosexual women. A 2004 population-based study demonstrated a 25% prevalence of cigarette use among lesbian women, 70% higher than that of heterosexual women in the same study (9).

Data from the 2000 National Alcohol Survey, a national population-based survey of adults (N = 7612), demonstrated that both lesbians and bisexual women had lower abstention rates and significantly greater odds of reporting alcohol-related social consequences, alcohol dependence, and past help-seeking for an alcohol problem (10). Higher alcohol use is theorized to be the result of community norms, bars as places for social connection with other women, and as a stress response to societal discrimination and resultant poor self-esteem. Many urban areas have recovery programs, such as Alcoholics Anonymous, specifically for lesbian, gay, and bisexual persons.

Depression/Suicide

Studies of lesbian and bisexual women have consistently shown increased prevalence of depressive symptoms, history of suicide attempts, and greater use of mental health services. Now, several population-based studies using the Youth Behavioral Risk Factor Survey demonstrate that GLB (gay, lesbian, or bisexual) youth who self-identify during high school report disproportionate risk for a variety of health disorders and problem behaviors, including suicide attempts and victimization (11). The data are less clear regarding depressive symptoms and suicidal tendencies among adult lesbian women, but studies are ongoing.

Medico-Legal Issues

Same-sex couples are not afforded the same legal protections that married heterosexual couples receive regarding issues that frequently arise in the medical setting, including:

- Healthcare durable power of attorney
- Health insurance coverage of spouse unless explicitly allowed by one partner's employer
- Hospital visitation
- Ability to serve as a foster parent or to adopt

Parental rights, such as visitation, ability to authorize medical treatment, and child-support payment for non-biologic parents. Although some local municipalities allow non-biologic parental adoption and other protections through domestic partnership legislation, most do not. Lesbian couples should be counseled to consult with an attorney familiar with local law as it pertains to same-sex couples. In doing so, couples and families can establish their wishes regarding inheritance, healthcare durable power of attorney, advanced directives, and parental rights.

References

1. **Edward O, Laumann John H, Gagnon Robert T, et al.** The Social Organization of Sexuality in the United States. Chicago: University of Chicago Press, 1994.
2. **Smith EM, Johnson SR, Guenther SM.** Health care attitudes and experiences during gynecologic care among lesbians and bisexuals. Am J Public Health. 1985;75:1085-7.
3. **Mravcak SA.** Primary care for lesbians and bisexual women. Am Fam Physician. 2006;74:279-86, 287-8.
4. **Diamant AL, Schuster MA, et al.** Lesbians sexual history with men: implications for taking a sexual history. Arch Intern Med. 1999;159:2730-6.
5. **Marrazzo JM.** Barriers to infectious disease care among lesbians. Emerg Infect Dis [serial on the Internet]. 2004 Nov [3/10/2008]. Available from http://www.cdc.gov/ncidod/EID/vol10no11/04-0467.htm
6. **Tjaden P, Thoennes N.** Extent, Nature, and Consequences of Intimate Partner Violence: Findings from the National Violence Against Women Survey. Washington, D.C., U.S. Department of Justice, National Institute of Justice, July 2000. NCJ181867. http://www.gaydata.org/02_Data_Sources/ds025_VAWS/ds025_VAWS_Report.pdf
7. **Gates GJ, Macomber JC, et al.** Adoption and Foster Care by Gay and Lesbian Parents in the United States. Williams Institute, UCLA School of Law. March 2007. Available from http://www.law.ucla.edu/williamsinstitute/publications/FinalAdoptionReport.pdf

8. **Patterson CJ.** Children of Lesbian and Gay Parents. Child Development. 1992Oct;63:1025–42.
9. **Tang H, Greenwood GL, Cowling DW, et al.** Cigarette smoking among lesbians, gays, and bisexuals: how serious a problem? Cancer Causes Control. 2004Oct;15:797–803.
10. **Drabble L, Midanik LT, Trocki K.** Reports of alcohol consumption and alcohol-related problems among homosexual, bisexual and heterosexual respondents: results from the 2000 National Alcohol Survey. J Stud Alcohol. 2005;66:111–20.
11. **Garofalo R, Wolf RC, Wissow LS, et al.** Sexual orientation and risk of suicide attempts among a representative sample of youth. Arch Pediatr Adolesc Med. 1999May;153:487–93; 66:111–20.

L. Primary Care of Women with Disabilities

Deborah Dreyfus and Sarina B. Schrager

KEY POINTS

- There are over 30 million women with disabilities in the U.S., representing approximately 20% of the female population.
- Many conditions are more prevalent in women with disabilities, including bladder and bowel difficulties, decubitus ulcers and pressure sores, chronic pain and arthritis, vaginitis, and migraines (1,2).
- Transportation and financial difficulties, as well as lack of knowledge on the part of both healthcare providers and patients, make it difficult to provide effective care.
- The medical home (a close partnership between the family and the primary healthcare practitioner) can reduce barriers to healthcare among women with disabilities, allowing the primary care provider to have greater knowledge of all of the medical complexities of the individual.

Definitions and Epidemiology

"Disability" is defined as a physical or mental impairment that substantially limits one or more major life activities (Americans with Disabilities Act of 1990) (3). Disabilities can include either physical or mental impairments. Several terms are used to describe mental impairment;

one often used is ID, or Intellectual Disabilities. Women with ID are characterized by limitations in cognitive and adaptive behavior that starts prior to the age of 18 (4). Women with physical disabilities are characterized by at least 1 functional limitation such as difficulty walking, and include a subset of women with lifelong severe disabilities, who often have specific needs. (5). Many of the health care needs of women with both physical and intellectual disabilities are not met currently by healthcare providers. Additionally, these individuals often require more services than an individual without disabilities (6). Over 30 million women in the U.S. have disabilities, representing about 20% of the female population (1).

Primary Care

Physicians need to provide regular health maintenance and disease-specific screening, with special awareness for conditions more prevalent in women with disabilities. Such conditions include bladder and bowel difficulties, decubitus ulcers and pressure sores, chronic pain and arthritis, vaginitis, and migraines (1,2). These issues should be discussed regularly at annual visits.

Screening for Violence

A 2000–2001 study performed in North Carolina, consisting of 5000 women over the age of 18 years, found that women with disabilities were 4 times as likely to be sexually assaulted within the past year as compared to those without disabilities (7). In this sample, the prevalence of physical (as opposed to sexual) assault was not higher in women with disabilities. However, women with disabilities were more likely to be abused for longer periods of time and were abused by a wider variety of people, such as caregivers, strangers or attendants, in addition to partners or family members (5,7).

Screening questions for violence may need to be modified for women with disabilities. For instance, appropriate questions include, "Has anyone ever prevented you from using a wheelchair, cane, or other assistive device?"; or, "Has anyone you depend on ever refused to help you with an important personal need, such as taking your medicine, getting to the bathroom, getting out of bed, bathing, getting dressed, or getting food or drink?" (1).

Advance Directives

Beginning at age 18 years, a discussion about resuscitation, power of attorney, and living wills should occur. In addition, a plan needs to be made for women with disabilities who reside in a community setting, be it a group home or alternate living arrangement, in case a care provider is no longer able to perform tasks needed for the patient. These documents should be updated annually.

Cardiovascular Screening

Heart disease is increasingly prevalent in women with any form of disability (2). Some developmental syndromes (such as Down Syndrome (DS)) are associated with an increased risk of structural heart disease like endocardial cushion defects. Women with physical disabilities also have an increased prevalence of hypertension, hyperlipidemia, inactivity, obesity, and diabetes, which increases the risk of heart disease (2,4) Smoking, another risk factor for heart disease, is asked about less frequently but appears to be just as common in women with disabilities as in women in the general population (4).

Screening for cardiovascular disease should occur regularly in women with disabilities and entails annual monitoring of risk factors, examining for signs/symptoms, and performing routine hypertension, cholesterol, obesity, diabetes, and smoking screening (5). A total cholesterol or fasting lipid panel should be checked at least once every 5 years, more frequently if elevated, in women over the age of 45 years. An annual fasting glucose should be obtained in women with hypertension or hyperlipidemia and every 3 years in women with ID (4,6). Many women with ID are on second generation antipsychotic medications, which can increase risk of diabetes and should be screened accordingly. A physician should calculate a BMI every year, and, if elevated, should counsel the individual on diet changes. Additionally, individuals with physical disabilities should be seen by a physical therapist and taught disability-specific exercises. Women with DS also have a higher risk of acquired valvular heart disease, and should have echocardiograms every 5 years (7).

Reproductive Health

Premenstrual syndrome (PMS) in women with ID may manifest as aggression, tantrums, or crying spells, especially if the patient is nonverbal. (8). A woman may need to use protective gear, such as a helmet, to keep from harming herself. Ways to decrease discomfort include using hormonal contraception or nonsteroidal anti-inflammatory drugs (NSAIDs) to help with dysmenorrhea and irregular bleeding (8).

Women with physical disabilities are less likely to be asked about contraception. In one study of 881 women between the ages of 18 and 65 years, 94% of women who described themselves as having physical disabilities were sexually active (9). Available forms of contraception may be limited in women with disabilities, depending on several factors, including other medications (interactions between some hormonal methods of contraception and disability-related medications such as anticonvulsants) and placement of devices (which may be difficult to position due to lack of manual dexterity). The provider should work with each individual woman to find a method that works best for her.

In the past, women with disabilities have had hysterectomies performed at a higher rate than women without disabilities (1). Obtaining consent for surgical procedures becomes more complicated when working with a woman with ID. In many states, a recommendation from the patient's physician is required. Additionally, informed consent from the legal guardian must be obtained, whether the patient is her own legal guardian or the guardian is a family member. The doctor needs to review the risks and benefits in a way that adapts to the guardian's level of understanding. Alternatives, such as hormonal contraception, need to be discussed. Court approval is sometimes required in these situations, and guardians must show that the procedure is in the best interests of the patient (8). Laws may vary from state to state.

Cervical Cancer Screening

Women with physical disabilities are less likely to have a Pap smear performed than women who do not have disabilities (8). The decision to screen a woman with disabilities, especially those with ID, should be individualized to that woman's risk. If a woman has not been sexually active, Pap smears do not need be performed annually. However, a woman with multiple sexual partners should be routinely screened for cervical cancer and for sexually transmitted infections (STIs).

When performing a pelvic exam, the clinician should determine the patient's level of understanding and explain the procedure at a level that she can comprehend. Discovering a patient's risk may be complicated in a woman with ID, since it may be difficult for her to communicate this information (10). In women who have never been sexually active, pelvic exams may be performed when she is having anesthesia for other procedures (i.e., dental exams). Another option would be to check a vaginal HPV test and if negative, being reassured that the risk of cervical cancer is low.

The examination needs to be individualized as well because many women with disabilities may find the exam uncomfortable. If a patient has a visual impairment, she should be oriented to the equipment, the staff, and the procedure. Staff should identify themselves when they enter or leave a room and should stand at the head of the bed to allow the woman to know what is happening while conserving her privacy. Many women with physical disabilities cannot comfortably lie in the traditional lithotomy pelvic exam position. Therefore, other positions may be more comfortable (Figure 4-2) (9).

If a speculum exam cannot be tolerated even with these alternative positions, additional screening modalities are available and are presented in Figure 4-3.

Breast Cancer

Self-breast exams (SBEs) are difficult if a woman lacks the manual dexterity to allow for effective screens. If a woman is unable to perform the exam herself, a partner may be trained to perform it. Annual breast exams performed by a physician provides the opportunity to teach the patient and/or partner how to perform a breast exam on her. Assistive devices such as breast models with lumps also may be educational (9).

Position	Description	Picture
The knee-chest position	Lying on one side, the woman bends both knees (or bends the top leg and straightens the bottom one). The speculum is placed with the handle pointed in the direction of the abdomen or directed to the back. The bills of the speculum should be angled toward the small of the woman's back. No footrests are needed.	The Knee-Chest Position
The diamond-shaped position	Lying on her back with her knees bent so that both legs are spread flat and her heels meet at the foot of the table, the speculum is inserted with the handle up. No need for footrests. The woman must be able to lie on her back.	The Diamond-Shaped Position
The M-shaped position	Lying on her back, the patient's knees are bent apart and her feet rest on the table close to her buttocks. An assistant may need to support the patient's feet or knees if the legs are not completely stable on the exam table. The speculum is inserted with the handle up. No footrests are needed.	The M-Shaped Position
The V-shaped position	Lying, on her back, the patient's legs are straightened and spread out wide to either side of the table (or one foot is placed in a foot rest and one leg straight is held straight). The speculum is inserted with the handle up.	The V-Shaped Position
The OB-rests position	Lying on her back near the foot of the table, the patient's legs are supported under the knees with the obstetrical knee-rests. The speculum is inserted with the handle down.	The OB Stirrups Position

Figure 4-2   Alternate positions for pelvic examinations. (Adapted from Simpson K. Table manners and beyond: The gynecological exam for women with developmental disabilities and other functional limitations. The Women's Wellness Project. California Department of Developmental Services May, 2001. http://www.bhawd.org/sitefiles/TblMrs/cover.html. From Kathleen Lankasky and UPC of the Golden Gate; with permission.)

If a woman discovers a lump during the SBE or is of the age when screening is appropriate, mammograms should be performed. Mammograms should be performed once a year after the age of 50 years. Based on risk as well as patient preference, current recommendations require that women between 40 and 50 years be offered mammograms

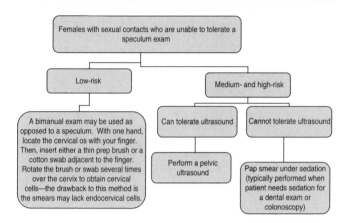

Figure 4-3   Algorithm for screening in women who are unable to tolerate a speculum exam. (Adapted from Grimes D. Reproductive healthcare for women with mental handicaps. The Contraception Report. 1997;8:1–11; with permission.)

annually or biannually. A clinician should attempt to choose a facility that provides wheelchair access, if available (4).

Colon Cancer

There has been little research into the risk of colon cancer and screening methodology in women with disabilities. Women with disabilities should be screened using the standard screening methods, with fecal occult blood cards, sigmoidoscopy, or colonoscopy as per routine (5).

Osteoporosis

Osteoporosis is more common in women with disabilities, probably due to a combination of factors, including immobility, medication use (*e.g.,* anticonvulsants), and decreased sunlight exposure (leading to a vitamin D deficiency) (10). Women with disabilities also are frequently unsteady due to imbalance and lower extremity weakness. Physical and occupational therapists may be able to maximize an individual's ability to remain steady by working on gait-training or teaching the individual how to use canes or shower chairs to aid in steadiness. Finally, calcium and vitamin D supplementation may improve vitamin deficiency-induced bone loss.

ID itself confers a risk of osteoporosis (11). This may be secondary to a genetic abnormality which causes low bone mineral density. DS is an independent risk factor for osteoporosis. In addition, women with DS experience menopause earlier than women in the general population, thereby exposing women to a low estrogen state at an earlier age (11). There is a high prevalence of seizure disorder in women with ID and antiepileptic medications are another risk factor for low bone density (11).

Osteoporosis screening recommendations in adults with ID vary from identifying and managing risk factors lifelong to performing routine bone density measurements at ages from 19 to 60 years (earlier than women in the general population due to multiple risk factors), depending on which guidelines are consulted (1,12). There is little evidence to guide clinicians. More research needs to be done to determine the ideal time of screening for these women. Screening is typically done via a DXA scan. However, it is often difficult for a woman with disabilities to lie flat on her back, as is required for accurate bone density measurement. An alternate form of screening may be used, such as a calcaneal ultrasound or peripheral DXA scanner.

Screening Recommendations for Neurological Functioning

Many women with disabilities have limitations in sensory function, and aggressive screening and management can help reduce further disability and risk of falls and injury (4,6) (Table 4-27).

Dental Screening

As in all adults, dental checks should occur every 6 months. Often, these exams need to occur under anesthesia in women with ID who may find it difficult to sit for the entirety of the exam (6).

Table 4-27   Screening Tests for Adults with ID

	Hearing	Vision	Neuro-psychological Testing	Swallowing
Office based-primary care	Yearly (perform otoscopic exam to look for impacted cerumen)	Yearly	Not needed	Ask about swallowing difficulties yearly
Exam with a licensed specialist	Every 5 y after age 45 (after age 30 in women with Down Syndrome)	Once before age 40 (before age 30 in women with Down Syndrome) and then rechecked every 2 y.	In women with ID at age 40	As needed (with a swallowing study)

From Wilkinson J, Culpepper L, Cerreto M. Screening tests for adults with intellectual disabilities. Journal of the American Board of Family Medicine. 2007;20:299–407 and Sullivan W, et al. Consensus guidelines for primary health care of adults with developmental disabilities. Canadian Family Physician. 2006;52:1410–18; with permission.

Thyroid Disease

Certain syndromes, such as DS, are associated with an increased risk for thyroid disease. Therefore, while in the general population screening for thyroid disease in asymptomatic women has not been recommended, among individuals with ID, all women should be screened for thyroid disease every 1–3 years, depending on risk factors such as other autoimmune diseases or family history of thyroid disease (5).

Depression

Depression is very common among women with physical disabilities, with a higher prevalence than in the general population (7). Additionally, women with ID are less able to verbalize their depression and may instead "act out" in terms of biting, hitting, or undressing, for instance. Screening for depression should occur annually.

Vaccinations

Women with disabilities should receive all routine vaccinations. Additionally, women who live in group homes, nursing homes, or institutions should receive influenza, hepatitis B, and pneumococcal vaccines at the same ages as women in the general population (1). Women with ID who are at risk for aspiration should have current *Haemophilus influenzae* and *Streptococcus pneumoniae* vaccinations (6).

Health Disparities

Women with disabilities have substantial healthcare needs but reduced healthcare access. This failure in prevention is often multifactorial. Transportation issues, inaccessible facilities (both in terms of location as well as handicapped access), financial constraints for both patient and provider (including attendant services and healthcare costs for the patient; productivity requirements for the provider), and lack of knowledge on the part of both healthcare providers (misunderstanding as to how to treat effectively) and patients (not knowing the diseases for which they are at risk), make it difficult to provide effective care (4).

To reduce these barriers to healthcare, the concept of a Medical Home was developed (12). This idea, championed by the American Academy of Pediatrics for children with special needs, appears to be equally replicable in other populations, including women with disabilities. The concept of a medical home is a partnership between the family and the primary healthcare practitioner, who work together to provide the health needs required for the individual to remain at her optimal level of functioning. A medical home maintains a central record of all pertinent medical information, allowing for continuity of care (12). If both practitioner and woman feel comfortable providing and receiving medical care, and if financial and transportation difficulties are addressed, then these healthcare disparities may be significantly reduced.

References

1. **Smeltzer S, Sharts-Hoko N.** "A provider's guide for the care of women with physical disabilities and chronic health conditioning." North Carolina Office on disability and Health in collaboration with Villanova University College of Nursing, September, 2005 http://www.fpg.unc.edu/~ncodh/pdfs/providersguide.pdf.
2. Persons with Disabilities and Health. CCSD's Disability Information Sheet Number 13. 2004 http://www.ccsd.ca/drip/research/drip14/index.htm
3. American with Disabilities Act of 1990, available at www.ada.gov
4. **Wilkinson J, Culpepper L, Cerreto M.** Screening tests for adults with intellectual disabilities. Journal of the American Board of Family Medicine. 2007;20:299-407.
5. **Martin S, et al.** Physical and sexual assault of women with disabilities. Violence against Women. 2006;12:823-37.
6. **Sullivan W, et al.** Consensus guidelines for primary health care of adults with developmental disabilities. Canadian Family Physician. 2006;52:1410-18.
7. **Cohen WI.** Down Syndrome Preventive Medicine Check List. Down Syndrome Quarterly 1999;4(3), available at http://www.ndsccenter.org/resources/healthcare.pdf.
8. **Grimes D.** Reproductive healthcare for women with mental handicaps. The Contraception Report. 1997;8:1-11.
9. **Nosek M.** "National Study of Women with Physical Disabilities: Final Report 1992-1996." Center for Research on Women with Disabilities Department of Physical Medicine and Rehabilitation, Baylor College of Medicine. 16 April 2001 http://www.bcm.edu/crowd/?pmid = 1408
10. **Simpson K.** Table Manners and Beyond: The Gynecological Exam for Women with Developmental Disabilities and other Functional Limitations. The Women's Wellness Project. California Department of Developmental Services May, 2001. http://www.bhawd.org/sitefiles/TblMrs/cover.html
11. **Schrager S.** Osteoporosis in women with disabilities review. Journal of Women's Health. 2004;13:431-7.
12. **Dickens M, Green J, Kohrt A, Pearson H.** The Medical Home. Pediatrics, Ad Hoc Task Force on Definition of the Medical Home, 1992;90:774.

5

Behavior/Mood Disorders

A. Depression

Joan E. Hamblin and Howard K. Gershenfeld

KEY POINTS

- ◆ Depression is common in women and is often under-diagnosed.
- ◆ Untreated depression represents a significant burden for a woman and her family.
- ◆ Clinicians must have a low threshold to screen for depression.
- ◆ Depression is a chronic disease with a high relapse rate.
- ◆ Clinicians should follow depressed patients closely with depression scales to assess treatment effectiveness.
- ◆ The goal of treatment is for patients to get completely well, not just improved.
- ◆ Clinicians should treat and monitor for relapse prevention and detection.
- ◆ Compliance with medication is more important than choice of medicine.

Epidemiology

The World Health Organization (WHO) estimates that by 2020 major depression will be second to ischemic heart disease as a cause of illness burden worldwide and will be the leading cause of disability (1). The lifetime prevalence of depression is reported to be 15–20%, with women having higher rates than men : 1 in every 3 women will experience depression in her lifetime (2). Depression in women is often different than in men (Table 5-1). In special populations, such as nursing home residents, prevalence rates have been reported to be as high as 20%. Without treatment, major depression lasts 6–13 months (10 months is average), compared to 3 months with treatment. By the end of 1 year, two thirds of patients will recover, while one third will relapse. However, long-term relapse rates are high, and depression for many may be considered a chronic, recurring illness. Although an individual's course is highly variable, patients have an average of 5 depressive episodes in their lifetime. The etiology of depression is not clearly established, although at least 25% of episodes are associated with a precipitating event. Risk factors for depression include past history, genetic predisposition, hormonal states, multiple medical conditions, certain medications and life stressors (3) (Table 5-2).

Relapse after an acute depressive episode is common, especially without treatment. Fifty to eighty percent of all untreated patients will have a second episode of depression, usually within 6 months. Risk of suicide is

Table 5-1   Differences between Women and Men with Depression

Lifetime Prevalence Rates	Women (33%) to Men (15%)
Incidence (Westernized nations)	Women (4.5–9.3%) to Men (2.3–3.2%)
Suicide attempt	Higher in women
Suicide completion rates	Higher in men
Previous childhood trauma/ sexual abuse	Counseling more effective in women
Atypical depression	More common in women
Antidepressants and counseling treatment	More effective preventing relapse in women
Hormone states: pregnancy, postpartum postmenopausal	Incidence (8–10%)

increased if the patient is male, has more severe depression, has concurrent alcohol abuse, is older, and has a painful medical condition (4).

Depression is associated with poor outcomes from a variety of medical conditions, including cardiac disease, neurologic disorders, chronic pain, fracture, and children's mental health (Box 5-1).

Table 5-2   Risk Factors for Depression

Risk Factors	Association
Personal history of depression	50–80% relapse
One parent with depression (3)	2.7 OR
Both parents with depression (3)	3.0 OR
Spouse with depression (4)	2.1 OR
Being bullied (5)	5.1 OR
Abused/neglect as child (6)	1.6 OR
Pregnancy, postpartum, spontaneous abortion (7)	2.5 OR
Peri- and postmenopausal (8)	2.5 OR
Past alcohol dependence (9)	4.2 OR
Smoking cessation (10)	40% depression
Chronic pain (11)	4.0 OR
Hearing impairment (12)	4.5 × depression rates
Sleep related breathing disorder (13)	1.6–2.6 × proportionate to severity
Caregivers of demented elderly (14)	32% depression
Grandparents becoming caretakers of grandchildren (15)	2 × depression rates
Stroke (16)	3.5 OR
Coronary artery disease—post MI/CABG (17)	75% depression
Dementia (18)	3 × depression rates
Head trauma (19)	1.5 OR
Stressful events (divorce, job loss, assault, etc.) (20)	2.3–25 OR

OR = odds ratio

Box 5-1   Depression and Associated Comorbidities (depression worsens outcomes)

- Coronary-artery disease/myocardial infarction/mortality after CABG
- Heart-failure mortality at 3 mo and 1 y
- Mortality in community-dwelling elderly
- Long-term mortality in hospitalized elderly
- Stroke and stroke mortality
- Unprovoked seizures
- Physical decline and disability in elderly
- Disabling back pain
- Low bone-mineral density/fractures
- Unemployment/loss of family income in subsequent 5 years
- Increased rate of children's mental-health disorders (maternal depression)

Clinical Features

Most patients with depression are initially seen by primary care providers. Depression is the 10th most common diagnosis made during family physician visits. However, 1 out of every 4 patients diagnosed with depression does not accept the diagnosis (3). These patients tend to take a lot of a physician's time because of various somatic complaints and may not follow medical recommendations.

The diagnosis of depression, according to DSM-IV criteria, requires that a patient have 5 or more of 9 symptoms and that the symptoms must be present during the same 2-week period of time, nearly every day, represent a change from previous functioning, and at least one of the symptoms must be either depressed mood or loss of interest or pleasure (Box 5-2). Ninety-seven percent of depressed patients complain of decreased energy, almost 80% have sleep disturbance, and 90% have anxiety. Many

Box 5-2   DSM-IV Criteria for Depression Diagnosis

- *Depressed mood
- *Loss of interest or pleasure
- Weight loss or gain or appetite loss or gain
- Sleep disturbance
- Fatigue
- Psychomotor retardation or agitation
- Trouble concentrating or indecisiveness
- Low self-esteem or guilt
- Thoughts of death or suicidal ideation

Must have at least 1 of the symptoms with asterisk *
Must have at least 5 of the symptoms above

depressed patients, especially the elderly, commonly present with physical complaints. In addition to the above DSM-IV criteria, somatic complaints of depression may include weakness, dizziness, gastrointestinal disturbances, various pain complaints (e.g., head, abdominal, back, and pelvic), as well as anxiety, agitation, or anger "attacks." Depressed patients may have multiple office visits for many somatic complaints, have problematic work or family relationships, and complain of anxiety.

Unipolar depressive disorders include the subtypes of anxious depression, atypical depression, seasonal affective disorder (SAD), and postpartum depression. Anxious depression may present with panic attacks, worrying, tension, restlessness, phobias, or compulsions. Response to treatment is often slower in these patients, with poorer overall treatment response and a higher rate of suicide in the first year. Atypical depression is more common in women, with earlier onset, more frequent mood swings, and a more chronic course. It can include increased appetite, weight gain, hypersomnia, or sensitivity regarding interpersonal rejection. Over 36% of depressed patients have atypical depression (5).

Although many screening tests are available, easy to administer, and have good sensitivity and specificity, routine screening in nonpsychiatric settings has not resulted in improved outcomes. Improved outcomes occur when the diagnosis is coupled with close management (6). Hence, the United States Preventive Services Task Force (USPTF) recommends screening adults for depression if systems are in place to assure accurate diagnosis, effective treatment, and follow-up. A number of free screening tests are available to diagnose and follow depression symptoms.

Screening and treatment are recommended in high-risk patients. For example, screening for depression should occur one month after coronary revascularization surgery, because as many as 75% of patients become depressed at that point after their procedure (8). The American Academy of Family Physicians recommends universal screening for postpartum depression, since some symptoms may be mistakenly perceived as normal in the postpartum period (9). Patients with early dementia should be screened for concomitant depression. Behavioral treatments help caregivers of demented patients and can reduce depressive symptoms in both patients and caregivers.

Depression is under-diagnosed and missed because the diagnosis is not sought for a variety of reasons: time, avoidance on the part of the patient and physician due to stigma of "depression," other "more pressing medical problems," overwhelming social factors, lack of follow-up, lack of available mental health services, or a belief held by both patients and physicians that depression is expected with many comorbidities like terminal illness.

Once depression is diagnosed, comorbidities (e.g., an anxiety disorder or substance dependence) should be evaluated. If present, the clinician must determine whether depression is primary or a symptom of another medical condition. A number of disorders increase a woman's risk for depression, including cancer, coronary artery disease, cerebral vascular accident, and both hypo- and hyperthyroidism. The medical condition can cause depression, as in the case of hypothyroidism, or trigger the onset of depression because of the perceived severity of the medical illness, such as cancer (3).

A complete medication history must be obtained, because many medications (prescription, over-the-counter, and/or herbal) can cause depression. Some medications that can cause depression include clonidine, methyldopa, reserpine, corticosteroids, sedatives/hypnotics, estrogens/progesterones, anti-Parkinsonian medicines, anticonvulsants, and interferons (3).

Treatment of Depression

The goal of treatment is 3-fold: 1) reduce all signs and symptoms of depression; 2) restore psychosocial and occupational function; and 3) reduce the likelihood of relapse or recurrence. Four types of treatment for depression include psychotherapy, pharmacologic therapy, electroconvulsive therapy (ECT), or a combination. If a woman has a clear suicidal or homicidal plan, has lost touch with reality, has significant psychosis, or a prolonged inability to work or care for self/family, then treatment should involve hospitalization or emergency behavioral health evaluation. Although "no suicide contracts" are common, there is no evidence to support or refute their effectiveness. Behavioral referral may be appropriate for comorbid diagnoses of mania, obsessive-compulsive disorder, eating disorder, alcohol or substance abuse, psychosis, lack of improvement with medications, or uncertain diagnosis.

Psychotherapy is particularly useful for mild-to-moderate depression related to issues associated with a clear trigger, such as a role transition and relationship disputes, and complicated bereavement or other losses (postpartum, perimenopausal, and retirement). Empirically validated therapies (interpersonal and cognitive, behavioral therapies) have been shown to be effective in both short-term (4-6 months) and longer-term follow-ups. Anti-depressant medications and counseling have been shown to be equally effective, although anti-depressants are associated with faster recovery than counseling. Combination treatments may be more effective, especially with recurrent depression in women and in patients with an early childhood history of abuse. Anti-depressants have been useful in mild, moderate, and severe depression; cognitive treatment in mild or moderate depression; and interpersonal psychotherapy in mild or moderate depression. Exercise may reduce symptoms, while pain may inhibit treatment efficacy. ECT is generally reserved for severe depression unresponsive to medication. Active clinical management is critical in depressed patients who have low energy, low motivation, noncompliance, and often lack of understanding of their disease.

Treatment is divided into 3 phases:

Acute phase (12 weeks): Three contacts between the patient and a health care provider are recommended during this phase. A telephone call or appointment within the first week should be made to determine if the patient is taking medications and to check for adverse side effects. Noncompliance is common regardless of the type of medication prescribed during this period. Compliance with a therapeutic dose is more important than the specific drug selected. Anti-depressants must be taken for 2–4 weeks to produce any improvement and for 6–8 weeks to achieve substantial benefit. Management should include a measurement-based evaluation such as A Quick Inventory of Depression (QIDS) (http://www.ids-quids.org/) or Center for Epidemiologic Studies Depression (CES-D) Scales (http://www.chcr.brown.edu/pcoc/cesdscale.pdf). Symptoms must be measured and monitored for complete, not partial, reduction in symptoms. Similar to managing a chronic disease like hypertension, for example, the provider must continually monitor depression and adjust medications until the treatment goal is reached. If symptoms are partially resolved (30% or more), then the dose may be increased to the maximally tolerated dose and compliance must be ensured before switching to a different anti-depressant or adding a second medication. Once depression has resolved, visits can be stretched out to every 4–12 weeks.

Continuation therapy (6–9 months to prevent relapse): This period is critical since relapse is as high as 50%, especially if treatment is <6 months in duration. Up to one third of patients discontinue drugs or take medications erratically during the first 6 months. Patients should be encouraged to continue to take their medicines even if they are feeling better. Patients should be encouraged to not discontinue anti-depressants without checking with their provider. Patients need to make and keep follow-up appointments. If a woman is at risk for relapse and recurrence (e.g., older age, chronic episodes, history of psychotic episodes, severe or life-threatening bouts, difficult to treat) has 2 or more recurrent episodes, or 2 or more episodes in five years, treatment should continue for at least two years, if not lifelong. If a woman is at low risk for relapse (e.g., few residual symptoms, single episode), treatment should be tapered slowly over 4–6 weeks to avoid discontinuation symptoms. If SSRIs (selective serotonin reuptake inhibitors), with the exception of fluoxetine which has a long half-life, are discontinued abruptly, withdrawal effects may occur, including nervousness, anxiety, irritability, electric shock sensations (sharp, nerve-type pains), crying, dizziness, lightheadedness, insomnia, confusion, trouble concentrating, nausea, vomiting.

Maintenance therapy: This phase lasts from one year to the patient's entire lifetime to prevent relapse. Maintenance doses are the same as acute phase treatment. Continuous anti-depressant treatment reduces the risk of relapse 1–3 years after recovery. Cognitive therapy reduces recurrence and relapse rates in depression (number needed to treat = 2) (10). In particular, patients with recurrent depression who are at a high risk of recurrence may benefit most from continuous therapy and frequent monitoring for early signs of relapse.

All anti-depressants have similar efficacy; 30% of patients will go into remission with the first agent given, and 50% will achieve remission with the second (11). If a woman has a personal or family history of response to a given anti-depressant without side effects, that medication should be tried first. SSRIs are often the first choice anti-depressant, because they are well tolerated and are relatively safe. Since no single SSRI is more effective than another, the decision is often made based on cost; for instance, fluoxetine, citalopram, and sertraline are generic and cost less. Since effectiveness is similar, an anti-depressant selection may be based on side effect profiles. SSRIs can be switched directly from one to another without tapering. Patients using fluoxetine should wait 4–7 days before starting other SSRIs because of the long half-life of this medication. Checking for compliance prior to switching anti-depressants is also helpful. An adequate trial of an anti-depressant means an adequate dose for an adequate duration, which may be as long at 8–12 weeks (though 80% of patients respond by 5 weeks).

All anti-depressants can induce mania in patients with bipolar illness. Prior to starting an anti-depressant, clinicians should check for a history of baseline hypomanic episodes or a family history of bipolar disorder. Providers should closely monitor for worsening depression or suicidal thoughts in *all* patients receiving anti-depressants, especially at the beginning of therapy or when the dose is changed (12). Patients need to be informed of the uncommon possibility of suicide.

Special Populations

Pregnancy and Postpartum Period

See Section D.

Perimenopausal/Postmenopausal Women

In addition to anti-depressants and counseling, estrogen replacement (oral or skin patches) appears effective in treating depressive symptoms in perimenopausal woman (13). However, other side effects of HRT preclude its use for this indication in most cases.

Geriatric Patients

In patients over 60 years, effective treatment modalities include anti-depressants, ECT, cognitive behavior therapy, interpersonal psychotherapy, and exercise. Although depression itself causes an increased risk of hip fractures, probably because of an increase in falls (14), both tricyclic antidepressants and SSRIs are associated with a greater than 2-fold increase in risk of hip fracture in patients >66 year olds (14).

Patients with Alcohol and Drug Addictions

In patients abusing alcohol or drugs, detoxification should be undertaken first, and re-evaluation should occur after 2 weeks, because the two thirds of patients who screen positively for depression on admission decreases to 13% after detoxification and 2 weeks of abstinence.

Seasonal Affective Disorder

All or most depressive episodes occur from November through April (in the Northern hemisphere), with most patients suffering from hypersomnia, increased appetite, carbohydrate craving, and weight gain (15). Effective treatments include light therapy, sleep deprivation, SSRIs, and monoamine oxidase inhibitors (MAOIs).

Summary

Major depression is common, often undiagnosed, and frequently not treated, causing significant burden on the woman, her children, and her family. Providers must screen high-risk patients and suspect depression in the setting of a multitude of symptoms. Like other chronic diseases, once depression is diagnosed, the provider must pursue active management: monitoring and treating until complete resolution of symptoms and close follow-up to prevent or treat relapses and recurrences throughout the lifespan.

References

1. **Murray VJ, Lopez AD.** Alternative project of mortality and disability by cause 1990–2020. Global Burden of Disease Study. Lancet. 1997;349:1498–504.
2. **Kessler RC, Berglund P, Demler O, et al.** Lifetime Prevalence and age-of-onset distributions of DSM-IV disorders in the National Co-morbidity Survey Replication. Arch Gen Psychiatry. 2005;62:593–602.
3. **Remick RA.** Diagnosis and management of depression in primary care: a clinical update and review. CMAJ. 2002;167:1253–60.
4. **Nemeroff CB, Compton MT, Berger J.** The depressed suicidal patient. Assessment and treatment. Ann N Y Acad Sci. 2001;932:1–23.
5. **Matza LS, Revicki DA, Davidson JR, et al.** Depression with atypical features in the national comorbidity survey classification, description, and consequences. Arch Gen Psychiatry. 2003;60:817–26.
6. **Nutting PA, Gallagher K, Riley, K, et al.** Care management for depression in primary care practice: findings from the respect-depression trial. Annals of Family Medicine. 2008;6:30–7.
7. **Mitchel AJ, Coyne JC.** Do ultra-short screening instruments accurately detect depression in primary care? A pooled analysis and meta-analysis of 22 studies. Br J Gen Pract. 2007;57:144–51.
8. Behav Modif 2003;27(1):26 in AHRQ Research Activities 2003; 276:4.
9. **Penfetti J, Clark R, Follmore C.** Postpartum depression: identification, screening and treatment. WI Med J. 2004;103:56–63.
10. **Vittengl JR, Clark LA, Dunn TW, et al.** Reducing relapse and recurrence in unipolar depression: A comparative meta-analysis of cognitive-behavioral therapy's effects. J Consult Clin Psychol. 2007;75: 475–88.

11. **Sussman D.** Prim Care Companion. Translating science into service: lessons learned from sequenced treatment alternatives to relieve depression (star*d) study. J Clin Psychiatry. 2007;9:331-7.

12. FDA Release, FDA MedWatch 2007. May 2.

13. **Cláudio de Novaes Soares, Almeida OP, Joffe H, et al.** Efficacy of estradiol for the treatment of depressive disorders in perimenopausal women a double-blind, randomized, placebo-controlled trial. Arch Gen Psychiatry. 2001;58:529-34.

14. **Liu B, Anderson G, Mittmann N, et al.** Use of selective serotonin-reuptake inhibitors or tricyclic antidepressants and risk of hip fractures in elderly people. Lancet. 1998;351:1303.

15. **Lurie SJ, Gawinski B, Pierce D, et al.** Seasonal affective disorder. Am Fam Physician. 2006;74:1521-2.

B. Panic Disorder

Rebecca O'Bryan, Andrew Goddard, and Anantha Shekhar

KEY POINTS

- Panic disorder is seen in 1–2% of the population, is more common in females, and generally presents in adolescence or early adulthood.
- Panic disorder is often complicated later by comorbid psychiatric disorders and may be a significant risk factor for cardiovascular disease.
- Panic attacks and panic disorder are separate diagnostic entities in the DSM-IV.
- A panic attack as an isolated event may be a normal response to acute stress.
- Panic disorder presents with spontaneous panic attacks in the absence of danger.
- Extensive work-up should be done only in the presence of compelling risk factors elicited during the history and physical examination.
- If possible, cognitive behavioral therapy (CBT) is first-line treatment for panic disorder.
- In the primary care setting, CBT is generally beyond the scope of most providers, and SSRIs are first-line treatment because of their proven safety and efficacy.
- Benzodiazepines may be used for short-term stabilization in conjunction with an SSRI for long-term management and control.
- SSRIs also may be helpful in treatment of comorbid psychiatric conditions.

Epidemiology

The anxiety disorders are among the most common psychiatric syndromes, affecting about 15% of the population during their lifetime (1). Panic disorder (PD), a particularly severe anxiety disorder commonly seen in general medical settings, is characterized by recurrent panic attacks which eventually lead to significant morbidity. It usually begins with spontaneous attacks that can eventually become associated with contextual cues (e.g., previous panic attacks occurred associated with bridges, crowded spaces, or situations in which rapid exit is difficult) (2). Thus, the initial pathology in these patients appears to be an alteration somewhere in the central neural pathways regulating normal panic response, thus rendering them susceptible to unprovoked panic symptoms (3). The disorder occurs in 1–2% of the population, first presenting during adolescence or early adulthood. Its prevalence is nearly 2-fold higher in females. It tends to be chronic and persistent and is later often complicated by other psychiatric disorders, especially agoraphobia, major depression, and substance use disorders (4). Panic disorder may be a significant risk factor for cardiovascular diseases, such as coronary artery disease, hypertension, and strokes (5).

Clinical Features or Presentation

The Diagnostic and Statistical Manual of Mental Disorders, fourth edition (DSM-IV), provides separate definitions for panic attacks and panic disorder. This is significant because a majority of individuals (approximately 80%) who meet criteria for other anxiety disorders also present with secondary panic attacks (6). The panic attack criteria require a sudden episode of distress with at least 4 of 13 key panic symptoms that must occur and peak within ten minutes. The 13 key symptoms of a panic attack, primarily due to autonomic overactivity, are heart palpitations/pounding, sweating, trembling/shaking, shortness of breath, feeling of choking, chest pain/discomfort, nausea/abdominal distress, dizziness/unsteadiness, derealization, fear of losing control/going crazy, fear of dying, paresthesias, and chills/hot flushes. With this separate definition, panic attacks are viewed as symptoms that can occur in the context of a perceived imminent, severe threat; thus, they may be diagnosed as occurring within any anxiety disorder, or, if occurring in isolation, may be a normal response to acute stress in 20% of adults in the community.

Panic disorder presents initially with the occurrence of spontaneous panic attacks in the absence of any objective danger. This false alarm may arise from genetic, biological, and life stress vulnerabilities. For the person who is experiencing the false alarm, however, the phenomenon is inexplicable. The absence of an external source of danger to associate with the alarm results in an internal scanning for the threat. The person then misperceives the occurrence of the alarm as an indication of an internal danger, such as heart attack, loss of control, or fainting. Further focus on the perception that the attacks themselves are dangerous results in a secondary process that worsens the panic attacks and anxiety (a phenomenon labeled anticipatory anxiety).

Diagnosis and Differential Diagnosis

A DSM-IV diagnosis of panic disorder is usually accomplished in the clinical interview by eliciting the typical pattern of initial spontaneous attacks, followed by the developing fear of the attacks, such as worrying about the attacks, about the implications or consequences of the attacks, or a significant behavioral change due to the attacks (Box 5-3). If seen in an emergency room during or immediately following an acute panic attack, it is important to elicit the sudden onset, rapid peaking, and multisystem symptoms (cardiac, respiratory, neurological, gastrointestinal, and psychological) of the attack in the absence of other serious medical conditions. Common signs observed on physical examination of a subject during an acute panic attack, most often in the emergency room, include sinus tachycardia, hyperventilation, and mild systolic hypertension. Patients seen in outpatient settings with typical history suggestive of panic disorder may show mild resting tachycardia or tachypnea.

Differential diagnoses for panic disorder are usually suggested by a good history and physical examination. Typically, the patient is a healthy young individual with very few cardiovascular risk factors. Therefore, any further work-up beyond basic chemistries, EKG, and urine toxicology should only be done if there are compelling risk factors elicited in the history or physical (Box 5-4). Similarly, beyond baseline thyroid functions in women, an extensive endocrine work-up should only be undertaken if indicated by physical signs. About 10% of patients with panic disorder also may have a mild mitral valve prolapse (MVP), resulting in a systolic

---

Box 5-3   Panic Disorder—DSM IV Diagnostic Criteria

- Recurrent, unexpected panic attacks
- Attack followed by at least 1 month of:
    a) Concern about further attacks
    b) Worry about consequences
    c) Significant behavioral change
- Panic attacks are not due to organic causes
- Panic attacks are not better accounted for by another psychiatric disorder

---

Box 5-4   Panic Disorder—Basic Workup

- Workup is guided by a good physical exam
- Tests such echocardiogram, EEG, or MRI, urinary catecholamines, upper GI endoscopy, etc., should be done only if there is compelling clinical evidence
- Reasonable baseline work-up:
    a) Basic chemistries
    b) EKG
    c) Thyroid-function tests

murmur (mid-systolic click), usually without hemodynamic instability. Additional work-ups, such as an echocardiogram, may be indicated if the murmur is thought to be clinically significant. Neurological evaluation with EEG and MRI may be indicated if the history is suggestive of seizures (such as loss of consciousness, loss of sphincter control, or prolonged dissociative episodes) but should not be done routinely for neurological symptoms of dizziness, numbness, tingling, or brief depersonalization that may occur during the peak of a panic attack but completely subside along with the other symptoms.

Treatment and Clinical Care

Panic disorder is highly treatable and responds to a number of treatment modalities (Box 5-5). The first-line treatment for uncomplicated panic disorder is cognitive behavior therapy (CBT), a type of stress management training, which is a brief, symptom-focused psychotherapy that enables the patient to learn a range of coping strategies to manage her anxiety (7). Unfortunately, the expertise for this treatment is not uniformly available and is often beyond the scope of a traditional medical office. Therefore, pharmacological treatments tend to be the most commonly utilized approach to treat panic disorder (8). Currently, the selective serotonin reuptake inhibitors (SSRIs), such as paroxetine, sertraline, or citalopram, are considered first-line medications for panic disorder because of their demonstrated efficacy and safety. In addition, SSRIs also treat many of the comorbid conditions associated with panic disorder, including depression, social phobia, generalized anxiety disorder (GAD), and post-traumatic stress disorder (PTSD) (see Section E). One drawback to SSRIs is initial exacerbation of panic symptoms in a subset of patients during the initiation of these medications. Newer serotonin norepinephrine reuptake inhibitors (SNRIs), such as venlafaxine XR and duloxetine, appear to be similarly effective to the SSRIs for panic management. Another effective drug class that is less often utilized now is the tricyclic antidepressants (TCAs). However, unlike the SSRIs and SNRIs, TCAs can produce greater weight gain and anticholinergic side effects, as well as dangerous cardiovascular toxicity in overdoses.

Box 5-5   Panic Disorder—Treatment

Cognitive Behavioral Therapy (CBT)
- A systematic, multimodal, time-limited treatment preferred in uncomplicated cases

Pharmacological Treatment
- Selective serotonin reuptake inhibitors (SSRIs) are the first-line drugs recommended
- Benzodiazepines (alprazolam, clonazepam or lorazepam) for acute episodes or for short periods during initiation of treatment

For resistant cases, use tricyclic antidepressants or monoamine oxidase inhibitors

Benzodiazepines are also effective in treating panic disorder. They are still a widely used treatment option, and the short half-life, high-potency benzodiazepines, like lorazepam, alprazolam, and clonazepam, are preferred now in clinical practice because of their simpler metabolism and fewer active metabolites. These benzodiazepines have the benefits of a favorable side effect profile and a rapid onset of action, showing improvement within a week in one study (9). Drawbacks to benzodiazepines, however, include the development of physiologic dependence with sustained use and the risk of abuse in persons predisposed to substance abuse. In contrast, SSRIs have very low abuse or dependence potential. Recent work has shown that co-administration of a benzodiazepine, such as clonazepam or alprazolam, with SSRIs, such as sertraline, accelerates the response of patients with moderate to severe panic disorder and may reduce early antidepressant-related stimulation. Thus, benzodiazepines may be effectively used for short-term stabilization and SSRIs for longer-term management/control of symptoms (9). In particularly resistant cases, a tertiary option is the use of monoamine oxidase (MAO) inhibitors.

A standard course of treatment for uncomplicated panic disorder is generally for 9–12 months before a trial of tapering of effective medications. Approximately 50% of patients will experience a full remission following effective treatment without further illness episodes. The remaining 50% of patients are prone to recurrence or a chronic persistent course. Patients who have had 3 or more illness episodes may benefit from long-term (5 years or more) maintenance treatment. A small subgroup of patients with infrequent panic and minimal agoraphobia may only require conservative treatment (reassurance, education about their condition, and monitoring of symptoms).

References

1. **Kessler RC, McGonagle KA, Zhao S, et al.** Lifetime and 12-month prevalence of DSM-III-R psychiatric disorders in the United States. Results from the National Comorbidity Survey. Arch Gen Psychiatry. 1994;51:8–19.
2. **Wilson KA, Hayward C.** A prospective evaluation of agoraphobia and depression symptoms following panic attacks in a community sample of adolescents. J Anxiety Disord. 2005;19:87–103.
3. **Vickers K, McNally RJ.** Respiratory symptoms and panic in the National Comorbidity Survey: A test of Klein's suffocation false alarm theory. Behav Res Ther. 2005;43:1011–18.
4. **Magee WJ, Eaton WW, Wittchen HU, et al.** Agoraphobia, simple phobia, and social phobia in the National Comorbidity Survey. Arch Gen Psychiatry. 1996;53:159–68.
5. **Weissman MM, Markowitz JS, Ouellette R, et al.** Panic disorder and cardiovascular/cerebrovascular problems: results from a community survey. Am J Psychiatry. 1990;147:1504–8.
6. **Sanderson WC, DiNardo PA, Rapee RM, et al.** Syndrome comorbidity in patients diagnosed with a DSM-III-R anxiety disorder. J Abnorm Psychol. 1990;99:308–12.

7. **Roberge P, Marchand A, Reinharz D, et al.** Cognitive-behavioral treatment for panic disorder with agoraphobia: a randomized, controlled trial and cost-effectiveness analysis. Behav Modif. 2008;32:333–51.
8. **van Apeldoorn FJ, van Hout WJ, Mersch PP, et al.** Is a combined therapy more effective than either CBT or SSRI alone? Results of a multicenter trial on panic disorder with or without agoraphobia. Acta Psychiatr Scand. 2008;117:260–70.
9. **Pollack MH, Simon NM, Worthington JJ, et al.** Combined paroxetine and clonazepam treatment strategies compared to paroxetine monotherapy for panic disorder. J Psychopharmacol. 2003;17:276–82.

C. Premenstrual Syndrome and Premenstrual Dysphoric Disorder

Sarina B. Schrager

KEY POINTS

- Premenstrual syndrome (PMS) symptoms affect up to 90% of all reproductive aged women.
- There is a vast assortment of symptoms associated with PMS.
- The diagnosis of PMS is a clinical one and requires documentation of cyclic symptoms that are present during the luteal phase of the menstrual cycle and resolve after the onset of menses.
- All women with PMS should exercise, eat a low fat diet, and take a calcium supplement.
- Ovulation suppression with oral contraceptive pills or depot medroxyprogesterone acetate are helpful in reducing physical symptoms of PMS.
- Women with severe psychological symptoms of PMS should consider luteal phase administration of an SSRI medication.

Epidemiology

PMS describes a constellation of physical, emotional, and cognitive symptoms that have been associated with the luteal phase (second half) of the menstrual cycle. Premenstrual dysphoric disorder (PMDD) is a more severe form of PMS, including mostly psychiatric symptoms and significantly interfering with daily life. The list of symptoms associated with either PMS or PMDD is vast (Table 5-3).

It is estimated that up to 90% of all reproductive aged women experience some menstrual related symptoms. About 40–50% of those

Table 5-3   Symptoms Associated with PMS

Behavioral	Psychological	Physical
Fatigue	Irritability	Headaches
Insomnia	Anger	Breast tenderness
Dizziness	Depressed mood	Back pain
Changes in sexual interest	Crying and tearfulness	Abdominal pain and
Food cravings or overeating	Anxiety	bloating
	Tension	Weight gain
	Mood swings	Edema
	Confusion	Water retention
	Forgetfulness	Nausea
	Restlessness	Muscle and joint pain
	Loneliness	
	Decreased self esteem	

women are classified as having premenstrual syndrome, and only 5–10% are classified as having PMDD (1). PMS symptoms usually present between ages 25 and 35 and increase in severity with age. However, some studies demonstrate that PMS can occur as early as adolescence or 2–3 years after menarche (2). Twin and mother–daughter studies have suggested that there is a genetic component to PMS, though the exact inheritance pattern is unclear. There is no ethnic predominance of PMS symptoms. A study of over 1400 women found that the prevalence of childhood sexual abuse and other traumatic events increased the risk of PMDD (3).

The etiology of PMS remains unclear. Several theories have been postulated, including hormonal changes in the luteal phase, nutritional deficiencies, decreased beta endorphin levels in the luteal phase, and stress. Most experts now believe that the etiology is multifactorial and that the symptoms are triggered by normal hormonal changes that occur during the luteal phase.

Diagnosis of Premenstrual Syndrome and Premenstrual Dysphoric Disorder

Three elements are required for the diagnosis of PMS: 1. Symptoms must occur during the luteal phase of the menstrual cycle; 2. Symptoms must resolve within a few days after the onset of menses; and 3. Symptoms must NOT be present during the follicular phase of the menstrual cycle. In order to distinguish PMS from an exacerbation of an underlying disease, women are asked to complete a symptom diary for 2–3 months to document the cyclic nature of their symptoms (4). There are no confirmatory blood tests or specific physical findings that are correlated with PMS.

The diagnosis of PMDD is described in the DSM-IV. It includes the requirement for the cyclic nature of the symptoms and also adds the requirement that the symptoms must significantly interfere with daily life (work, school, relationships, etc.). The DSM-IV criteria also require that a woman complete a symptom diary to document the symptoms for at least 2 months (5).

Several underlying medical disorders, including depression, asthma, irritable bowel syndrome, migraines, and eczema, can be exacerbated by menstrual cycle changes. This is a distinct phenomenon from PMS and underlies the importance of documenting that the symptoms of PMS are present in the luteal phase of the menstrual cycle but resolve within a few days after the onset of menses. All women with PMS symptoms should be screened for depression and dysthymia, disorders, which would be present throughout the entire month.

Treatment of Premenstrual Syndrome and Premenstrual Dysphoric Disorder

Although there is limited evidence documenting the benefit of education about PMS, exercise, or stress management in the treatment of PMS symptoms, these interventions can improve overall health and should be recommended to all women. Some specific stress management techniques, such as biofeedback, guided imagery, and yoga, have shown promise in controlled studies in reducing symptoms of PMS. Psychological counseling also can be helpful if stress symptoms are severe. Aerobic exercise may be helpful through increasing levels of endogenous endorphins (6).

Theories of management of PMS include interrupting ovulation and changing the neurotransmitter substrate. Ovulation suppression with either oral contraceptive pills (taken monthly or on an extended cycle regimen) or depot medroxyprogesterone acetate are effective ways to reduce physical symptoms of PMS. New research on the oral contraceptive pill containing drospirenone shows promise in controlling psychological symptoms as well (7).

It is recommended that women with PMS follow a diet low in sodium and avoid caffeine, based on observational studies showing that women with the most severe PMS symptoms consume more of these substances. Low fat and high fiber diets may help decrease endogenous estrogen levels and decrease PMS symptoms. Simple carbohydrate drinks have shown benefit in improving mood and decreasing food cravings (7).

Well-designed studies have shown that calcium supplementation can decrease both physical and emotional symptoms of PMS. Magnesium supplementation shows promise in reducing depressive symptoms and water retention associated with PMS. Vitamin B6 may improve the emotional symptoms of PMS, but the evidence is conflicting. Vitex (chasteberry) and Ginkgo biloba are 2 herbs used commonly for PMS symptoms. Studies have shown that use of alprazolam and other benzodiazepines can be effective luteal phase treatments for patients with PMS with predominantly anxiety symptoms (8). Nonsteroidal anti-inflammatory agents and spironolactone are sometimes used for physical symptoms. Other diuretics have not been shown to be effective in reducing water retention symptoms of PMS (4).

The gold standard for treating severe psychological symptoms of PMS or PMDD is an SSRI, which can be dosed only during the luteal phase of the menstrual cycle. In contrast to use for depression, these medications take effect within 1–2 days of administration which enables their cyclic use (9) (Table 5-4).

All treatments should be followed for at least 3 months before adding new therapy.

Table 5-4   Treatment of PMS Symptoms

Medication	Dose	Efficacy	Level of Evidence
Magnesium	200–800 mg/d	Likely reduces negative mood and water retention	Level B (small trials)
Vitamin B6	500–100 mg/d	Likely improves emotional symptoms	Level B (small trials, systematic review)
Calcium	1200 mg/d	Reduces physical and emotional symptoms	Level A (large trials, systematic review)
Vitamin E	400 IU/d	Likely improves both physical and emotional symptoms	Level B (small trials)
Chasteberry	20 mg/d	Reduces PMS symptoms	Level B (small trials)
Ginkgo	80 mg twice during the luteal phase	Likely improves breast tenderness, depressed mood, and water retention	Level B (small trials)— caution regarding drug interactions
St. John's Wort	300 mg TID	Likely improves depressed mood	Level B (small trials)— caution regarding drug interactions
SSRIs		Improve depressed mood and anxiety symptoms	Level A (large trials)
Alprazolam	0.25 mg up to QID during the luteal phase	Improves anxiety symptoms	Level A (large trial)—caution regarding addictive potential
Spironolactone	25–100 mg/d	Improves water retention and breast tenderness	Level B (small trials)
NSAIDs		Improves physical symptoms (but not breast tenderness)	Level B (small trials)

From Dickerson LM, Mazyck PJ, Hunter MH. Premenstrual syndrome. American Family Physician. 2003;67:1743–52 and Braverman PK. Premenstrual syndrome and premenstrual dysphoric disorder. Journal of Pediatric and Adolescent Gynecology. 2007;20:3–12; with permissioin.

References

1. **Mishell DR.** Premenstrual disorders: Epidemiology and disease burden. American Journal of Managed Care. 2005;11:S473-9.
2. **Cleckner-Smith CS, Doughty AS, Grossman JA.** Premenstrual symptoms: Prevalence and severity in an adolescent sample. Journal of Adolescent Health. 1998;22:403-8.
3. **Perkonigg A, Yonkers KA, Pfister H, et al.** Risk factors for premenstrual dysphoric disorder in a community sample of young women: the role of traumatic events and posttraumatic stress disorder. Journal of Clinical Psychiatry. 2004;65:1314-22.
4. **Dickerson LM, Mazyck PJ, Hunter MH.** Premenstrual syndrome. American Family Physician. 2003;67:1743-52.
5. American Psychiatric Association: Diagnostic and Statistical Manual of Mental Disorders, 4th ed, DSM-IV-Text Revision. American Psychiatric Association DSM-IV-TR, Washington, DC, 2000.
6. **Steege JF, Blumenthal JA.** The effects of aerobic exercise on premenstrual symptoms in middle-aged women: a preliminary study. Journal of Psychosomatic Research. 1993;37:127-33.
7. **Braverman PK.** Premenstrual syndrome and premenstrual dysphoric disorder. Journal of Pediatric and Adolescent Gynecology. 2007;20:3-12.
8. **Freeman EW, Rickels K, Sondheimer SJ, et al.** A double blind trial of oral progesterone, alprazolam, and placebo in treatment of severe premenstrual syndrome. JAMA. 1995;274:51-7.
9. **Steiner M, Pearlstein T, Cohen LS, et al.** Expert guidelines for the treatment of severe PMS, PMDD, and comorbidities: the role of SSRIs. Journal of Women's Health. 2006;15:57-69.

D. Postpartum Mood Disorders

Jo Marie R. Reilly

KEY POINTS

◆ Postpartum mood disorders are a spectrum of mood disturbances, which include postpartum "blues," postpartum depression (PPD), and postpartum psychosis (PSS).

◆ Early screening at prenatal and postpartum clinical visits is essential for the detection and early intervention of these conditions.

◆ Risk factors include a prior history of depression or bipolar disorder, history of a postpartum mood disorder after a previous pregnancy, unplanned pregnancy, and lack of partner and family support.

◆ Treatment options include psychotherapy, family support, and medications.

◆ Women with PPD are at increased risk for suicide and infanticide.

Epidemiology

There are significant differences in the psychiatric illnesses of women compared to men. Women suffer from depressive disorders at twice the rate of men (1). Factors contributing to the higher rates of depression in women may include fluctuations in gonadal hormones (estrogen and progesterone), higher rates of neuroendocrine disorders, such as thyroid dysfunction, and the increased and multiple psychosocial roles and demands of women in modern society (2,3).

Postpartum mood disorders are a spectrum of depressive mood disturbances on a continuum of severity and include postpartum blues, PPD, and PSS.

Postpartum blues affects 50–70% of women within 10–14 days postpartum and is self-limited. PPD affects 10–22% of all postpartum women and is serious and disabling. The average time of onset is 4 weeks postpartum. PSS affects 1 in 500–1000 women. Seventy percent have an underlying affective disorder (bipolar disorder or depression). It is considered a medical emergency. One in 50 000 women with this disorder is at risk for infanticide (4).

Clinical Features or Presentation

Postpartum blues begins in the first several days after delivery. Common clinical features include general anxiety, irritability, tearfulness, sleep and appetite disturbances, emotional lability, sadness, and confusion. Symptoms can begin as early as the first day postpartum but typically do not present until 3–5 days after delivery (5).

Risk factors for postpartum blues include a prior personal history of depression or bipolar disorder, depressive symptoms during pregnancy, unplanned pregnancy, maternity blues or euphoria, marital discord/lack of partner support, recent adverse life events, family history of affective disorders, premenstrual dysphoric disorder (PMDD), or pregnancy loss (6).

PPD typically begins in the first 4 weeks after delivery. Common maternal clinical features include those associated with DSM-IV major depression, such as depressed mood, anhedonia, low energy, guilt, profound anxiety, disturbances in sleep and eating patterns, obsessional thoughts of harming the infant, and suicidal ideation (7). Sometimes a woman's thought of harming her infant can become so severe that she is unable to care for the baby (8).

Studies of infants of mothers suffering from PPD indicate that their infants are more hyperactive, distractable, and have higher levels of behavioral disturbances than do the infants of mothers without PPD (9). These symptoms appear to be worse in children born into economically depressed families, and in boys (10). These children also have been found to have higher rates of major depression, poor social functioning, and school performance later in life (11). Additionally, women who suffer from PPD may have increased risk for preterm, small-for-gestational-age, and low birth-weight infants compared to women without PPD (12).

The risk factors for PPD include a prior history of depression, antenatal depression, inadequate social support, and a prior history of PPD (5). Thirty to fifty percent of all women who suffer from PPD may have a relapse in subsequent pregnancies (13).

PSS is the most extreme manifestation of the postpartum mood disorders. It may be characterized by an abrupt onset within the first week after delivery or up to 6 weeks postpartum. Symptoms initially include insomnia, restlessness, anxiety, hyperactivity, and depressed or elated mood. The mood disturbances may increase in severity to include bizarre behavior, disorientation, cognitive disorganization, and impaired insight. Tactile, olfactory, or visual hallucinations are some of the more unusual features of PSS (14).

The risk factors for PSS include a prior history of PSS, a personal history of bipolar disorder, and a family history of bipolar disorder. As with PPD, the recurrence risk of PSS is very high, often making decisions to plan another pregnancy very difficult (14).

Diagnosis and Differential Diagnosis

The differential diagnosis of all postpartum psychiatric complications includes postpartum blues, PSS, and PPD (Table 5-5). Decreased energy, excessive somnolence, and changes in appetite are common features of depression. These symptoms also can be mimicked by both anemia and hypothyroidism (15). The latter conditions are fairly common in the postpartum period and must be excluded when making the diagnosis of any of the postpartum mood disorders. A simple thyroid panel and complete blood count, with particular attention to the hemoglobin, hematocrit, and MCV, aids in the diagnosis of both hypothyroidism and anemia, respectively. Additionally, a physical examination with specific attention to the thyroid gland and color of the buccal mucosa, conjunctivae, and nail beds is important when considering a diagnosis of hypothyroidism and anemia, respectively.

Prevention and Clinical Care

Prevention

Mood disorders in women often go undiagnosed. Because new mothers may feel guilt or shame at their feelings of hurting their infants, they may not share their disturbing thoughts or fears. As a result, they may not get the necessary interventions or support needed to avoid the extreme and tragic cases of suicide or infanticide.

Depression Risk Assessment

The best preventive clinical care is rendered by assessing a women's risk for depression at her first prenatal visit. This may include having a women complete an antenatal depression risk scale or assessing her risk factors for depression (16). Physicians should monitor a patient's mood throughout her pregnancy at her prenatal visits. Women with depression

Table 5-5   Differential Diagnosis of Postpartum Mood Disorders

	Incidence	Time of Onset	Duration	Symptoms
Baby Blues	80% of mothers	First few days postpartum	Hours to 10th postnatal day	Crying spells, sadness, confusion, insomnia, and anxiety
Postpartum Depression	10–22% of mothers	Within 4 wk postpartum	Med treatment recommended for 6 mo–1 y.	At least five of the following every day for 2 wk**: • Depressed mood • Diminished pleasure or interest in activities • Sleep disturbance • Weight loss or gain • Loss of energy • Psychomotor agitation or retardation • Decline in social and/or occupational functioning • Feelings of worthlessness or inappropriate guilt • Decrease concentration or indecisiveness • Frequent thoughts of death or suicide
Postpartum Psychosis	0.2% of new mothers	First month postpartum	Med treatment recommended for 6 mo–1 y.	• Insomnia • Agitation • Irritable mood • Hallucinations/delusions (often involve infant) • Mania and depression

** See the DSM-IV for a more detailed description of the diagnostic criteria and symptoms of depression.
Adapted from Flores DL, Hendrick VC. Etiology and treatment of postpartum depression. Current Psychiatry Reports. 2002:4:461–6 and Jennings, KD, Ross S. Popper S, et al. Thought of harming infants in depressed and not depressed mothers. J Affect Disorde. 1999;54:21–8; with permission.

have increased risks of poor self-care, nutrition, and sleep, in addition to tobacco, alcohol, and drug use. These may be the first indicators for care providers to screen their patients more extensively for depression.

Patients should be screened for PPD at their 4–6 week visit after delivery by their obstetric provider or sooner if they are "at-risk." This is best done by using the Edinburgh Postnatal Depression Scale (Box 5-6) (17). A family physician or pediatrician may note a mother's depression at one of her children's well-child visits and institute an intervention or referral at that time.

Suicide and Infanticide Risk Assessment
All patients with a postpartum mood disorder should have a suicide risk assessment because of their increased risks of suicidality. A suicide risk

---

Box 5-6   Edinburgh Postnatal Depression Scale

The Edinburgh Postnatal Depression Scale (EPDS) has been developed to assist primary care health professionals to detect mothers suffering from postnatal depression; a distressing disorder more prolonged than the "blues" (which occur in the first week after delivery) but less severe than puerperal psychosis. Previous studies have shown that postnatal depression affects at least 10% of women and that many depressed mothers remain untreated. These mothers may cope with their baby and with household tasks, but their enjoyment of life is seriously affected and it is possible that there are long-term effects on the family. The EPDS was developed at health centers in Livingston and Edinburgh. It consists of ten short statements. The mother underlines which of the 4 possible responses is closest to how she has been feeling during the past week. Most mothers complete the scale without difficulty in less than 5 minutes. The validation study showed that mothers who scored 13 or more were likely to be suffering from a depressive illness of varying severity. Nevertheless the EPDS score should not override clinical judgment. A careful clinical assessment should be carried out to confirm the diagnosis. The scale indicates how the mother has felt during the previous week and in doubtful cases it may be usefully repeated after 2 weeks. The scale will not detect mothers with anxiety neuroses, phobias or personality disorder.
Instructions for users:

- The mother is asked to underline the response which comes closest to how she has been feeling in the previous 7 days.
- All ten items must be completed.
- Care should be taken to avoid the possibility of the mother discussing her answers with others.
- The mother should complete the scale herself, unless she has limited English or has difficulty with reading.
- The EPDS may be used at 6–8 weeks to screen postnatal women. The child health clinic, postnatal check-up or a home visit may provide suitable opportunities for its completion.

Name: _____

Address: _____

Baby's Age: _____

cont'd

Box 5-6   Edinburgh Postnatal Depression Scale (cont'd)

Edinburgh Postnatal Depression Scale (EPDS)

As you have recently had a baby, we would like to know how you are feeling. Please UNDERLINE the answer which comes closest to how you have felt IN THE PAST 7 DAYS, not just how you feel today.

1. I have been able to laugh and see the funny side of things.
   - As much as I always could
   - Not quite so much now
   - Definitely not so much now
   - Not at all
2. I have looked forward with enjoyment to things.
   - As much as I ever did
   - Rather less than I used to
   - Definitely less than I used to
   - Hardly at all
3. * I have blamed myself unnecessarily when things went wrong.
   - Yes, most of the time
   - Yes, some of the time
   - Not very often
   - No, never
4. I have been anxious or worried for no good reason.
   - No, not at all
   - Hardly ever
   - Yes, sometimes
   - Yes, very often
5. * I have felt scared or panicky for no very good reason.
   - Yes, quite a lot
   - Yes, sometimes
   - No, not much
   - No, not at all
6. * Things have been getting on top of me.
   - Yes, most of the time I haven't been able to cope at all
   - Yes, sometimes I haven't been coping as well as usual
   - No, most of the time I have coped quite well
   - No, I have been coping as well as ever
7. * I have been so unhappy that I have had difficulty sleeping.
   - Yes, most of the time
   - Yes, sometimes
   - Not very often
   - No, not at all
8. * I have felt sad or miserable.
   - Yes, most of the time
   - Yes, quite often
   - Not very often
   - No, not at all
9. * I have been so unhappy that I have been crying.

- Yes, most of the time
- Yes, quite often
- Only occasionally
- No, never

10. * The thought of harming myself has occurred to me.
- Yes, quite often
- Sometimes
- Hardly ever
- Never

Response categories are scored 0, 1, 2, and 3 according to increased severity of the symptoms. Items marked with an asterisk are reverse scored (i.e., 3, 2, 1, and 0). The total score is calculated by adding together the scores for each of the ten items. © 1987 The Royal College of Psychiatrists. The EPDS may be photocopied by individual researchers or clinicians for their own use without seeking permission from the publishers. The scale must be copied in full and all copies must acknowledge the following source: Cox, J.L., Holden, J.M., & Sagovsky, R. (1987). Detection of postnatal depression. Development of the 10-item Edinburgh Postnatal Depression Scale. *British Journal of Psychiatry*, **150**, 782–786. Written permission must be obtained from the Royal College of Psychiatrists for copying and distribution to others or for republication (in print, online or by any other medium). Translations of the scale, and guidance as to its use, may be found in Cox, J.L. & Holden, J. (2003) *Perinatal Mental Health: A Guide to the Edinburgh Postnatal Depression Scale*. London: Gaskell.

From Cox JL, Holden JM, Sagovsky R. Detection of postnatal depression. Development of the 10-item Edinburg Depression Scale. Br J Psychiatry. 1987;150:782–6.

assessment should include questions about both passive suicide ideation and active intent. A standard question for inquiring about suicide ideation is, "Have you ever felt so sad that you felt your life was not worth living?" Standard questions for inquiring about suicidal intent are: "Have you ever thought about ending your life?" and, if so, "What types of things have you considered doing?"

A health care provider who is concerned about a woman's suicide risk should admit her to the hospital for psychiatric evaluation. If a patient refuses and is thought to be truly at risk to herself or others, she can be committed involuntarily to the hospital.

Women with postpartum mood disorders also are at increased risk for infanticide (8). These women should be screened for their concerns about hurting their infants and their guilt and confusion about these feelings. This screening is essential to protect the life of the woman's infant and family.

Treatment (Table 5-6)

Postpartum Blues

Treatment of postpartum blues is supportive (see Table 5-6). Postpartum blues usually resolves spontaneously within 2 weeks after delivery.

Table 5-6   Treatment of Postpartum Mood Disorders

	Psychosocial Support	Medications	Hospitalization	Other Treatment Options
Postpartum Blues	• Reassurance • Education • Family Support	None needed	None	None

Postpartum Depression	• Reassurance
	• Education
	
	• Family Support
		• Selective
		  Serotonin
		  Reuptake
		  Inhibitors*
		• Tricyclic antidepressants
		* drugs of choice
			Only if suicidal or
			homicidal
				• Behavioral counseling
				• Cognitive therapy
				• Individual therapy
				• Group therapy
				• Electroconvulsive therapy, if severe

Postpartum Psychosis	• Reassurance
	
	• Education
	• Family
	
	• Support
		• Lithium
		• Valproate
		• Selective
		  Serotonin
		  Reuptake
		  Inhibitors*
		• Anxlyotics
		* may exacerbate mania
			Yes, is a medical
			emergency
				• Behavioral counseling
				• Cognitive therapy
				• Individual therapy
				• Group therapy
				• Electroconvulsive therapy, if severe

Adapted from Flores DL, Hendrick VC. Etiology and treatment of postpartum depression. Current Psychiatry Reports. 2002;4:461–6; with permission.

Medication is not usually necessary. These women should be carefully monitored to ensure that their postpartum blues does not evolve into a more serious and sustained postpartum mood disorder (5).

Postpartum Depression

First-line treatment for PPD includes education, reassurance, and support. Psychosocial assistance with the support of family members, religious community, or local aid agencies is essential to reducing the stressors for caring for a new infant. Psychotherapy, whether individual, cognitive, supportive, or group therapy, is also of benefit (18).

Anti-depressant therapy is often necessary for more severe cases of PPD. The medication and timing of dosing are very important, particularly if the mother is breast-feeding her infant, since all psychotropic medications are excreted into breast milk (19). Factors involved in appropriate medication choice must take into consideration a mother's personal depression history, her prior use of drugs during the current pregnancy and lactation, the severity of her illness, and the side-effect profile of each potential medication. No decision is risk-free.

While tricyclic antidepressants are occasionally used in treating PPD, the anti-depressants of choice in pregnancy and lactation are the selective serotonin re-uptake inhibitors (SSRIs) (20). Sertraline is the best studied and favored SSRI during breast-feeding, because, while there are detectable serum drug levels in some infants, no adverse effects of infant exposure have been noted. Fluoxetine, venlafaxine, and paroxetine also have been used successfully in women with PPD (18,19). The dosing of all medications should start at the lowest level necessary to achieve euthymia. Medication treatment may be required for up to a year to avoid depression relapse (5). Hospitalization and electro-convulsive therapy may be necessary for the most extreme and refractory cases of PPD (21).

Researchers have evaluated the benefit of giving prophylactic SSRIs antenatally to at-risk women. Although SSRIs are Category C drugs, studies have indicated that mothers who take them during pregnancy have rates of neonatal and congenital malformations within the normal range (22). Some newborns exposed antenatally to SSRIs develop seratonergic central nervous system adverse effects (withdrawal symptoms) during the first 4 days of life. Infants should be monitored after birth for symptoms, including tremors, irritability, seizures, and abnormal crying (23).

Postpartum Psychosis

Postpartum psychosis is a psychiatric emergency and requires hospitalization. Women with PSS often require mood stabilizers, such as lithium or valproate, anti-depressants, and/or anxiolytic and antipsychotic medications to treat their affective disorders (14). Hospitalization and electroconvulsive therapy may be required for the most extreme and refractory cases of PSS (14). These women are at very high risk of having a recurrence in subsequent pregnancies.

Infants

Infants of mothers with mood disorders must be carefully monitored, since these women may have trouble with parenting and bonding with their infants. As a result, these infants and children may grow up having attachment problems, behavioral problems, lower activity levels, delays in language development, and challenges later in school (24).

References

1. **Weissman MM, Klerman GI.** Sex differences and the epidemiology of depression. Arch Gen Psychiatry. 1977;34:98-111.
2. **Wisner K, Stowe Z.** Psychobiology of postpartum mood disorders. Semin Reprod Endocrinol. 1997;15:77-89.
3. **Harris B, Lovett L, Newcombe RG, et al**. Maternity Blues and major endocrine changes. BMJ. 1994;308:949-53.
4. **Jones HW, Vwnis JA.** Identification and classification of postpartum psychiatric disorders. J Psychol Nursing. 2001;39:23-9.
5. **Rapkin AJ, Mikacich JA, Moatakef-Imani B.** Reproductive mood disorders. Primary Psychiatry. 2003;10:31-40.
6. **Flores DL, Hendrick VC.** Etiology and treatment of postpartum depression. Current Psychiatry Reports. 2002;4:461-6.
7. American Psychiatric Association. Diagnostic and Statistical Manual of Mental Disorders, Fourth Edition. Washington, DC: American Psychiatric Association; 1994:317-91.
8. **Jennings, KD, Ross S, Popper S, et al.** Thought of harming infants in depressed and not depressed mothers. J Affect Disord. 1999;54:21-8.
9. **Zuckerman, B, Bauchner H, Parker S, et al.** Maternal depressive symptoms during pregnancy, and newborn irritability. Developmental and Behavioral Pediatrics. 1990;114:190-4.
10. **Sincalir D, Murray L.** Effects of postnatal depression on children's adjustment to school: Teacher's report. Br J Psychiatry. 1998;172:58-66.
11. **Weissman MM, Gammon GD, John K, et al.** Children of depressed parents: Increased psychopathology and early onset of major depression. Arch Gen Psychiatry. 1987;44:847-53.
12. **Chung, TH, Lau, TK, Yip, ASK, et al.** Antepartum Depressive Symptomatology is associated with adverse obstetrical outcomes. Psychosomatic Medicine. 2001;63:830-4.
13. **Garvey M, Tueran V, et al.** Occurrence of depression in the postpartum state. J Affect Disord. 1983;5:91-101.
14. **Rohde A, Marneros A.** Postpartum psychosis: onset and long term course. Psychopathology. 1993;26:203-9.
15. **Hendrick V, Altshuler L, Suri H.** Hormonal change in postpartum and amplification for postpartum depression. Psychosomatics. 1998;39:93-101.
16. **Posner NA, Unterman RR, Williams KN, et al.** Screening for postpartum depression: an antepartum questionnaire. J Reprod Med. 1997;42:207-15.
17. **Cox JL, Holden JM, Sagovsky R.** Detection of postnatal depression. Development of the 10-item Edinburg Postnatal Depression Scale. Br J Psychiatry. 1987;150:782-6.
18. **Atshuler LL, Cohen LS, Moline ML, et al.** Treatment of depression in women: a summary of the Expert Consensus Guidelines. J Psychiatr Pract. 2001;7:185-208.

19. **Whitby DH, Smith KM.** The use of tricyclic antidepressants and selective serotnonin reuptake inhibitors in women who are breastfeeding. Pharmacotherapy. 2005;25:411–25.
20. **Parry BL.** Management of depression and psychoses during pregnancy and the puerperium. In RK Creasy et al., eds. Maternal-Fetal Medicine: Principles and Practice, 5th edition., pp. 1193–200. Philadelphia: Saunders 2004.
21. **Berle JO.** Severe post-partum depression and psychosis-when is electro-convulsive therapy the treatment of choice? Tidsskr Nor Laegeforen. 1999;30:3000–3.
22. **Hendrick V, Smith L, Suri R, et al.,** Birth outcomes after prenatal exposure to antidepressant medication. Am J Obstet Gynaecol. 2002;3:193–9.
23. **Moldovan A, Kozer E, Ho T, et al.** Perinatal Outcome following third trimester exposure to paroxetine. Arch Pediatr Adolesc Med. 2002;156: 1129–32.
24. **Wisner KL, et al.** Postpartum depression. New England Journal of Medicine. 2002;347:194–9.

E. Post-Traumatic Stress Disorder

Smitha Patibandla, Jeffrey Lightfoot, and Anantha Shekhar

KEY POINTS

- Post-traumatic stress disorder (PTSD) is a chronic, severe anxiety disorder.
- The incidence is about 8% of the general population.
- PTSD is twice as common in women as in men.
- It can affect over 25% of combat veterans and 50% of victims of abuse.
- Diagnostic criteria for PTSD require traumatic experiences.
- Key symptoms are increased arousal, re-experiencing the trauma, and avoidance of trauma-related stimuli.
- Differential diagnosis includes other anxiety disorders, dissociative disorder, or seizures due to traumatic brain injury.
- Workup may include neuroimaging, EEG, and neuropsychiatric test battery.
- Treatment approaches include serotonergic antidepressants, anticonvulsants, and psychotherapy.
- Complications and comorbid conditions include depression, substance abuse, cognitive difficulties, and worsened prognosis for many concomitant medical conditions.
- Early diagnosis and interventions are the key to preventing complications and comorbidities.

Epidemiology

The anxiety disorders are among the most common psychiatric syndromes and consist of a group of specific syndromes with characteristic clinical courses. PTSD is a severe anxiety disorder that develops following exposure to a traumatic event. In the general population, the lifetime rate of PTSD is approximately 8% (1). However, in high-risk populations, such as military veterans with combat exposure or victims of sexual assault, the incidence of PTSD is estimated to be 25% to 50%, respectively (2). The incidence of PTSD is about 2-fold higher in females than in males. The disorder has a chronic course lasting many years in about 30% of the subjects.

Clinical Features or Presentation

The Diagnostic and Statistical Manual of Psychiatric Disorders, Edition IV (DSM-IV), provides separate definitions for "trauma" and the 2 psychiatric syndromes arising from a traumatic experience: the more common and short-duration anxiety disorder known as acute stress disorder (ASD), and PTSD, the longer-lasting, more severe anxiety syndrome. The concept of "trauma" needed to be defined because, while most subjects develop ASD or PTSD following the experience of an actual threat of death or physical injury to oneself, these conditions can also arise from a perceived threat or witnessing harm to someone else, which arouses a severe experience of horror (DSM-IV). Subjects who have experienced trauma will report transient distressing reactions, usually some form of re-experiencing of the trauma (images, thoughts, dreams, flashbacks); symptoms of dissociation (numbing of emotion, reduction in awareness, derealization, depersonalization, and amnesia); increased arousal (difficulty sleeping, irritability, exaggerated startle response, motor restlessness, poor concentration); and avoidance of stimuli associated with the trauma. If such responses last a few days, but resolve within 4 weeks, a diagnosis of ASD is given. However, if these symptoms last longer than 4 weeks, a diagnosis of PTSD would be made based on the specific criteria noted in Box 5-7.

Etiology and Pathophysiology

A number of brain homeostatic mechanisms are disrupted following a severe traumatic experience resulting in the different symptoms of PTSD. Several neurotransmitter pathways, such as norepinephrine, serotonin, and corticotrophin-releasing factor (3), have been implicated in the pathophysiology of the disorder. Recent neuroimaging studies have revealed significant disruptions of normal recovery processes of fear-extinction in subjects with PTSD (4). A variety of risk factors also have been identified that predispose a person to developing PTSD (5). These include age, gender (children and women are more vulnerable), family history of anxiety and depressive disorders, and the type of trauma experienced (e.g., sexual assaults have the highest likelihood, while natural disasters have much lower likelihood, of causing PTSD).

Box 5-7   PTSD–DSM IV Diagnostic Criteria

The diagnostic criteria for PTSD, per the *Diagnostic and Statistical Manual of Mental Disorders IV (Text Revision)* (DSM-IV-TR):

A. Exposure to a traumatic event
B. Persistent re-experience (e.g., flashbacks, nightmares)
C. Persistent avoidance of stimuli associated with the trauma (e.g., inability to talk about things even related to the experience; avoidance of things and discussions that trigger flashbacks and re-experiencing symptoms; fear of losing control and harming another person)
D. Persistent symptoms of increased arousal (e.g., difficulty falling or staying asleep, anger, hypervigilance)
E. Symptoms have a duration of >1 month
F. Significant impairment in social, occupational, or other important areas of functioning (e.g., problems with work and relationships)

Note: The definition of "trauma" exposure consists of 2 parts: 1) the person experienced, witnessed, or was confronted with an event or events that involved actual or threatened death, serious injury, or a threat to the physical integrity of self or others; and 2) the person's response involved intense fear, helplessness, or horror.

Diagnosis and Differential Diagnosis

DSM-IV diagnosis of PTSD is usually made by eliciting the typical features in a clinical interview: the occurrence of a traumatic experience followed by symptoms of re-experiencing, hyperarousal, emotional numbing, and avoidance (6). If the symptoms have lasted <4 weeks, then a diagnosis of ASD can be made. Diagnosis of PTSD requires persistence of symptoms for at least 4 weeks. If seen in an emergency room during or immediately following an acute traumatic event, it is important to enquire about acute dissociation or numbing, since these may predict a greater likelihood of developing PTSD. Such subjects should be referred to appropriate follow-up facilities to treat any emerging symptoms of ASD and, if possible, prevent the development of PTSD.

The differential diagnoses for PTSD are usually suggested by atypical features in either the history or physical examination. Beyond basic chemistries, a neurologic workup with EEG and MRI may be indicated if the history is suggestive of head trauma or seizures (Box 5-8). More extensive evaluations with sleep studies or neuroendocrine tests may be indicated in some patients.

Treatment and Clinical Care

Subjects with PTSD are relatively difficult to engage in treatment, with <50% of them entering treatment. A variety of barriers to treatment have been noted (7). The first and the most important step in successfully treating a subject with PTSD is the development of a trusting relationship with the health professional. Cognitive behavioral therapy (CBT), especially

---

Box 5-8   PTSD—Basic Workup

- Workup is guided by a good history and physical examination
- Tests such as sleep studies, endocrine studies and neuropsychological battery should be done if clinically indicated
- Reasonable baseline workup (especially when there is evidence of head trauma or loss of consciousness) including basic chemistries and
  - EEG
  - MRI

---

when instituted soon after trauma, may be a very effective treatment (8). Currently the selective serotonin reuptake inhibitors (SSRIs), such as paroxetine (Paxil®) and sertraline (Zoloft®), are approved by the FDA and are considered first-line medication treatments for PTSD (9). Also, SSRIs can be used to treat many of the comorbid conditions, such as depression, panic, and generalized anxiety disorder. Unfortunately, a substantial number of patients respond only partially to SSRIs, while others may develop intolerable side effects during the initiation of these medications. There is evidence that adding alpha-adrenergic receptor antagonists, such as prazocin, may be helpful in treating symptoms of hyperarousal and sleep disturbances (10). Another effective drug group, which is used less often now but could become second-line drugs, are the tricyclic antidepressants (TCAs). The TCAs cause greater weight gain and anticholinergic side effects but, of greater concern is their lethal toxicity in overdose.

Some anticonvulsant drugs, such valproate (Depakote®) and gabapentin (Neurontin®), also are employed to treat some symptoms of PTSD (11). Benzodiazepines and hypnotics are still widely used medications for short periods of symptomatic relief, but they need to be closely monitored for potential dependence. In particularly resistant cases, some studies have reported benefits from the use of atypical antipsychotic drugs, such as olanzapine (Zyprexa®), as adjuncts to standard treatments (12). Box 5-9 summarizes the potential treatment options available for PTSD.

Box 5-9   Post-Traumatic Stress Disorder—Treatment

Psychotherapy
- Cognitive Behavioral Therapy: A systematic multimodal treatment with gradual desensitization to the trauma experience

Pharmacological Treatment
- Selective serotonin reuptake inhibitors (SSRIs) are the first-line drugs recommended
- Anticonvulsants (divalproate, gabapentin, or carbamazepine) for severe symptoms of re-experiencing
- Alpha-adrenergic antagonists for hyperarousal symptoms
- For resistant cases, consider:

Tricyclic antidepressants, atypical antipsychotics drugs

In summary, PTSD is a severe, chronic psychiatric disorder that can develop following a serious traumatic experience. It is important to recognize the potential for this long-term complication while evaluating patients in emergency rooms for trauma or in the office setting after a recent experience of trauma. There are a variety of existing and emerging treatments that can be effective in reducing the morbidity associated with this disorder.

References

1. **Kessler RC, Sonnega A, Bromet E, et al.** Posttraumatic stress disorder in the National Comorbidity Survey. Arch Gen Psychiatry. 1995Dec; 52:1048–60.
2. **Seal KH, Bertenthal D, Miner CR, et al.** Bringing the war back home: mental health disorders among 103,788 US veterans returning from Iraq and Afghanistan seen at Department of Veterans Affairs facilities. Arch Intern Med. 2007;167:476–82.
3. **Southwick SM, Krystal JH, Bremner JD, et al.** Noradrenergic and serotonergic function in posttraumatic stress disorder. Arch Gen Psychiatry. 1997;54:749–58
4. **Phan KL, Britton JC, Taylor SF, et al.** Corticolimbic blood flow during nontraumatic emotional processing in posttraumatic stress disorder. Arch Gen Psychiatry. 2006Feb;63:184–92.
5. **Nemeroff CB, Bremner JD, Foa EB, et al.** Posttraumatic stress disorder: a state-of-the-science review. J Psychiatr Res. 2006;40:1–21.
6. **Nakell L.** Adult post-traumatic stress disorder: screening and treating in primary care. Prim Care. 2007;34:593–610
7. **Hoge CW, Castro CA, Messer SC, et al.** Combat duty in Iraq and Afghanistan, mental health problems, and barriers to care. N Engl J Med. 2004;351:13–22
8. **Sijbrandij M, Olff M, Reitsma JB, et al.** Treatment of acute posttraumatic stress disorder with brief cognitive behavioral therapy: a randomized controlled trial. Am J Psychiatry. 2007Jan;164:82–90.
9. **Stein DJ, Ipser JC, Seedat S.** Pharmacotherapy for post traumatic stress disorder (PTSD). Cochrane Database Syst Rev. 2006Jan25;(1): CD002795.
10. **Raskind MA, Peskind ER, Hoff DJ, et al.** A parallel group placebo controlled study of prazosin for trauma nightmares and sleep disturbance in combat veterans with post-traumatic stress disorder. Biol Psychiatry. 2007Apr15;61:928–34.
11. **Berlin HA** Antiepileptic drugs for the treatment of post-traumatic stress disorder. Curr Psychiatry Rep. 2007;9:291–300.
12. **Stein MB, Kline NA, Matloff JL.** Adjunctive olanzapine for SSRI-resistant combat-related PTSD: a double-blind, placebo-controlled study. Am J Psychiatry. 2002;159:1777–9.

F. Child Abuse: The Basics for *All* Healthcare Providers

Antoinette L. Laskey

KEY POINTS

- Child abuse affects millions of children annually; over 1000 children die each year as a result of abuse.
- All 50 states have mandated reporter laws that require healthcare providers to report their *suspicion* of child abuse or neglect to the proper state child welfare agency.
- In homes with intimate partner violence (IPV), also known as domestic violence (DV), there is a 50% or higher co-occurrence rate of child abuse.
- Proper evaluation and documentation by healthcare professionals can help protect children from further injury; the absence of either proper evaluation or documentation can lead to repeated abuse and possibly death.
- Children of both genders, all races and ethnicities, all socioeconomic backgrounds, and in all types of families are at risk for abuse.

Epidemiology

In 2005, 899 000 children were found to be victims of child abuse or neglect in the U.S., equivalent to 12.1 per 1000 children. Nearly two-thirds of cases were due to neglect, 17% were physically abused, and 9% were sexually abused. Frequently, children were the victims of more than one type of abuse. Approximately 4 children die every day in the U.S. due to abuse or neglect, resulting in almost 1500 fatalities a year. Sadly, these numbers are all likely underestimates due to problems with reporting and investigations of child fatalities. The cost to society is estimated to be $258 million *each day* (in 2001 USD) or the equivalent of $1,461.66 per U.S. family annually (www.preventchildabuse.org). These staggering numbers clearly speak to the need for a concerted effort on behalf of healthcare providers to identify, report, and treat abuse in children.

Clinical Features or Presentations

Child physical abuse can present with any number of injuries (Table 5–7). The key for the healthcare provider is to consider:

1. The developmental capabilities of the child;
2. The history provided by the caregiver (or the lack of history in a child who should reasonably be expected to be supervised by an adult);
3. The type of injury, location of injury, and the severity of the injury.

Bruises in non-ambulatory infants are uncommon. With ambulation, the likelihood of finding bruises on a child significantly increases. Likewise, fractures in children <18 months of age are more often inflicted than not; however, accidental fractures can occur in this age group. The American Academy of Pediatrics (AAP) recommends a complete skeletal survey in children <2 years of age who are undergoing evaluation for physical abuse (1). It is a commonly held myth that infants and children with fractures will have overlying swelling or bruising, so it is not uncommon that on evaluation with a skeletal radiological survey, multiple occult fractures may be identified. Inflicted burns in the U.S. are most commonly scalds or immersion-type burns and are commonly associated with potty training. Healthcare providers should be alert to certain clinical features, including burns in a "stocking-and-glove" distribution (i.e., those involving the feet and hands), burns with clear lines of demarcation, or burns in unusual locations. Pattern burns may indicate that a hot item was held to the child's skin.

Abusive head trauma (sometimes referred to as "Shaken Baby Syndrome") is the leading cause of inflicted traumatic death in children <4 years of age. While the peak age is in children <6 months, it can occur in older infants and toddlers. A frequently cited trigger is crying, followed by potty training accidents, or disciplinary issues. Children who suffer from abusive head trauma may be shaken or shaken and impacted and can present within a wide clinical spectrum of symptoms, ranging from vomiting, lethargy, and irritability to unconsciousness, coma, seizing, or death. Head CT may reveal subdural or subarachnoid hemorrhage, cerebral edema, skull fractures, and/or soft tissue swelling. A dilated funduscopic exam may reveal retinal hemorrhages. As in other forms of physical abuse, a skeletal survey is important to delineate the extent of the injuries. Rib fractures, skull fractures, and metaphyseal corner fractures are commonly found in children who have suffered from abusive head trauma (2). It has been shown that doctors miss the diagnosis of abusive head trauma nearly one-third of the time, more often when the patient presents with symptoms such as vomiting, lethargy, or irritability, when the child is from a white, intact family (e.g., the parents are married), or when the child is from a higher socioeconomic status. Clinicians must remain vigilant to this diagnosis, since the likelihood of further injury or death, if the child is returned to the abuser, is high.

Child sexual abuse can present acutely or be removed in time from the event. It is essential that the healthcare provider be aware of the following:

- Children *rarely* present with injuries or physical scars from sexual abuse.
- It is a myth that doctors can tell if a child has been "penetrated" on examination.
- The disclosure a child makes often is the most important component of a sexual abuse evaluation, and the absence of injury does **not** mean that sexual contact/abuse did not occur.

Children frequently present weeks, months, and even years after they have been assaulted. Sexual abuse is often perpetrated by someone the child knows. Sometimes, threats are used to silence the child, while other times an elaborate obfuscation process occurs that allows the abuse to continue undiscovered for an extended period of time. The medical evaluation plays an important role in reassuring children that they are physically "OK," since they often worry that something is wrong with them or they are damaged from the abuse (3). However, the likelihood of identifying either forensic evidence or injury is very rare. An acute exam should be arranged for a child who discloses assault within 72 hours of the event, because the likelihood of recovery of forensic evidence or documentation of an injury is highest in this time-frame. Beyond 72 hours, a non-acute evaluation can be arranged with a local provider skilled in the assessment of child sexual abuse (Table 5-7).

In all forms of abuse, documentation is essential to successful team collaboration. Multiple professionals outside of the medical field rely on the medical record to aid in their investigation. It is essential that the healthcare provider write *legibly, with minimal jargon, and precisely*. Objective facts, as opposed to subjective speculations, are important to include in a thorough note. Histories should be taken using open-ended questions and avoiding yes/no or leading questions. Follow-up questions to understand the details of the history are necessary. Paraphrasing should not be used, and direct quotes should be utilized when recording information obtained from caregivers. Illegible notes have little value to others caring for potentially abused children. Photodocumentation should be used whenever there are visible injuries. Digital photography is acceptable, as is film photography. All photos should include the patient's name, date and time of photo, name or initials of photographer, and a size standard in at least one shot of each injury. Photos should be taken first with an overall view, including landmarks to identify location, and followed up with close-up views. The photography and location of the pictures should be documented in the medical record.

Prevention and Clinical Care

Primary prevention of abuse has been an elusive topic for decades. Recently, research has identified some promising prevention programs, including education for parents on crying (see www.dontshake.com, PURPLE Period of Crying). Community support for parents through programs such as Healthy Families also has been successful in reducing child abuse. Unfortunately, money for prevention programs is often limited, and outcomes research on such programs is limited. Healthcare providers play an essential role in recognizing the abused child and preventing further injury and death of the index child and other children in the care of the abuser. While this is the least effective form of the 3 types of prevention (primary, secondary, and tertiary), it is the type of prevention in which healthcare providers can excel.

When the healthcare provider evaluates a child and is concerned that the child may be the victim of abuse or neglect, the provider is required by law to report these concerns to the proper state authorities.

Table 5-7   Diagnosis and Differential Diagnosis

Type of Abuse	Diagnostic Testing/ Documentation	Differential Diagnoses
Physical Abuse	**Children ≤2y with concerns of physical abuse needs a skeletal survey**	
• Bruising	Complete blood count Consider PT/PTT Photodocument bruises	Consider bleeding disorders (inherited, acquired).
• Fractures	Calcium, phosphorus, magnesium, alkaline phosphatase, Vitamin D Consider nuclear medicine bone scan. Consider 2-wk follow-up skeletal survey	Consider rickets, inherited bone dysplasias, immobility due to disability.
• Burns	Photodocument burns	Consider chemical burns mimicking immersion burns.
Abusive Head Trauma	Head CT Consider MRI. Skeletal survey PT/PTT Complete blood count Dilated eye exam Complete skin exam, documenting injuries Consider genetic screens for metabolic diseases.	Consider inherited conditions (glutaric aciduria). Consider venous malformations. Consider accidental trauma. Consider infectious diseases.
Sexual Abuse	If <72 h since contact: Consider forensic evidence collection by qualified medical personnel Consider testing for STIs and pregnancy, if indicated. Photodocument genital injuries *If greater than 72 h since contact*: Consider testing for STIs and pregnancy, if indicated Refer for forensic interview by qualified personnel if not done already. Photodocument any genital injuries or scars	Consider whether behavior is normal sexual development. Consider whether any "abnormal" findings are actual normal variants. Consider conditions such as prolapsed urethra, labial adhesions or lichen sclerosis as causes of genital bleeding. Consider non-sexual transmission of infections such as herpes or genital warts.

All 50 states have mandated reporter laws (refer to your local phone book for "how to report child abuse"), and these laws protect the reporter from civil litigation when they make a good faith report, even if the child is not found to be abused or neglected. Failure to report your concerns to those who are able to conduct a thorough investigation into the child's individual circumstances can result in criminal prosecution or civil litigation. It is also important to know that HIPAA does *not* prevent the healthcare provider from discussing a case of suspected abuse or neglect with Child Welfare authorities or law enforcement.

References

1. **Kellogg ND,** and the Committee on Child Abuse and N. Evaluation of Suspected Child Physical Abuse. 2007:1232–41.
2. Shaken baby syndrome: Rotational cranial injuries-technical report. Pediatrics. 2001;108:206–10.
3. **Kellogg N.** The evaluation of sexual abuse in children. Pediatrics. 2005;116:506–12.
4. http://www.cdc.gov/std/treatment/

G. The Effect of Stress on Health

Kiet A.T. Ton and Helen Luce

KEY POINTS

- One third of Americans live with major daily stress.
- Chronic stress can weaken the immune system.
- Stress can worsen cardiac and pulmonary diseases.
- Chronic stress correlates with depression, post-traumatic stress disorder (PTSD), and anxiety disorders.
- Relaxation, mindfulness meditation, and biofeedback are promising alternatives to medications in the treatment of chronic stress.

Epidemiology

Stress has a big impact in our society. Half of the U.S population has conflicts with their loved ones due to stress. One third of Americans live with extreme stress on a daily basis, and the number continues to rise. Stress can lead to divorce and separation, as well as health problems such as fatigue, obesity, and heart disease (1,2). Long-term psychological consequences of stress can include depression, PTSD, and anxiety disorder. Almost half

(48%) of Americans report lying awake at night due to stress, according to a survey conducted by the American Psychological Association (APA) (3).

Stressfulness is a natural physiologic state that helps an individual cope with changes in everyday life. However, when stress overwhelms the coping mechanism of the individual, psychological and physical health problems can develop.

Acute stress is the response to a stressful situation and does not cause health concerns as much as chronic stress. Chronic stress includes the repeated exposure to stressful situations or a prolonged response to past acute stressful events (e.g., sexual assault).

Although ethical concerns preclude conducting randomized controlled trials to study the relationship between chronic stress and disease, many observational studies support such a relationship. There are 3 theoretical models which explain a possible mechanism for such a relationship (2):

1. Stress can affect the immune system, which, in turn, can cause worsening of underlying disease.
2. Stress can cause depression, which in turn can affect underlying illness.
3. Stress can cause behavioral changes (e.g., decreased adherence to medications, less sleep, poor eating habits) that compromise health (2).

The Physiology of the Stress Response

To better understand stress, a brief review of the physiologic mechanism of stress is essential. The human body has an intrinsic physiologic response to stress that is delivered by the autonomic nervous system, which is comprised of the parasympathetic and sympathetic nervous systems (3). In a stressful state, the sympathetic nervous system (SNS) initiates a "fight-or-flight" response by increasing cortisol and adrenaline production from the adrenal gland via the hypothalamic-pituitary-adrenocortical axis (HPA) (1,2). In addition, the recently discovered corticotropin releasing hormone-1 (CRH_1) receptor system serves as a third pathway of stress response. While cortisol increases blood sugar secretion from the liver for energy, epinephrine, the primary adrenaline from the adrenal medulla, causes vasoconstriction and increase in heart rate. This stress response is advantageous for acute stress (2).

The biological pathway in chronic stress involves the recently discovered stresscopin-related substances known as urocortin II and III (stresscopin) peptides. These substances bind to corticotrophin releasing hormone-2 (CRH_2) receptors and are released from the hypothalamus. The CRH_2 receptor system dysregulation leads to the maladaptation and ineffective coping mechanisms seen in chronic stress (4).

Stress and the Immune System

The effect of stress on health can also be explained by understanding its effects on the immune system. The link between stress and the immune system occurs in 2 ways: 1) The SNS exerts its immunologic effects via the adrenergic receptor present on all the lymphocytes (e.g., β_2 receptors on NK, B cells, and T cells) and 2) The hypothalamic-pituitary-adrenal axis, the sympathetic-adrenal-medullary axis, and the hypothalamic-pituitary-ovarian axis secrete epinephrine, norepinephrine, and cortisol from the adrenal gland, prolactin and growth hormone (GH) from the pituitary, and melatonin, β-endorphin, and enkephalin from the brain, all of which bind to receptors on lymphocytes and other white blood cells (5).

There is a biphasic relationship between stress and the immune system: acute stress enhances, while chronic stress suppresses, the immune response. Acute stress only recruits the natural immunity for a rapid and nonspecific response. This is the response of "fight-or-flight" activation of the adrenergic pathway and increased cortisol production. Chronic stress, on the other hand, exhibits a more long-term immunologic response. Chronic stress promotes cytokine release in the humoral arm of the specific immune system, at the same time that stress suppresses the cellular arm of immunity. Meanwhile, the elevated T-helper 2 (Th-2) cell cytokines explain the exacerbation of allergy and autoimmune diseases often seen in stress-induced states. The recruitment of the humoral response is stimulated by cortisol secretion in the chronic stress state (5).

Stressful events appear to affect the immune system in a specific pattern. Acute stress leads to solicitation of natural immunity, a quick type of response, to accommodate for the "fight-or-flight" response, and to shift away from specific immunity, which takes longer to assemble and respond to injuries. Bereavement, trauma, and PTSD elicit a less clear immunologic response, a combination of natural and specific immunity. Chronic stress causes a more global immunosuppression, decreasing almost all functioning immunity. This suppression leads to a decreased potential to fight infections and an overall decline in health (5).

Stress and Disease

Chronic stress has been shown to influence the progression of depression, infection, autoimmune disease, and coronary artery disease (CAD) (2). A major life event or stressor 3–6 months before the onset of depression is seen in 60–80% of depressed individuals, while only 20–30% of the non-depressed have a preceding stressor (2). Stress also increases the relapse rate of depressive episodes in those with underlying depression. Chronic stress also can lead to sleep disturbances, smoking, decreased physical activity, unhealthy diet, metabolic abnormalities, decreased heart rate variability and vagal tone, early atherosclerosis, impaired inflammatory and immune response, and accelerated cellular aging (6).

Chronic stress also can increase the risk of developing insulin resistance, central obesity, essential hypertension, and dyslipidemia. The metabolic syndrome is mediated by several pathways that are activated by stress. Hypertension is mediated by the excess sympathetic activation seen in chronic stress. Similar mechanisms lead to cardiovascular disease. Cortisol hypersecretion plays an important role in obesity, diabetes, and dyslipidemia (4).

There are significant cardiovascular effects of stress. A systematic review and meta-analysis of prospective cohort studies linking work stress and coronary heart disease (CHD) found that there was a 50% increased risk of CHD in people with work stress (6). This finding is consistent with prior work relating work stress and CHD. Stress itself has also been shown to increase the risk of acute cardiovascular events and long-term CAD. This could be due to a combination of persistent adrenergic activation and glucocorticoid secretion (4).

The course of chronic obstructive pulmonary disease (COPD) and asthma is also affected by stress. Anxiety and stress have been linked to asthma exacerbations. Anxiety and depression also worsen asthma-associated symptoms. Poor asthma control and asthma-related quality of life have been found in patients with a coexisting psychiatric disorder. A recent study of Vietnam veterans found a relationship between the most severe PSTD and the rate of asthma (7). The group with the most severe PTSD had a 2.3 times greater risk of asthma. Other studies also have shown that patients with asthma have worse health status due to concurrent anxiety and depression and higher risk of re-hospitalization (8,9). Stress is associated with cancer survival, HIV/AIDS outcomes, and autoimmune disease outcomes (2).

Stress and Psychiatric Comorbidities

While stress can lead to the decline of health via biological pathways and long-term changes in the immune system, it also has psychological effects that lead to detrimental behaviors that ultimately affect health. Many studies and observations have linked stress to psychological disorders such as PTSD, depression, anxiety, and panic. Chronic and acute stress has been found with PTSD. In PTSD, the HPA pathways are modified in such a way that there is a heightened and exaggerated response to subsequent stressors. Symptoms may develop to cope with the newfound stressors, including chronic headaches, back pain, or gastrointestinal discomfort. PTSD also leads to changes in mood, behavior, and learning capacity (4).

Depression has been associated with stress and has been extensively examined for the last 15 years. Stressful major life events account for 80% of cases of depression. The stressors-to-onset-of-depression time usually range from 3 to 6 months, but can present within the first month after the inciting event (10). The pathways linking stress and depression involve the interplay of the abnormally functioning HPA, high cortisol levels, and disruption of normal endocrine rhythms.

The extra-hypothalamic CRH secretion controls adaptive behaviors associated with chronic stress. The CRH_1 system, in particular, controls anxiety and depression-like behaviors. Depression is a CRH over-drive state, causing hyperactivity of the adrenergic system and excess circulating glucocorticoid hormones as a consequence of stress induction (11). Depression is often associated with chronic stress, and, with this comorbidity, health suffers via non-productive behaviors. Depression commonly leads to decreased motivation for self-care and nutritional maintenance. Nutritional deficiencies lead to decreased ability to fight infections, among other health problems. Decreased physical activity is often seen leading to obesity and long-term complications of a sedentary life. Depression also increases risk of CAD by causing increased serotonin-mediated platelet activation and hyperactive platelet 5-HT_{2A} receptor, thereby increasing the risk of thromboembolic events (4).

Bereavement can affect health in a significant way, causing physical symptoms such as headaches, dizziness, indigestion, and chest pain. Disability and illness also can occur, including hypertension and functional impairment associated with significant activity-limiting pain (10).

Stress commonly precedes panic disorder. Panic disorder is associated with other disorders, including major depression, social phobia, generalized anxiety disorder, obsessive compulsive disorder (OCD), and increased risk of drug and alcohol abuse. Panic disorder also is associated with increased risk of attempted suicide and decreased social and occupational functioning (12).

Stress-induced behavioral changes include addiction to tobacco and alcohol. Recently, the APA task force reported in an adverse childhood experiences (ACE) study that childhood trauma is strongly correlated with tobacco and alcohol abuse and that there is a 46-fold increase in risk of IV drug use later in life. Childhood traumatic stress, according to the study, is linked to depression, PTSD, and medical morbidity and mortality (13).

Stress Management

While randomized studies of the management of stress are lacking, the mental and somatic disorders that coexist with stress mentioned above have been more extensively reviewed. Similarly, pharmacologic treatment of stress focuses on treating the coexisting anxiety, depression and insomnia that contribute to the symptoms of stress. Studies have shown that multiple modalities, such as progressive muscle relaxation (PMR), electromyogram (EMG) biofeedback, relaxation, and so forth, have potential for treatment of somatic disorders associated with stress.

Lifestyle modification and awareness are often overlooked as the focus for the management of stress. Many women and men turn to over-the-counter (OTC) medications, alcohol, or hypnotic medications to help them cope with anxiety. These substances often do not help the stressful situation and actually may make the symptoms worse.

Physical exercise is a simple but effective treatment for stress and associated comorbidities. Cardiovascular exercise has the potential to release endogenous endorphins, which can improve mood. Stretching and yoga also have a relaxation benefit. Relaxation exercises serve equally well to decrease stress. Additionally, social support, whether from family and friends or community and religious groups, is a pivotal option for anyone with stress (4)

The coexisting somatic and mental illnesses associated with chronic stress often require more intensive treatment than insight and exercise. For example, autogenic training and functional relaxation are 2 modalities that have been shown to decrease beta-agonist use in asthma.

Relaxation can improve lung function and decrease asthma triggers (8). Cancer patients have benefited from stress reduction, often improving their mood, coping better with their cancer, and reducing their anxiety while adding years to their lifespan (8). Stress management decreased mortality after 6 years. Supportive-expressive group therapy may be effective in reducing anxiety and improving mood (4).

The technique with the most impressive record is mindfulness meditation-based stress reduction (MBSR). Recent studies have shown decrease in depression, anxiety, anger, and confusion symptoms, along with increased vigor, fewer stress and somatic symptoms, from only 7 weeks of an MBSR. Similarly, breast and prostate cancer patients benefit from improved sleep and reduced stress, fatigue, and mood disturbances after MBSR (4).

Sleep disorders are very common, with 30–40% prevalence in the general population, and are even higher when stress is a comorbidity. Mood disorders and anxiety cause insomnia as well. The role of behavioral therapy, for example, stimulus control and sleep hygiene, continues to be an effective treatment for insomnia. Pharmacologic management of insomnia ranges from short term treatment with sedative hypnotic medications (i.e., benzodiazepines) to long term treatment with some antidepressants (14).

Gender Differences: "Tend and Befriend versus Fight-or-Flight"

Some new research explores the idea that women respond differently to acute stress (14). Whereas the traditional model describes a fight-or-flight response to acute stress that is mediated by the SNS, women's reactions to acute stress seem to be more socially mediated or "tend and befriend" (15). This model contends that a woman's response to stress is focused on maximum survival of herself and her offspring by tending to her children and creating social networks for resource sharing and protection. In women, this response is mediated by oxytocin, estrogen, and endogenous opioids. These 3 hormones work together to down regulate the SNS and the HPA in response to acute stress.

Conclusion

Stress is very common among primary care patients. Clinicians should screen for increased stressful conditions and discuss stress management on a regular basis.

References

1. **Jeremy WS.** Stress at Work: management and prevention, Elsevier 2005.
2. **Cohen S, et al.** Psychological stress and disease. JAMA. 2007; 298:1685–87.
3. http://apahelpcenter.org/articles/article.php?id = 141
4. **Paul ML, et al.** Principles and Practice of Stress Management, 3rd ed, NY, London, The Guilford Press 2007.

5. **Sergerstrom SC, Miller GE.** Psychological stress and the human immune system: A Meta-Analytic Study of 30 Years of Inquiry, NIH, Psychological Bulletin, 2004July;130:601–30.

6. **Kivimaki M, Virtanen M, Elovainio M, et al.** Work stress in the etiology of coronary heart disease–a meta-analysis. Scand J Work Environ Health. 2006;32:431–42.

7. **Goodwin RD, et al.** A twin study of post-traumatic stress disorder symptoms and asthma. Am J Resp Crit Care Med. 2007;176:983–7.

8. Primary Care Update, Asthma and COPD Complicated by Anxiety and Depression: Implications for care, Consultant, July2006; 885–86.

9. **Goodwin RD, Jacobi F, Thefeld W.** Mental disorders and asthma in the community. Archives of General Psychiatry. 2003;60:1125–30.

10. **Stroebe S, Schut H, Strobe W.** Health Outcomes of Bereavement. Lancet. Dec 8, 2007;370:1960–69.

11. **Herman M.van Praag, et al.** Stress, the Brain and Depression, United Kingdom, the Press Syndicate of the University of Cambridge 2004.

12. **Hawgood J, DeLeo D.** Anxiety disorders and suicidal behaviour: an update. Current Opinion in Psychiatry. 2008;21:51–64.

13. **Nancy Walsh.** Early trauma tied to adult mental, physical health. Family Practice News. 2006Nov;16:34.

14. **Ramakrishnan K, Scheid DC.** Treatment options for insomnia. American Family Physician. 2007;76:517–26, 527–8.

15. **Taylor SE et al.** Biobehavioral response to stress in women: tend and befriend, not fight or flight. Psychological Review. 2000;107:411–29.

6

Musculoskeletal Disorders

A. Osteoarthritis
   Rafael Grau, MD

B. Sports-Related Conditions
   Sarah Fox, MD; Emily Porter, MD; Sarina B. Schrager, MD, MS

C. Rheumatoid Arthritis
   Nighat Tahir, MD; Rafael Grau, MD

D. Systemic Lupus Erythematosus
   Rose S. Fife, MD, MPH

E. Back Pain
   Ann M. O'Connor, PA-C

F. Fibromyalgia
   Rose S. Fife, MD, MPH

A. Osteoarthritis

Rafael Grau

KEY POINTS

- Osteoarthritis (OA) is the most common form of joint disease.
- The majority of persons over the age of 65 years have radiographic evidence of OA.
- Obese individuals are at increased risk of developing OA in the knees and hips.
- Primary OA is most prevalent in the distal interphalangeal (DIP) joints and proximal interphalangeal (PIP) joints of the hands, the first carpometacarpophalangeal joint, spine, knees, and hips.
- Pain is the most prominent symptom and is a major determinant of disability.
- Secondary OA occurs in previously injured individual joints, or systemically, in the presence of endocrine, metabolic, or heritable forms of connective tissue disease.
- Non-pharmacological modalities include patient education, weight reduction, physical and occupational therapy.
- Pharmacological management options include analgesic and nonsteroidal anti-inflammatory agents, as well as intra-articular corticosteroids and visco-supplementation.

Epidemiology

Osteoarthritis (OA) is the most common form of joint disorder and is present in populations throughout the world. In the U.S., OA is found in over 50% of people over the age of 65 years. Before age 50, men have a higher prevalence of OA than women, but after age 50 women are more likely to suffer from this condition (1). OA is a common cause of disability in men over age 50, second only to ischemic heart disease. As the population ages, OA is becoming an ever increasing source of expenditure.

The pathology of OA is similar in all affected joints and is marked by the presence of osteophytes, or bony outgrowths, thickening of the subchondral bone, and eventual destruction of articular cartilage. The risk factors for OA may be systemic or local, and their influence varies according to joint location. Systemic risk factors include genetic susceptibility, sex hormones, and age. Local risk factors include excess weight, injury, occupation, developmental deformities, muscle strength, and joint laxity (2).

Pathophysiology

The integrity of the articular cartilage is maintained by the chondrocytes, which fulfill the dual role of synthesizing components of articular cartilage (collagen and proteoglycans) and facilitating the turnover of these components through the production of proteases. An imbalance in degradation and repair of the extracellular matrix is the central problem in OA. While OA is classified as a non-inflammatory disease, inflammatory cytokines are present and provide the signals promoting the release of cartilage-degrading enzymes. Other mediators play an important role and include prostaglandins, nitric oxide, and matrix degradation products (2).

Primary OA is the most common form of the disease and can involve the DIP and PIP joints, the first carpometacarpal joint (base of the thumb), knees, hips, and spine (Figure 6-1). Although involvement of

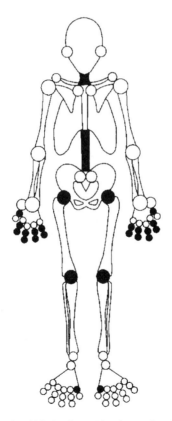

Figure 6-1   Distribution of joint involvement in primary osteoarthritis.

Table 6-1   Conditions Associated with Secondary Forms of Osteoarthritis

Local	Systemic
• Joint trauma	• Hyperparathyroidism
• Osteonecrosis	• Acromegaly
• Neuropathic arthropathy	• Diabetes mellitus
• Fracture	• Hemachromatosis
• Developmental deformities	• Ochronosis
• Inactive rheumatoid arthritis	• Wilson's disease
	• Hypermobility syndrome

all joints increases with age, not all individuals develop the same joint distribution. Secondary forms of OA can appear in previously damaged joints or in a more generalized pattern, in conjunction with endocrine, metabolic, and heritable forms of connective tissue disease (Table 6-1). In the latter, the pattern of involvement is different from the primary variant in that the metacarpophalangeal (MCPs) joints, wrists, elbows, shoulders, and ankles may be involved.

Clinical Features

Pain is usually the feature that brings patients to the attention of a physician. However, not all patients with OA have substantial pain, and functional impairment may be a primary reason for the consultation. Mechanisms that underlie joint pain are poorly understood. Joint pain may originate from periosteal irritation, subchondral fractures, synovial inflammation, periarticular structures, sensory nerve endings, elevated intraosseous pressure, and neuromuscular changes. It is of interest that there is little or no correlation between the presence or severity of joint pain and the structural damage of the affected joint as seen on radiologic examination.

Joint pain is usually of gradual onset. Typically, it is present with activity and is relieved by rest. As structural changes become more severe, joint pain may persist during rest and throughout the night. Because cartilage itself has no pain receptors, joint pain must arise from non-cartilaginous intra-articular tissues or the adjacent bone and periarticular structures. OA patients may suffer sudden periods of pain, redness, and swelling, indicating acute bouts of inflammation. This has been attributed to microtrauma or, perhaps, is the consequence of the presence of calcium-associated crystals in the joint. Joint stiffness upon awakening is limited to the affected joints and usually lasts 30 minutes or less. In the knee joints, a giving way or "buckling" sensation may occur and cause great alarm. Involvement of the carpometacarpal joint at the base of the thumbs can severely affect pinch and grasp. Hip pain is localized to the groin with occasional radiation to the anterior thigh.

On examination of the musculoskeletal system, affected joints appear enlarged and are often firm to compression, with variable degrees of tenderness. There is little or no warmth. Range of motion may be limited, with exacerbation of pain at the extreme positions. Erythema is rare and, when present in the DIP and PIP joints of the hands, it is associated with a peculiar subset of OA called erosive (inflammatory) OA. Crepitus, which is felt on passive range of motion of a joint, is most easily detected in the knees and results from cartilage loss and irregularity of the bony margins. Joint fluid is most commonly identified in the knees. Malalignment can be seen in the DIP and PIP joints of the hands, first metatarsal joints of the feet, and knees. Because of the depth of the hip joint, findings are usually limited to painful and/or restricted range of motion of the coxofemoral joint.

OA of the spine is very common and usually affects the lower cervical spine and the lumbar region. Often it is asymptomatic but can present with pain and limited range of motion. Radiologic findings include degenerative changes of the intervertebral fibrocartilaginous discs, spur formation, or osteophytes, especially in the anterior and lateral portions of the vertebral bodies. Oblique views of the lumbar spine show sclerosis and joint space narrowing of the apophyseal joints similar to those seen in peripheral joints. An exaggerated form of spinal OA with large exuberant osteophytes is called diffuse idiopathic skeletal hypertrophy or DISH.

Radiographic and Laboratory Findings

The radiologic features of OA are very characteristic and serve to confirm the diagnosis. The classic findings include joint space narrowing, bony proliferation at the margins of the joint, and remodeling of the subchondral bone. Subchondral cysts with sclerotic margins can be seen in advanced disease. Inflammatory erosive OA, which involves the DIP and PIP joints of the hands, is accompanied by central erosions and cortical collapse. Chondrocalcinosis, or calcification of the articular cartilage, is associated with OA of the knees. Magnetic resonance imaging (MRI) and bone scintigraphy add little to the evaluation of OA but can be helpful when the diagnosis is uncertain (3).

OA of the spine is very common and usually involves the lower cervical and lumbar regions. Spinal OA is often asymptomatic but can present with pain and limited range of motion. Radiologic findings include flattening of the intervertebral discs, spur formation, or osteophytes on anteroposterior views. Oblique images of the lumbar spine show sclerosis and joint space narrowing of the apophyseal joints, similar to that seen in peripheral joints. As noted above, an exaggerated form of spinal OA called DISH can occur and is more often seen in elderly persons with insulin-resistant diabetes mellitus (4).

The diagnosis of OA is made by history and clinical findings. No specific laboratory abnormalities exist. Routine laboratory tests such as blood count, erythrocyte sedimentation rate, blood chemistries, and urinalysis are normal but are helpful in ruling out inflammatory forms of arthritis. They also serve as a baseline to monitor the effects of treatment on blood, kidney, and liver.

If the distribution of joint involvement suggests a secondary form of OA, measurement of serum calcium, phosphorus, magnesium, ferritin, and parathyroid hormone are useful. Caution is in order if one obtains a rheumatoid factor and antinuclear antibodies, since these are positive in 5–10% of normal individuals and can be found in as many as 20% of persons over the age of 70 years regardless of OA (5).

Synovial fluid analysis from osteoarthritic joints, usually the knees, reveals a white blood cell count of <2000 cells, with mononuclear cell predominance. Crystals of calcium pyrophosphate dihydrate (CPPD) or cholesterol can be found in the synovial fluid. The former can be associated with periodic inflammatory monarthritis (pseudogout); the latter appears to be an incidental finding (6).

Treatment

The primary goals of OA treatment include pain relief, maintaining and improving function, and limiting physical disability. Effective treatment is multifaceted and requires a multidisciplinary approach (Table 6-2). Emphasis must be placed on all aspects of therapy. For the patient, understanding the illness and developing realistic expectations are very important. The Arthritis Foundation and its local chapters have printed material and classes in self-management that are very helpful for patients. Recommendations and guidelines (7–9) are available from organizations such as the American College of Rheumatology (ACR), Osteoarthritis Research International (OARSI), and the European League Against Rheumatism (EULAR).

Non-Pharmacological Interventions

Non-pharmacological modalities are the first-line therapy in OA and cannot be overemphasized. Physical therapy is primarily aimed at

Table 6-2   Management of the Most Common Forms of Osteoarthritis

Type of Osteoarthritis	Patient Education & Support*	Nonpharma-cological Therapy	Pharma-cological Therapy	Initial Interventional Therapy
Hands	Education Self Management programs Social support	OT	Analgesics/NSAIDs	Alignment and stabilization
Knees		Weight reduction PT		Intra-articular injection
Hips		Weight reduction PT		Rarely intra-articular injection

*http://www.rheumatology.org

strengthening and improving function in the lower extremities, as well as teaching transfer skills. Aerobic exercise programs and strength training have been demonstrated to fulfill these goals (10). Orthotics can stabilize the joint and promote pain control. Assistive devices (canes, crutches, elevated toilet seats, shower stools, etc.) are only a few of the many ingenious modalities available. Pain-relieving modalities are available as well. Upper extremity function is the primary responsibility of occupational therapists and is particularly helpful for those who have OA of the hands. A thorough evaluation of hand function, with particular attention to activities of daily living (ADLs), and use of splints and assistive devices, can help stabilize the joints and reduce pain in the hands.

Obesity aggravates OA symptoms in weight-bearing joints, and weight loss in conjunction with strengthening exercises is very beneficial. This is the most important non-pharmacological intervention available for lower extremity OA. Benefit appears quickly and with a modest loss of weight. In addition, weight reduction lowers perioperative morbidity and mortality and accelerates recovery when total joint replacements are indicated.

Pharmacological Interventions

Pain relief is the primary goal, and non-narcotic analgesics are recommended as initial therapy for OA because of a lower toxicity profile. Acetaminophen can be used intermittently or regularly, but the total dose should be <4 g a day. Tramadol, not catalogued as a narcotic but with narcotic-like action and addictive potential, also can be used. Concern about its effect to induce seizures appears unwarranted. Narcotic analgesics are reserved for severe pain unresponsive to initial measures and are more likely to be employed for advanced OA. Management of chronic pain is a difficult problem and is best handled with a narcotic contract.

Inflammation plays a role in the symptoms of OA, and non-steroidal anti-inflammatory drugs (NSAIDs) have been shown to be helpful. They can be added when acetaminophen alone is ineffective. Different NSAIDs are about equally effective in relieving pain, so cost, toxicity profiles, and frequency of dosing are factors that should be considered in choosing a particular drug. A major concern is gastrointestinal toxicity, particularly upper gastrointestinal bleeding and gastric and duodenal ulcers. Renal toxicity (fluid retention, reversible renal failure, and hyperkalemia) may occur. For these reasons, baseline studies should include a complete blood cell count and laboratory tests for liver and renal function. Every 4–6 months thereafter, blood pressure, urinalysis, and stools for occult blood should be obtained. Present guidelines recommend the addition of gastroprotective agents, such as misoprostol or proton pump inhibitors, in the elderly or in those with a prior history of gastric or duodenal ulcers (11).

NSAIDs inhibit both the cyclooxygenase-1 and -2 (COX-1 and COX-2) enzymatic pathways, the former performing important physiologic roles in gastroprotection and platelet function. Selective COX-2 inhibitors attempt to respect this physiologic role, but, by so doing, have altered the balance in platelet function leading to increased incidence of myocardial infarctions and strokes due to thrombotic tendencies. Celecoxib, the remaining selective COX-2 inhibitor available, has not been shown conclusively to have this effect, but a dose-related increase in risk for cardiovascular events and death was found in the adenomatous polyp prevention trial and led to a suspension of the study (12).

Interventional Therapy

Intra-articular corticosteroid injections can be helpful but almost always have only a temporary effect. They can be beneficial for controlling acute bouts of pain and should be used in conjunction with other treatment modalities. Repeat injections can be performed, up to 3–4 times a year, without evidence of detrimental effect. They are not recommended in the months preceding orthopaedic surgery and may accelerate damage to the coxofemoral joint. Visco-supplementation is the intra-articular injection of hyaluronan and its derivatives. This has led to reduced symptoms in some patients, but no long-term benefit has been demonstrated (13).

For those patients who fail to gain relief from medical therapy and who have significant physical dysfunction, orthopaedic surgery is an option. Total joint replacements for knees and hips have provided excellent pain relief and, sometimes, improved function. Infection, thromboembolic disease, and loosening are the primary complications of surgery of the hip and knee. Thumb function and pain may improve with partial or complete resection of the trapezium, with interposition of tendinous structures or a silicone rubber implant.

Non-Traditional Alternatives

Alternative and complementary therapies are very popular among patients with OA. Almost a quarter of patients try many of the non-traditional modalities available. Glucosamine and chondroitin sulfate preparations have been available in over-the-counter formulations for over 10 years. While manufacturer-sponsored studies have shown that these nutriceuticals relieve OA pain and may slow the rate of structural progression of OA, a recent clinical trial sponsored by the NIH failed to show any substantial benefit of these nutritional supplements for patients with knee OA (14).

Summary

OA is a widespread rheumatic condition that causes considerable suffering and substantial cost to our health care system. Effective management of OA requires a multifaceted approach to relief of joint pain and ensures preservation of function. Although initial research on disease-modifying agents for OA have been promising, we are still years away from pharmacological interventions that will modify the course of the disease, as has happened recently with rheumatoid arthritis.

References

1. **Felson DT.** Epidemiology of osteoarthritis. In Brandt KD, Doherty M, Lohmander S (eds): Osteoarthritis. New York: Oxford University Press; 2003. pp. 9–16.
2. **Berenbaum F.** Osteoarthritis—Pathology and Pathogenesis. In Klippel JH, Stone JH, Crofford LJ, White PH (eds): Primer on the Rheumatic Diseases. New York: Springer Science; 2008. pp. 229–34.
3. **Duer A, Ostergaard M, Horsley-Petersen, et al.** Magnetic resonance imaging and bone scintigraphy in the differential diagnosis of unclassified arthritis. Ann Rheum Dis. 2008;67:48–51.
4. **Forgacs SS.** Diabetes mellitus and rheumatic diseases. Clin Rheum Dis, 1986; 12:729–53.
5. **Juby AG, Davis P, McElhaney JE, et al.** Prevalence of selected autoantibodies in different elderly subpopulations. Br. J Rheumatol. 1994;33:1121–4.
6. **Jaovisidha K, Rosenthal AK.** Calcium crystals in osteoarthritis. Curr Opin Rheumatol. 2002;14:298–302.
7. **Altman RD, Hochberg MC, Moskowitz RW, et al.** Recommendations for the medical management of osteoarthritis of the hip and knee. Arthritis Rheum, 2000;43:1905–15.
8. **Zhang W, Doherty M, Leeb L, et al.** EULAR evidenced based recommendations for the management of hand osteoarthritis: report of a task force of the EULAR Standing Committee for International Clinical Studies Including Therapeutics. Ann Rheum Dis. 2007;66:377–88.
9. **Zang W, Moskowitz RW, Nuki Ga, et al.** OARSI recommendations for the management of hip and knee osteoarthritis, Part II OARSI evidence-based, expert consensus guidelines. Osteoarthritis and Cartilage. 2008;16:137–62.
10. **Van Baar ME, Assendelft WJ, Dekker J, et al.** The effectiveness of exercise therapy in patients with osteoarthritis of the hip or knee. Arthritis Rheum. 1999;42:1361–9.
11. **Zullo A, Hassan C, Campo SM, et al.** Bleeding peptic ulcer in the elderly: risk factors and prevention strategies. Drugs & Aging. 2007;24:815–28.
12. **Solomon SD, Pfeffer MA, McMurray JJ, et al.** Effect of celecoxib on cardiovascular events and blood pressure in two trials for the prevention of colorectal adenomas. Circulation. 2006;114:1028–35.
13. **Lo GH, LaValley M, McAlindon T, et al.** Intra-articular hyaluronic acid in treatment of knee osteoarthritis: a meta-analysis. JAMA. 2003;290:3115–21.
14. **Clegg DO, Reda DJ, Harris CL, et al.** Glucosamine, chondroitin sulfate, and the two in combination for painful knee osteoarthritis. N Engl J Med. 2006;354:795–808.

B. Sports-Related Conditions
Sarah Fox, Emily Porter, and Sarina B. Schrager

KEY POINTS

♦ Some musculoskeletal health problems are more common in women, and gender can influence outcomes and treatment.

♦ Anterior knee pain is a common presenting complaint and is most amenable to physical therapy (PT) to improve patellar alignment.

♦ Knee anterior cruciate ligament (ACL) injuries are more common in women because of anatomic, strength, and hormonal differences, and are preventable with conditioning programs.

♦ Female athlete triad is a combination of low energy availability, menstrual dysfunction, and impaired bone health, and should be screened for in active female patients.

♦ Adhesive capsulitis (frozen shoulder) is relatively common in women, and good outcomes can be obtained with steroid injections combined with PT.

Background

It is increasingly common for women to be involved in athletic pursuits and hold active jobs, a situation that has increased the numbers of women suffering injuries and overuse musculoskeletal conditions. Anterior knee pain is a common presenting complaint of women to primary care offices and can often be successfully treated with PT. ACL injury is a very common orthopedic condition that occurs more frequently in women for a variety of reasons; treatment and prevention must focus on the factors that put women at risk for injury, and further research is needed to better elucidate potential treatment options. Female athlete triad is common in an athletic population, and its early recognition is key to prevention of long-term adverse bone and endocrine effects. Finally, adhesive capsulitis, or frozen shoulder, is a common orthopedic problem in women that has an unclear etiology.

Anterior Knee Pain

Women commonly present to primary care physicians with the complaint of anterior knee pain, which can be a frustrating problem for patients and physicians alike. The most common cause, termed patellofemoral pain syndrome or patellofemoral stress syndrome, manifests as a painful knee without internal derangement, usually presenting without a history of injury (1). The pain is typically generalized around the patella and is precipitated by activities that heavily load the knee joint during its usual range of motion (ROM), that is, walking up or down stairs. Often a patient will report a recent sudden increase in activity, such as starting a running program for weight loss, as precipitating the pain, but it can have a more insidious onset as well (2). Its incidence is up to 20% in women, compared with 5–10% in men (1,2).

The difference in incidence is often attributed to relative weakness in the quadriceps muscle in women, delayed firing of the vastus medialis oblique (VMO), and a wider pelvis, leading to increased quadriceps, or "q," angle (2). This more lateral pull of the quadriceps on the patella leads to distracted tracking of the patella during knee flexion and extension, causing friction and potentially degenerative changes in the patellofemoral compartment. Physical exam typically reveals no ligamentous laxity or meniscal signs. Patients may have pain with palpation of the underside of the patella or a positive patellar grind test (pain and/or crepitus with downward compression of the patella during flexion/extension). The alignment and tracking of the patella with relation to the femur and tibia should be noted; this is accomplished most easily with a single leg squat test, which also assesses overall core strength and balance (2). It is important to note any valgus deformity at the knees and the presence of pes planus (flat feet). There may be evidence of quadriceps atrophy or weakness, particularly if the knee pain is unilateral (1). Knee x-rays often will be normal, but views of the patellofemoral compartment, either by a lateral view or a sunrise view, may show abnormal position of the patella, or, less commonly, degenerative changes like bone spurring and loss of joint space.

PT can be an effective treatment. Therapy usually focuses on quadriceps (particularly VMO) and hip external rotator strengthening, hamstring stretching, and proprioception and balance training (1–3). Some patients find knee braces and foot orthotics to be effective, though their utility is not clearly demonstrated in longitudinal studies, and they can be quite expensive. Taping of the patella to encourage proper tracking is often just as effective for pain relief as a custom brace, is much more cost effective, and can be easily taught by a qualified physical therapist (2). If, despite these conservative measures for at least a 6-month period, the patient continues with significant symptoms, there are surgical options that an orthopedist may recommend, including lateral release, tibial tubercle transfer, or patellar realignment to improve patellar tracking (1).

ACL Injury

ACL injury is one of the most common and devastating injuries affecting athletes. An estimated 100 000–250 000 ACL tears occur each year in the U.S., resulting in missed work and athletic participation, along with significant surgery and rehabilitation-related costs (4,5). In addition to the acute injury and possible need for surgery, many ACL tears result in chronic instability and secondary injury to menisci and articular surfaces, leading to OA later in life. In one 12-year follow-up study, 51% of women who had suffered an ACL injury had radiographic evidence of osteoarthritis; the average age of the women at the time of follow-up was 31 years (4). This suggests that increasing numbers of women will present with early OA related to ACL injuries unless we can improve preventive efforts (4,6). Women are 2–10 times more likely than men to suffer ACL tears, particularly the non-contact variety, which occur during a sudden deceleration combined with landing and pivoting (4). Women participating in sports such as volleyball, basketball, and soccer are at greatest risk (5,7). Some estimates put the risk of tear at 5% per player per year participating at a collegiate level in these high-risk sports (4). The reasons that women are more severely affected are complex and incompletely understood. The injuries are caused by a loading force on the ligament that exceeds its tensile strength. In women, the loading forces put on the ACL are greater due to angles of force related to wider hips (7). There is also decreased ACL tensile strength because of relative decreased tendon diameter, relative hamstring weakness, and varying laxity, depending on sex hormone concentrations throughout the menstrual cycle (4,8). Although studies have shown increased laxity during the ovulatory and luteal phases of the cycle, increased ACL injury has been temporally linked to the follicular phase, with the difference possibly related to turnover time of collagen bundles (8,9).

The strongest evidence for ACL injury prevention is in proprioceptive and neuromuscular training programs, with reported reductions in serious ACL injury of 60–89% (4). This effect was particularly strong in women, since the injuries are typically non-contact and are related to high-risk movements and positions that can be prevented with training (4,8). There is no evidence that prophylactic bracing prevents ACL injury (4). The recovery time for a typical ACL injury requiring surgery is 6–9 months, during which PT and rest from activities that put stress on the ACL are imperative. Prevention of these injuries in a high-risk population by enrolling athletes in an ACL-tear prevention program is very effective (4,8).

Female Athlete Triad

The female athlete triad (also known as the Triad) was officially recognized as a disorder by the American College of Sports Medicine (ACSM) in 1992. It consists of three interrelated issues: low energy availability, menstrual dysfunction, and impaired bone strength. The ACSM published a position paper in 1997 which emphasized the endpoint of these issues, namely eating disorders, amenorrhea, and osteoporosis (10). This position paper was revised in 2007 to emphasize that each of these three issues exists as a spectrum from optimal health to a pathologic state (11). Low energy availability often arises from disordered eating patterns, which may range from restriction of calories or certain food groups to a more serious eating disorder, such as anorexia or bulimia nervosa. Menstrual dysfunction may range from oligomenorrhea to complete amenorrhea. Impaired bone strength may range from low bone density and stress fractures to osteoporosis. It is thought that the triad often originates as the result of a female athlete restricting her diet, increasing her physical activity, or both, in hopes of improving performance or appearance. This low energy availability state then contributes to menstrual dysfunction, which in turn brings about low bone mineral density (12).

The exact prevalence of the triad is unknown, since many studies have yielded unreliable results. Estimates may be affected by the secretive nature of disordered eating and the belief that athletic amenorrhea is normal. It has been estimated that 15–62% of female college athletes may be affected (11). Amenorrhea occurs in 3.4–66% of female athletes, compared with 2–5% of the general population (12).

Athletes who participate in sports that emphasize a lean physique, such as gymnastics, figure skating, ballet, and distance running, are at higher risk for the triad. Disordered eating, eating disorders, and amenorrhea have been shown to occur more frequently in these sports (11). Other risk factors include poor self-image, frequent required weigh-ins, overly controlling parents or coaches, early start of sport-specific training and dieting, injury, sudden increase in training volume, a restrictive eating pattern (such as vegetarianism), and social isolation.

Screening for the triad should be included in pre-participation physicals for female athletes beginning in adolescence. It also should be a part of acute visits for fractures, weight changes, disordered eating, and menstrual abnormalities. Screening begins with a thorough menstrual, diet, and exercise history. Height, weight, and vital signs should be recorded. Physical findings may include bradycardia, orthostatic hypotension, cold/discolored hands/feet, lanugo, or parotid gland enlargement; however, physical exam may be entirely normal. A diagnosis of one part of the triad should trigger work-up for the other components.

Athletic amenorrhea is a diagnosis of exclusion. Causes of amenorrhea that should be ruled out include pregnancy, hypothalamic and pituitary dysfunction, ovarian and uterine dysfunction, and endocrine disease. Evaluation of amenorrhea should begin within the first 3 months of diagnosis in order to prevent long-term bone density loss.

Loss of bone density may present along a continuum from stress fracture to frank osteoporosis. Stress fractures commonly present as insidious-onset focal bony pain and tenderness that worsens with activity, usually in the lower extremity. Plain x-rays are often normal, and further imaging with a bone scan or MRI may be necessary for diagnosis. Osteoporosis screening should include a DEXA scan after any stress or low-impact fractures. Screening also should be considered after a total of 6 months of amenorrhea or oligomenorrhea, since bone mass may be compromised after this period of time without regular menses (12).

Treatment of the triad requires a team approach, including the primary care physician, dietician, mental health provider, coach, and athletic trainer. Initial measures should focus on lifestyle changes. A goal weight should be agreed on between the athlete and primary care physician; however, the target should be determined based on optimal health and performance instead of weight per se. A period of relative rest, cross-training, or non-weight-bearing status may be required in the setting of stress fractures to allow bone healing to occur.

The main pharmacologic treatment for the triad includes calcium supplementation and possible use of oral contraceptive pills (OCPs) or other combined hormonal preparation (hormone patch or ring). All females between the ages of 11 and 24 should ingest 1200–1500 mg of calcium and 400–800 IU of vitamin D daily (13). OCPs may be used to treat amenorrhea; however, increases in bone mineral density are more associated with increases in weight than with OCP administration. OCPs should be considered in athletes with functional hypothalamic amenorrhea who are older than 16 years of age if bone mineral density is decreasing with non-pharmacologic management despite adequate nutrition and body weight (13). Bisphosphonates should be avoided due to unproven efficacy in women of child-bearing age and possible teratogenicity. Clomiphene citrate to induce ovulation may be considered in an athlete seeking pregnancy. These athletes also should be counseled about the importance of adequate weight gain throughout pregnancy. A selective serotonin reuptake inhibitor (SSRI) may be considered for athletes with eating disorders.

Athletes should not return to play until they are agreeable to treatment. They must comply with treatment strategies, agree to be closely monitored, place treatment over competition, and modify their activity and diet. A written contract may be helpful.

Adhesive Capsulitis

Adhesive capsulitis, also termed "frozen shoulder," is a clinical condition of uncertain etiology, characterized by shoulder pain and limited passive and active range of motion. It is relatively common, affecting 2% of the general population. Females are more commonly affected by this condition, with women representing 50–75% of study populations (14). The cause is unclear, and there is debate regarding whether it is a primarily inflammatory or degenerative condition with fibrosing features. Women may be affected more due to increased ligamentous laxity and shoulder joint instability, with resultant degenerative changes and fibrosis (15). Many possible etiologies, including autoimmune, endocrine, biochemical, and others, have been postulated, but no specific evidence currently supports any of these theories. An increased incidence has been noted in those with diabetes mellitus, hyperthyroidism, and hypertriglyceridemia, and it is a disease that primarily affects people over age 40 (14,15).

There are 4 clinical stages in the progression of the adhesive capsulitis, and treatment may depend on the stage at which the patient presents.

Stage 1 includes the first 3 months after symptoms begin and is defined primarily by pain, with little impairment of ROM. Stage 2, the "freezing stage," occurs during months 3–9 of the condition and is characterized by chronic pain and progressive loss of active and passive ROM. Stage 3, the "frozen stage," seen during months 9–15, is characterized by significant loss of ROM, with very little pain at rest. Stage 4, the "thawing stage," shows progressive improvement in ROM until complete resolution (14). The natural history of the disease is self-limited, with most people observing complete resolution within 2 years of onset of symptoms. In 10–15% of the population, there is persistent pain and functional limitation, described in the literature as taking up to 10 years to recover (15).

Treatment is based on decreasing pain and optimizing function while the natural history described above plays itself out. Nonsteroidal anti-inflammatory drugs (NSAIDs) and PT are considered mainstays of the treatment, but it is difficult to perform PT during stage 1 of the disease because of severe pain. Often, steroid injections are used as an adjunct to PT, and there is evidence that those treated with this combination have the best short-term results and improved pain and function (14,15). Regardless of treatment or "observed neglect," results were equivalent at 2 years. Long-term data do not support the benefits of any one modality over another. For cases more resistant to conservative treatment, surgical intervention is an option, although it is not recommended as first-line therapy. Closed manipulation under anesthesia, manipulation under anesthesia combined with arthroscopy, and open surgical release of the capsule all have been described in the management of this condition. Of the three, arthroscopy combined with manipulation has the best safety profile and has the advantage of visualizing the pathology in the capsule at the time of surgery (14). None of the surgical options show improvement over conservative care at 2 years, although some short-term improvement in ROM has been noted (14,15).

References

1. **Ivkovic A, Miljenko F, Bojanic I, et al.** Overuse injuries in female athletes. Croat Med J. 2007;48:767–78.
2. **Brukner P, Crossley K, Morris H, et al.** Recent advances in sports medicine. The Med J of Australia. 2006;184:188–93.
3. **Arendt E.** Dimorphism and patellofemoral disorders. Orthop Clin N Am. 2006;37:593–99.
4. **Silvers HJ, Mandelbaum BR.** Prevention of anterior cruciate ligament injury in the female athlete. Br J Sports Med. 2007;41:i52–59.
5. **Prodromos CC, et al.** A meta-analysis of the incidence of anterior cruciate ligament tears as a function of gender, sport, and a knee injury–reduction regimen. Arthroscopy: The J of Arthr and Rel Surg. 2007Dec;23:1320–5.
6. **O'Connor MI.** Osteoarthritis of the hip and knee: Sex and gender differences. Orthop Clin N Am. 2006;37:559–68.
7. **Yu B, Garrett WE.** Mechanisms of non-contact ACL injuries. Br J Sports Med. 2007;41:47–51.

8. **Dugan SA.** Sports related knee injuries in female athletes: What gives? Am J of Physical Medicine and Rehabilitation. 2005;84:122–30.
9. **Zazulak BT, Paterno M, Myer GD, et al.** The effects of the menstrual cycle on anterior knee laxity. Sports Med. 2006;36:847–62.
10. **DiPietro L, Stachenfeld NS.** The female athlete triad. Med Sci Sports Exerc. 1997;29:1669–71.
11. **Nattiv A, et al.** American College of Sports Medicine Position Stand: The female athlete triad. Med Sci Sports Exerc. 2007;39:1867–82.
12. **Beals KA, Meyer NL.** Female athlete triad update. Clin Sports Med. 2007;26:69–89.
13. **Hobart JA, Smucker DR.** The female athlete triad. Am Fam Physician. 2000;61:3357–64.
14. **Sheridan MA, Hannafin JA.** Upper extremity: Emphasis on frozen shoulder. Orthop Clin N Am. 2006;37:531–9.
15. **Tasto JP, Elias JW.** Adhesive Capsulitis. Sports Med Arthrosc Rev. 2007;15:216–21.

C. Rheumatoid Arthritis

Nighat Tahir and Rafael Grau

KEY POINTS

- Rheumatoid arthritis (RA) is the most common form of inflammatory arthritis and is present throughout the world.
- RA occurs in women approximately 3–4 times more often than in men.
- Onset of disease can be sudden or insidious, and the subsequent course can be variable.
- Important prognostic factors include elevated rheumatoid factor (RF), positive anti-cyclic citrullinated peptide (anti-CCP), poor initial response to treatment, early onset, and low socioeconomic class.
- The arthritis is characterized by symmetric proximal small joint involvement of hands and feet and can involve wrists, elbows, shoulders, cervical spine, hips, knees, and ankles, too.
- Laboratory tests include elevated acute phase reactants, anemia of chronic disease, and positive RF and anti-CCP in approximately 75% of patients.
- Radiologic studies show periarticular osteopenia and marginal erosions without osteophytes or subchondral sclerosis.
- Early treatment is essential to limit articular damage and functional loss.

- Disease-modifying drugs should be initiated within 6 months of onset of disease.
- Inadequate response to disease-modifying drugs can be followed by biological agents, including anti-tumor necrosis factor agents, B cell depletion drugs, and other modalities.
- Coordinating management with a rheumatologist will optimize care.

Epidemiology

RA is a chronic systemic autoimmune inflammatory disease that affects people throughout the world. It is the most common form of inflammatory arthritis and primarily affects the diarthrodial joints. The prevalence in the general population is between 1% and 2%, and the incidence is highest after the age 50 years, continuing into the seventh decade. The female predominance in prevalence is 3–4-fold that of males in this period. Differences in prevalence among some ethnic groups exist. In the U.S., Native Americans, such as members of the Pima, Yakima, and Chippewa tribes, have a prevalence of disease of approximately 5%, while RA is rare among rural African Americans (1).

The greater female prevalence of RA suggests an influence of hormonal factors in the appearance and severity of the disease. The influence of pregnancy on the immune system is also significant and may participate in the modulation of disease onset and severity. Hormones influence T-cell subsets, with distinct cytokine profiles. Other factors that are likely to contribute to RA include genetic components and possibly exogenous exposure to various bacterial and viral products as the result of infection. Environmental factors such as tobacco appear to increase the risk for RA (2). Numerous factors contribute to a poor outcome, including severity of disease, seropositivity, low socioeconomic and educational status, and poor functional status.

While RA is usually thought of as a form of arthritis, it is a multisystem disorder that affects many extra-articular tissues, including skin, blood vessels, heart, lungs, and muscles. Such involvement can be found in as many as 35–40% of patients (3).

Clinical Presentation

The onset of symptoms occurs over weeks to months (4,5). Pain and swelling usually appear slowly, but less common presentations include an abrupt polyarthritis or monarthritis. The subsequent course can be monocyclic, intermittent, remittent, or, on occasions, unrelenting. Early disease involves the small joints of the extremities, that is, metacarpophalangeal (MCP), proximal interphalangeal (PIP), and metatarsophalangeal (MTP), but spares the distal interphalangeal (DIP) joints. The distribution is symmetrical but does not need to be a mirror image on both sides of the body. Morning stiffness reflects active disease and is present upon rising; it may last from 30 minutes to several hours. In addition, constitutional symptoms may be present, including fatigue, malaise, myalgias, and diminished appetite.

Examination reveals localized swelling over the PIP and MCP joints and tenderness on compression of affected joints. Sometimes the swelling is not visibly apparent, but tenderness is elicited. Pain is exacerbated by range of motion. Persistent disease leads to joint deformities, including ulnar deviation of the fingers, hyperextension of the PIP joints (swan-neck deformity) and hyperflexion of the PIP joints (boutonniere deformity) and indicate destructive disease. Involvement of the MTP joints leads to cocking-up deformities and hallux valgus subluxation. The knee joints are commonly involved, and both swelling and fluid can be identified. The shoulders and hips are very difficult to palpate but manifest their involvement by pain on motion and limited range of motion. Simplified criteria for the diagnosis of RA are presented in Table 6-3.

Extra-articular manifestations are found in nearly half of all patients (Table 6-4). They are usually associated with more aggressive disease. Rheumatoid nodules are present in a quarter of patients. They are usually located over the olecranon and along the extensor surface of the forearm. They are firm, non-tender, and can be mobile or attached to the deeper tissues. They may appear on pressure points. Almost all patients with nodules are RF-positive. Other extra-articular manifestations include dryness of the eyes (keratoconjunctivitis sicca) and mouth (and xerostomia), pleural effusions, pulmonary fibrosis, pericarditis, and anemia of chronic disease. Vasculitis of small- and occasionally medium-sized blood vessels can appear, usually after years of aggressive disease (6).

Table 6-3   Simplified Criteria for the Diagnosis of Rheumatoid Arthritis

Item	Description
Morning stiffness	Lasting ≥1 h before maximal improvement
Arthritis of 3 or more peripheral joints	The 14 possible areas including the right and left PIP, MCP, wrist, elbow, knee; ankle, and MTP joints
Arthritis of hand joints	At least 1 area involved from the wrist, MCP, or PIP joints
Symmetric arthritis	Simultaneous involvement of same joint group on both sides of the body
Rheumatoid nodules	Over bony prominences (e.g., olecranon) or extensor surfaces (e.g., forearms)
Serum rheumatoid factor	Present in 75% of patients with rheumatoid arthritis
Radiographic changes	On anteroposterior view of hand and wrist radiographs

MCP: metacarpophalangeal; PIP: proximal interphalangeal; MTP: metatarsophalangeal.
From the 1987 revised criteria for the classification of rheumatoid arthritis. Arthritis and Rheumatism. 1988;31:315–24; with permission.

Table 6-4   Common Extra-Articular Manifestations of Rheumatoid Arthritis

Organ System	Comment
Integument	Rheumatoid nodules (25–50%)
Hematologic	Normocytic normochromic anemia, neutropenia (Felty's syndrome)
Pulmonary	Pleural effusions, interstitial lung disease
Cardiovascular	Pericarditis, accelerated atherosclerotic disease
Ophthalmologic	Dryness of eyes and mouth (secondary Sjogren's syndrome)
Vascular	Small vessel vasculitis, polyarteritis nodosa-like vasculitis (10%)

Of great concern is the increased incidence of accelerated athero-sclerosis, as manifested by myocardial infarctions and strokes related to the state of chronic inflammation (7). Common factors associated with atherosclerosis (smoking, hyperlipidemia, obesity) must be monitored and managed, but good control of the inflammatory state is equally important for prevention of coronary events (8,9).

Laboratory Studies

Laboratory tests are important in the diagnosis of RA, for the assessment of severity of inflammation, and as a baseline for following response to treatment. Erythrocyte sedimentation rate (ESR) and C-reactive protein (CRP) are important inflammatory markers (10). The severity and type of anemia and liver and renal function are important as a baseline for subsequent management. Other common findings include low albumin levels and polyclonal gammopathy.

RF is present in approximately 75% of patients with RA. Titers are quite variable, but higher titers are associated with more aggressive ero-sive disease and correlate with poor outcomes (11). On the other hand, low-titer RF is commonly found in healthy normal individuals (5%), in those with chronic inflammatory states such as infections, and in those with other autoimmune conditions, such as systemic lupus erythemato-sus and chronic liver disorders. With increasing age, RF becomes more common. The sensitivity and specificity of RF for the diagnosis of RA are 69% and 85%, respectively.

Anti-CCP antibody is a recent addition to the diagnostic armamen-tarium for RA (12). Citrullination of the arginine amino acid occurs in RA patients. Anti-CCP has a similar sensitivity to that of RF but is more specific (95%). Antinuclear antibodies (ANA) are found in up to 40% of patients with RA (13). Clinically, these patients do not have features of systemic lupus erythematosus, and complement levels are usually normal or elevated, since the latter can behave as acute phase reactants. Synovial fluid usually shows an inflammatory profile, with white cells above 2000 cells/mm^3 with a polymorphonuclear predominance. It is helpful in ruling out infection, crystal arthropathy, and non-inflammatory arthropathies, such as osteoarthritis.

Imaging Studies

Typical features of RA include periarticular osteopenia, marginal erosions, and joint space narrowing on routine radiographs. Unfortunately, these findings reflect irreversible damage, and radiographs should be obtained as early as possible to serve as a baseline for subsequent management decisions. Subluxation and loss of alignment represent laxity or rupture of the periarticular structures. Patients with very late disease may develop secondary osteoarthritis, radiographically manifested by osteophytes and sclerosis.

Early diagnosis and intervention are the goals for reducing the potentially devastating consequences of RA. Such early recognition and treatment can greatly influence the outcome of the disease. Newer imaging techniques, including magnetic resonance imaging (MRI) and ultrasonography, detect synovial proliferation and early erosions and allow quicker diagnosis. Periarticular disease, including tenosynovitis and tendon rupture, also can be seen. Evaluation of clinically difficult joints, such as shoulders and ankles, can be performed, and obese patients, for example, can be confidently evaluated with these techniques.

Treatment

Effective management goals of RA include prevention or control of joint damage, preservation of function, and reduction of pain. Focus is on early aggressive treatment of synovitis to prevent accrual damage and disability during the first several years of the disease.

Treatment should be individualized for each patient. Disease activity markers as Disease Activity Score (DAS)-28, is calculated from the number of tender and swollen joints (28-joint count), and Health Assessment Questionnaire-Disability Index (HAQ-DI) can be used to supplement clinical impression. Non-pharmacologic therapy is also very important in the effective management of RA and includes patient education, exercise programs tailored to the patient's level of function and extent of joint damage, and physical and occupational therapy to improving function. Efforts should be made for psychosocial stress reduction, and the physician should ensure that preventive health measures, such as discontinuation of smoking, weight management, and treatment of comorbid conditions, are pursued.

Pharmacologic Treatment (Figure 6-2).

Traditionally, drugs for treatment of RA have been divided into two groups: those used primarily for control of joint pain and swelling, and those used as disease-modifying anti-rheumatic drugs (DMARDs).

Anti-Inflammatory Drugs

Non-steroidal anti-inflammatory drugs (NSAIDs)
These drugs reduce inflammation and pain; however, they do not prevent tissue injury or joint damage. Commonly used agents include aspirin,

ibuprofen, and cyclooxygenase-2 (COX-2) inhibitors (14). Patients should be monitored for gastrointestinal, renal, and cardiovascular side effects.

Corticosteroids

Steroids are potent suppressors of inflammation, and there is some evidence that steroids in low doses may slow joint damage. These agents should be used in low doses, preferably <10 mg of prednisone per day. Their use is limited by side effects, including, but not limited to, weight gain, osteoporosis, hypertension, hyperlipidemia, and cataracts.

DMARDs

The American College of Rheumatology (ACR) RA guidelines state that initiation of DMARD therapy should not be delayed beyond 3 months for any patient with established RA who continues to experience joint pain, active synovitis, radiographic joint damage, or elevation in acute phase reactants, such as C-reactive protein (CRP) or erythrocyte sedimentation rate (ESR). DMARDs are further divided into conventional agents and the newer biologic agents.

- Methotrexate

Methotrexate (MTX) (14) inhibits purine biosynthesis, in addition to other effects, and traditionally is used as the standard first-line DMARD. It can be used as a single therapy, as well as in combination with other agents. It has a well-established long-term efficacy and toxicity profile and the lowest long-term discontinuation rate of any DMARD.

MTX can be taken orally or by subcutaneous injection. Initial doses of MTX range from 7.5 to 15 mg weekly and may be escalated to 25 mg/week. Side effects include stomatitis, nausea, hepatic fibrosis, pneumonitis, cytopenias, and hair loss. Patients need to be checked routinely with blood tests while taking MTX and should avoid alcohol intake. It should not be used in pregnant or lactating patients.

- Leflunomide

Leflunomide (14) is a pyrimidine synthetase inhibitor and has been shown to reduce the rate of progression of erosive disease. It is taken once a day orally in doses of 10 or 20 mg. It can be used in combination with other agents. Side effects include rash, alopecia, diarrhea, elevated blood pressure, and thrombocytopenia, and it has the potential for teratogenicity. Patients should have regular blood counts and liver enzyme monitoring.

- Hydroxychloroquine

This antimalarial agent has a favorable toxicity profile. It is particularly useful in early or mild disease or in combination with other medications. Patients should have eye exams every 6 months to monitor for retinopathy.

- Sulfasalazine

Sulfasalazine (14) was designed as a drug that linked an antibiotic, sulfapyridine, with an anti-inflammatory agent, 5-aminosalicylic acid

(5-ASA). It is used in the treatment of early or mild RA or in combination with other agents. Side effects can include gastrointestinal (GI) upset and myelosuppression

- Other Anti-Rheumatic Agents

Gold compounds are rarely used now because of frequent toxicity and the availability of other agents with better tolerability. Gold is available in oral and parenteral formulations (15,16).

Cyclosporine has been shown to reduce the progression of RA in clinical trials; however, its use is limited by its renal side effects and availability of other effective agents (17). Immunosuppressive agents, such as azathioprine and cyclosporine, are employed when the disease does not respond to other agents. These drugs were more commonly used in the past but still have a place in treatment today.

Biologic Agents

The therapeutic armamentarium for effective treatment of RA has expanded significantly with the advent of biologic agents (18). These are divided into Tumor Necrosis Factor (TNF) Inhibitors and newer biologics targeting other sites.

- TNF Inhibitors

Etanercept, infliximab, and adalimumab are approved by the FDA for the treatment of RA (18) (Figure 6-2). These drugs were engineered to

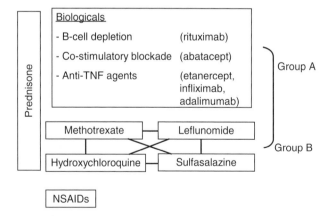

Figure 6-2   Summary of treatment of rheumatoid arthritis. NSAIDs are for symptomatic relief; Group B can be used individually or in combination up to three; Group A should not be combined among themselves but can be used with members of group B; prednisone or other corticosteroids can be used with any of the above combinations. (Reprinted from Wiley-Liss, Inc., a subsidiary of John Wiley & Sons, Inc.; with permission)

specifically inhibit TNF, which is a pivotal proinflammatory cytokine (18). Etanercept is a soluble receptor fusion protein that binds to soluble TNF and neutralizes it. It is administered as a subcutaneous injection once or twice weekly. Infliximab is a chimeric monoclonal antibody that binds to both soluble and membrane-bound TNF and is administered as an intravenous infusion every 6–8 weeks. Adalimumab is a fully human monoclonal antibody with a mechanism of action similar to infliximab and is administered as a subcutaneous injection every 2 weeks.

Use of TNF inhibitors has been associated with several side effects, which range from minor injection site reactions to infusion reactions, especially with infliximab. There is also an increased risk of development of serious bacterial and opportunistic infections, including reactivation of latent tuberculosis. Patients have an increased risk of lymphoproliferative disorders, namely lymphoma, and other malignancies, including non-melanoma skin cancers. These drugs may exacerbate heart failure and should not be used in patients with NYHA Class III or IV heart disease, although more research is needed (19).

- Anakinra

Anakinra (20) is a human recombinant anti-IL-1 (anti-interleukin-1) receptor antagonist. It is administered as a daily subcutaneous injection. Its use is limited to selected patients with refractory disease because of lower efficacy.

- Rituximab and Abatacept

These are newer biologics used to treat moderate-to-severe RA in patients who have had an inadequate response to other DMARDs or have failed an anti-TNF agent (21,22). Rituximab is a chimeric anti-CD20 monoclonal antibody that selectively depletes B cells (Figure 6-2). It is given as an infusion (21).

Abatacept is a recombinant fusion protein consisting of the extracellular domain of the human CTLA-4 and the Fc domain of human IgG1 (22).

Health Maintenance

Osteoporosis is a major comorbidity in patients with RA and can result from the disease itself and/or the use of corticosteroids. Most patients benefit from daily calcium and vitamin D supplementation. Patients with risk factors should undergo bone densitometry, and, if indicated, bisphosphonates should be initiated.

RA is a risk factor for cardiovascular disease (23). Attempts should be made to reduce risk factors in these individuals, including avoidance or cessation of smoking, regular exercise, cholesterol monitoring, and control of chronic illnesses, such as hypertension, diabetes, and obesity.

References

1. **Spector TD.** Rheumatoid arthritis. Rheum Dis Clin North Am. 1990;16:513.
2. **Odegard S, Kvien TK, Uhlig T.** Incidence of clinically important 10-year health status and disease activity levels in population-based cohorts with rheumatoid arthritis. J Rheumatol. 2008;35:54–60.
3. **Hochberg MC, Johnston SS, John AK.** The incidence and prevalence of extra-articular and systemic manifestations in a cohort of newly diagnosed patients with rheumatoid arthritis between 1999 and 2006. Curr Med Res. 2008;24:469–80.
4. **Lee DM, Weinblatt ME.** Rheumatoid arthritis. Lancet. 2001;358:908.
5. **Lineker S, Badley E, Charles E, et al.** Defining morning stiffness in rheumatoid arthritis. J Rheumatol. 1999;26:1052.
6. **Genta MD, Genta RM, Gabay C.** Systemic rheumatoid vasculitis: a review. Semin Arthritis Rheum. 2006Oct;36:88–98. Review
7. **Solomon DH, et al.** Patterns of cardiovascular risk in rheumatoid arthritis. Ann Rheum Dis. 2006;65:1608–12.
8. **Doornum SV, McColl G, Wicks IP.** Accelerated Atherosclerosis an extra-articular feature of rheumatoid arthritis. A & R. 2002Apr;46:862–73.
9. **Albano SA, Santan-Sahagyn E, Weisman MD.** Cigarette smoking and rheumatoid arthritis. Semin Arthritis Rheum. 2001Dec;31:146–59.
10. **Wu JF, Yang YH, Wang LC, et al.** Comparative usefulness of C-reactive protein and erythrocyte sedimentation rate in juvenile rheumatoid arthritis. Clin Exp Rheumatol. 2007Sep-Oct;25:782–5.
11. **Shmerling RH, Delbanco TL.** The rheumatoid factor: an analysis of clinical utility. Am J Med. 1991Nov;91:528–34.
12. **Nishimura K, et al.** Meta-analysis: Diagnostic accuracy of anti-cyclic citrullinated peptide antibody and rheumatoid factor for rheumatoid arthritis. Ann of Intern Med. 2007;146:797–808.
13. **Agrawal S, Misra R, Aggarwal A.** Autoantibodies in rheumatoid arthritis: association with severity of disease in established RA. Clin Rheum. 2007Feb;26:201–4. Epub 2006 Mar 30.
14. **O'Dell JR.** Therapeutic strategies for rheumatoid arthritis. N Engl J Med. 2004;350:2591–602.
15. **Abruzzo JL.** Auranofin: A new drug for rheumatoid arthritis. Ann Intern Med. 1986;105:274.
16. **Jones G, Brooks PM.** Injectable gold compounds: An overview. Br J Rheumatol. 1996;35:1154.
17. **Olsen NJ, Stein CM.** New drugs for rheumatoid arthritis. N Engl J Med. 2004;350:2167.
18. **Scott DL, Kingsley GH.** Tumor necrosis factor inhibitors for rheumatoid arthritis. N Engl J Med. 2006;355:704–12.
19. **Kwon HJ, Cote TR, Cuffe MS, et al.** Case reports of heart failure after therapy with a tumor necrosis factor antagonist. Ann Intern Med. 2003;138:807.
20. **Fleischmann RM, Schechtman J, Bennett R, et al.** Anakinra, a recombinant human interleukin-1 receptor antagonist (r-metHuIL-1ra), in patients with rheumatoid arthritis: A large, international, multicenter, placebo-controlled trial. Arthritis Rheum. 2003;48:927.

21. **Cohen SB, Emery P, Greenwald MW, et al.** Rituximab for rheumatoid arthritis refractory to anti-tumor necrosis factor therapy. Arthritis Rheum. 2006;54:2793.
22. **Kremer JM, Westhovens R, Leon M, et al.** Treatment of rheumatoid arthritis by selective inhibition of T-cell activation with fusion protein CTLA4Ig. N Engl J Med. 2003;349:1907.
23. **Turesson C, Jarenros A, Jacobsson L.** Increased incidence of cardiovascular disease in patients with rheumatoid arthritis: results from a community based study. Ann Rheum Dis. 2004;63:952.

D. Systemic Lupus Erythematosus

Rose S. Fife

KEY POINTS

- Systemic lupus erythematosus (SLE) is a systemic, autoimmune disorder that affects women 10 times more often than men and is more common in African American women than in white women.
- SLE occurs throughout the lifespan but is most common during the child-bearing years.
- SLE can flare during the third trimester of pregnancy and in the postpartum period.
- SLE can cause congenital heart block or transient rashes in infants born to mothers with the disease.

Epidemiology

SLE is much more common in women than men (10:1 ratio). While some of its most devastating consequences occur when it presents in women of child-bearing age, it can occur throughout the lifespan, from childhood to old age (1). SLE has been estimated to have an incidence of 90.5/100 000 among white women and 280/100 000 among African American women in the U.S. (2).

Etiology

As is true with most connective tissue diseases, the etiology of SLE remains unknown. It is an autoimmune disease, highly associated with elevated antinuclear antibody titers and other autoantibodies (e.g., anti-double-stranded

[ds] DNA, anti-ribonucleoprotein, anti-Smith, anti-phospholipid, rheumatoid factor, and others). Biologic false-positive tests for syphilis are not uncommon and are usually associated with anti-phospholipid antibody (3).

Immunofluorescence staining of skin and kidney biopsies may show a pattern consistent with immune complex deposition (such as mesangial deposition in the kidneys) (4) and has led to the theory that SLE is an immune complex deposition disease. The tendency of SLE to cluster in some families, along with other autoimmune disorders like rheumatoid arthritis, Sjogren's syndrome, scleroderma, and others, and associations with various HLA antigens, have led some researchers to consider a genetic basis for the disorder. Associations with virus infections and other exposures, such as ultraviolet light, have been observed over the years and have suggested a role for environmental factors (5,6). However, to date, the cause of this condition remains speculative.

Clinical Manifestations

In 1982, the American College of Rheumatology (ACR) published revised criteria for the diagnosis of SLE (7), with an additional update in 1997 (8). The latest criteria are shown in Table 6-5 (3).

SLE can range from a very mild disease, often consisting of mainly arthralgias, rash, fatigue, and occasional low-grade fevers, to a severe and sometimes fatal condition with involvement of various visceral organs, including the heart, lungs, kidneys, central nervous system, and blood vessels (3). Vasculitis is a prominent feature of many manifestations of SLE, affecting mainly small vessels and causing various patterns of disease.

Certain laboratory tests are commonly abnormal in lupus. Approximately 95% of all patients with SLE have a positive and significant (>1:640) ANA (antinuclear antibody) titer. Erythrocyte sedimentation rates (ESR) and/or C-reactive protein (CRP) titers, both acute phase reactants, are often elevated during or just before the onset of an active phase of the disease. Patients with lupus can be cytopenic with respect to any of the blood cell components (9). Rheumatoid factor (RF) titers may be positive, since some ANAs actually function as RFs, binding to immunoglobulins as well as to nuclei. Elevated anti-phospholipid antibody titers can be associated with lupus (10). Urine should be analyzed in all patients with lupus, since the various forms of lupus nephritis may present with a variety of abnormalities in a urinalysis, including proteinuria, hematuria, leukocytes, other cells, casts, and so forth (3). Levels of creatinine and blood urea nitrogen vary depending on the type and severity of the renal involvement.

Renal lesions seen on biopsy range from none (Class I) through mesangial hypertrophy and immune complex deposits (Class II) to involvement of the mesangium and endothelium (Class III), diffuse proliferative glomerulonephritis (Class IV), membranous glomerulonephritis (Class V), and finally sclerosis (Class VI) (4). Any individual patient does not necessarily progress through all of these phases; indeed, some may present with Class I and not progress, while others may present with sclerosis.

Table 6-5 Classification of Systemic Lupus Erythematosus

Criterion	Definition
1) Malar rash	Fixed erythema, flat or raised, over the malar eminences, tending to spare the nasolabial folds
2) Discoid rash	Erythematous raised patches with adherent keratotic scaling and follicular plugging; atrophic scarring may occur in older lesions
3) Photosensitivity	Skin rash as a result of unusual reaction to sunlight, by patient history or physician observation
4) Oral ulcers	Oral or nasopharyngeal ulceration, usually painless, observed by a physician
5) Arthritis	Nonerosive arthritis involving 2 or more peripheral joints, characterized by tenderness, swelling, or effusion
6) Serositis	a) Pleuritis: convincing history of pleuritic pain or rub heard by a physician or evidence of pleural effusion OR b) Pericarditis: documented by EKG, rub, or evidence of pericardial effusion
7) Renal disorder	a) Persistent proteinuria >0.5g/d or >3+ if quantitation not performed OR b) Cellular casts, which may be red cell, hemoglobin, granular, tubular, or mixed
8) Neurologic disorder	a) Seizures: in the absence of offending drugs or known metabolic derangements (e.g., uremia, ketoacidosis, or electrolyte imbalance) OR b) Psychosis: in the absence of offending drugs or known metabolic derangements (e.g., uremia, ketoacidosis, or electrolyte imbalance)
9) Hematologic disorder	a) Hemolytic anemia, with reticulocytosis OR b) Leukopenia: <4000/mm^3 total on 2 or more occasions OR c) Lymphopenia: <1500/mm^3 on 2 or more occasions d) Thrombocytopenia: <100,000/mm^3 in the absence of offending drugs
10) Immunologic disorder	a) Anti-DNA: antibody to native DNA in abnormal titer OR b) Anti-Sm: presence of antibody to Sm nuclear antigen OR c) Positive finding of antiphospholipid antibodies based on 1) an abnormal serum level of IgG or IgM anti-cardiolipin antibodies, 2) a positive test result for lupus anticoagulant using a standard method, or 3) a false-positive serologic test for syphilis known to be positive for at least 6 months and confirmed by *Treponema pallidum* immobilization or fluorescent treponemal antibody absorption test

cont'd

Table 6-5   Classification of Systemic Lupus Erythematosus (cont'd)

Criterion	Definition
11) Antinuclear antibody	An abnormal titer of antinuclear antibody (ANA) by immunofluorescence or an equivalent assay at any point in time and in the absence of drugs known to be associated with "drug-induced lupus" syndrome

Modified from Classification of SLE from Harris EN, et al. Kelley's Textbook of Rheumatology. Vol 2. 7th Ed., 2005. p. 1205. Elsevier; with permission.

In asymptomatic patients, chest radiographs may be normal or may show a variety of lesions, including pneumonitis, nodules, pleural or pericardial effusions, or calcifications, requiring appropriate evaluation. Cardiomegaly may be present because of pericardial effusion or other cardiac abnormalities. Electrocardiograms (EKGs) may be abnormal due to blocks resulting from localized vasculitis in the heart, elevated ST segments associated with pericarditis, etc. (11,12). Sterile valvular vegetations, called Libman-Sacks lesions, can affect the mitral and aortic valves and be asymptomatic or cause flow abnormalities (13,14).

Thromboembolic phenomena occur in SLE, especially in association with anti-phospholipid antibodies. These were originally detected as so-called biological false-positive serologic tests for syphilis but are now known to be due to autoantibodies (15–17). Their presence can be associated with neurologic abnormalities, fetal loss, recurrent miscarriages, and other specific conditions (18–20).

As is true with most organ involvement by SLE, neuropsychiatric manifestations may range from mild to life-threatening. Patients may present with an enormous diversity of symptoms, including psychological/psychiatric disorders, headaches, vasculitis, myelitis, meningitis, organic brain syndrome, cognitive dysfunction, neuropathies, and cerebrovascular accidents, among others (3).

Musculoskeletal involvement by SLE can include arthralgias, myalgias, nonerosive arthritis, or an arthropathy (referred to as Jaccoud's arthropathy) with distribution similar to rheumatoid arthritis (see Differential Diagnosis below). In most individuals, musculoskeletal lesions are mild and transient (21).

A multitude of skin lesions may be seen with SLE. These can range from malar erythema, a rash across the cheeks and bridge of the nose that is responsible for the name of the disease, since it reminded physicians of the "lupoid" features of a wolf, to diffuse skin rashes, usually vasculitic in origin, which can become ulcerated and infected (22). Other cutaneous manifestations include livedo reticularis, alopecia, photosensitivity, periungual erythema, discoid lupus, and so forth (3).

SLE can be associated with Raynaud's syndrome, a condition in which the digits are very sensitive to stimuli such as cold or stress and go through a reproducible series of color changes from white to blue to red when the individual is exposed to such factors. This can result in digital ulcerations, gangrene, and even loss of digits in rare, very severe cases.

Some patients may have findings similar to those of scleroderma, including telangiectases and sclerodactyly (see Differential Diagnosis below).

Differential Diagnosis

As can be surmised from the enormity of the scope of symptoms that may be associated with SLE, the disease can mimic a multitude of systemic and focal disorders. Indeed, SLE can mimic many diseases and must be considered in the differential diagnosis of diseases as diverse as tuberculosis, metastatic cancer, and endocarditis, etc. SLE may include such substantial features of many other rheumatologic disorders (e.g., Raynaud's, scleroderma, rheumatoid arthritis, and the vasculitides) that these must often be considered in the differential diagnosis of SLE. It also should be borne in mind that the classification schema for SLE are only applicable to populations and not to individual patients, so a combination of symptoms and signs, classification criteria, and common sense must be applied to arrive at the correct diagnosis.

Another important caveat regarding the diagnosis of SLE is that diagnosis should be based on clinical features supported by laboratory findings. Many patients have found themselves in the midst of a major, and often negative but expensive, medical evaluation because their physician sent samples for ANA testing, for instance, as part of a work-up of nonspecific symptoms and findings, and the ANA was "positive." Many autoantibodies, including ANA and RF, may be mildly elevated in older individuals, for example. Healthcare providers should obtain such tests when there is a significant suspicion of SLE or other diseases associated with these markers. However, they should beware that a positive result should be analyzed in the context of the clinical setting. There are no absolute cutoffs for "significant" ANA levels, for instance. However, levels of 1:320 (and possibly greater) and below should not trigger a major work-up in the absence of other evidence suggestive of SLE or another connective tissue disease. Watchful waiting and even repetition of the ANA in the near future is probably a preferable approach.

SLE is an extremely complex disease and, when suspected, early referral to a rheumatologist is recommended.

Treatment

Comprehensive treatment of SLE is beyond the scope of this book. As noted above, patients suspected of or diagnosed with SLE should be referred to a rheumatologist as soon as possible. Therapy can be started by the specialist, and the patient can be subsequently followed and managed, in most cases, by the primary care provider with periodic follow-up by the rheumatologist.

A snapshot of treatment modalities for SLE is shown in Figure 6-3 (23).

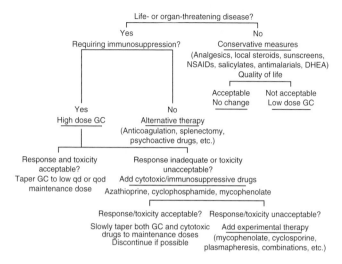

Figure 6-3   Algorithm for treatment for SLE. (From Harris EN, et al. Kelley's Textbook of Rheumatology. Vol 2. 7th Ed. Pp.1225–1247, 2005. Figure 76.1, p 1226. Elsevier; with permission.)

References

1. **Jonsson H, et al.** Estimating the incidence of SLE in a defined population using multiple sources of retrieval. Br J Rheumatol. 1990;29:185–88.
2. **Fessel WJ.** SLE in the community. Arch Intern Med. 1974;134:1027–35.
3. **Edworthy SM.** Clinical manifestations of SLE. In: Harris ED, et al. Kelley's Textbook of Rheumatology. Vol 2. 7th Ed. pp. 1201–24, 2005.
4. **Weening JJ, et al.** The classification of glomerulonephritis in SLE revisited. Kidney Int. 2004;65:521–30.
5. **Sontheimer RD.** Photoimmunology of lupus erythematosus and dermatomyositis: A speculative review. Photochem Photobiol. 1996;63:583–94.
6. **Cohen MR, Isenberg DA.** Ultraviolet irradiation in SLE: Friend or foe? Br J Rheumatol. 1996;35:1002–07.
7. **Tan EM, et al.** The 1982 revised criteria for the classification of SLE. Arthritis Rheum. 1982;25:1271–77.
8. **Hochberg MC.** Updating the American College of Rheumatology revised criteria for the classification of SLE. Arthritis Rheum. 1997;40:1725.
9. **Keeling DM, Isenberg DA.** Haematological manifestations of SLE. Blood Rev. 1993;7:199–207.
10. **Alarcon-Segovia D, et al.** Antiphospholipid antibodies and the antiphospholipid syndrome: Clinical relevance in neuropsychiatric SLE. Ann NY Acad Sci. 1997;823:279–88.
11. **Bruce IN, Gladman DD, Urowitz MB.** Detection and modification of risk factors for coronary artery disease in patients with SLE: A quality improvement study. Clin Exp Rheumatol. 1998;16:435–40.

12. **Manzi S, et al.** Age-specific incidence rates of myocardial infarction and angina in women with SLE: Comparison with the Framingham Study. Am J Epidemiol. 1997;145:408-15.

13. **Ames DE, et al.** SLE complicated by tricuspid stenosis and regurgitation: Successful treatment by valve transplantation. Ann Rheum Dis. 1992;51:120-2.

14. **Chartash EK, et al.** Aortic insufficiency and mitral regurgitation in patients with SLE and the antiphospholipid syndrome. Am J Med. 1989;86:407-12.

15. **Boey ML, et al.** Thrombosis in SLE: Striking association with the presence of circulating lupus anticoagulant. Br Med J Clin Res Ed. 1983;287:1021-23.

16. **Hughes GR, et al.** Veno-occlusive disease in SLE: Possible association with anticardiolipin antibodies? Arthritis Rheum. 1984;27:1071.

17. **Harris EN, Gharavi AE, Hughes GR.** Anti-phospholipid antibodies. Clin Rheum Dis. 1985;11:591-609.

18. **Lavalle C, et al.** Transverse myelitis: A manifestation of SLE strongly associated with antiphospholipid antibodies. J Rheumatol. 1990;17:34-7.

19. **Martinez-Rueda JO, et al.** Factors associated with fetal losses in severe SLE. Lupus. 1996;5:113-9.

20. **Petri M.** SLE and pregnancy. Rheum Dis Clin North Am. 1994; 20:87-118.

21. **Cervera R, et al.** SLE: Clinical and immunologic patterns of disease expression in a cohort of 1,000 patients—The European Working Party on SLE. Medicine (Baltimore). 1993;72:113-24.

22. **McCauliffe DP, Sontheimer RD.** Dermatologic manifestions of rheumatic disorders. Prim Care. 1993;20:925-41.

23. **Hahn B.** Management of SLE. In: Harris EN, et al. Kelley's Textbook of Rheumatology. Vol 2. 7th Ed. pp. 1225-47, 2005.

E. Back Pain

Ann M. O'Connor

KEY POINTS

- Low back pain (LBP) is the second most common complaint seen by primary care providers in an outpatient setting, with lifetime incidence approaching 70% for all patients.
- Women and men both suffer from LBP, but the incidence is slightly higher in pregnant and older women.
- More dangerous conditions can mimic LBP in women, and these diagnoses should be identified as soon as possible.

> ◆ In the absence of "red flag" indicators of more serious problems, 4–6 weeks of conservative therapy is appropriate for most acute LBP episodes, and routine imaging is not recommended in the initial evaluation.
>
> ◆ Women have significantly more scoliosis, fibromyalgia, depression, and osteoporosis than men, all conditions that can contribute to LBP.
>
> ◆ Identifying risk factors for developing chronic back pain when seeing women with acute LBP may help to reduce progression of the condition.

Epidemiology

LBP is a very common complaint, affecting 70–80% of the population at some point in their lifetime. The annual prevalence of LBP for all patients is 15–45% (1,2). LBP is second only to upper respiratory infections for prompting visits to primary care providers. Although LBP is usually a benign and self-limited disorder, it can be frustrating for both the patient and the clinician, since the majority of acute LBP sufferers cannot be given a specific diagnosis. Seventy-five to ninety percent of those with an acute LBP episode will return to baseline in 4–6 weeks, but about 15% to 20% will develop chronic LBP. Spine conditions are the most common reason for lost work in the U.S., are responsible for 25% of all lost work days, and are the most common reason for young adults to limit activity. Direct and indirect costs attributable to LBP in the U.S. are estimated to be $80–100 billion per year, the majority of which is spent on the chronic LBP sufferers (1,2).

A large German study of a representative sample of people belonging to ages 20–64 showed that women had a LBP prevalence rate of 40% compared to 32% for men. Risk factors for increased LBP in this sample included being overweight, having higher somatization tendencies, lower social support or sedentary lifestyles, being a smoker, being elderly, unemployed, or a blue-collar worker (3). It is likely that these findings can be applied to other populations. In addition, work dissatisfaction, severe scoliosis, depression, and history of headache or drug abuse have been associated with increased risk of back pain (4).

Most of the literature reports that women and men suffer nearly equally from LBP, but pregnant women, elderly women, and women with other comorbidities have significantly higher rates of LBP. LBP is a common complaint during pregnancy, affecting 50–90% of women, depending on the subpopulation examined. Women with back pain prior to becoming pregnant are twice as likely to experience LBP with pregnancy, and 36% suffer from LBP that awakens them during their pregnancy (5).

Older women also have higher rates of LBP than men. In a recent large community-based study in Australia of women 70–85 years of age, rates for LBP approached 50%. Daily LBP was associated with a significantly reduced quality of life, lower mobility, and higher risk for coronary artery disease

(CAD) and mortality (6). Osteoporotic compression fractures affect 25% of postmenopausal women and can cause acute LBP (7). These vertebral fractures can be asymptomatic but can also cause significant pain (8).

Clinical Features (Table 6-6)

Definitive diagnosis cannot be determined in 85% of cases because of the weak association between symptoms, pathology, and imaging. Non-radiating LBP is generally thought to be due to musculoskeletal ligamentous injury, degenerative changes, or both. Increased strain on paraspinous muscles as a result of physical activity, such as lifting, may result in avulsion of tendinous attachments or injury to either muscle fibers or the muscle sheath. Overuse of a muscle can lead to pain and spasm. Radiating or radicular pain may be due to compression and inflammation of the spinal nerves. Referred pain may be multifactorial and include non-spinal, visceral disease, tumors, or infection (4).

Discogenic pain is worsened with sitting and flexion, which increases the weight on the anterior vertebral body and pushes the disc posteriorly towards the canal. Narrowing (stenosis) of the spinal canal may be caused by degenerative changes at the vertebral facets. Pain due to spinal stenosis typically radiates down the legs with walking and is relieved with rest, sitting, and slight flexion. Patients with stenosis have more pain with standing and walking, which unloads the vertebral bodies, loads the facets, and narrows the neuroforaminal canals slightly (1).

Table 6-6   Origins of Low Back Pain

97% are Mechanical	2% are Non-spinal or Visceral Disease
>70%–lumbar strains 10%–degenerative disc or facet disease 4%–herniated disc 4%–osteoporotic fractures 3%–spinal stenosis 2%–spondylolisthesis	**Pelvis**: pelvic inflammatory disease (PID), endometriosis, uterine fibroids, fibromyalgia **Renal**: nephrolithiasis, pyelonephritis **Vascular**: aortic aneurysm with or without dissection **Gastrointestinal**: pancreatitis, cholecystitis, peptic ulcer disease **Skin**: herpes zoster
1% are Non-mechanical Spinal Conditions tumors inflammatory arthritis infection	

From Devereaux M.W. Low back pain. Prim Care Clin Office Practice. 2004;31:33–51.
Kinkade, Scott. Evaluation and treatment of low back pain. Am Fam Phys. 15April2007.
Chou, Roger L, Huffman. Nonpharmacologic therapies for acute and chronic low back pain: a review of the evidence for an American Pain Society/American College of Physicians clinical practice guideline. Ann Intern Med. 2October2007;147:492–504; with permission.

Biomechanical stress, hormonal changes, and vascular changes of pregnancy all can contribute to LBP. Increased risk of LBP in pregnancy is correlated with LBP in previous pregnancies and with smoking. In the past, it was theorized that exaggerated lordosis in pregnant women caused LBP, but this has since been refuted. Increased overall weight and direct pressure of the gravid uterus can compress the lumbosacral plexus and cause radicular pain to the buttocks and legs (5).

Although osteoporotic compression fractures can be silent, they can be caused by a fall, sudden movement, or Valsalva-like event such as a cough. Pain from an acute fracture subsides in a few weeks, but the mechanical changes as a result of the fracture can cause sciatica, nerve root impingement, and kyphosis (10).

Diagnosis and Differential Diagnosis

A complete history and focused exam is central to differentiating between a self-limited episode of LBP and a more serious underlying problem. Patients reporting signs of cauda equina syndrome (a compression of the nerve roots of the lower lumbar spine that can cause permanent neurologic damage if not treated with surgery immediately), such as progressive neurologic deficits, bowel or bladder dysfunction, bilateral sciatica, leg weakness or numbness in a saddle distribution, require urgent surgical referral. Screening for a herniated disc using straight leg-testing and strength, sensation, and deep tendon reflex (DTR) testing in the lower extremities is helpful (9).

"Red flags" should warrant immediate investigation and treatment (11) (Box 6-1):

Box 6-1   History and Physical Examination Red Flags

Signs and Symptoms of Concern for Infection or Malignancy
- Age under 18 or over 50 y
- Pain lasting for more than 6 wk
- History of cancer
- Fever, chills, night sweats, weight loss
- Unremitting pain, night pain (may awaken patient from sleep)
- Intravenous drug use
- Immunocompromised subjects
- Fever

Signs and Symptoms of Concern for Epidural Compression
- Bowel or bladder incontinence
- Saddle anesthesia
- Decrease or loss of anal sphincter tone
- Severe or progressive neurologic defect
- Motor weakness

Signs and Symptoms of Concern for Fracture
- Major trauma
- Minor trauma in the elderly or osteoporotic subject

Table 6-7   Physical Examination Findings in Nerve Root Impingements

Herniation	Nerve Root Affected	Sensory Loss	Motor Weakness	Screening Examination	Reflex
L3–L4 disk	L4	Medial foot	Knee extension	Squat and rise	Patellar
L4–L5 disk	L5	Dorsal foot	Dorsiflexion ankle/great toe	Heel walking	None
L5–S1 disk	S1	Lateral foot	Plantar flexion ankle/toes	Walking on toes	Achilles

From Kinkade. Evaluation and treatment of low back pain. Am Fam Phys. 75:1181–8; with permission.

Sudden and severe onset of pain suggests a herniated disc, while slowly progressive symptoms are more likely related to degenerative changes. Localized pain is common with musculoskeletal injury, while radicular pain may be present with nerve root impingement. L5 and S1 radiculopathies account for 90–95% of all lumbar radiculopathies (4). Careful exam findings can localize the level of a disc herniation (Table 6-7). Sciatica is associated with L5–S1 radiculopathies and is often present with low back pain that radiates down the leg to the knee.

Spondylosis is a naturally occurring process of aging in the spine that produces degenerative changes of the vertebral bodies with development of osteophytes that can cause narrowing of the spinal canal and compression symptoms. By age 79, nearly 100% of individuals have some degree of spondylosis. By age 49, 60% of women and 80% of men have some evidence of spinal degenerative changes, such as osteophytes. Progressive spondylosis with osteophyte formation, ligament hypertrophy, and bulging discs can lead to spinal stenosis and, ultimately, compression of the individual nerve roots (4).

If no red flags are present in the initial history and physical exam of a person with acute low back pain, 4–6 weeks of conservative treatment can be initiated. Clinicians should not routinely obtain imaging in patients with nonspecific LBP, since significant radiological abnormalities may be found in completely asymptomatic patients and normal radiographs may be seen in those with severe disorders (9). Imaging should be reserved for those patients with severe or progressive neurologic deficits or if they do not improve with conservative therapy (12).

Prevention and Clinical Care

Ninety percent of patients with LBP seen in primary care will be pain-free in 3 months, and 90% of those will have recovered within 4 weeks. Evidence suggests that cognitive-behavioral therapy, exercise, and rehabilitation therapy are moderately effective in treating chronic or subacute

LBP. Some evidence supports using acupuncture, massage, yoga, and functional restoration (e.g., work hardening) for chronic LBP. For acute LBP, applying heat can also be helpful (13) (Table 6-8).

Nonsteroidal anti-inflammatory drugs (NSAIDs) and acetaminophen are effective first-line therapies for LBP. Muscle relaxants may be more effective in the first week or two of treatment, rather than long-term. Epidural steroid injections may be useful in short-term relief of symptoms in patients with radicular symptoms not responsive to conservative treatment (9,12). Consideration should be given to maximizing benefit while minimizing potential harm and side-effects when choosing medication.

Bedrest provides no benefits to patients with acute LBP, and, in fact, remaining modestly active reduces time lost from work, improves function, and reduces pain. Two to three days of bed rest, if any, should be the maximum for most individuals. General recommendations, such as staying active, avoiding heavy lifting, bending, twisting, and prolonged sitting, are helpful. Return to work on light duty is favored over waiting for full recovery.

Table 6-8   Treatment Recommendations in the Treatment of Low Back Pain

Medication/Measure	Recommendation
Exercise therapy	Effective
	Lack of quality data to support a particular therapy
	Core strengthening has been shown to have a 3-y benefit.
Manipulation	As effective as other conventional treatment
	Low complications for noncervical manipulation
Heat therapy	Effective
	Added benefit if combined with exercise
Cold therapy	Quality studies lacking
Tens	Lack of quality, consistent data
	Should be used with other treatment
Lumbosacral supports	Limited, inconclusive studies
Massage	More effective in patients with high pretreatment expectations
Acupuncture	More evidence for effectiveness in chronic low back pain
	Few trials for acute low back pain
Analgesics	Effective
	Small study showed no difference between opioid/ nonopiod/NSAIDs
Muscle relaxants	Effective
	Significant side effects
NSAIDs	Conflicting data, but generally effective
Antidepressants	Effective for both depressed and nondepressed patients

From McCamey K, Evans P. Low back pain. Primary Care: Clinics in Office Practice. 2007;34: 71–82; with permission.

Preventing acute LBP from progressing to chronic LBP may be accomplished by identifying psychosocial factors associated with chronic LBP: disputed compensation claims; fear avoidance (exaggerated pain or fear that activity will cause permanent damage); job dissatisfaction; pending or past litigation for LBP; psychological distress and depression; reliance on passive therapies rather than active participation and somatization (9).

Pregnant women can reduce LBP, sick time, and improve sleep by remaining active. Walking, swimming, or bicycling at low to moderate intensities and performing abdominal strengthening exercises may help prevent LBP in pregnant women. Trochanteric and sacroiliac support belts may reduce LBP in 71–82% of pregnant women. Any safe measure that can reduce the need for medication and improve the restorative sleep of a pregnant woman should be considered (5).

Similarly, early screening, diagnosis, and treatment of osteoporosis can reduce debilitating vertebral fractures and secondary LBP in elderly women (8).

References

1. **Harwood MI, Smith BJ.** Low back pain: A Primary care approach. Clinics in Family Practice. 2005;5:279–303.
2. **McCann M.** Rakel/Conn's Current Therapy, 59th Edition, Philadelphia, Saunders Elsevier, 2007, Spine Pain, pp. 40–5.
3. **Schneiders.** Why do women have back pain more than men? A representative prevalence study in the Federal Republic of Germany. Clin J Pain. 1October2006;22:738–47.
4. **Devereaux MW.** Low back pain. Prim Care Clin Office Practice. 2004;31:33–51.
5. **Sneag DJ, Bendo JA.** Pregnancy-related low back pain. Orthopedics. 2007;30:839–45.
6. **Barclay L, et al.** Daily back pain may have adverse health effects in elderly women. Spine. 2007;32:2012–18.
7. **Meleger AL.** Neck and Back Pain: Musculoskeletal Disorders. Neurologic Clinics. May2007;25.
8. Bone Health and Osteoporosis: A Report of the Surgeon General. 2004.
9. **Kinkade S.** Evaluation and treatment of low back pain. Am Fam Phys. 15April2007.
10. **Simon L.** Osteoporosis. Rheumatologic Diseases Clinics of North America. February2007;33,149–76.
11. **Rooks Y, Corwell B.** Common urgent musculoskeletal injuries in primary care. Primary Care: Clinics in Office Practice. September2006;33:751–77.
12. Diagnosis and Treatment of Low Back Pain: A Joint Clinical Practice Guideline from the ACP and APS. Annals of Internal Medicine. 2October2007;147,478–91.
13. **Chou R, Huffman L.** Nonpharmacologic therapies for acute and chronic low back pain: a review of the evidence for an American Pain Society/ American College of Physicians clinical practice guideline. Ann Intern Med. 2October2007;147:492–504.
14. **McCamey K, Evans P.** Low back pain. Primary Care. Clinics in the office. 2007;34:71–82.

F. Fibromyalgia

Rose S. Fife

KEY POINTS

♦ Fibromyalgia (FM) is a syndrome characterized by chronic pain in specific regions (tender points).

♦ FM is more common in women and is frequently associated with other syndromes, such as irritable bowel syndrome, chronic fatigue syndrome (CFS) (see below), temporomandibular pain disorders, depression, and post-traumatic stress disorder (PTSD).

♦ Treatment is difficult and should be multidisciplinary, including physicians, psychologists, physical therapists, and others.

Epidemiology

FM is more common in women than in men (1). It affects approximately 2% of the U.S. population, with a prevalence of about 3.4% in women and 0.5% in men (2). The most common age of presentation lies between 50 and 70 years, but FM may present as early as childhood, especially in individuals with other chronic diseases, such as juvenile rheumatoid arthritis. No racial or ethnic relationships have been noted. FM often is associated with other disorders, including irritable bowel syndrome, CFS, depression, post-traumatic stress disorder (PTSD), and temporomandibular pain (1–3). The cause of FM is not known, but the consensus opinion at present leans toward a response by the body to various significant stressors. Indications of this are its frequent association with other such conditions (Figure 6-4) (1–3).

Clinical Features

The diagnosis of FM requires that chronic pain be present for at least 3 months in a distribution of reproducible zones called "tender points." Pain in 11 of 18 of these regions is necessary for a diagnosis. These areas include symmetrical bilateral sites (Table 6-9) (4). Many patients also have "non-restorative sleep," that is, they awake from a night's sleep without feeling rested. Such sleep patterns have been associated with decreased periods of REM (rapid eye movement) sleep on polysomnography, but the role of REM sleep in FM is unknown (5).

Manifestations of FM are identical in males and females, but the condition is much more common in women. Blood and other laboratory studies are typically normal in subjects with FM.

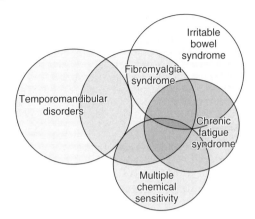

Figure 6-4   Overlap between fibromyalgia and other syndromes. (From Kelley's Textbook of Rheumatology, Vol. 1, Harris, Budd, Firestein, et al., Fibromyalgia: A Chronic Pain Syndrome, page 523, Copyright Elsevier, 2005; with permission.)

Diagnosis and Differential Diagnosis

Specific criteria for the diagnosis of FM were defined by the American College of Rheumatology (ACR) in 1990 as: 1) a minimum of 3 months of pain that is bilateral and above and below the waist; and 2) pain to palpation with approximately 4 kg of pressure at a minimum of 11 of the 18 sites noted above (4). It should be noted that, unlike many other conditions, the exclusion of other disorders is not required to permit the diagnosis of FM. It is *not* a diagnosis of exclusion by any means, but rather it is often associated with other comorbid conditions (1,3).

Other disorders producing chronic pain should be considered before making the diagnosis of FM. Obviously, as just noted, FM can coexist with such disorders, but the health care provider must be able to recognize the existence of other states that require different therapies. Rheumatoid arthritis, both juvenile and adult, can be present in those diagnosed with FM. Adult RA is diagnosed as described in Chapter 6C in this book, with its characteristic symmetrical synovitis and associated features. Complex regional pain syndromes, such as reflex sympathetic dystrophy, a condition manifested by pain in a specific isolated part of the body (e.g., a limb that may have sustained trauma), can be distinguished by their usually unilateral and focal location (Table 6-10).

The etiology of FM is not known, but association with various stressors, including conditions such as PTSD and depression, are frequent, as previously noted.

Table 6-9   The American College of Rheumatology 1990 Criteria for The Classification of Fibromyalgia*

---

1. History of Widespread Pain

Definition: Pain is considered widespread when all of the following are present: pain in the left side of the body, pain in the right side of the body, pain above the waist, and pain below the waist. In addition, axial skeletal pain (cervical spine or anterior chest or thoracic spine or low back) must be present. In this definition, shoulder, and buttock pain is considered as pain for each involved side. "Low back" pain is considered lower segment pain.

2. Pain In 11 Of 18 Tender Point Sites On Digital Palpation

Definition: Pain, on digital palpation, must be present in at least 11 of the following 18 tender point sites:

Occiput: bilateral, at the suboccipital muscle insertions
Low cervical: bilateral, at the anterior aspects of the intertransverse spaces at C5-C7
Trapezius: bilateral, at the midpoint of the upper border
Supraspinatus: bilateral, at origins, above the scapula spine near the medial border
Second rib: bilateral, at the 2nd costochondral junctions, just lateral to the junctions on upper surfaces
Lateral epicondyle: bilateral, 2 cm distal to the epicondyles
Gluteal: bilateral, in upper outer quadrants of buttocks in anterior fold of muscle
Greater trochanter: bilateral, posterior to the trochanteric prominence
Knee: bilateral, at the medial fat pad proximal to the joint line
Digital palpation should be performed with an approximate force of 4 kg.
For a tender point to be considered "positive" the subject must state that the palpation was painful. "Tender" is not to be considered "painful."

---

*For classification purposes, patients will be said to have fibromyalgia if both criteria are satisfied. Widespread pain must have been present for at least 3 months. The presence of a second clinical disorder does not exclude the diagnosis of fibromyalgia.
From Wolfe F, Smythe HA, Yunus MB, et al. The American College of Rheumatology 1990 Criteria for the Classification of Fibromyalgia: Report of the Multicenter Criteria Committee. Arthritis Rheum. 1990;33:160–72; with permission.

Prevention and Care

FM is difficult to treat. Comprehensive pain programs that include physical therapy, analgesics, and behavioral and/or psychological intercessions have been used, with response in some patients (6). Because of the presence of the sleep abnormality described earlier, agents such as tricyclic antidepressants (e.g., amitriptyline and its relatives) have been used in very low doses at bedtime to improve sleep, and some patients have reported a reduction in symptoms (7). However, many cannot tolerate the not uncommon side effects of fatigue and "hangover."

More recently, in clinical trials, agents such as duloxetine, a selective norepinephrine reuptake inhibitor (SNRI), and similar compounds have been examined for effectiveness and safety in subjects with FM, with some evidence of success (8). In 2007, pregabalin, a relative of

Table 6-10   Differential Diagnosis of FM (Not Inclusive)

Condition	Type	Differentiation
CFS	Unknown	Severe fatigue, pain without characteristic localization
Depression	Psychiatric disorder	Fatigue, flat affect, tearfulness
Hypothyroidism	Endocrine disorder	Fatigue, weight gain, low thyroxine levels, elevated TSH
Polymyalgia rheumatica	Rheumatologic disorder	Proximal muscle pain, elevated ESR, usually over age 60
Polymyositis	Rheumatologic disorder	Proximal muscle weakness, pain, elevated CPK
PTSD	Psychiatric disorder	Flashbacks, anger, fatigue, withdrawal
Regional pain syndromes	Neuropathic	Pain in usually 1 extremity or part thereof
Rheumatoid arthritis	Rheumatologic disorder	Symmetrical synovitis, elevated RF, ESR, CRP, other features
Seronegative spondyloarthropathies	Rheumatologic disorder	Involvement of spine, peripheral joints, inflammation, elevated ESR, CRP

From Burkham J, Harris ED. Fibromyalgia: A Chronic Pain Syndrome. In: Harris ED, Budd RC, Genovese MC, et al. Kelley's Textbook of Rheumatology. 7th Ed. Philadelphia: Elsevier Saunders, 2005; with permission.

gabapentin, became the first drug to receive official approval from the FDA for use in FM (9,10). However, we are still a long way from good control for most FM sufferers.

Because of its association with depression and presumptive stressors, participation of psychologists and/or psychiatrists and other mental health caregivers is a very important component in the treatment of many persons with FM.

There are no preventive measures for FM. Stressful lifestyles or events seem to be related, but they usually cannot be avoided by an individual, nor do we know which individuals might be likely to respond to such stressors by developing FM.

Chronic Fatigue Syndrome

This is one of the conditions that intersects with FM in the pseudo-Venn diagram in Figure 6-4. It is characterized by severe fatigue in the absence of a recognizable constitutional illness. However, patients frequently note a flu-like syndrome as an antecedent to the development of CFS, and they may have lymphadenopathy, fever, and headache. They have more generalized musculoskeletal discomfort than those with FM. CFS also may be associated with depression and some of the other comorbidities described for FM (1,3,11). Over the years, some have considered CFS as a possible form of "chronic Lyme disease" or Epstein-Barr virus-related disease, which should be ruled out by appropriate studies if suspicion is high. CFS is difficult to treat.

References

1. **Burkham J, Harris ED.** Fibromyalgia: A Chronic Pain Syndrome. In: Harris ED, Budd RC, Genovese MC, et al. Kelley's Textbook of Rheumatology. 7th Ed. Philadelphia: Elsevier Saunders, 2005
2. **Wolfe F, Ross K, Anderson J, et al.** The prevalence and characteristics of fibromyalgia in the general population. Arthritis Rheum. 1995;38:19–28.
3. **Weir PT, Harlan GA, Knoy FL, et al.** The incidence of fibromyalgia and its associated comorbidities. J Clin Rheumatol. 2006;12:124–28.
4. **Wolfe F, Smythe HA, Yunus MB, et al.** The American College of Rheumatology 1990 Criteria for the Classification of Fibromyalgia: Report of the Multicenter Criteria Committee. Arthritis Rheum. 1990;33:160–72.
5. **Moldofsky H, Scarisbrick P, England R, et al.** Musculoskeletal symptoms and Non-REM sleep disturbance in patients with "fibrositis syndrome" and healthy subjects. Psychosom Med. 1975;37:341–51.
6. **Hooten WM, Townsend CO, Sletten CD, et al.** Treatment outcomes after multidisciplinary pain rehabilitation with analgesic medication withdrawal for patients with fibromyalgia. Pain Med. 2007;8:8–16.
7. **Rooks DS.** Fibromyalgia treatment update. Curr Opin Rheumatol. 2007;19:111–7.
8. **Arnold LM.** Duloxetine and other antidepressants in the treatment of patients with fibromyalgia. Pain Med. 2007;8:S63–S74.
9. **Wu SC, Wrobel JS, Armstrong DG.** Assessing the impact of pharmacologic intervention on the quality of life in diabetic peripheral neuropathic pain and fibromyalgia. Pain Med. 2007;8:S33–S43.
10. **Arnold LM, Goldenberg DL, Stanford SB, et al.** Gabapentin in the treatment of fibromyalgia. Arthritis Rheum. 2007;56:1336–44.
11. **Whiting P, Bagnall A-M, Sowden AJ, et al.** Interventions for the treatment and management of chronic fatigue syndrome. JAMA. 2001;286:1360–68.

7

Neurological Disease

A. Stroke
Sabina Agrawal

KEY POINTS

◆ Stroke in women is a major public health burden with far-reaching consequences.

◆ Risk factors for stroke unique to women include oral contraceptive use, migraine, pregnancy, exogenous hormone therapy (EHT), and autoimmune disorders.

◆ EHT is not recommended for the primary or secondary prevention of stroke in women.

◆ Aspirin may be used as primary and secondary prevention of stroke in women.

◆ Carotid endarterectomy as a means of stroke prevention works better in men than in women.

◆ Further research is necessary to bridge gaps in knowledge of strokes in women.

Epidemiology

Stroke is one of the leading causes of disability and death in women. The estimated direct and indirect cost of stroke in 2007 was $62.7 billion (1). In 2004, women accounted for 61% of stroke deaths in the U.S. (1). The burden of stroke is higher in women than in men because they live approximately 10 years longer. Consequently, as the population ages, stroke incidence increases. In the U.S., the rate of stroke in White women is 0.6–0.8/1000 women/year at age 50–59 years, 2/1000 at age 60–64 years, 4.2/1000 at age 65–74 years, and 11.3/1000 at age 75–87 years (2). Blacks appear to have a risk of first-ever stroke that is almost twice that of Whites (1).

Although studies of stroke in women are limited, previous research suggests that women have poorer outcomes and higher total mortality than men (3,4). Under-recognition of stroke in women could be a potential cause of differences in stroke care. One study found that women with stroke present for medical care more frequently with non-traditional symptoms (e.g., pain, change in level of consciousness, disorientation, unclassifiable neurologic symptoms, and nonspecific symptoms) and complaints compared with men with stroke (5). Moreover, the type of stroke (i.e., ischemic vs. hemorrhagic) might affect the type of symptoms reported (Table 7-1). Another study found that women with stroke underwent fewer diagnostic tests than men, despite

Table 7-1   Clinical Features of Stroke

Clinical features—sudden onset of:	Clinical features in women that may be indicative of a stroke—sudden onset of:
• Numbness or weakness of the face, arm, or leg • Confusion, trouble speaking or understanding • Problem walking, dizziness, or loss of balance or coordination • Problem seeing in 1 or both eyes • Severe headache with no known cause	• Face and limb pain • Hiccups • Nausea • Generalized weakness and fatigue • Chest pain • Dyspnea • Palpitations • Seizure • Falls or accidents

From http://www.4women.gov/faq/stroke.htm. Accessed February 2, 2008.

adjusting for potential confounders, including stroke risk factors, stroke severity, insurance status, age, and ethnicity. This suggests that women may receive a different level of care and evaluation for stroke than men (6).

Risk Factors

General risk factors for stroke are described in Table 7-2.

Risk Factors Specific to Women

Oral Contraceptives : Oral contraceptive (OCP) use confers an increased risk of stroke, probably as a result of alterations in coagulation. However, in relatively healthy women under the age of 35 years, the benefits of OCPs probably outweigh the potential risk of stroke, after careful consideration of other risk factors (i.e., age, smoking, hypertension, migraine with

Table 7-2   Risk Factors for Stroke (In rank order)

Non-modifiable	Modifiable
• Age >55 y • Gender (men > women, when adjusted for age) • Race (African Americans and Hispanics > Caucasians) • Family history	• Atrial fibrillation • Carotid stenosis • Hypertension • Diabetes • Previous stroke/TIA • Hyperlipidemia • Smoking • **Obesity/physical inactivity**

From http://www.4women.gov/faq/stroke.htm. Accessed February 2, 2008.

aura, and history of venous thromboembolism, etc.). The absolute risk of stroke is 6.7/100 000 women/year in users of low-dose OCPs and 12.9 in users of high-dose OCPs (8). Progesterone-only OCPs are not associated with increased risk of stroke; however, data are limited (8).

Migraine: Migraine has been identified as a risk factor for stroke. Migraine with aura, specifically, has a higher risk of ischemic stroke than migraine without aura (9). The mechanism by which migraine increases the risk of stroke is unknown, but it may be related to vasospasm, endothelial dysfunction, and increased platelet aggregation (10).

Interestingly, the prevalence of migraine is higher in women than in men (11). Estrogen is considered to play a role in migraine headaches. In women, migraines decrease with advancing age and improve in many after menopause when estrogen levels stabilize (12). However, during pre-menopausal years, menstrual migraine is common, probably because of erratic estrogen secretion (12). Often, treatment of menstrual migraine includes OCPs, which alone appear to carry an independent risk for stroke. In fact, among women with migraine, the use of OCPs is associated with a 2- to 4-fold increased risk of stroke, compared to women who do not use OCPs (13). According to the World Health Organization (13), the use of OCPs as treatment for migraine depends on the presence of an aura. Low-dose OCPs pose an "unacceptable health risk" (13) if used in women who have migraine with aura, regardless of age, and if used in women over the age of 35 years who have migraine without aura. In women under the age of 35 years who have migraine without aura, OCPs may be used, but only after careful consideration of the risk-benefit ratio.

Finally, migraine with aura has been associated with cardiac abnormalities, such as patent foramen ovale (PFO). PFO has been implicated as a possible mechanism for the association between migraine and stroke (14). The mechanism is still unclear; however, it may be related to paradoxical brain embolism or the presence of a right-to-left shunt, which would enable venous blood containing activated platelets to reach the brain and trigger a migraine (15).

Pregnancy: Pregnancy is a hypercoagulable state that increases the risk of stroke in young women, although stroke occurrence remains infrequent in this cohort. Analysis of the Nationwide Inpatient Sample revealed an all-stroke incidence of 34.2/100 000 deliveries (16). According to the Baltimore-Washington Cooperative Young Stroke Study, the risk of ischemic stroke or intracerebral hemorrhage during pregnancy and the first 6 weeks postpartum was 2.4 times greater than for non-pregnant women of similar age and race (1). Risk factors for pregnancy-associated stroke and transient ischemic attack (TIA) include age >35 years, Black race, hypertension, heart disease, smoking, diabetes, lupus, sickle cell disease, migraine headaches, alcohol and substance abuse, Caesarean delivery, fluid/electrolyte/acid-base disorders, thrombophilia, multiple gestation, greater parity, postpartum infections, pre-eclampsia, and eclampsia (16,17). Many of the cases occur in women with pre-eclampsia or eclampsia; these conditions may lead to endothelial dysfunction and affect cerebral autoregulation. Fewer cases are attributable to venous thrombosis (i.e., cerebral venous sinus thrombosis and thrombophilic disorders).

Autoimmune disorders: Women experience a higher frequency of the following autoimmune disorders, which can have an impact on stroke: systemic lupus erythematosus, primary anti-phospholipid antibody syndrome, Takayasu's arteritis, and fibromuscular dysplasia.

Diagnostic Evaluation

The diagnostic evaluation of a woman with a possible stroke begins with a complete history and physical examination, as well as consideration of other states that may mimic stroke (Box 7-1).

The neurological exam should be thorough and document clearly any deficits that are apparent. In the acute setting, a CT scan is indicated to screen for acute intra-cerebral hemorrhage and masses. MRI has increased sensitivity for detection of embolic strokes compared to CT. Diffusion weighted imaging (DWI) can detect infarcts within 30 minutes of onset and can distinguish acute infarct from chronic ischemic changes. Perfusion weighted imaging (PWI) demonstrates regions of cerebral hypoperfusion. Areas demonstrating abnormal perfusion without restricted diffusion are called "mismatched." The presence of mismatch may allow for reperfusion therapies to be administered even beyond the traditional 3-hour window, although the evidence supporting this is mixed (18). Carotid artery duplex ultrasound assesses the integrity of the carotid vessels, while cerebral angiography, the gold standard, evaluates the cerebral vasculature. An EKG is indicated to evaluate for atrial fibrillation, and an echocardiogram is useful to assess for potential sources of emboli. Table 7-3 lists laboratory tests commonly ordered for evaluating stroke.

Box 7-1   Differential Diagnosis of Stroke

- Migraine accompaniment
- Seizure/Todd's paralysis*
- Hypoglycemia
- Encephalopathy (infectious, metabolic, hypertensive)
- Transient global amnesia
- Cerebral neoplasm
- Multiple sclerosis
- Conversion disorder
- Acute coronary syndrome

*Todd's paralysis is a transient period of paralysis after a seizure.

Table 7-3   Laboratory Evaluation of a Stroke

Laboratory evaluation:	Tests for hypercoagulability:
1. Chem 7	1. Lupus anticoagulant
2. CBC with platelets	2. Anticardiolipin antibodies
3. PTT and PT/INR	3. Anti-beta 2 glycoprotein I antibodies
4. Fasting lipid panel	4. Protein C and Protein S
5. Fasting glucose	5. Anti-thrombin III
6. Consider toxicology screen	6. Factor V Leiden mutation*
	7. Prothrombin gene mutation
	8. Homocysteine

*Or activated protein C resistance. The Leiden mutation results in APC resistance.

Prevention

Exogenous Hormone Therapy

The incidence of stroke increases in women after menopause, presumably resulting from a decline in endogenous estrogen and progesterone. Historically, EHT was prescribed to women for many putative health benefits, since EHT could enhance endothelial-dependent blood flow and had the potential to block or attenuate the secondary mechanism of injury after stroke (19). However, in recent years, such therapy has raised concerns about increased risk of cardiovascular disease, venous thromboembolism, stroke, and breast cancer, during use ranging from 1 to 5 years (20). The Women's Health Initiative primary prevention clinical trial of relatively healthy postmenopausal women found that estrogen plus progestin increased ischemic stroke by approximately 44% (20). The mechanism for increased stroke and other adverse outcomes may be related to an increase in the inflammatory response and a probable increase in the activation of the coagulation system (19).

Given the ambiguity and the incomplete understanding of the mechanism of action of EHT in humans, current recommendations are to not prescribe EHT for cerebrovascular benefits as primary or secondary prevention until further studies take place.

Primary Prevention of Stroke

Aspirin: There are differences in platelet activity induced by sex hormones: testosterone increases platelet activity, whereas estrogen inhibits it (21). Additionally, anti-platelet drugs can show variations in effectiveness in men and women, due to possible gender differences in metabolism and anti-aggregant activity (22). In the absence of high coronary disease risk, aspirin is not of proven value for the primary prevention of stroke in men; this is not true in women. There is conflicting evidence regarding the appropriate dose of aspirin for primary prevention of stroke in women.

of these
aspirin
ed with

...ined the 5 major trials involving aspirin use i
...nyocardial infarction and stroke. In summary,
...f stroke in women over the age of 50 years, the
...aspirin may be >100 mg/day, and for women
...ne dose is 325 mg/day. However, careful consid-
...ven the potential risk of gastrointestinal hemor-
...pirin dose of 50 mg/day (RR 1.40, 95% CI: 1.07 to

...ences
...g bet-
...may
...ts of
...h fat
...ent,
...ving
...cial
...en-
...tid
...at
...n
...of
...).

...risk factors: Treatment of hypertension, diabetes, and
...important in the prevention of stroke. A reduction in
...sure by 10 mm Hg is associated with a 33% reduction in
...egardless of the baseline blood pressure (25). Depending
...e blood pressure goal should be either <140/90 mm Hg
...Hg. Aggressive management of blood glucose and lip-
...vent stroke as well. All smokers should be encouraged to
...should also be counseled regarding limiting alcohol use,
...healthy weight, and increasing physical activity. The Nurse's
...found that physical activity reduces the risk of stroke, where
...sks for stroke in women with the lowest to the highest physi-
...vere 1.00, 0.98, 0.82, 0.74, and 0.66, respectively (1).

Prevention of Stroke

...ry prevention of another stroke starts with management of all
...pove modifiable risk factors. Several medications have an indica-
...secondary prevention as well.

...: The lowest effective dose of aspirin recommended for second-
...revention of stroke in women is 50 mg/day. In women with acute
...mic stroke, 160 mg/day of aspirin can significantly reduce the rate
...ecurrent stroke or death (23). Of note, although aspirin therapy has
...potential to increase the risk of hemorrhagic stroke, the cardiovascu-
...and cerebrovascular benefits outweigh the risk, which is estimated to
...e 0.2 events/1000 patient-years in both primary and secondary preven-
...ion studies (26).

Extended-release dipyridamole (ER-DP) and Aspirin: Two randomized control trials have demonstrated the benefit of combination therapy versus aspirin alone (27,28).

Clopidogrel: For those intolerant of aspirin (e.g., those with gastrointestinal distress or bleeding), with an aspirin allergy (e.g., those with nasal polyps, rhinorrhea, and bronchospasm), or who experience headaches with dypyridamole, clopidrogrel is an appropriate alternative. However, clopidogrel alone is not considered first-line therapy (29,30).

Clopidogrel and Aspirin: This combination of medications is not recommended in those with a history of stroke.

Warfarin: Warfarin is indicated for specific conditions that increase the propensity of stroke (i.e., atrial fibrillation and artificial cardiac valve).

It has a lesser role in the prevention of ischemic stroke outside
situations. Studies do not support the use of warfarin ove
given the high rate of mortality and major hemorrhage associa
warfarin (31).

Carotid Endarterectomy

Previous studies have established that there are gender diffe
in benefits from carotid endarterectomy (CEA), with men farin
ter than women (32). Possible explanations for this discrepanc
include: smaller plaque volume in women compared to men, effe
hormones on atherosclerosis, and plaque characteristics (i.e., hig
content, low structural components, high inflammatory cell con
and increased protease activity), with asymptomatic women ha
more stable plaques than men (32). Thus, CEA may be less benef
in women with asymptomatic carotid artery disease (primary prev
tion). Further support of this has come from the Asymptomatic Carc
Atherosclerosis Study (ACAS), where subgroup analysis suggested t
CEA was less effective in women. Men had an absolute risk reducti
of 8% versus 1.4% in women, probably due to a higher incidence
perioperative complications in women, 3.6% versus 1.7% in men (33
The operative complications in women may be a result of technical di
ficulty in handling anatomically smaller-sized vessels (34).

   For symptomatic carotid artery stenosis (secondary prevention), *post
hoc* analysis of the North American Symptomatic Carotid Endarterectomy
Trial (NASCET) study demonstrated that in subjects with 50–69% stenosis, the benefit of CEA was greater in men than in women. The number
needed to treat was 12 and 16 for men and 67 and 125 for women for
prevention of an ipsilateral stroke of any severity or for prevention of a
disabling stroke, respectively (35). In summary, CEA appears to be most
beneficial in women with symptomatic stenosis of 70–90%.

Socioeconomic Implications

There are significant socioeconomic and health care implications for
women who suffer from a stroke. First, since women live longer than men,
stroke poses a greater financial hardship for women and their families.
Second, although gender equality in American society has improved, the
responsibilities for the care of the home and family still fall to women
much of the time. Thus, should the woman of the family suffer from a
stroke, the illness and the recovery may pose far-reaching consequences.

References

1. Heart disease and stroke statistics. American Heart Association Heart
   and Stroke Statistics: 2007 Update.
2. **Lobo RA.** Menopause and stroke and the effects of hormonal therapy.
   Climacteric. 2007;10:27–31.
3. **Wyller TB.** Stroke and gender. J Gender Specific Med. 1999;2:41–5.

A recent review (23) examined the 5 major trials involving aspirin use i n primary prevention of myocardial infarction and stroke. In summary, for primary prevention of stroke in women over the age of 50 years, the lowest effective dose of aspirin may be >100 mg/day, and for women with atrial fibrillation the dose is 325 mg/day. However, careful consideration is necessary given the potential risk of gastrointestinal hemorrhage even with an aspirin dose of 50 mg/day (RR 1.40, 95% CI: 1.07 to 1.83; p=0.02) (24).

Control of modifiable risk factors: Treatment of hypertension, diabetes, and hyperlipidemia are important in the prevention of stroke. A reduction in systolic blood pressure by 10 mm Hg is associated with a 33% reduction in the risk of stroke, regardless of the baseline blood pressure (25). Depending on risk factors, the blood pressure goal should be either <140/90 mm Hg or <130/80 mm Hg. Aggressive management of blood glucose and lipids will help prevent stroke as well. All smokers should be encouraged to quit. Women should also be counseled regarding limiting alcohol use, maintaining a healthy weight, and increasing physical activity. The Nurse's Health Study found that physical activity reduces the risk of stroke, where the relative risks for stroke in women with the lowest to the highest physical activity were 1.00, 0.98, 0.82, 0.74, and 0.66, respectively (1).

Secondary Prevention of Stroke

Secondary prevention of another stroke starts with management of all of the above modifiable risk factors. Several medications have an indication for secondary prevention as well.

Aspirin: The lowest effective dose of aspirin recommended for secondary prevention of stroke in women is 50 mg/day. In women with acute ischemic stroke, 160 mg/day of aspirin can significantly reduce the rate of recurrent stroke or death (23). Of note, although aspirin therapy has the potential to increase the risk of hemorrhagic stroke, the cardiovascular and cerebrovascular benefits outweigh the risk, which is estimated to be 0.2 events/1000 patient-years in both primary and secondary prevention studies (26).

Extended-release dipyridamole (ER-DP) and Aspirin: Two randomized control trials have demonstrated the benefit of combination therapy versus aspirin alone (27,28).

Clopidogrel: For those intolerant of aspirin (e.g., those with gastrointestinal distress or bleeding), with an aspirin allergy (e.g., those with nasal polyps, rhinorrhea, and bronchospasm), or who experience headaches with dypyridamole, clopidrogrel is an appropriate alternative. However, clopidogrel alone is not considered first-line therapy (29,30).

Clopidogrel and Aspirin: This combination of medications is not recommended in those with a history of stroke.

Warfarin: Warfarin is indicated for specific conditions that increase the propensity of stroke (i.e., atrial fibrillation and artificial cardiac valve).

It has a lesser role in the prevention of ischemic stroke outside of these situations. Studies do not support the use of warfarin over aspirin given the high rate of mortality and major hemorrhage associated with warfarin (31).

Carotid Endarterectomy

Previous studies have established that there are gender differences in benefits from carotid endarterectomy (CEA), with men faring better than women (32). Possible explanations for this discrepancy may include: smaller plaque volume in women compared to men, effects of hormones on atherosclerosis, and plaque characteristics (i.e., high fat content, low structural components, high inflammatory cell content, and increased protease activity), with asymptomatic women having more stable plaques than men (32). Thus, CEA may be less beneficial in women with asymptomatic carotid artery disease (primary prevention). Further support of this has come from the Asymptomatic Carotid Atherosclerosis Study (ACAS), where subgroup analysis suggested that CEA was less effective in women. Men had an absolute risk reduction of 8% versus 1.4% in women, probably due to a higher incidence of perioperative complications in women, 3.6% versus 1.7% in men (33). The operative complications in women may be a result of technical difficulty in handling anatomically smaller-sized vessels (34).

For symptomatic carotid artery stenosis (secondary prevention), *post-hoc* analysis of the North American Symptomatic Carotid Endarterectomy Trial (NASCET) study demonstrated that in subjects with 50–69% stenosis, the benefit of CEA was greater in men than in women. The number needed to treat was 12 and 16 for men and 67 and 125 for women for prevention of an ipsilateral stroke of any severity or for prevention of a disabling stroke, respectively (35). In summary, CEA appears to be most beneficial in women with symptomatic stenosis of 70–90%.

Socioeconomic Implications

There are significant socioeconomic and health care implications for women who suffer from a stroke. First, since women live longer than men, stroke poses a greater financial hardship for women and their families. Second, although gender equality in American society has improved, the responsibilities for the care of the home and family still fall to women much of the time. Thus, should the woman of the family suffer from a stroke, the illness and the recovery may pose far-reaching consequences.

References

1. Heart disease and stroke statistics. American Heart Association Heart and Stroke Statistics: 2007 Update.
2. **Lobo RA.** Menopause and stroke and the effects of hormonal therapy. Climacteric. 2007;10:27–31.
3. **Wyller TB.** Stroke and gender. J Gender Specific Med. 1999;2:41–5.

4. **Holroyd-Leduc JM, Kapral MK, Austin PC, et al.** Sex differences and similarities in the management and outcome of stroke patients. Stroke. 2000;31:1833–7.

5. **Labiche LA, Chan W, Saldin KR, et al.** Sex and acute stroke presentation. Ann Emerg Med. 2002;40:453–60.

6. **Smith MA, Lisabeth LD, Brown DL, et al.** Gender comparisons of diagnostic evaluation for ischemic stroke patients. Neurology. 2005;65:855–8.

7. http://www.4women.gov/faq/stroke.htm. Accessed February 2, 2008.

8. **Wityk RJ, Llinas RF.** Stroke. American College of Physicians, 2007.

9. **Etminan M, Takkouche B, Isorna FC, et al.** Risk of ischaemic stroke in people with migraine: systematic review and meta-analysis of observational studies. BMJ. 2005;330:63.

10. **Tzourio C, Kittner SJ, Bousser MG, et al.** Migraine and stroke in young women. Cephalalgia. 2000;20:190–9.

11. **Lipton RB, Stewart WF, Diamond S, et al.** Prevalence and burden of migraine in the United States: data from the American Migraine Study II. Headache. 2001;41:646–57.

12. **Ashkenazi A, Silberstein SD.** Hormone-related headache pathophysiology and treatment. CNS Drugs. 2006;20:125–41.

13. World Health Organization. Medical eligibility criteria for contraceptive use. 2004;3rd edition.

14. **MacClellan LR, Giles W, Cole J, et al.** Probable migraine with visual aura and risk of ischemic stroke—The Stroke Prevention in Young Women Study. Stroke. 2007;38:2438–45.

15. **Anzola GP.** Patent foramen ovale and migraine. Cleveland Clinic Journal of Medicine. 2007;74:S114–7.

16. **James A, Bushnell CD, Jamison M, et al.** Incidence and risk factors for stroke in pregnancy and the puerperium. Obstet Gynecol. 2005;106:509–16.

17. **Lanska DJ, Kryscio RJ.** Peripartum stroke and intracranial venous thrombosis in the National Hospital Discharge Survey. Obstet Gynecol. 1997;89:413–8.

18. **Hacke W, Albers G, Al-Rawi Y, et al.** The Desmoteplase in Acute Ischemic Stroke Trial (DIAS): a phase II MRI-based 9-hour window acute stroke thrombolysis trial with intravenous desmoteplase. Stroke. 2005;36:66–73.

19. **Bushnell, Cheryl D.** Hormone replacement therapy and stroke: The current state of knowledge and directions for future research. Seminars in Neurology. 2006;26:123–30.

20. Writing Group for the Women's Health Initiative Investigators. Risks and benefits of estrogen plus progestin in healthy post-menopausal women: principal results from the Women's Health Initiative randomized controlled trial. JAMA. 2002;288:321–33.

21. **Emms H, Lewis GP.** Sex and hormonal influences on platelet sensitivity and coagulation in the rat. Br J Pharmacol. 1985;86:557–63.

22. **Montgomery PR, Berger LG, Mitenko PA, et al.** Salicylate metabolism: effects of age and sex in adults. Clin Pharmacol Ther. 1986;39:571–6.

23. **Dalen JE.** Aspirin to prevent heart attack and stroke: What's the right dose? American Journal of Medicine. 2006;119:198–202.

24. **Ridker PM, Cook NR, Lee IM, et al.** A randomized trial of low-dose aspirin in the primary prevention of cardiovascular disease in women. N Engl J Med. 2005;352:1293–304.

25. **Lawes CMM, Bennett DA, Feigin VL, et al.** Blood pressure and stroke. an overview of published reviews. Stroke. 2004;35:776–85.

26. **Gorelick PB and Weisman SM.** Risk of hemorrhagic stroke with aspirin use: an update. Stroke. 2005;36:1801–7.

27. **Diener HC, Cunha L, Forbes C, et al.** European Stroke Prevention Study. 2. Dipyridamole and acetylsalicylic acid in the secondary prevention of stroke. J Neuro Sci. 1996;143:1–13.

28. **Halkes PH, van Gijn J, Kappelle LJ, et al.** for the ESPRIT Study Group. Aspirin plus dypyridamole versus aspirin alone after cerebral ischaemia of arterial origin (ESPRIT): randomized controlled trial [Published correction appears in Lancet 2007;369:274]. Lancet. 2006;367:1665–73.

29. **Sacco RL, Adams R, Albers G, et al.** Guidelines for prevention of stroke in patients with ischemic stroke or transient ischemic attack: a statement for healthcare professionals from the American Heart Association/ American Stroke Association Council on Stroke: co-sponsored by the Council on Cardiovascular Radiology and Intervention: the American Academy of Neurology affirms the value of this guideline. Stroke. 2006;37:577–617.

30. **Albers GW, Amarenco P, Easton JD, et al.** Antithrombotic and thrombolytic therapy for ischemic stroke: the Seventh ACCP Conference on Antithrombotic and Thrombolytic Therapy. Chest. 2004;126: S483–512.

31. **Algra A.** The Esprit Study Group. Medium intensity oral anticoagulants vs. aspirin after cerebral ischemia of arterial origin (ESPRIT): a randomized controlled trial.

32. **Hellings WE, Pasterkamp G, Verhoeven BAN, et al.** Gender-associated differences in plaque phenotype of patients undergoing carotid endarterectomy. Journal of Vascular Surgery. 2007;45:289–97.

33. Endarterctomy for asymptomatic carotid artery stenosis. Executive Committee for the Asymptomatic Carotid Atherosclerosis Study. JAMA. 1995;273:1421.

34. **Krejza J, Arkuszewski M, Kasner SE, et al.** Carotid artery diameter in men and women and the relation to body and neck size. Stroke. 2006;37:1103.

35. **Chaturvedi S, Bruno A, Feasby T, et al.** Carotid endarterectomy—An evidence-based review. Neurology. 2005;65:794–801.

B. Multiple Sclerosis

David H. Mattson

KEY POINTS

- Multiple sclerosis (MS) is a presumed autoimmune disease that results in lymphocytic inflammatory demyelination and subsequent dropout of axons in the white matter of the brain.

- MS is twice as common in women as in men and typically begins between the ages of 20 and 40 years.

- MS usually starts with a relapsing and remitting course and then frequently becomes relentlessly progressive with neurologic symptoms and signs referable to white matter pathways in the brain.

- MS can be diagnosed clinically by documenting 2 different clinical attacks involving 2 different locations in the white matter of the brain, or by demonstrating the occurrence of new typical white matter lesions on brain MRI over time.

- There are several partially effective FDA-approved first- (interferon-betas and glatiramer) and second- (natalizumab) generation immunotherapies proven to decrease MS exacerbating activity, progression, and MRI activity.

- MS immunotherapies should be initiated upon diagnosis to decrease further brain damage.

- First-generation immunotherapies are FDA-approved and are recommended for those experiencing a first episode of demyelination with an abnormal brain MRI, which increases the risk that they will go on to develop MS.

- Recovery from MS relapses can be hastened by treatment with pulse corticosteroids.

- Quality of life in MS can be enhanced by comprehensive treatment of common symptoms including fatigue, depression, spasticity, neurogenic bladder and bowel, neuropathic pain, and tremor.

Epidemiology

MS is twice as common in women as in men. This sex difference could reflect as yet undefined hormonal or neuroendocrine-immunologic factors. MS typically begins in young adulthood, between the ages of 20 and 40 years, and uncommonly begins before menarche or after menopause. There is a higher incidence of MS further north of the equator, where there is less exposure to sunlight and people have lower relative vitamin D levels. The Boston Nurses Health Study suggests that women who take supplements containing 400 MIU of vitamin D daily have a 40% lower risk of developing MS.

Clinical Features or Presentation (1,2)

Most patients with MS start out with a first attack of inflammatory demyelination, which raises the possibility of this condition. This first attack is called a clinically isolated syndrome (CIS), if it involves a single white matter pathway. Classic examples include visual deficits from optic neuritis; paraparesis, bladder problems, and leg sensory symptoms from transverse myelitis (spinal cord); or diplopia from an internuclear ophthalmoplegia (medial longitudinal fasciculus). Other common initial symptoms and involvements include hemiparesis (corticospinal tract); sensory symptoms such as numbness and tingling (spinothalamic tract in spinal cord or subcortical white matter); double vision (sixth cranial nerve), ataxia and tremors (cerebellar pathways); vertigo (vestibular pathways); facial weakness (seventh cranial nerve); and facial numbness or trigeminal neuralgia (fifth cranial nerve). Initial attacks involving more than one of these pathways are termed acute disseminated encephalomyelitis (ADEM), which, classically, was considered fulminant and severe but, more recently, has come to include milder attacks of even 2 of these pathways. MS attacks are typically incomplete, patchy, stuttering in onset, and last at least 24 hours, but usually days to weeks. Recovery from the initial attack is typically complete, but any attack of demyelination can leave a fixed static deficit. For an attack of demyelination to be considered a separate relapse and not part of the initial stuttering bout of demyelination, it must be separated from the first event by at least a month. Typical MS during the first several years involves 1 clinical attack per year, and 5–10 new MRI lesions for each clinical attack. With the second clinical attack, also called a relapse, exacerbation, or bout, the course is described as relapsing-remitting, and 90% of MS begins in this manner. By about 10 years, on the average, approximately half of relapsing-remitting MS becomes secondary progressive, with baseline neurologic deficits that continually get worse at a variable rate. Attacks can still occur on top of this progression but are often more blunted and harder to recognize. Eventually, no discrete attacks are discernible, and the MS becomes purely progressive. At this stage, neurogenic bladder and bowel symptoms, sexual dysfunction, tremors, and cognitive dysfunction become more prominent. In women, sexual dysfunction typically involves decreased libido, decreased or unpleasant vaginal sensations, and decreased ability to achieve orgasm. The other 10% of patients with MS begin with insidious progression from the outset, typically with a spastic paraparesis, progressive sensory disturbance of the legs followed by arms, neurogenic bowel and bladder, sexual dysfunction, and optic atrophy. This is termed primary progressive MS.

Fatigue is a prominent feature of MS exacerbations, but it also can be relentless and disabling throughout the course of MS. Depression is common and typically occurs early in the disease as a young adult in the "prime of life" confronts a new diagnosis of a potentially disabling disease with an unpredictable course.

MS does not affect fertility or cause birth defects, and an MS diagnosis should have minimal impact on family planning decisions. If a woman is significantly disabled in a way that may affect her ability to care for children, or has significant fatigue that may make caring for a newborn difficult, then it is more critical than usual to have a supportive spouse and family. It is probably preferable not to conceive a child during an MS exacerbation, since the fatigue and disabilities may make the early pregnancy difficult. As with so many other putative autoimmune diseases, MS tends to be less active during pregnancy, especially in the third trimester. In the 6 months postpartum, there is approximately a 35% chance of an exacerbation, presumably as the putative protective effects of some pregnancy hormones are lost. One candidate for such a protective pregnancy hormone is estriol, which has shown some clinical and MRI benefits in preliminary clinical trials (3). Breast-feeding may continue the protective effects of pregnancy on MS, perhaps through elevation of the potentially immunosuppressive hormone prolactin. This is one more reason to encourage breast-feeding, provided that a supportive spouse or family can help prevent fatigue.

Several studies suggest that oral contraceptives may have a protective effect on MS disease activity (4). Some forms of estrogen may decrease MS clinical and MRI activity (3).

Menopause appears to have no positive or negative effect on MS disease course.

Diagnosis and Differential Diagnosis (5,6)

The classical clinical criteria for diagnosing MS require 2 attacks referable to 2 different white matter pathways separated in time and space, with objective evidence on neurologic exam for each episode. Evoked potential testing can be used to objectively "capture" lesions in optic nerve, vestibular, or somatosensory pathways from attacks that were not documented at the time they occurred, and CSF demonstrating oligoclonal IgG bands not seen in serum can be used to objectively document dissemination over time (Box 7-2) (5,6). More recently, the so-called McDonald criteria (6) have standardized the use of MRI lesion count and characteristics to support an MS diagnosis when 1 of the 2 clinical attacks is not objectively documented, or they can be used to make an MS diagnosis if a second MRI a month or more after a baseline MRI shows definite evidence of a new lesion, even in the absence of a new clinical event. In this way, MS can be diagnosed earlier than by waiting for a second clinical attack to occur, which is important in the era of aggressively initiating immunotherapy as soon as MS is diagnosed to decrease further brain damage.

Box 7-2   MS Diagnostic Criteria

Clinically definite MS—2 attacks, 2 time points, objective evidence of each attack on neurologic exam or evoked potential testing or MRI scans, or CSF showing oligoclonal IgG bands not present in serum

McDonald criteria definite MS—at least 1 typical clinical attack with objective evidence on neurologic exam, and new lesions occurring on MRI brain done at least 1 mo apart

Probable MS (this category is NOT recognized by the McDonald criteria)—2 clinical attacks, 1 of which cannot be confirmed by any objective evidence for clinically definite MS, or 1 attack (CIS) with abnormal MRI of the brain consistent with demyelination or CSF showing oligoclonal IgG bands

Possible MS—single or multiple attacks but without objective evidence meeting criteria for probable or definite MS, typically with normal or minimally abnormal MRI brain and CSF studies

No other diagnosis fits better (see Box 7-3)

Box 7-3   Differential Diagnosis of MS

- Clinically isolated demyelinating syndrome or acute disseminated encephalomyelitis
- Multiple strokes
- Multiple brain metastases
- Central nervous system lymphoma
- Systemic lupus erythematosus
- Anticardiolipin antibody syndrome
- Sjogren's syndrome
- Vasculitis/connective tissue disease
- Vitamin B12 deficiency
- Neurosyphilis
- Lyme disease
- HIV or HTLV-I infection
- Whipple disease
- Thyroid disease
- Cervical spondylosis or disc disease (for primary progressive MS)
- Complicated migraine

Any diagnosis of MS requires that no better diagnosis fits and requires selectively ruling out a series of other mimics, some of which are other autoimmune diseases that can affect the central nervous system (Box 7-3).

Prevention and Clinical Care (1,7)

A National Multiple Sclerosis Society consensus statement advocates for the initiation of treatment with first-generation immunotherapy as soon as a definite diagnosis of MS is made, and an active course (clinically or on MRI scanning) is established. The recommendations do not differentiate between the first-generation injectable interferon-beta or glatiramer therapies, allowing physician and patient preference regarding route (IM or SQ) and frequency (weekly, three times a week, every other day, or daily) of administration, and side effect issues and concerns (flu-like side effects, depression, menstrual irregularity, and need for checking liver functions and white cell count for interferon-beta, and more injection site reactions for glatiramer) to be factored into decision-making (Box 7-4). These treatments are all partial, decrease clinical and MRI activity by approximately one-third, and there is some evidence that interferon-beta-1a IM weekly is slightly less effective than higher-dose, higher-frequency interferon-beta-1a SQ 3 times a week or interferon-beta-1b SQ every other day. Recent studies suggest similar efficacy for both SQ interferon-beta products and glatiramer. For failures of these first-generation therapies, either because of continued clinical or MRI activity, or intolerance of side effects, there are 2 current FDA-approved second-generation options. One is infusions of natalizumab, which appears to be more effective than first-generation therapies but has a known, but not well-defined, risk of 1 in 1000 cases of fatal brain infections or progressive multifocal leukoencephalopathy. The other is switching to 2-year "rescue" therapy with mitoxantrone, administered every 3 months, with a poorly defined but definite risk of cardiotoxicity, that limits lifetime dose to 3 years maximum, and also a poorly defined risk of blood dyscrasias, including leukemia. If these approaches are not successful, then a variety of off-label treatments can be attempted, either by themselves or in combination (except in the case of natalizumab, where combination therapy is expressly discouraged) (see Box 7-4). For exacerbations or subacute progressions that occur despite maintenance or rescue immunotherapy, pulses of oral or IV corticosteroids can be used. In some patients, monthly pulses of IV corticosteroids are used as an off-label maintenance therapy for up to 3 years and also can be used in the transition among first- and second-generation therapies.

Box 7-4 Immunotherapies for MS

Acute exacerbations—pulse oral or intravenous corticosteroids

First-generation maintenance immunotherapy:
    Less aggressive—interferon-beta-1a (Avonex) IM weekly
    More aggressive—interferon-beta-1a (Rebif) SQ thrice weekly, interferon-beta-1b
       (Betaseron) SQ every other day, glatiramer (Copaxone) SQ daily

Second-generation immunotherapy for first-generation failures:
    Rescue—every 3 monthly IV mitoxantrone (Novantrone) for 2–3 y
    Maintenance—natalizumab (Tysabri) IV every 4 wk

Box 7-5   Symptomatic Treatments for Common MS Symptoms

1. Fatigue—amantadine, modafanil, methylphenidate, fluoxetine
2. Depression—any of the SSRI or SNRI or tricyclic antidepressants
3. Spasticity—baclofen, tizanidine, benzodiazepines
4. Neurogenic bladder—oxybutinin, tolteridine, trospium, solifenacin, tamsulosin
5. Constipation—bowel regimen, fiber/liquid, bulking agents, suppositories, enemas
6. Tremor—benzodiazepines, amantadine, beta-blockers, a variety of anticonvulsants
7. Neuropathic pain—tricyclic antidepressants, carbamazepine, tizanidine, baclofen, gabapentin, pregabalin, topical lidocaine, capsaicin

None of the MS immunotherapies is recommended during pregnancy. Interferon-betas are category C and glatiramer is category B, though none of these are known to be teratogenic or to reduce fertility. Interferon-betas can increase the chances of a miscarriage, even if stopped as soon as a pregnancy is confirmed. The general recommendation is to discontinue interferon-betas or glatiramer 1 or 2 menstrual cycles before trying to conceive. Mitoxantrone is contraindicated in pregnancy. Natalizumab is category C.

Beyond appropriate attention to initiating immunotherapies to decrease further MS clinical activity and disability, attention to comprehensively treating all of the various episodic or persistent symptoms of MS can markedly improve quality of life (Box 7-5). For major or disabling episodes, inpatient rehabilitative care can be critical.

References

1. **Nosew orthy JH, Lucchinetti C, Rodriguez M, et al.** Multiple sclerosis. N Engl J Med. 2000;343:938–52.
2. **Mattson DH.** Multiple sclerosis. In Neurologic Disorders and Pregnancy. Continuum. 2000;6:64–78.
3. **Sicotte NL, Liva SM, Klutch R, et al.** Treatment of multiple sclerosis with the pregnancy hormone estriol. Ann Neurol. 2002;52:421–8.
4. **Alonso A, Jick SS, Olek M, et al.** Recent use of oral contraceptives and the risk of multiple sclerosis. Arch Neurol. 2005;62:1362–5.
5. **Mattson DH.** Update on the diagnosis of multiple sclerosis. Expert Rev Neurotherapeutics. 2002;2:319–28.
6. **McDonald WI, Compston A, Edan G, et al.** Recommended diagnostic criteria for multiple sclerosis:Guidelines from the international panel on the diagnosis of multiple sclerosis. Ann Neurol. 2001;50:121–7.
7. **Goodin DS, Frohman EM, Garmany GP, et al.** Disease modifying therapies in multiple sclerosis. Report of the Therapeutics and Technology Assessment subcommittee of the American Academy of Neurology and the MS Council for Clinical Practice Guidelines. Neurology. 2002; 58:169–78.

C. Headache

Charles C. Flippen II

KEY POINTS

♦ Women suffer from a disproportionate burden of headache.
♦ Accurate diagnosis is essential to treatment success.
♦ Secondary headache must be considered with first presentation of headache.
♦ Abortive medications should be prescribed with each attack and with weekly limits of use.
♦ Consider early use of preventive medications when indicated.

Epidemiology

Headache is one of the most common presenting complaints to primary care physicians. It accounts for 1–2% of emergency department visits and 4% of physician office visits (1,2).

In American Migraine Study I, Lipton, *et al.* (3) found that 47% of migraine sufferers who had consulted physicians about their headaches sought help first from family physicians. Only 12% of sufferers consulted neurologists initially, and ongoing care was provided most frequently by family physicians (3). Women suffer from a disproportionate share of the burden of primary headache disorders. Migraine headache affects 12% of Americans, approximately 18% of women and 7% of men, translating into approximately 21 million women with significant physical and social/economic burdens from this cause. Reasons for this gender disparity lie in the effect of female sex hormones on migraine headache, with 60% of women sufferers noting a relationship between migraine and menstruation (4).

Clinical Features

A useful headache history includes a full description, including manner of onset, location, associated symptoms, duration, and frequency of occurrence. Additional information includes family history of headache, relieving/exacerbating factors, and response to prior treatment attempts. The history should be followed by thorough general physical and neurologic examinations. All components of the neurologic system should be assessed, including a funduscopic examination. Initial evaluation for headache warrants particular attention to the presence of "red flags" (Box 7-6). The presence of these historical and physical signs indicates the likely existence of secondary headache and the

---

Box 7-6   Headache "Red Flags"

- Abnormal vital signs
- Altered consciousness/cognition
- Meningeal irritation
- Visual field defect
- New onset
- Change in headache duration and/or character

---

subsequent need for diagnostic testing to determine headache etiology. Most primary headaches are gradual in onset. A particularly worrisome presentation for headache is the sudden onset of head pain described as a "thunderclap." The presence of a headache with rapid onset and accompanied by focal neurological symptoms suggests a diagnosis of subarachnoid hemorrhage and should be pursued until disproved. In the absence of these indicators, a primary headache disorder is a much more likely diagnosis.

Tension-Type Headache

The tension headache is the most common type of primary headache disorder, and its clinical features are described in Box 7-7 (5). In general patients usually do not seek medical attention for this type of headache, which commonly responds to over-the-counter medications. Chronic tension-type headache (more than 15 days of headache, as defined by the International Classification of Headache Disorders, Second Edition, ICHD-2) may prompt consultation, but many of these patients, if followed over time, may actually suffer from migraine.

Migraine

Migraine comes in many varieties; the most common is migraine without aura (MOA), followed by migraine with aura (MA). The diagnostic

---

Box 7-7   ICHD-II Diagnostic Criteria for Tension Type Headache

- Headache lasting from 30 min to 7 d
- At least 2 of the following:
    - pressing/tightening quality
    - mild or moderate intensity
    - bilateral location
    - no aggravation with movement
- Both of the following:
    - no nausea or vomiting
    - no photo- or phonophobia
- At least 10 prior similar episodes

Box 7-8 ICHD-2 Diagnostic Criteria for Migraine Headache without Aura

- Headache lasting 4–72 h
- Two of the following:
  - unilateral location
  - pulsating quality
  - moderate or severe intensity
  - aggravation by routine physical activity
- At least 1 of the following:
  - nausea and/or vomiting
  - photophobia and phonophobia
  - At least 5 prior similar episodes

Box 7-9 ICHD-2 Diagnostic Criteria for Migraine Headache with Aura

- Aura consisting of at least 1 of the following without motor weakness:
  - fully reversible visual symptoms including positive features
  - fully reversible sensory symptoms including positive features and/or negative features
  - fully reversible dysphasic speech
- At least 2 of the following:
  - homonymous visual symptom and/or unilateral sensory symptom
  - 1 symptom that progresses gradually over ≥ 5 min and/or different aura symptoms occur in succession over ≥ 5 min
  - each symptom lasts ≥5 min and ≤60 min
- Headache fulfilling migraine without aura criteria begins during the aura or follows aura within 60 min

---

criteria for each of these are found in Boxes 7-8 and 7-9. Migraine has a variable presentation, but its main distinguishing features are its relatively long episodic duration and associated disabling features. Recurrent headaches lasting hours to days in duration that are accompanied by behavior-altering symptoms are likely migraine. Behavior-altering implies that the symptom causes the patient to actively avoid circumstances that worsen the discomfort (covering eyes, retreating to a quiet room) or impairs a person's normal functioning.

Menstrual Migraine and Menstrually Related Migraine

Women, as previously stated, exhibit a strong relationship between their sex hormones and headaches. A variety of migraines specific to women are menstrual migraine and menstrually-related migraine. The diagnostic criteria for each migraine variant are listed in Box 7-10. The prevalence of menstrually-related migraine is approximately 60%, and the prevalence of pure menstrual migraine ranges from 3.5% to 21.3% of women migraine sufferers (4). The clinical characteristics of menstrual

---

Box 7-10   Diagnostic Criteria for Menstrual and Menstrually Related Migraine

ICHD-2 Diagnostic Criteria for Menstrual Migraine without Aura
- Attacks in a menstruating woman meeting criteria for MOA
- Attacks occur exclusively on day 1 (+2) of menstruation in at least 2 of 3 cycles
  - Day 1 = first day of menstruation
  - Menstruation = endometrial bleeding
ICHD-2 Diagnostic Criteria for Menstrually Related Migraine
- Attacks in a menstruating woman meeting criteria for MOA
- Attacks occur exclusively on day 1 (+2) of menstruation in at least 2 of 3 cycles and at other times of the cycle

---

migraine may differ from non-menstrually-related migraine in that the former are more severe in intensity, of longer duration, more likely to be accompanied by significant nausea and vomiting, are less responsive to treatment, and are associated with greater disability (6).

Chronic Daily Headache

Chronic daily headache is a general term for a number of headache types sharing the feature of frequent occurrence (Box 7-11). The prevalence is about ~4% of the adult and elderly population, and these headaches are twice as common in women as in men. They may account for 75% of tertiary headache patients and are associated with habitual snoring/sleep problems, obesity, and stressful life events. Episodic headache disorders may become daily events as a result of analgesic medication overuse (MO). It appears that frequency of use, as opposed to dose of medication, is the key factor in developing daily headache (7). Medication overuse headache (MOH) has been defined by the ICHD-II according to class of medication and duration of use (Box 7-12). MOH is thought to be highly prevalent, with studies estimating daily analgesic use for headache ranging from 1% to 3% of the population.

Chronic migraine is thought to represent an evolution from episodic migraine due to increased severity and frequency. A similar evolution is

---

Box 7-11   Chronic Daily Headaches

- Chronic migraine
- Chronic cluster headache
- Chronic tension-type headache
- Hemicrania continua
- Chronic paroxysmal hemicrania
- Chronic post-traumatic headache
- New daily persistent headache

> **Box 7-12**   ICHD-II Medication Overuse Headache Diagnostic Criteria
> _____
> 1. >15 d of HA/month
>   • Headache has developed or worsened during MO
> 2. Ergotamine, triptan, combination analgesic, and opioid use >10 d/mo; simple analgesic use >15 d/mo
>   • Minimum of 3 mo misuse

felt to be responsible for chronic tension-type headache. Chronic cluster headache, chronic paroxysmal hemicrania, and hemicrania continua, are rare headache disorders and beyond the scope of this chapter. New-onset persistent daily headache differs from chronic tension-type headache in that from the onset or within 3 days of onset, the headache is daily and unremitting. A diagnosis of any primary daily headache disorder must exclude the presence of abortive MO.

Prevention and Clinical Care

General principles of treatment for primary headache disorders include the appropriate choice of abortive medication and assessment of the need for preventive medication. All patients who have a primary headache disorder need an abortive medication. The choice of abortive medication should be directed by the type of headache disorder, comorbid conditions/risk factors, and social demands (e.g., workplace safety issues, child care, etc.), matched with individual medication characteristics (potential side effects, efficacy data, interaction potential with existing medication(s) taken by the patient).

It is considered best to choose the most likely effective medication initially and dose at an effective level as opposed to a "stepped care" approach. Abortive medications should be prescribed with limits both on doses taken in 1 day and number of days of use per week. This practice helps to mitigate the chance of patients falling into MO and subsequent chronic daily headache.

Preventive medications are prescribed to decrease the frequency and severity of headache attacks. The decision to start preventive treatment usually takes into account the patient's headache frequency (>2 severe headaches/month) and/or the degree of functional disability in relation to the responsibilities that must be met by the patient (childcare, work, social). Successful preventive therapy includes several key components, such as the initiation of treatment with the lowest effective dose, titrating to best clinical effect, patient education of the intended goal of treatment, appropriate length of treatment (6–8 weeks at least), and written records of treatment effect (headache diary). The choice of medication should be made considering comorbid conditions that could benefit from the right medication.

Tension-Type Headache

The choices available for abortive treatment of tension-type headaches are principally from the classes of simple analgesics or non-steroidal anti-inflammatory drugs (NSAIDs), basically over-the-counter therapies. In general, there is no clear difference in efficacy among these drugs; response cannot be predicted for a given patient.

Tricyclic antidepressants are the most commonly used preventive medications for tension-type headaches. Serotonin selective reuptake inhibitors (SSRIs) also are used for tension-type headache prevention.

Non-pharmacological therapies for tension-type headaches include biofeedback, relaxation therapy, and cognitive behavioral therapy. Unproven methods of prevention include physical therapy, massage, and heat or cold application.

Migraine

Abortive treatment of migraine headache includes drugs from the classes of simple analgesics, NSAIDs, combination analgesics, dihydro-ergotamine, and serotonin agonists. To date, the data necessary for a singular, hierarchical ranking of medications does not exist. These medications have been critically evaluated by the U.S. Headache Consortium, a group of representatives from primary care, neurology, and headache specialty and subspecialty organizations, on their effectiveness for migraine abortive therapy (Table 7-4) (8).

Preventive treatment includes avoidance of trigger factors, substances and/or circumstances that induce a migraine attack, and other nonpharmacological techniques and medications.

Migraine preventive medications include drugs from several classes, such as beta- adrenergic blockers, tricyclic antidepressants, and others. Again, preventive medications should be chosen based on efficacy, comorbid conditions, and potential side effects. The U.S. Headache Consortium also evaluated these medications based on available evidence to rank them for efficacy. These rankings are a useful guide as a starting point for a given patient but do not guarantee treatment success. Nonpharmacological treatments that have a favorable recommendation by the Consortium include thermal or electromyographic biofeedback, cognitive behavioral therapy, and relaxation therapy.

Chronic Daily Headache

Management of chronic daily headache starts with identification of the presence of MO. Preventive medication use will not be effective if abortive MO exists. If the patient has MO, then the first step is withdrawal of the offending medication. This is the most difficult step in treatment. Patients must understand that taking any abortive medication on a daily or near daily basis will continue the cycle of daily head pain. Depending on the offending medication, some may be quickly stopped or tapered (simple analgesics, NSAIDs, ergots, triptans), while others require longer

Table 7-4 Evidence Based Ranking of Abortive Migraine Medications

Group 1: Proven pronounced statistical and clinical benefit, on the basis of at least 2 double-blind, placebo-controlled studies plus clinical impression of effect	Group 2: Moderate statistical and clinical benefit, on the basis of 1 double-blind, placebo-controlled study plus clinical impression of effect	Group 3: Statistically effective but not proven clinically effective OR clinically effective but not proven statistically effective, on the basis of conflicting or inconsistent evidence
Acetaminophen plus aspirin plus caffeine, orally	Acetaminophen plus codeine, orally	Butalbital plus aspirin plus caffeine, orally
Aspirin, orally	Butalbital plus aspirin plus caffeine plus codeine, orally	Ergotamine, orally
Butorphanol, IN	Butorphanol, IM	Ergotamine plus caffeine, orally
Dihydroergotamine, SC, IM, IV	Chlorpromazine, IM, IV	Metoclopramide, IM, rectally
Dihydroergotamine, IV plus antiemetic	Diclofenac-K, orally	**Group 4: Proven to be statistically or clinically ineffective, on the basis of failed efficacy versus placebo**
Dihydroergotamine, IN	Ergotamine plus caffeine plus pentobarbital plus bellafoline, orally	Acetaminophen, orally
Ibuprofen, orally	Flurbiprofen, orally	Chlorpromazine, IM
Naproxen sodium, orally	Isometheptene compound, orally	Granisetron, IV
Naratriptan, orally	Ketorolac, IM	Lidocaine, IV
Prochlorperazine, IV	Lidocaine, IN	**Group 5: Clinical and statistical benefits unknown, on the basis of insufficient evidence available**
Rizatriptan, orally	Meperidine, IM, IV	Dexamethasone, IV
Sumatriptan, SC, IN, orally	Methadone, IM	Hydrocortisone, IV
Zolmitriptan, orally	Metoclopramide, IV	
	Naproxen, orally	
	Prochlorperazine, IM, rectally	

From Ramadan NM, Silberstein SD, Freitag FG, et al. US Headache Consortium. Evidence-based guidelines for migraine headache in the primary care settting: pharmacological management for perevention of migraine. Copyright © by American Academy of Neurology; with permission.

periods of tapering (opioids, barbiturate-containing medications, benzodiazepines), possibly over as long as 12 weeks, depending on the dose/duration of chronic overuse.

If MO has occurred over a long period of time (>1 year), with use of barbiturate-containing or opioid medications, or outpatient withdrawal has been unsuccessful, then a short inpatient stay may be more effective. During hospitalization, intravenous fluid support may be used in cases of frequent nausea/emesis with scheduled intravenous dihydroergotamine 1–2 mg every 8 hours for 2–3 days (9). Opioid withdrawal may be treated with clonidine 0.1–0.2 mg 3 times a day. Upon discharge, patients should keep a medication diary, and if headache recurs >3 days a month, preventive therapy should be started. Preventive medications that may not have worked previously may be effective in the non-overuse state and are worth revisiting.

References

1. **Leicht MJ.** Non-traumatic headache in the emergency department. Ann Emerg Med. 1980Aug;9:404–9.
2. **Frishberg BM.** The utility of neuroimaging in the evaluation of headache in patients with normal neurologic examinations. Neurology. 1994Jul;44:1191–7.
3. **Lipton RB, Stewart WF, Simon D.** Medical consultation for migraine: Results from the American Migraine Study. Headache. 1998;38:87–96.
4. **Granella F, Sances G, Zanferrari C, et al.** Migraine without aura and reproductive life events: a clinical epidemiological study in 1300 women. Headache. 1993;33:385–9.
5. Headache Classification Subcommittee of the International Headache Society, The International Classification of Headache Disorders, 2nd edition. Cephalalgia, 24:Suppl 1, 2004.
6. **Granella F, Sances G, Allais G, et al.** Characteristics of menstrual and nonmenstrual attacks in women with menstrually related migraine referred to headache centres. Cephalalgia. 2004;24:707–16.
7. **Mathew NT, Kurman R, Perez F.** Drug induced refractory headache—clinical features and management. Headache. 1990;30:634–8.
8. **Matchar DB, Young WB, Rosenberg JH, et al.** Evidence-Based Guidelines for Migraine Headache in the Primary Care Setting: Pharmacological Management of Acute Attacks. 2000.American Academy of Neurology Website, www.aan.org.
9. **Raskin NH.** Repetitive intravenous dihydroergotamine for intractable migraine. Neurology. 1986;36:995–7.
10. **Morey SS.** Guidelines on Migraine: Part 2. General principles of drug therapy. American Family Physician. 2000;62:1915–7.
11. **Morey SS.** Guidelines on Migraine: Part 4. General principles of preventive therapy. American Family Physician. 2000;62:2359–63.

D. Screening for Dementia

Melissa M. Stiles

KEY POINTS

- Dementia is a clinical diagnosis.
- Alzheimer's dementia is the most common form of dementia.
- It is important to distinguish dementia from other conditions which can cause cognitive changes.
- The Mini-Mental Status Examination is the most studied screening test.
- There are limitations in the current screening tests for dementia.

Epidemiology of Disease

The prevalence of dementia in the U.S. varies with age. For patients between 60 and 69 years of age, the prevalence is 1%. The prevalence doubles every 5 years peaking at 39% for patients between 90 and 95 years old. Increasing age is the strongest risk factor for development of dementia. Other risk factors are hypertension, stroke, and a positive test for the Apoprotein E genotype. Protective factors include moderate alcohol intake, higher levels of education, and physical activity (1–3). Since definitive diagnosis of some of the dementias can only be made by pathological examination of brain tissue, the probable diagnosis is made by clinical history, examination, selected laboratory tests and, in some cases, radiological imaging. The Diagnostic and Statistical Manual of Mental Disorders, Fourth Edition (DSM IV) (4), bases its definition of dementia on the following criteria:

- Memory impairment
- Impairment in another area of cognitive function, such as agnosia, apraxia, aphasia, or executive functioning
- Impairment severe enough to cause decline in social and/or occupational functioning

The 4 major types of dementia are Alzheimer's dementia (50–80%), vascular dementia (10–20%), frontotemporal dementia (12–25%), and Lewy body dementia (5–10%). Mixed dementias account for 10–30% of the total. The clinical history can aid in differentiating the types of dementia. The hallmarks of Alzheimer's disease are inability to develop new memory and early loss of visual-spatial skills. Vascular dementia is characterized by a stepwise decline in cognition and function. Frontotemporal dementias are differentiated by early behavioral disturbances, disinhibition, and changes in personality. Lewy body dementia is characterized by fluctuating cognitive impairment with 1 or more of the following: visual and/or auditory hallucinations, spontaneous extrapyramidal features or marked sensitivity to neuroleptics, repeated unexplained falls, and/or transient clouding or loss of consciousness. Dementia should be distinguished from normal cognitive changes of aging, mild cognitive impairment, delirium, and depression. Normal changes of aging include slower information processing and acquisition speeds. However, the ability to learn new information is not impaired. Mild cognitive impairment is defined as cognitive changes not associated with aging, which do not impact social or occupational functioning. Delirium is characterized by an acute onset of cognitive dysfunction with a fluctuating course. Depression and dementia often coexist, but generally depression is manifested by shorter duration of onset, difficulty with concentration, and impairment of both short and long-term memory (1–3).

Screening

The US Preventive Services Task Force (USPSTF) does not recommend for or against routine screening of dementia (5). There are dozens of screening tests for dementia, but few are well studied in primary care settings. The most commonly used and studied test is the Mini-Mental Status Examination (MMSE). The MMSE tests a number of areas, including orientation, registration, attention, calculation, and visual-spatial skills (6). The sensitivities range from 71% to 92%, and the specificities range from 56% to 96%, depending on the cut-point used in the particular study. The MMSE is best at identifying patients with at least moderate dementia, but not as good at identifying patients with early dementia. The limitations of the MMSE include variable accuracy in patients of different ages, ethnicities, and educational levels (1–3,5). The Mini-Cog is another potential screening test, which had similar sensitivity (76% vs. 79%) and specificity (89% vs. 88%) to the MMSE in one retrospective study (8). The test involves a clock drawing test (CDT) and an uncued 3-item recall of 3 non-related items. The CDT is considered normal if all numbers are present in the correct sequence and position, and the hands readably display the requested time. In a review of studies testing the CDT, the mean sensitivity and specificity was 85%, but a significant weakness of the studies was that they were not performed in either primary care or community settings (9). Because of the limitations in screening instruments, clinicians should consider formal neuropsychological testing in patients whom they suspect of having dementia despite normal screening tests (1–3).

Summary

Dementia is extremely common among the elderly. Primary care providers should screen patients in the office setting and refer for neuropsychological testing if the diagnosis is unclear.

References

1. **Holsinger T, Deveau J, Boustani M, et al.** Does this patient have dementia? Journal of the American Medical Association. 2007;297:2391–402.
2. **Geldmacher D, Whitehouse P.** Evaluation of Dementia. The New England Journal of Medicine. 1996;335:331–6.
3. **Boustani M, Peterson B, Harris R, et al.** Screening for dementia. Systematic evidence review. Rockville (MD); Agency for Healthcare Research and Quality; 2003 Jun. (Systematic evidence review; no. 20).
4. American Psychiatric Association Diagnostic and Statistical Manual, 4th ed, APA Press, Washington DC, 1994.
5. **Boustani M, Peterson B, Hanson L, et al.** Screening for dementia in primary care: a summary of the evidence for the U.S. Preventive services task force. Ann Internal Med. 2003;138:927.
6. **Folstein MF, Folstein SE, McHugh PR.** "Mini-mental state." A practical method for grading the cognitive state of patients for the clinician. J Psychiatr Res. 1975;12:189–98.
7. **Brodaty H, Low L, et al.** What is the best dementia screening instrument for General Practioners to use? American Journal of General Psychiatry. 2006;14:391–400.
8. **Borson S, Scanlan JM, Chen P, et al.** The mini-cog as a screen for dementia; validation in a population-based sample. J Am Geriatr Soc. 2003;51:1451.
9. **Schulman K.** Clock-drawing: is it the ideal cognitive screening test? International Journal of Geriatric Psychiatry. 2000;15:548–61.

8

Substance Use and Abuse

A. Alcohol
   Sean O'Connor, MD

B. Substance Abuse
   Lee T. Dresang, MD; Linnea Williams, DO

C. Weight Loss and Over-the-Counter Diet Products
   Joanne E. Williams, MD, MPH

A. Alcohol

Sean O'Connor

KEY POINTS

♦ Younger women are becoming alcohol dependent at rates approaching those of men.
♦ The genetic influence on the risk for alcoholism is the same in men and women.
♦ Women have lower thresholds for alcohol complications.
♦ Women's livers are more vulnerable to the harmful effects of alcohol.
♦ Telescoping of physiological damage attributable to alcohol occurs in women.
♦ Alcohol consumption by pregnant women can result in the fetal alcohol syndrome.

Epidemiology

Thirty-five percent of women in the U.S. did not consume any alcohol in the last year. Most of those who did probably enjoyed some health benefits by drinking in moderation (1 drink a day; half an ounce of alcohol in any beverage).[1] However, about 1 in 3 women who drink at all will abuse alcohol at some point in their lives: putting drinking ahead of some other important value (e.g., family, friends, opportunity, education, health, responsibility, etc.). About half of those who abuse alcohol will progress to psychological dependence: the simultaneous preference for continued drinking in favor of 3 or more important life values. About 20% of those women who ever abuse alcohol will manifest symptoms of physiologic dependence (e.g., tolerance, loss of control, alcohol withdrawal syndrome followed by intense cravings for alcohol, and repeated relapses). The number of women in the U.S. who were dependent on alcohol (DSM-IV criteria) in the last year approximates 3 million, and another 3.7 million were abusing alcohol (1). Nearly half of women who remain physiologically dependent on alcohol will eventually die as a result of a medical manifestation of alcohol toxicity or the synergistic influence of alcohol on some other disease.

---

[1]But not an average of 1 drink a day achieved by drinking more on fewer occasions

Clinical Features or Presentation

Frequency

More than 6 million American women currently abuse or depend on alcohol, accounting for one-third of the total cases (2). American women are catching up to men: the Epidemiologic Catchment Area (ECA) Study, conducted in the early 1980s, found an overall male:female ratio of alcohol use disorders of 5.2:1 (3). The National Comorbidity Survey, conducted in the early 1990s, found an overall male:female ratio of 2.4:1, but in the early 21st century the ratio is only 1.9:1 (4) (Figure 8-1).

The progression of prevalence rates of alcohol dependence among women during the last 30 years is significant. No hypothesis based on disparities in sampling, study methodologies, or diagnostic instruments used have explained this increase. Decreasing stigma associated with women's drinking may account for some of these changes (5,6).

Genetic Influence on the Risk for Alcoholism

Early family and adoption studies concluded that the heritable influence on the future development of alcohol dependence differed in men and women, but early twin studies suggested comparable hereditability of the influence of alcoholism on morbidity and mortality (7). The former discrepancy is now beginning to disappear as the prevalence of alcoholism in women catches up to that of men; due to the increase in the fraction of women using alcohol to excess, sample sizes are now sufficient to detect the same ~50% influence of the interaction of many genes on the risk for alcoholism. This same trend is apparent in studies of genetic influence on the susceptibility to lung cancer attributable to smoking (8).

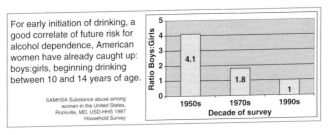

Figure 8-1   For early initiation of drinking, a good correlate of future risk for alcohol dependence, American women have already caught up: boys:girls beginning drinking between 10–14 y of age. (SAMHSA Substance abuse among women in the United States; Rockville, MD, USD-HHS 1997 Household Survey.)

Impact of Alcohol on Women

Alcohol is a toxin that is lethal to any living tissue at concentrations above 12.5% by volume. Thus, many studies have documented increased morbidity and mortality associated with elevated lifetime alcohol exposure in diseases of the digestive tract. These include cancers of the oropharynx, esophagus, stomach, pancreas, small and large intestines, and the rectum. The liver, however, is particularly susceptible to damage attributable to alcohol, and drinking is the most common cause of hepatitis. All of the alcohol absorbed anywhere in the digestive tract is conveyed to the liver before it is distributed to the body. Worse, the liver is the principal organ for metabolizing alcohol, and the first step is conversion of ethanol to acetaldehyde. The aldehyde is extremely toxic; its metabolism occurs solely in hepatocyte mitochondria and is usually completed there, rarely escaping the liver before oxidation to acetate. Transient elevation of hepatic transaminases, detected after a ten-fold dilution in venous blood, occurs after a single exposure to alcohol that raises the blood alcohol concentration above 0.3 g/L, indicating reversible inflammation. However, repeated exposures lead to fatty liver, also reversible with abstinence, but this eventually can result in irreversible scarring, hepatic failure, and esophageal varices associated with portal hypertension (9) (Figure 8-2).

The livers of women are the same size as those of men of the same body weight. On the other hand, as shown above, the volume of distribution of alcohol (total body water, TBW) is smaller in men than in women of the same body weight. Thus, if a man and a woman have achieved the same concentration of alcohol in their TBW, the alcohol elimination rate will be greater in women, who also have a greater rate of acetaldehyde production. Many studies also have demonstrated that the livers of women are more vulnerable to insults of many kinds, compared to men, possibly associated with a differential exposure to estrogen (Figure 8-3).

Telescoping appears to be true for the onset of many of the diseases that are directly attributable to excessive and prolonged consumption of alcohol. A recent neuroimaging study in Germany (12) found a significantly shorter interval between onset of heavy drinking and detection of significant brain atrophy in women compared to men.

Common Symptoms

Early: Early symptoms include: habitual use of alcohol to relieve stress, decreased tolerance for anxiety, frequent absence from work or neglect of social obligations in order to drink, craving for any substance, denial of the obvious relative importance of drinking in one's daily routine, drinking early in the workday, complaints of depression, irritability, fatigue, poor sleep, or persistent dysphoria.

Late: Memory loss, confusion, daily anxiety, irritability, shakiness, loss of social and sexual interest, malnutrition, numbness of extremities, gastrointestinal distress, blackouts.

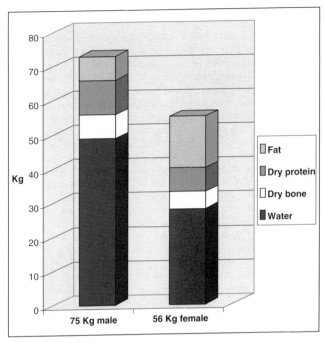

Figure 8-2   On average, women have higher blood alcohol levels than men after ingestion of the same amount of alcohol. Women are smaller than men and, pound-for-pound, there is a substantially lower total body water in women; usually ~51% of body weight in women and ~65% in men. Since alcohol is distributed in body water, the same dose will be diluted less in women, and reach all of the target organs, brain, liver, etc., at higher concentrations. (From Becker et al. Prediction of risk of liver disease by alcohol intake, sex and age: a prospective population study. Hepatology. 1996;23:1025–9. Reprinted from Wiley-Liss, Inc., a subsidiary of John Wiley & Sons, Inc.; with permission)

Common Signs

Early: Early signs include: elevated transaminase enzyme concentrations, macrocytic anemia, hypertension, and tachycardia.

Late: Jaundice, coma, seizures, auditory hallucinations, fatty liver, cirrhosis, congestive heart failure, pancreatitis, esophageal varices, uncontrolled diabetes, difficulty controlling the effective dose of medications metabolized by the liver, and failure of anti-depressants to alleviate depression.

The most common comorbidity of alcoholism is depression, and the odds ratio of this comorbidity is nearly twice as high in women as it is in men (13).

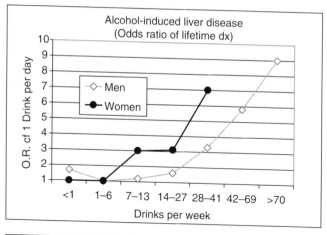

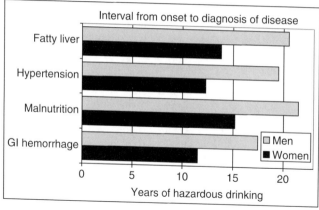

Figure 8-3   While the pathophysiology is not clear, the time interval between the onset of excessive alcohol consumption and other milestones of alcohol dependence such as the appearance of the first sign of physiologic harm attributable to alcohol is substantially shorter in women than in men; a phenomenon called "telescoping." (Top: From Becker et al, Prediction of risk of liver disease by alcohol intake, sex and age: a prospective population study. Hepatology. 1996;23:1025–9; with permission. Bottom: From Ashley MJ et al, Morbidity in alcoholics: evidence for accelerated development of physical disease in women. Arch. Int. Med. 1977; 137:883–7. Copyright (c) (1977), American Medical Association. All Rights reserved; with permission.)

Women and Fetal Alcohol Syndrome

Alcohol consumed by the mother crosses the placental barrier with ease. The developing head, including the brain, is sensitive to the adverse effects of alcohol exposure at all stages of pregnancy; damage to other organs occurs more often in the first 2 months of pregnancy. There is no confirmatory test for fetal alcohol syndrome (FAS), and the relevant history of alcohol exposure may be uncertain or denied. On the other hand, irreversible consequences include microencephaly, characteristic facial features including epicanthal folds, long smooth philtrum, short palpebral fissures, depressed nasal bridge, delayed speech, and learning disability. Growing evidence suggests that there is no lower limit to the potential for toxicity to the fetus attributable to alcohol exposure during pregnancy (14).

Prevention and Clinical Care

Prevention of alcohol dependence depends on recognizing increased risk based on a careful history and diagnosis of early signs and symptoms, followed by education of the patient. A biological familial history of alcohol dependence increases the risk for future problems tenfold, compared to the general population, but more than half of those from such families will not become dependent. Those at high risk who do not drink cannot become dependent. The increased risk conferred by genetic and familial influences is expressed early in life; the peak rate of onset of alcohol dependence occurs at age 19 and the rate declines to that of the general population by age 40. A brief educational intervention by a medical clinician is effective in reducing future risk if signs and symptoms of early disease are identified and tracked and continued attention to reduction in consumption of alcohol is provided.

Once psychological or physiological dependence is diagnosed, treatment by any one clinician is often not effective, and engagement of the patient *and the patient's family* in care provided by a team-based, professionally dedicated system is the best treatment decision. The knowledge of, and willingness to, use a growing number of FDA-approved medications that reduce craving is one hallmark of such systems. That care is as expensive as it is necessary to prevent progression of the illness, and clinical care of consequent or comorbid illness should be thoroughly coordinated with that system. On the other hand, combining treatment with free membership in Alcoholics Anonymous (AA) or other similar programs for adolescents and families enhances the chances of sustained recovery (15).

Helpful Links

www.niaaa.nih.gov: National Institute on Alcohol Abuse and Alcoholism

http://pubs.niaaa.nih.gov/publications/brochurewomen/Woman_ English.pdf

www.samhsa.gov: Substance Abuse and Mental Health Services
   Administration
Alcoholics Anonymous (AA) World Services www.aa.org
Al-Anon Family Group Headquarters www.al-anon.alateen.org

References

1. **Grant BF, Dawson DA, Stinson FS, et al.** The 12-month prevalence and trends in DSM-IV alcohol abuse and dependence: United States, 1991–1992 and 2001–2002. Drug Alcohol Depend. 2004;74:223–34.
2. **Cyr M.** Alcohol use disorders in women. Postgraduate Medicine. 2002;112:31–47.
3. **Regier D.** Comorbidity of Mental Disorders with Alcohol and Other Drug Abuse Results from the Epidemiologic Catchment Area Study. Journal of the American Medical Association. 1990;264:2511–8.
4. **Degenhardt L, Chiu WT, Sampson N, et al.** Epidemiological patterns of extra-medical drug use in the United States: evidence from the National Comorbidity Survey Replication, 2001–2003. Drug Alcohol Depend. 2007;90:210–23.
5. **Fuchs CS.** Alcohol consumption and mortality among women. New England Journal of Medicine. 1995;332:1245–50.
6. **Greenfield.** Women and alcohol use disorders. Harvard Review Psychiatry. 2001;10:76–86.
7. **Medlund P, Cederlöf R, Flodérus-Myrhed B, et al.** A new Swedish twin registry containing environmental and medical base line data from about 14,000 same-sexed pairs born 1926-58. Acta Med Scand Suppl. 1976;600:1–111.
8. **Wodarz N, Bobbe G, Eichhammer P, et al.** The candidate gene approach in alcoholism: are there gender-specific differences? Arch Womens Ment Health. 2003;6:225–30.
9. **Kwo PY, Ramchandani VA, O'Connor S, et al.** Gender differences in alcohol metabolism: relationship to liver volume and effect of adjusting for body mass. Gastroenterology. 1998;115:1552–7.
10. **Becker et al.** Prediction of risk of liver disease by alcohol intake, sex and age: a prospective population study. Hepatology. 1996;23:1025–9.
11. **Ashley MJ et al.** Morbidity in alcoholics: evidence for accelerated development of physical disease in women. Arch Int Med. 1977;137:883–7.
12. **Mann K, Ackermann K, Croissant B, et al.** Neuroimaging of gender differences in alcohol dependence: are women more vulnerable? Alcohol Clin Exp Res. 2005 May;29:896–901.
13. **Dixit AR, Crum RM.** Prospective study of depression and the risk of heavy alcohol use in women. Am J Psychiatry. 2000;157:751–8.
14. **Henderson J, Kesmodel U, Gray R.** Systematic review of the fetal effects of prenatal binge-drinking. J Epidemiol Community Health. 2007 Dec;61:1069–73.
15. **Dawson DA, Grant BF, Stinson FS, et al.** Estimating the effect of help-seeking on achieving recovery from alcohol dependence. Addiction. 2006;101:824–34.

B. Substance Abuse

Lee T. Dresang and Linnea Williams

KEY POINTS

♦ In general, women abuse drugs less often, start at a later age, become addicted more quickly, and suffer more medical complications than men.

♦ The social stigma of substance abuse in women leads to delayed diagnosis and treatment and a lack of research.

♦ There is a strong link between mental health problems and substance abuse in women.

♦ In the case of prescription drugs, teenage girls are more likely to abuse stimulants and sedatives, while adult women are more likely to abuse pain relievers and anxiolytics.

♦ Screening for substance abuse is recommended for all pregnant women.

Definition

Substance abuse is defined as "a maladaptive pattern of substance use leading to clinically significant impairment or distress" (1). This should be manifested by one (or more) of the following, within the preceding year: 1) failure to fulfill major role obligations at work, school, or home; 2) use in situations in which such agents are physically hazardous; 3) recurrent substance-related legal problems; or 4) continued use despite persistent or recurrent social or interpersonal problems caused or exacerbated by the effects of the substance (1).

Epidemiology

In the U.S. 3.1 million women regularly use illicit drugs, and 3.5 million women intentionally misuse prescription drugs (2). Approximately one-third of people abusing illicit drugs are women (2). This gender gap is closing (3). During pregnancy, 3% of women use illicit drugs, most commonly marijuana (4). Ten percent of women under the age of 35 years report marijuana use in the previous month (3). In some large urban centers, urine testing at the time of labor reveals substance use rates >20% (5). Substance abuse transcends racial and socioeconomic divisions.

Clinical Features or Presentation

The clinical presentation of female substance abusers is often challenging for the healthcare professional to decipher. A list of common signs and symptoms of drug abuse is found in Table 8-1. Biological differences have been implicated in the accelerated course to abuse and dependence that women often experience, with estrogen and decreased enzymatic activity in the gut as possible mechanisms documented in the literature (2). Women's drug use levels strongly correlate with those of their partner or husband (3). Female addicts are usually introduced to drugs by a man (3).

Diagnosis and Differential Diagnosis

Diagnosis of substance abuse is mainly based on history. Laboratory testing, imaging, and other testing may be indicated for screening or assessment of end-organ damage. A toxicology screen (urine or serum) can confirm the presence of a substance. Some substances, such as cocaine, leave the body within hours of usage, whereas others, such as marijuana, may be detectable for weeks. With cocaine abuse, a cardiac stress test, echocardiogram, or cardiac catheterization may demonstrate cocaine-related atherosclerosis or myocardial damage. Cocaine toxicity in women, as in men, is due primarily to vasospasm. Cocaine can result in myocardial infarction, cardiomyopathy, and sudden death (3).

Diagnosis of substance abuse in women is often not considered in the differential diagnosis, and, therefore, many women are missed simply because the physician has discounted the possibility. Mental health issues are in the differential diagnosis for, and often co-exist with, substance abuse. All mental health diagnoses are more frequent among women and men with substance abuse (3).

Female and male abusers tend to engage in more risky behaviors, increasing their chances of acquiring HIV, hepatitis B, and other sexually

Table 8-1   List of Common Signs/Symptoms of Substance Abuse in Women

Fatigue	Sleepiness	Change in appetite	Depression	Anxiety
Headaches	Body aches	Memory problems	Irritability	Needle marks
Skin lesions	Frequent ED visits	Frequent infections	Malnutrition	Family history of substance abuse
Personal history of sexual or physical abuse	Significant other who abuses substances	Other psychiatric disorders	Pathologic heart murmur	Jitteriness

From the National Institute of Drug Abuse (NIDA); with permission.

transmitted infections (STIs) (6). STIs should be considered in women with substance abuse and vice versa. Since substance abuse occurs across racial and economic lines, questions concerning it should be asked of all women and men.

Evidence-Based Screening Recommendations

The US Department of Health and Human Services (DHHS) Substance Abuse & Mental Health Services Administration (SAMHSA) recommends the evidence-based *Screening, Brief Intervention, Referral, and Treatment (SBIRT)* program (7).

Several substance abuse screening tools that have been validated and reported, including AUDIT, CAGE, T-ACE, TWEAK, National Institute on Alcohol Abuse and Alcoholism (NIAAA) questionnaire (6). AUDIT, CAGE and TWEAK are described on the CORK website (http://www.projectcork.org/) (8). Women with substance abuse disorders can be difficult to identify, primarily due to accompanying psychiatric illness and/or somatic disorders.

Prevention and Clinical Care

Treatment of substance abuse in women must be multifaceted to be successful in reversing the behavior. A review of 38 studies, 7 of which were randomized clinical trials (RCTs), found 6 key components that positively influenced outcomes for women substance abusers: child care, prenatal care, women-only programs, women-focused supplemental services and workshops, mental health services, and comprehensive programming (9). Improved outcomes included increased completion of treatment, better birth outcomes, better employment and health status, fewer mental health symptoms, decreased substance use, and reduced risk of HIV (9). Evaluation of treatment programs for pregnant women found a substantial savings, attributed to decreased complications in the neonate and reduced need for neonatal intensive care services (10). A Cochrane review of 6 studies and 709 women found that home visits for pregnant or postpartum substance abusers did not decrease continued illicit drug use, alcohol use, or failure to enroll in a drug treatment program, and did not increase breast-feeding at 6 months, vaccination rates at 6 months, or non-accidental injury and non-voluntary foster care (4). A Cochrane review of 5 studies and 346 women found that contingency management, that is, providing positive incentives such as money or employment, was effective in maintaining women in treatment programs but was ineffective in decreasing their drug usage (10). Review of 4 studies and 266 women found that motivational interviewing did not improve enrollment in treatment programs or neonatal outcomes (10).

Women receive 10–25% less outpatient and total lifetime care for substance abuse than men; the reasons for this are unclear and likely multifactorial (11). Though male substance abusers may be parents, treatment of substance abuse in women is more likely to be impacted by lack of child care or support services for the family (9).

Because heroin cessation rates are low and criminal activity is fairly high with heroin dependence, outpatient treatment with long-acting opioids can help men and women with opioid dependence to function in society (2). A Cochrane review of 13 RCTs found that methadone and buprenorphine are more effective than placebo in heroin suppression, but that buprenorphine is not more effective than methadone (12).

Websites with helpful resources in treating substance abuse in women include: the National Institute on Drug Abuse (13), Project CORK (8), Screening, Brief Intervention, Referral, and Treatment (7), and Substance Abuse & Mental Health Services Administration (14).

Special Populations

Substance Abuse in Young Women

In young girls, marijuana use is often preceded by alcohol or tobacco use, and marijuana is often a "gateway" drug leading to experimentation with other illicit drugs (2). Teen girls are more likely to abuse prescription medications, choosing stimulants and sedatives over pain relievers (15).

Substance Abuse in Pregnancy

Pregnant substance abusers require special consideration, particularly because of the impact that their drug use may have on the developing fetus. Preterm delivery, low birth-weight infants, placental abruption, neonatal abstinence syndrome (NAS), and Neonatal Intensive Care Unit (NICU) admission are all associated with illicit drug use in pregnancy (10). Table 8-2 provides a summary of maternal and fetal effects of classes of illicit drugs in pregnancy. It can be difficult to isolate the effect of a single drug on pregnancy from the effects of other drugs being abused, as well as from psychosocial factors (5).

Cocaine use during pregnancy is associated with placenta previa, placental abruption (6–8%), intrauterine growth restriction (25–30%), premature rupture of membranes (20%), and preterm delivery (25%) (2,5). Studies are conflicting regarding the long-term effects of *in utero* cocaine exposure (2). Marijuana use in pregnancy is associated with preterm delivery, placental abruption, congenital anomalies, low birth-weight, newborn neurologic abnormalities, and attention deficit hyperactivity disorder (ADHD) later in childhood (2). Opioid use in pregnancy is associated with ante-partum hemorrhage, preterm delivery, low birth-weight, and perinatal mortality (2). Rates of stillbirth, fetal growth retardation, prematurity, and neonatal mortality are 3–7 times higher among heroin addicts than in the general population (5). In one study, women enrolled in a methadone program had outcomes similar to those of non-opioid abusers (5). Newborns of women abusing opioids in pregnancy often need to be slowly weaned from methadone in order to avoid the withdrawal syndrome that can include tremor, high-pitched cry, increased muscle tone, poor feeding, yawning, seizures, emesis, fever, and death (2,5).

Table 8-2   Maternal and Fetal Effects of Illicit Drugs in Pregnancy

Drug	Maternal Obstetric Effects	Fetal Effects
Cannabinoids (hashish, marijuana)	Preterm delivery Placental abruption	Congenital anomalies Low birth weight Increase in perinatal mortality Newborn neurologic abnormalities ADHD in later childhood
Depressants (barbiturates, benzodiazepines)	No significant obstetrical effects	No anomalies Depression of interactive behavior Withdrawal symptoms possible.
Dissociative anesthetics (ketamine, PCP and analogs)	Possible increase in miscarriage rate	Dysmorphic face Increase in behavioral problems
Hallucinogens (LSD, mescaline, Psilocybin)	Possible increase in miscarriage rate	Dysmorphic facies Increase in behavioral problems Chromosomal breakage (LSD)
Opioids and morphine derivatives (codeine, fentanyl, heroin, methadone, morphine, opium, oxycodone, hydrocodone)	Ante-partum hemorrhage Preterm delivery Increase in meconium stained amniotic fluid	Low birth weight Increased perinatal mortality Opioid dependence, requiring weaning after birth Increased rates of still birth (heroin) Fetal growth retardation (heroin)
Stimulants (amphetamine, cocaine, methylphenidate, nicotine)	Placental abruption Placenta previa Preterm delivery Preterm, premature rupture of membranes Increase in meconium stained amniotic fluid (cocaine) Increased miscarriage rates (cocaine) Adverse pregnancy outcomes (nicotine)	Low birth weight Increase in perinatal mortality Cerebral infarction (cocaine) Increase risk of SIDS (cocaine) Congenital anomalies Depression of interactive behavior Neonatal necrotizing enterocolitis Fetal growth retardation (cocaine)
Inhalants	Preterm labor	Fetal growth retardation Impaired heme synthesis Increased risk of leukemia in childhood

Adapted from the National Institute of Drug Abuse (NIDA) (Ref. 2,5,12); with permission.

The subject of substance use often is not discussed during prenatal visits. Consequently, physicians fail to uncover this obstetrical risk, increasing the likelihood of complications and reducing the chance of successful intervention (3). Urine toxicology can be helpful in certain circumstances, including monitoring of women with a history of illicit drug use, but universal screening is not recommended (5). Antenatal testing has not been shown to improve outcomes in substance-abusing women with normal fetal growth (5).

Substance Abuse in Older Women

Although substance abuse has been increasing in women over 65 years of age in the U.S. (3), stigma and shame keeps these women from disclosing their drug use and seeking treatment. Unintentional misuse of pain relievers and anxiolytics can progress to addiction in elderly women (15).

Conclusions

Substance abuse in women will continue to be a public health issue for many years to come. Primary care physicians are frequently the only health care professionals from whom such women seek care throughout their lives. Physicians and other healthcare professionals must be diligent about identification and treatment of substance use disorders in women, recognize the unique characteristics of female abusers, and offer them the resources necessary for successful intervention. All women should be screened for substance abuse, no matter their age, socioeconomic, or reproductive status.

References

1. Diagnostic and Statistical Manual of Mental Disorders, Fourth Edition, Text Revision. Washington, DC, American Psychiatric Association, 2000.
2. **Greenfield S, Manwani S, Nargiso J.** Epidemiology of substance use disorders in women. Obstet Gynecol Clin North Am. 2003;30:413–46.
3. **Stein M, Cyr M.** Women and substance abuse. Med Clin North Am.1997;81:979–98.
4. **Doggett C, Burrett S, Osborn D.** Home visits during pregnancy and after birth for women with an alcohol or drug problem. Cochrane Database Syst Rev. 2005;19:CD004456.
5. Substance abuse in pregnancy. ACOG Technical Bulletin Number 195—July 1994 (replaces No. 96, September 1986). Int J Gynaecol Obstet. 1994;47:73–81.
6. ACOG Committee on Ethics. ACOG Committee Opinion. Number 294, May 2004. At-risk drinking and illicit drug use: ethical issues in obstetric and gynecologic practice. Obstet Gynecol. 2004;103:1021–31.
7. US Department of Health and Human Services. Screening, Brief Intervention, Referral, and Treatment (SBIRT). http://sbirt.samhsa.gov/index.htm. Site last visited March 27, 2008.
8. Project CORK. http://www.projectcork.org/ Site last visited March 27, 2008.

9. **Ashley O, Marsden M, Brady T.** Effectiveness of substance abuse treatment programming for women: a review. Am J Drug Alcohol Abuse. 2003;29:19–53.

10. **Terplan M, Lui S.** Psychosocial interventions for pregnant women in outpatient illicit drug treatment programs compared to other interventions. Cochrane Database Syst Rev. 2007;4:CD006037.

11. **Westermeyer J, Boedicker A.** Course, severity, and treatment of substance abuse among women versus men. Am J Drug Alcohol Abuse. 2000;26:523–35.

12. **Mattick R, Kimber J, Breen C, et al.** Buprenorphine maintenance versus placebo or methadone maintenance for opioid dependence. Cochrane Database Syst Rev. 2003;2:CD002207.

13. National Institute on Drug Abuse. http://www.nida.nih.gov/ Site last visited March 27, 2008.

14. US Department of Health and Human Services. Substance Abuse & Mental Health Services Administration (SAMHSA). http://www.samhsa.gov/. Site last visited March 27, 2008.

15. **Nolen-Hoeksema S, Hilt L.** Possible contributors to the gender differences in alcohol use and problems. J Gen Psychol. 2006;133:357–74.

16. **Bolnick J, Rayburn W.** Substance use disorders in women: special considerations during pregnancy. Obstet Gynecol Clin North Am. 2003;30:545–58.

C. Weight Loss and Over-the-Counter Diet Products

Joanne E. Williams

KEY POINTS

- Prevention of obesity should begin in childhood.
- Effective treatment of obesity includes reducing calories and increasing exercise. The specific diet does not matter.
- A modest weight loss of 5–15% of one's body weight can have a significant health impact.
- Women spend billions of dollars each year on over-the-counter diet aids, many of which are not effective.

Obesity has reached epidemic proportions in the U.S. The problem exists globally, even in developing countries. There is documentation that obesity has been increasing for at least a century in the U.S., with a sharp rate of increase noted over the past 30–40 years (1). This chapter will examine specific strategies and over-the-counter products for weight loss (see Chapter 3D).

The Role of Prevention

Efforts to curb or address the problems of an overweight or obese society, nationally or globally, must begin at the level of the pediatric patient. Currently, 19% of U.S. children between 6 and 12 are classified as overweight or obese (2). Children who are obese are at much higher risk of being overweight in adulthood (2). Of course, prevention works best when the entire family is required to participate and be involved in the daily nutrition and physical activity plans and activities. Every aspect of society, including schools and the healthcare arena, has an important role to play, and a vested interest, in the outcome of these efforts. Prevention is the best way to make significant inroads toward a solution for this growing epidemic.

Several countries, and even many school systems in the U.S., have tried to recapture control of school nutrition programs by only allowing healthy food on the menu and in schools (2). Removing candy, salty snacks, and soft drinks from the schools, re-introducing physical activity into the curriculum, planning, developing, and restructuring communities, and reassessing individual, family, and community priorities are some of the other measures that must be taken if significant changes are to be made in order to prevent further morbidity (2).

Effective Treatments of Obesity

The components of effective weight loss regimens include (3)

- Focusing on lowering calories and increasing activity/exercise. Generally, diets are successful when calories are limited to 1200–1500 per day, which creates a calorie deficit of 500–1000 cal/day. Recommended energy expenditure via exercise ranges from 1000 cal/week (minimum) to 2000 cal/week (optimally).
- Education and help with stimulus control, self-monitoring, strategies for eating in restaurants and social eating, making healthy food choices, portion control, emotional eating, stress management, assertiveness, motivation, and appropriate goal-setting. Limiting food choices or groups, decreasing portions, and counting calories work best.

Caloric balance is the main determinant of weight loss; all low-calorie diets result in loss of body weight and body fat. Optimally, women should eat 1400–1500 kcal/day at baseline with increases in calories depending on physical activity. Moderate fat reduction (to a level of 20–30% of daily intake) is nutritionally adequate. Very low-fat diets may be deficient in vitamin E, vitamin B12, and zinc. There does not appear to be an optimal diet for reducing hunger (3). Ketogenic diets (generally high-fat, low-carbohydrate diets like the Atkins diet) work because followers consume fewer calories (3). In a head-to-head trial of the Atkins diet, Ornish diet (very low-fat), Weight Watchers (calorie measurement with peer support), and the Zone diet (moderately low-carbohydrate), there was no significant difference among study participants in overall weight loss at 1 year (4). In this study, the main determinant of weight loss was adherence to the specific diet (4).

All weight loss methods should be considered as "first steps" in the continuum toward making more permanent nutritional, behavioral, and lifestyle changes. The group approach provides education, structure, and support, encourages or instructs participants in limiting food intake, promotes exercise and healthy lifestyle, and demands client accountability through meetings and weigh-ins. An example of the group approach is "Weight Watchers."

Prepackaged food plans allow for a specific number of calories per day, meeting the client's food preferences and dietary needs. There is a market for the "easy fix" to the food preparation problem, with the public often having limited time to shop or cook, or choosing not to prepare their own meals. "Nutri-System" and "Jenny Craig" are examples of this method. Fast foods are generally not included on a weight loss plan, although fast food restaurants are currently offering healthier choices.

Some patients choose a very low calorie (800 calories) physician-supervised liquid diet supplied by high protein drinks. These programs can cause rapid weight loss, which may be necessary before surgery, but they may be expensive, and the client, as in all programs, still has the challenge of maintaining the new (lower) weight and/or of continuing to lose the remainder of the excess weight after the period of rapid weight loss. "OptiFast" and "MediFast" are examples of these programs.

Support groups are an important adjunct to any diet program. "Overeaters Anonymous," which uses the 12-step program to fight food and other negative behavior addictions, and "take off pounds sensibly" (TOPS) are low cost examples of these programs. Online support is available through various Web sites.

Personal trainers, circuit training, walking, any form of increased physical activity or increased energy expenditure, are an integral part of the weight loss and maintenance regimen. Wellness programs at many workplaces encourage employees to take the stairs, participate in walking clubs, and offer on-site gyms or subsidized gym memberships.

Medications for Weight Loss

It is commonly agreed that obesity is a chronic illness, and recent discussions have entertained the notion that, as such, it requires chronic medications. Currently available bariatric medications include drugs in 1 of 2 categories: appetite suppression and decreased fat absorption (5). Orlistat is a pancreatic lipase inhibitor that inhibits fat absorption from the colon. Sibutramine inhibits serotonin and norepinephrine re-uptake in the hypothalamus, thereby decreasing one's appetite. They are approved for individual or combined long-term treatment and have shown moderate efficacy (loss of about 5% of initial weight) after 1 year of use (5). Other appetite suppressants approved for short-term use (up to 12 weeks) are benzphetamine, diethylproprion, phendimetrazine, and phentermine (5). Some medications, such as fluoxetine, sertraline, buproprion, topiramate, metformin, exenatide, and somatostatin, have been used off-label for obesity treatment, with mixed results and with varied adverse effects. Clinical trials are underway for new medications (5).

Many physicians using these medications require the patient to have attempted lifestyle changes before they will prescribe these medicines. The patient must also have a BMI >30 if there are no other comorbidities, or a BMI >27 if there are obesity-related health problems (6).

Mental Health Concerns

Psychiatric disorders can play a significant role in a patient becoming obese and in an individual's efforts to lose weight or to maintain weight loss. In many situations, it is unclear to what extent the psychiatric diagnosis preceded and caused the obesity, or vice versa. Excessive weight can exacerbate a patient's depression, low self-esteem, obsessive behaviors, and eating disorders (binging, cravings, anorexia, and bulimia) (7).

Maintenance of Weight Loss

Regardless of the method used to lose weight, the harder task is *not regaining the weight*. There is no set "formula for success," but there are certain actions that have repeatedly been proven to assist those who have been successful in keeping off unwanted pounds. Ongoing participation in support groups, food diaries and journaling, regular weigh-ins with a plan of action if the weight increases by more than a set number of pounds, daily exercise or activity from 30–60 minutes a day have all been beneficial (3). Maintenance of successful, long-term weight loss is its own reward.

Over-the-Counter Medications for Weight Loss

There are more than 200 non-proprietary weight loss medications on the market. This is a multi-billion dollar industry. Medications containing ephedrine were removed from the market in 2004. Table 8-3 lists some of the over-the-counter medications for weight loss.

Other substances frequently found in weight-loss preparations include milk thistle, inositol, collagen hydrolysate, citirn K, aminogen, pyruvate, and various amino acids. Individual studies have not been published for these substances (8).

Complementary and Alternative Medicine Therapies for Weight Loss

Acupuncture/acupressure—Four studies were reviewed; 2 showed some decrease in hunger. Overall, there was no evidence that these methods were effective for reducing body weight (7).

Ayurvedic preparations—One double-blind study showed that patients in treatment groups receiving ayurvedic preparations plus *Triphala guggul* experienced significant weight loss averaging 8 kg (7).

Table 8-3 Complementary Therapies and Over-the-Counter Treatments for Obesity

Name of Drug	Brand Names	Mechanism of Action	Results/Evidence/ Studies	Source	Risks/Adverse Effects
Garcinia cambogia/ indica	Brindleberry, Brindleslim; Medislim; Slim Life, Beer Belly Busters	↓s lipogenesis de novo; ↓appetite through glucostatic mechanisms	Six studies reviewed; no strong support for weight loss found	Rind of exotic citrus fruit (Malabar tamarind); hydroxycitric acid	
Capsaicin	Optislim 2000	↑s metabolism; may ↑ secretion of epinephrine. ↓s appetite	No support for thermogenic effect; ↓d food intake in 1 study	Major pungent ingredient of hot chilies and peppers	Pain from spicy foods
Caffeine/ Guarana	Slim Life, Beer Belly Busters; Body Lean	↑Alertness; ↓ fatigue; lipolytic effect; ↑d availability of FFA for oxidation.	Weight loss effects not proven by studies; possible effects on energy balance		Large doses can cause nervousness, GI discomfort, anxiety, insomnia, cardiac arrhythmias, and mild hallucinations; may lead to dependence
L-Carnitine	Fat metaboliser, ProteCol, Pro-Sport L-carnitine	↑s fat metabolism	No evidence of weight loss; no controlled studies		Possible diarrhea
Chitosan		↓s fat absorption; binds to dietary fat preventing digestion and storage	Evidence doubtful	Crustaceans	Constipation, flatulence
Chromium picolinate		A co-factor to insulin	Reduction of 1.1–1.2 kg during 6–14 wk intervention		Possible tissue accumulation and DNA damage; renal damage after chronic large ingestion

E. sinica		Ephedrine, with and without caffeine		Evergreen shrub native to central Asia	↑ psychiatric, autonomic, and GI sx and heart palpitations
Fucus vesiculosus (seaweed)	Cellasene; Medex; Bioslim diet patches	Iodine in Fucus vesiculosis ↑ thyroid response	No proven effect on weight loss	Seaweed	Iodine ↑ thyroid response. ↑energy expenditure. Possible hyperthyroidism if taken in excess
Garcinia cambogia	Hydroxycitric acid	Inhibits citrate cleavage enzyme, suppresses fatty acid synthesis	Results vary but are encouraging	From extracts of *Garcinia cambogia*	Headache, URI sx, GI sx
Gingko biloba	Cellasene; Cellusense	Reduction in adrenal peripheral benzodiazepine receptors; ↓d corticosteroid response to stress	May help with stress and anxiety, but no evidence to prove this	Leaves of the maidenhair tree (*Ginkgo biloba*)	Possible "serotonin syndrome" if combined with antidepressants or other non-Rx meds
Glucomannan			Significantly larger weight loss in 1 double blind RCT in pats >20% IBW	Component of konjac root, *Amorphophallus konjac*; like galactomannan, from guar gum. Polysaccharide chain of glucose and mannose	None
Guar gum				Dietary fiber from *Cyamopsis tetragonolobus*	

cont'd

Table 8-3 Complementary Therapies and Over-the-Counter Treatments for Obesity (cont'd)

Name of Drug	Brand Names	Mechanism of Action	Results/Evidence/ Studies	Source	Risks/Adverse Effects
Grapeseed extract	Cellasene	Not specified	No rational presented	Grape seeds	None known
5-HTP		May ↑serotonin and help to regulate appetite	Four small studies; short duration; 3 by same author; all showed effective for weight loss	An intermediate metabolite in biosynthesis of serotonin to L-tryptophan	Do not mix with carbidopa; rarely associated with EMS and eosinophilia; possible interaction with SSRIs; could have N, V, D, ↓ appetite
Hydroxy-methyl-butyrate		Anti-catabolic actions through inhibition of protein breakdown	Two double-blind RCTs	Metabolite of leucine	Not reported in trial
Lecithin		Prevents deposition of fat in fat cells	No support for weight loss	Phospholipid in soybeans, egg yolks; also made in the intestines.	None known
Horse chestnut (escin)	Cellasene	Aids circulation; prevents edema	None	Seed extract from horse chestnut	None known
Pectin	Zellulean, Beer Belly Busters, Exofat, Fatsorb	↓energy density; ↓food intake; lower chol; delay gastric emptying/↑satiety	Little to no effect on weight loss	Soluble fiber from fruit	Low to none
Plantago psyllium				Water soluble fiber from the ripe seeds of Plantago psyllium	

Supplement	Description	Evidence	Source / What it is	Adverse effects
Pyruvate	Enhances exercise performance; improves body composition measures	Weak evidence	Generated in the body via glycolysis	None or not reported
Cellasene — Sweet clover / Soy beans (isoflavones)	Not specified	One study—no effect on weight	Phytoestrogens from soybeans and sweet clover	None known for adults
Beer Belly Busters — St. John's wort	Not specified; antidepressant effects may ↓ depression eating	No studies proving weight loss	Is an herb	Not known
Yohimbine	An alpha-2 receptor antagonist is main ingredient in the ground bark of the *Pausinystalia yohimbe* tree	Studies done on the bark. Three relevant double-blind RCTs reviewed; conflicting results	Tall evergreen native to Central Africa	Few adverse events reported; impaired sleep, nervousness, joint pains, headache

RCT—randomized control trials.

From Pittler MH, Ernst E. Complementary therapies for reducing body weight: a systematic review. International Journal of Obesity. 2005;29:1030–8 and Egger G, Cameron-Smith D, Stanton RT. The effectiveness of popular, non-prescription weight loss supplements. The Medical Journal of Australia. 1999;171:604–8; with permission.

Homeopathy—Two RCTs were studied. One used *Helianthus tuberosus* D1; patients lost an average of 7.1 kg after 3 months. The other study looked at the effectiveness of a single dose of thyroidinum 30cH, which did not prove to be effective (7).

Hypnotherapy—A meta-analysis examined 6 RCTs and found that hypnotherapy directed at stress reduction improved weight loss, as did, to a much lesser extent, hypnotherapy added to cognitive-behavioral therapy (7).

Because of the serious nature of the comorbidities and the sequelae of chronic obesity, it is important to identify, acknowledge, and inform the patient of any weight issues and their consequences. Healthcare providers must become, and remain, sensitized about obesity and overweight issues. Their involvement needs to be on the individual, family, and community levels.

A woman's BMI should be recorded at each visit. If it is elevated, she should be informed, and a plan of action should be put in place with an early follow-up visit scheduled. The patient's family history, past medical history, and medications should be reviewed annually or more often, with regard to possible complications of obesity.

Assessment should be made of the stresses facing the obese patient, especially with regard to eating behaviors, food temptations, and support from other family members and persons living in the home. Resources should be identified and utilized (e.g., dietician, outside weight management groups, personal coaches, and exercise facilities). Consideration of hiring a dietician to work in a physician's primary care office may increase the effectiveness of weight loss efforts (9). A goal of therapy should be initially a weight loss of 5–15% of the patient's body weight, which can effect significant health benefits (10).

Healthcare providers have a responsibility to educate and train patients to read food labels, to be aware of portion sizes, to encourage healthy food choices for their children in the schools, and to make healthy food choices for themselves and their family. All family members should be involved in the food and meal planning that is necessary for the success of the lifestyle changes. There is a responsibility to the greater community to be involved in the legislation and community planning efforts that may affect the nutrition and lifestyle of the areas in which their patients live, work, and attend school.

Each patient encounter should motivate the patient to change to a healthier behavior. The provider should not pre-judge or give up on the patient but should treat the obese patient with empathy (10). The practitioner must align him/herself with the patient to fight this individual and public health problem on all fronts and on all levels.

References

1. **Keith SW, et al.** Putative contributors to the secular increase in obesity: exploring the roads less traveled. International Journal of Obesity. 2006;30:1585-94

2. **Lobstein T, Baur L, Uauy R.** for the IASO International Obesity Task Force. Obesity in children and young people: a crisis in public health. International Association for the Study of Obesity. Obesity Reviews. 5:4–85.

3. **Boucher J, et al.** Weight loss, diets, and supplements: does anything work? Diabetes Spectrum. 2001;14:169–75.

4. **Dansinger ML, Gleason JA, Griffith JL, et al.** Comparison of the Atkins, Ornish, Weight Watchers, and Zone diets for weight loss and heart disease risk reduction: a randomized trial. JAMA. 2005 Jan 5;293:43–53.

5. **Bray GA.** Medical therapy for obesity – current status and future hopes. Medical Clinics of North America. November 2007;91:1225–53.

6. Disease Management. Pharmacotherapy for the treatment of obesity has only modest benefits and should be used in combination with lifestyle modifications. Drugs Therapy Perspectives. 2006;22:1.

7. **Pittler MH, Ernst E.** Complementary therapies for reducing body weight: a systematic review. International Journal of Obesity. 2005;29:1030–8.

8. **Egger G, Cameron-Smith D, Stanton RT.** The effectiveness of popular, non-prescription weight loss supplements. The Medical Journal of Australia. 1999;171:604–8.

9. **Welty FK, Nasca MM, Lew NS, et al.** Effect of onsite dietitian counseling on weight loss and lipid levels in an outpatient physician office. The American Journal of Cardiology. 2007;100:73–5.

10. **Hainer V, Toplak H, Mitrakou A.** Treatment modalities of obesity: what fits whom? Diabetes Care. 2008;31:S269–77.

9

Dermatologic

A. Acne Vulgaris and Steroid Acne
   Kimberly A. Bauer, MD; Bethanee Schlosser, MD, PhD;
   Ginat W. Mirowski, DMD, MD

B. Atopic Dermatitis
   Richard H. Huggins, MD; Bethanee Schlosser, MD, PhD;
   Dennis P. West, PhD; Amy S. Paller, MD, PhD;
   Ginat W. Mirowski, DMD, MD

A. Acne Vulgaris and Steroid Acne

Kimberly A. Bauer, Bethanee Schlosser, and Ginat W. Mirowski

KEY POINTS

- Acne vulgaris is a common skin disorder.
- Pathogenesis of acne vulgaris involves 4 factors: increased sebum production, abnormal keratinocyte shedding, colonization by *Propionibacterium acnes*, and inflammation.
- Acne vulgaris has an equal gender prevalence in adolescence; women have a higher prevalence than men in adulthood.
- Diagnosis is based on the presence of characteristic clinical findings that include open and closed comedones, papules, pustules, nodules, and cysts, in various stages of development.
- Treatment consists of a multi-pronged approach, potentially consisting of both topical and systemic agents.
- Early intervention is essential to minimize scarring and residual hyperpigmentation.

Epidemiology

Acne vulgaris is one of the most common skin disorders, affecting up to 50 million individuals in the U.S. (1). The highest prevalence is seen in individuals between the ages of 12 and 24, with up to 85% of this population affected (1). Although typically viewed as a problem of the teen population, post-adolescent acne is increasingly recognized. Twelve percent of women and 3% of men, 25–58 years of age, continue to suffer with acne (2).

Clinical Features

Acne vulgaris may involve the face, upper chest, and back, in descending order of frequency. The pathogenesis of acne vulgaris involves increased sebum production, abnormal keratinocyte differentiation at the follicular epithelium, colonization of the pilosebaceous unit with *Propionibacterium acnes*, and inflammation. Clinically, acne is characterized as mild, moderate, or severe (Figure 9-1). Individual lesions are categorized as non-inflammatory or inflammatory. The initial lesion of acne, the comedo, may be either closed or open and is not inflamed. A closed comedo, or whitehead, is a collection of sebum, keratinocytes, and microorganisms, which blocks a dilated follicular opening but does not open onto the skin surface. A closed comedo appears as a fine, skin-colored papule

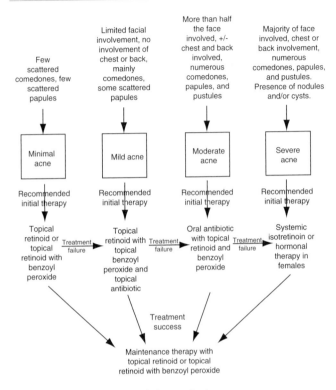

Figure 9-1   Approach to treatment of acne vulgaris.

which may be better appreciated by palpation than by visual inspection. An open comedo, or blackhead, opens onto the skin surface with oxidation of sebum imparting the characteristic and easily recognized central gray/black plug.

Inflammatory lesions of acne include papules, pustules, nodules, and cysts. Acne papules are erythematous and may be tender to palpation. Acne nodules can be markedly inflamed and tender and are located deep in the dermis. As the severity of acne increases, greater numbers of nodules are often present. Acne cysts are deeper, fluctuant nodules that are filled with a combination of purulent and serosanguinous fluid. Lesions at different stages of development and resolution are a typical feature of acne vulgaris (Figure 9-2). Early intervention, in conjunction with limiting traumatic manipulation of lesions, is crucial in order to minimize scarring and residual hyperpigmentation caused by inflammatory acne lesions (Figure 9-3).

In the adolescent population, males and females have similar prevalence, distribution, and severity of acne vulgaris (3). In contrast, in adults,

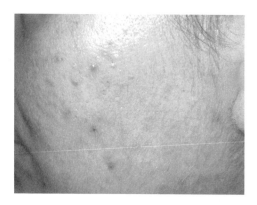

Figure 9-2   Mild comedonal and inflammatory acne on the face of a young woman. (Courtesy of Dennis West, Ph.D.)

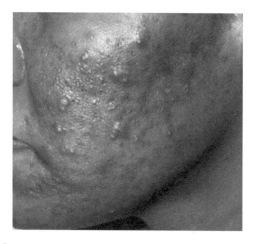

Figure 9-3   African American female with acute acne lesions and residual acne scars. Active lesions consist of pustules, inflammatory papules, and a single excoriated papule. Scarring includes post-inflammatory hyperpigmented macules, some hyperpigmented pitted scars, particularly on the chin, and some non-hyperpigmented pitted scars. (Courtesy of Dennis West, Ph.D.)

women have a higher prevalence of clinical facial acne than men (2). In some patients, acne that began in adolescence may persist into adulthood, or beyond the age of 25 years. Late-onset acne identifies those persons whose initial onset of acne occurs after age 25, in the absence of recognizable acne during the teen years. Women with persistent acne may exhibit deep, tender, inflammatory papules and nodules that are distributed on the lower third of the face, particularly along the jaw-line and neck. Late-onset acne may present as peri-menstrual flares involving the chin and perioral regions. Alternatively, late-onset acne may demonstrate sporadic acne with no clear temporal association with the menstrual cycle (4).

Diagnosis and Differential Diagnosis

A diagnosis of acne vulgaris is made based on the clinical features and age at onset of the disease. Microbiologic testing is not necessary unless one suspects gram-negative folliculitis (Table 9-1). Serologic studies are only indicated when patients also exhibit signs of androgen excess, such as hirsutism, irregular periods, deepening of the voice, muscular habitus, or androgenic alopecia.

The differential diagnosis of acne includes acne rosacea, staphylococcal folliculitis, gram-negative folliculitis, drug-induced acne (5) (Table 9-2),

Table 9-1   Differential Diagnosis of Acne Vulgaris

Disease	Diagnostic Clues
Acne rosacea	No comedones. Erythematous papules and pustules often superimposed on diffuse erythema. Discrete telangiectases. Symmetric distribution at cheeks, forehead, nose, chin. Ocular symptoms may include stinging, foreign body/gritty sensation, lid crusting, and photophobia. Flushing with environmental triggers.
Drug-induced acne, including steroids (see Table 9-2)	Temporal relationship to initiation of medication. Monomorphous pustules.
Gram-negative folliculitis	Follicular pustules + /– abscesses around mouth or cheeks, upper chest. Most often in patients with long-term antibiotic use (i.e., tetracyclines).
Keratosis pilaris	Slightly rough, firm papules with follicular plugs + /– erythema involving cheeks, shoulders, upper arms, buttocks, and thighs. Atopic diathesis.
Pityrosporum folliculitis	Itchy, small follicular papules and pustules at middle to lower back, upper arms. No comedones. Negative bacterial culture.
Polycystic ovary syndrome	Recalcitrant acne in patient with signs of androgen excess, including central obesity, hirsutism, oligomenorrhea, infertility, acanthosis nigricans, androgenic alopecia. Elevated levels of DHEAS and/or total/free testosterone.
Sebaceous hyperplasia	Soft, yellow-pink, dome-shaped, shiny papules + /– central umbilication in sun-exposed areas of face.
Staphylococcal folliculitis	Pustules and red follicular papules. No comedones. Bacterial culture positive for *Staphylococcus* species.

Table 9-2 Agents that Cause Acneiform Eruptions

Drug class	Specific agents
Androgens	Fluoxymesterone, methyltestosterone, stanozolol, testosterone
Anesthetics	Chloral hydrate, halothane
Antibiotics	Ceftazidime, ciprofloxacin, clofazimine, ethionamide, grepafloxacin, **isoniazid**, pyrazinamide, rifampin, trovafloxacin
Anticonvulsants	Felbamate, fosphenytoin, gabapentin, lamotrigine, mephenytoin, paramethadione, phenobarbital, **phenytoin**, primidone, tiagabine, topiramate, trimethadione, valproic acid
Anti-inflammatory agents	Fenoprofen, mesalamine, nabumetone, olsalazine
Antimalarials	Quinidine, quinine
Antipsychotics	Haloperidol, risperidone
Antiretrovirals	Ritonavir, saquinavir, tizanidine, zalcitabine, zidovudine
Antivirals	Acyclovir, foscarnet, ganciclovir
Anxiolytics	Alprazolam, buspirone, diazepam, estazolam
Beta blockers	Betaxolol, bisoprolol, carteolol, propranolol
Bromides	Propantheline bromide
Calcium channel blockers	Diltiazem, nimodipine, nisoldipine, verapamil
Chemotherapeutics	Dactinomycin, methotrexate, pentostatin, vinblastine
Corticosteroids	Systemic or topical
Hormonal agents	**ACTH**, clomiphene, danazol, medroxyprogesterone, nafarelin, **oral contraceptives**
Immunosuppressants	**Azathioprine, cyclosporine**
Iodides	**Potassium iodide**, radiopaque contrast
Selective serotonin reuptake inhibitors	Fluoxetine, fluvoxamine, paroxetine, sertraline
Tricyclic antidepressants	Amitriptyline, amoxapine, clomipramine, desipramine, maprotiline
Tyrosine kinase inhibitors	Dasatinib, erlotinib, **gefitinib**, imatinib, leflunomide, sorafenib

Bold indicates most common causative agents.

polycystic ovary syndrome and other androgen excess disorders, keratosis pilaris, and sebaceous hyperplasia (see Table 9-1).

Prevention and Clinical Care

Treatment of acne vulgaris consists of various topical and systemic therapies, often used in combination (see Figure 9-1 and Table 9-3). The choice of therapeutic regimen depends on the severity of the disease, the side effect profile, as well as patient and physician preferences (4,6–9).

Topical retinoids target the microcomedo and are the first-line treatment of mild to moderate acne. Retinoids may cause significant irritation, particularly in adults and in patients with a history of "sensitive" skin or an atopic diathesis. To minimize such irritation, the formulation (creams, microspherules, gels, solutions), as well as the potency, should be considered. Tolerability may be enhanced by initiating treatment with short application times on alternate days and gradually increasing frequency and duration of use as tolerated. Topical retinoids should not be used in women who are actively trying to conceive or those who are pregnant (see Table 9-3 for pregnancy categories).

Topical antibiotic therapies, such as clindamycin or erythromycin, should not be used alone because monotherapy is associated with development of bacterial resistance. The formulation chosen (lotions, solutions, or gels) is based on the patient's skin type and preference. Benzoyl peroxide, a powerful antimicrobial topical agent, is very effective in combination with other antibacterial agents and has been shown to reduce the development of antibiotic resistance by *Propionibacterium acnes* (6). Retinoids used in combination with topical or oral antimicrobial agents achieve a greater reduction in acne lesions than do the individual agents used alone (7).

Systemic antibacterial agents, such as tetracyclines, are indicated for the treatment of moderate to severe acne. Second-generation tetracyclines, including minocycline, doxycycline, and lymecycline, show quicker patient responses than does tetracycline (7,8). Due to increasing bacterial resistance, the macrolides, such as erythromycin, are typically reserved for cases where tetracyclines are contraindicated, such as in women who may be pregnant or breast-feeding. Trimethoprim/sulfamethoxazole (TMP/SMX) or trimethoprim alone may be considered as a third-line agent, but one should be vigilant about adverse drug effects, including Stevens–Johnson syndrome. Regardless of the treatment regimen, notable improvement may require 6–8 weeks of therapy. After initiation of either topical or systemic therapies, it is not uncommon for patients to note an increase, or flare, of acne lesions. This typically occurs 2–3 weeks into therapy.

For patients with severe inflammatory acne or moderate to severe acne that is unresponsive to systemic antibiotic therapy, oral isotretinoin may be indicated. The use of isotretinoin, a well-recognized teratogen, is highly regulated. In March, 2006, a mandatory pregnancy risk management program, the iPLEDGE program, was instituted. Physicians and patients both must register with iPLEDGE in order to

Table 9-3   Treatment Options

Treatment Class	Available Therapies within Treatment Class	Pregnancy Class*
Topical retinoids	Tretinoin: 0.01–0.1% gel or cream	C
	Adapalene: 0.1% cream, 0.1% or 0.3% gel	C
	Tazarotene: 0.05% or 0.1% gel or cream	X
Topical anti-bacterial agents	Benzoyl peroxide: 2.5–10%, various formulations	C
	Clindamycin, erythromycin: 1 to 4%, cream or lotion	B
	Azelaic acid: 15% gel or 20% cream	B
	Sodium sulfacetamide/sulfur: 10% /5% lotion or cleanser	C
Combination topical agents	Benzoyl peroxide/clindamycin: 5%/1% gel	C
	Benzoyl peroxide/erythromycin: 5%/3% gel	C
	Clindamycin/tretinoin: 1.2%/0.025% gel	C
Systemic antibiotics	Doxycycline: 100–200 mg daily	D
	Minocycline: 100–200 mg daily	D
	Lymecycline: 300–600 mg daily	D
	Oxytetracycline: 500 mg twice daily	D
	Erythromycin: 500 mg twice daily	B
	Trimethoprim (TMP): 200–300 mg twice daily	C
	TMP/sulfamethoxazole: 80/400–160 mg/800mg daily	C
Systemic isotretinoin	0.5–2 mg/kg/day as tolerated	X
	Total cumulative dose goal: 120–150 mg/kg	
	Pregnancy testing at baseline and monthly	
	CBC, liver enzymes, and lipid profile at baseline and monthly	
Hormonal therapies	Combination oral contraceptive pills	X
	Flutamide: 250 mg daily	D
	Spironolactone: 25–200 mg per day	D
Other	Salicylic acid: over-the-counter, up to 2%, various formulations	C
	Intralesional triamcinolone acetonide injections: 2–5 mg/ml, maximum volume per lesion <0.1 ml.	C
	Systemic corticosteroids: prior to initiation of systemic isotretinoin in severe nodulocystic acne or acne fulminans	C

*FDA categories: "A = Adequate and well-controlled studies have failed to demonstrate a risk to the fetus in the first trimester of pregnancy (and there is no evidence of risk in later trimesters); B = Animal reproduction studies have failed to demonstrate a risk to the fetus and there are no adequate and well-controlled studies in pregnant women; C = Animal reproduction studies have shown an adverse effect on the fetus and there are no adequate and well-controlled studies in humans, but potential benefits may warrant use of the drug in pregnant women despite potential risks; D = There is positive evidence of human fetal risk based on adverse reaction data from investigational or mareting experience or studies in humans, but potential benefits may warrant use of the drug in pregnant women despite potential risks; X = Studies in animals or humans have demonstrated fetal abnormalities and/or there is positive evidence of human fetal risk based on adverse reaction data from investigational and/or marketing experience, and the risks involved in the use of the drug in pregnant women clearly outweigh potential benefits." From: http://depts.washington.edu/druginfo/Formulary/Pregnancy.pdf, accessed 11/9/2008.

prescribe or obtain prescriptions (www.iPledgeProgram.com, 1-866-495-0654). All women of child-bearing potential are required to adhere to 2 forms of contraception and to undergo monthly pregnancy testing beginning 1 month prior to initiation of isotretinoin, throughout the treatment course, and for 1 month following cessation of treatment. A complete blood count, liver function tests, and a fasting lipid profile should be obtained prior to initiation of therapy and should be repeated monthly throughout treatment in order to identify any potential adverse effects as quickly as possible (9). Common side effects of isotretinoin include cheilitis, xerosis, pruritus, mild epistaxis, irritation and dryness of the eyelids and eyes, joint and muscle aches, hair thinning, rash, intestinal symptoms, headache, photosensitivity, decreased night vision, depression, and suicidal ideation. Isotretinoin also may contribute to early epiphyseal closure. Increases in liver function tests and hypertriglyceridemia may reveal a rare complication seen in some patients on isotretinoin, pancreatitis. The average duration of isotretinoin treatment is 6 months, but, more importantly, a total cumulative dose of isotretinoin of 120–150 mg/kg should be obtained in order to reduce the risk of recurrence of acne.

Women who report significant perimenstrual flaring of acne lesions, or who exhibit signs or laboratory evidence of hyperandrogenemia, may benefit from hormonal therapies. Combination oral contraceptives reduce ovarian androgen production and may have a positive impact on acne. However, progestin-only pill formulations (i.e., Minipill) have been shown to worsen acne. Oral contraceptive pills that have been approved for the treatment of acne in the U.S. include ethinyl estradiol 35 mcg/norgestimate (Ortho Tri-Cyclen), ethinyl estradiol 20–35 mcg/ norethindrone acetate (Estrostep), and ethinyl estradiol 20 mcg/drosperinone (YAZ), although there is good evidence that other combination oral contraceptives are equally efficacious (8). GnRH agonists and low-dose glucocorticoids block ovarian and adrenal androgen production and may be effective in the treatment of women with either persistent or late-onset acne. Anti-androgens or androgen receptor blockers, such as spironolactone or flutamide, work by opposing androgen effects on the sebaceous glands and may be used in conjunction with oral contraceptives in the treatment of these women, too. The significant teratogenicity of these agents requires strict counseling of patients and contraception use.

An endocrine evaluation should be considered in women who fail to respond to conventional therapy or who demonstrate signs of androgen excess, including central obesity, hirsutism, oligomenorrhea, infertility, acanthosis nigricans, or male- or female-pattern androgenic alopecia. Such laboratory investigations also are indicated for prepubertal children with acne, as well as body odor, axillary or pubic hair, or clitoromegaly. Laboratory tests which may be helpful in these settings include total and free testosterone, dehydroepiandrosterone sulfate (DHEAS), luteinizing hormone, and follicle-stimulating hormone. Radiologic evaluation of the ovaries may be indicated in patients who demonstrate elevated serum total testosterone, since polycystic ovary syndrome is seen with increasing frequency in the setting of serum testosterone levels ranging from 150–200 ng/dl. Numerous adrenal disorders, including congenital adrenal hyperplasia, late-onset adrenal hyperplasia, and Cushing's syndrome, result in androgen excess and should prompt further endocrine evaluation. Testosterone levels above 200 ng/dl or DHEAS levels above 8 mcg/ml should prompt evaluation for an androgen-secreting tumor of the ovary or adrenal gland, respectively.

Steroid acne is induced by the use of anabolic steroids, including intravenous dexamethasone and high-dose corticosteroids, as well as inappropriate use of topical corticosteroids. In contrast to acne vulgaris, steroid acne is characterized by an abrupt onset of papules and pustules that are uniform in evolution and appearance (Figure 9-4). Resolution of lesions is seen shortly after discontinuation of the offending agent.

Acne fulminans, a rare and severe form of cystic acne that typically affects adolescent males, is characterized by the acute onset of suppurative nodules and cystic lesions (Figure 9-5). Erythema nodosum also has been associated with acne fulminans. Systemic symptoms, including fever, arthralgias, myalgias, and weight loss, are common. Laboratory abnormalities include elevated erythrocyte sedimentation rate, proteinuria, leukocytosis, and anemia. Use of anabolic steroids and testosterone, as well as the use of isotretinoin (9), ironically, also have been documented as triggers of acne fulminans. Oral corticosteroids should be instituted for 4–6 weeks prior to initiation of isotretinoin in order to reduce the inflammatory response and exacerbation of skin and systemic symptoms that may occur in these patients. Corticosteroids are tapered after oral isotretinoin is introduced.

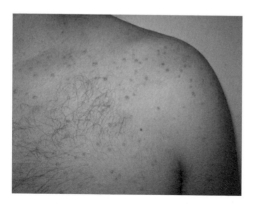

Figure 9-4   Steroid acne consisting of monomorphous papules and pustules that are 1–3 mm in size over the chest and shoulder of a young man.

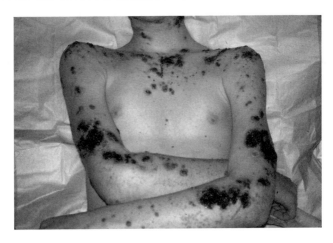

Figure 9-5   Acne fulminans in a 16-year-old male who presented with acute onset of necrotic and hemorrhagic lesions on the neck, chest, and arms.

References

1. **White GM.** Recent findings in the epidemiologic evidence, classification, and subtypes of acne vulgaris. J Am Acad Dermatol. 1998;39:S34–7.

2. **Goulden V, Stables GI, Cunliffe WJ.** The prevalence of facial acne in adults. J Am Acad Dermatol. 1999;41:577–80.

3. **Cunliffe WJ, Gould DJ.** Prevalence of facial acne vulgaris in late adolescence and in adults. BMJ. 1979;1:1109–10.

4. **Williams C, Layton A.** Persistent acne in women: implications for the patient and for therapy. Am J Clin Dermatol. 2006;7:281–90.

5. Litt's Drug Eruption Reference Manual, 13th edition, by Jerome Z. Litt. 2007.

6. **Cunliffe WJ, Holland KT, Bojar R, et al.** A randomized, double-blind comparison of a clindamycin phosphate/benzoyl peroxide gel formulation and a matching clindamycin gel with respect to microbiologic activity and clinical efficacy in the topical treatment of acne vulgaris. Clinical Therapeutics. 2002;24:1117–33.

7. **Gollnick H, Cunliffe W, Berson D, et al.** Management of acne: a report from a global alliance to improve outcomes in acne. J Am Acad Dermatol. 2003;49:S1–37.

8. **Strauss JS, Krowchuk DP, Leyden JJ, et al.** American Academy of Dermatology/American Academy of Dermatology Association. Guidelines of care for acne vulgaris management. J Am Acad Dermatol. 2007:56:651–63.

9. **Layton AM.** A review on the treatment of acne vulgaris. Int J Clin Pract. 2006;60:64–72.

B. Atopic Dermatitis

Richard H. Huggins, Bethanee Schlosser, Dennis P. West, Amy S. Paller, and Ginat W. Mirowski

---

KEY POINTS

- Atopic dermatitis is a common, chronic, relapsing skin condition that begins most often in infancy, though all age groups may be affected.
- It is characterized by pruritus and dry skin with flaking and redness.
- Exacerbating factors include exposure to an irritant, infection, skin barrier disruption, emotional stress, and seasonal/climate change.
- Atopic dermatitis results from a complex interplay of skin barrier dynamics and genetic and immunologic factors.
- Atopy describes the predisposition of certain individuals to develop atopic dermatitis, asthma, and/or allergic rhinitis.

Epidemiology

Atopic dermatitis (AD) is one of the most common skin disorders, with a worldwide prevalence in adults of 7.1% (1). In 60% of patients with AD, onset occurs in infancy. The disorder resolves by adulthood in 50% of individuals (2). AD has an equal prevalence in males and females. AD is the most common dermatosis of pregnancy, and 60–80% of women with AD experience their first episode during pregnancy. Of women diagnosed with AD prior to pregnancy, more than 50% experience a worsening of their disease during gestation and/or during the postpartum period (3).

Clinical Features

Patients with AD complain of dry, itchy, and/or painful skin. Pruritus may precede any visible eruption. Scratching, which patients may be able to suppress while awake, also occurs during sleep. The "itch-scratch cycle," in which scratching leads to increasing degrees of pruritus, is disruptive to a patient's quality of life. There is a strong predisposition for individuals with AD to develop asthma and/or allergic rhinitis, a phenomenon termed atopy. AD is typically the first to present in the "atopic march" (4).

Clinically, there are 3 stages of AD. One or more stages may present sequentially or simultaneously. Acute AD is characterized by patches or plaques with erythema and/or scale (Figure 9-6). Erythematous papules with excoriations, erosions, and serous exudate may be noted. Subacute AD lesions present as erythematous, excoriated, scaling papules (Figures 9-7 and 9-8). Chronic AD lesions include lichenified papules and plaques. Lichenification is characterized by thickening and accentuation of skin markings. Associated reversible changes in pigmentation, either hypo- or hyperpigmentation, are commonly seen. Hypopigmented patches also are found in pityriasis alba, which some consider to be a variant of AD.

Chronologically, AD exhibits a characteristic distribution of involvement. In infancy, from birth to age 2 years, the cheeks, forehead, and scalp are affected initially. Involvement of the extensor aspects of the extremities may occur next. After teething begins, facial AD may worsen on the medial cheeks and chin exacerbated by repeated exposure to salivary drool. Childhood AD, from 2 years of age to puberty, characteristically affects the face, wrists, ankles, hands, feet, and the antecubital and

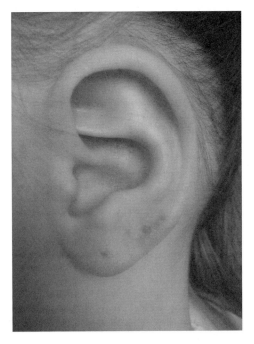

Figure 9-6   Young girl with eczematous patches of her ear. Note the fine scale and erythematous papules.

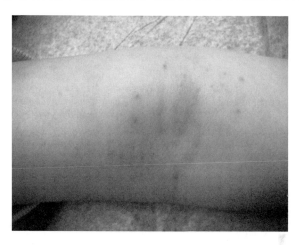

Figure 9-7 Erythematous papules and mild lichenification of the antecubital fossa in a young girl with atopic dermatitis.

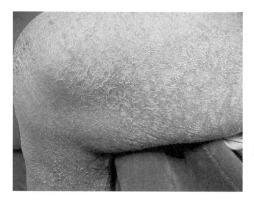

Figure 9-8 Extensive erythema and fine scale in an adult with severe atopic dermatitis.

popliteal fossae. The periorbital and perioral regions are the most common sites of facial involvement. In adults, AD lesions are often localized to flexural areas of the arms and legs, the face, neck, back, hands, and feet. The eyelids also may be affected (4). The vulva and perianal areas may be involved, but these sites typically present as pink, pruritic patches with minimal or no scale, with or without excoriation. Nipple eczema presents with erythema, scaling, weeping, crusting, fissuring, vesiculation, erosions, excoriations, and lichenification. Both nipples may be affected, and extension onto or beyond the areolae may occur (Figure 9-9) (5). Nipple eczema occurs in non-lactating women and in men less often than in nursing women.

Patients with AD are prone to frequent and/or more severe superficial bacterial and viral infections which can alter the lesion morphology. Clues to infection include increased warmth, erythema, tenderness, edema, and/or worsening pruritus. Secondary bacterial infection often is caused by *Staphylococcus aureus* and *Streptococcus pyogenes*. Honey-colored crust with or without pustules is highly suggestive of bacterial infection (impetigo). Ninety-three percent of AD patients are colonized by *S. aureus,* which has been attributed to a deficiency of endogenous antimicrobial peptides (4). Infection with *Herpes simplex* virus may result in the explosive development of a widespread, painful, vesiculopustular eruption called eczema herpeticum. This medical emergency requires immediate systemic antiviral therapy, particularly in pregnancy to limit vertical transmission.

Diagnosis and Differential Diagnosis

The diagnosis of AD is based on history and clinical evaluation of essential and associated findings (Table 9-4). High total and specific IgE levels in the context of clinical AD support the diagnosis. Serum tests for allergen-specific IgE (RAST) and skin-prick testing may be helpful. A biopsy may differentiate AD from other chronic dermatoses, infections, and metabolic, genetic, and immunologic disorders (Table 9-5).

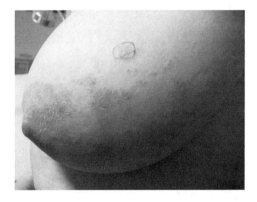

Figure 9-9   Ill-defined erythematous coalescing papules with mild scale on the lateral breast and areola. Biopsy performed and revealed no evidence of Paget's disease.

Table 9-4   Atopic Dermatitis Diagnostic Criteria

Essential features	• Morphology and distribution typical of AD • Chronic or relapsing dermatitis
Important features	• Early age of onset • Atopy (IgE reactivity) • Pruritus • Xerosis
Associated features	• Facial pallor or erythema • Ichthyosis vulgaris • Keratosis pilaris • Ocular and periorbital changes (infraorbital folds, recurrent conjunctivitis, anterior-subcapsular cataracts) • Palmar hyperlinearity

Adapted from Paller A. Eczematous eruptions in childhood. In Hurwitz Clinical Pediatric Dermatology, 3rd ed, eds: Paller AS, Mancini AJ. Philadelphia: Elsevier Saunders; 2006. pp. 49–82; with permission.

Table 9-5   Differential Diagnosis of Atopic Dermatitis in Adults

Inflammatory skin disorders	• Allergic contact dermatitis • Asteatotic eczema • Irritant contact dermatitis • Lichen simplex chronicus • Nummular dermatitis • Psoriasis
Infections and infestations	• Scabies • Superficial fungal infection (tinea corporis)
Metabolic and genetic disorders	• Familial keratosis pilaris • Nutritional deficiencies (zinc deficiency, biotin deficiency, pellagra)
Immunologic disorders	• Dermatitis herpetiformis • Dermatomyositis • Graft-versus-host disease • Immunodeficiency (combined variable immunodeficiency) • Lupus erythematosus • Pemphigus foliaceus
Others	• Cutaneous T-cell lymphoma • Drug eruption • Paget's disease of the breast or vulva • Photoallergic contact dermatitis

Prevention and Treatment

No current therapy offers complete cure. The goal of AD treatment is to control symptoms and limit signs while minimizing the development of potential adverse reactions. Both pharmacologic and non-pharmacologic interventions have shown efficacy in the management of AD and its sequelae (Table 9-6).

Table 9-6   Recommended Atopic Dermatitis Interventions

Class/Category	Agent	Pregnancy Category
Topical therapy		
	Corticosteroids	C
	Calcineurin inhibitors	C
	Doxepin	B
Systemic therapy		
	Cyclosporine (2–5 mg/kg per d)	C
	Interferon gamma (50 ug/m² nightly (8))	C
	Sedating antihistamines	B or C
	Corticosteroids	C
	Efalizumab (0.7 mg/kg followed by 1.0 mg/kg weekly (7))	C
	Methotrexate (5–25 mg/wk)	X
	Azathioprine (50–200 mg/d)	D
	Mycophenolate mofetil (1 g BID × 4 wk, then 500 mg BID × 4 wk (9))	D
Phototherapy		
	Broad-band UVB/UVA	NA (Safe)
	Narrow-band UVB	NA (Safe)
	UVA1	NA (Safe)
	PUVA	C
Secondary infection therapy		
	Topical mupirocin, retapamulin	B
	Oral antibiotics	Variable
	Acyclovir, valacyclovir, famciclovir	B
Non-pharmacologic interventions		
	Psychotherapy	NA (Safe)
	Emollients	NA (Safe)
	Daily baths	NA (Safe)
	Irritant avoidance	NA (Safe)

Non-Pharmacologic Interventions

Emollients are the standard of care in AD and create a barrier to evaporative water loss. Thicker, greasier emollients, because of their higher oil-to-water ratios, are more effective than creams or lotions. Daily lukewarm baths followed by an appropriate emollient improve skin hydration. If needed, cleansers should be limited to mild bar soaps (e.g., Dove® or Basis®) or soapless cleansers (e.g., Cetaphil® or Aquanil®). Bubble baths and body gels should be avoided (4).

Measures to minimize pruritus should be emphasized. Exposure to a variety of irritants, infectious agents, and/or environmental or emotional factors results in the worsening of AD (Box 9-1). Irritant triggers, such as sweating and overheating, should be avoided. Wool and other rough materials should be replaced when possible with cotton or silk.

Box 9-1 Exacerbating Factors in Atopic Dermatitis

- Temperature changes, particularly in winter
- Low humidity
- Perspiration
- Excessive washing
- Wool or other harsh clothing materials
- Irritating chemicals
- Food or environmental allergens
- Emotional stress

Scented detergents, fabric softeners, and other scented products should be avoided. Known allergens also should be avoided. Because dust mites may be a trigger, encasing mattresses and pillows in fabric coverings, washing bedding in hot water on a weekly basis, vacuuming living areas frequently, removing or cleaning carpets regularly, and eliminating pets may be beneficial (4). Psychotherapy, including behavior modification and stress reduction, is effective in reducing the pruritus of AD (6).

Topical Therapies

Topical corticosteroids (CS) are first-line agents in AD treatment (Table 9-7). Steroids directly down-regulate inflammatory mediators. CS are available in various formulations, the use of which varies by body site and patient preference. Ointments penetrate more effectively and are more potent than creams or lotions. However, ointments may occlude eccrine sweat ducts, thereby exacerbating pruritus. Cream and lotion formulations are cosmetically elegant and more acceptable for use during hot weather and in intertriginous areas. However, creams and lotions may contain irritants or allergens. Gel preparations penetrate well, and their significant desiccating effect make these ideal for wet or weeping lesions. CS oils are useful, particularly when applied to a wet scalp for 1 hour to overnight. Topical CS are applied twice daily, with tapering as control of AD is achieved. Long-term therapy necessitates monitoring for cutaneous complications such as striae, atrophy, and telangiectasia (6). These can be minimized by intermittent dosing and utilization of the least potent CS necessary to control AD (4,6).

The topical calcineurin inhibitors (TCI), pimecolimus (Elidel®) and tacrolimus (Protopic®), effectively reduce the pruritus and inflammation of AD by suppressing T-cell activity. These agents are ideal for use on the head, neck, and intertriginous areas, or in lesions that responded poorly to topical CS. Local immunosuppression by TCI is achieved by the reduction of cytokines necessary for T-cell activation (4). The most common side effect of TCI is burning or stinging at the site of application. TCI-induced local immunosuppression may predispose to the development of skin infections, especially by *Herpes simplex* virus. The side-effect profile is otherwise excellent. Long-term safety information (beyond 5 years) is not yet available.

Table 9-7   Available Topical Corticosteroids

Super high potency	
Betamethasone diproprionate	0.05% gel/ointment (Diprolene®)
Clobetasol propionate	0.05% cream/ointment (Temovate®)
	0.05% foam (OLUX®)
	0.05% lotion (Clobex®)
Diflorasone diacetate	0.05% ointment (Psorcon®)
Halobetasol propionate	0.05% cream/ointment (Ultravate®)
High potency	
Amcinonide	0.1% ointment (Cyclocort®)
Betamethasone diproprionate	0.05% ointment (Diprosone®)
Desoximetasone	0.25% cream/ointment, 0.05% gel (Topicort®)
Fluocinonide	0.05% cream/ointment (Lidex®)
Halcinonide	0.1% cream (Halog®)
Betamethasone diproprionate	0.05% cream (Diprosone®)
Mid potency	
Betamethasone valerate	0.1% ointment (Valisone®)
Fluticasone propionate	0.005% ointment (Cutivate®)
Mometasone furoa	0.1% ointment (Elocon®)
Triamcinolone acetonide	0.5% cream (Aristocort®)
Betamethasone valerate	0.12% foam (Luxiq®)
Clocortolone pivalate	0.1% cream (Cloderm®)
Desoximetasone	0.05% cream (Topicort LP®)
Fluocinolone acetonide	0.2% cream (Synalar-HP®)
	0.025% ointment (Synalar®)
Flurandrenolide	0.05% ointment (Cordran®)
Triamcinolone acetonide	0.1% cream (Aristocort®)
	0.1% ointment (Kenalog®)
Low potency	
Betamethasone diproprionate	0.05% lotion (Diprosone®)
Betamethasone valerate	0.1% cream/lotion (Valisone®)
Fluocinolone acetonide	0.025% cream (Synalar®)
Flurandrenolide	0.05% cream (Cordran®)
Fluticasone propionate	0.05% cream (Cutivate®)
Hydrocortisone butyrate	0.1% cream (Locoid®)
Hydrocortisone valerate	0.2% cream (Westcort®)
Prednicarbate	0.1% emollient cream (Dermatop®)
Triamcinolone acetonide	0.1% cream/lotion (Kenalog®)
Alclometasone diproprionate	0.05% cream/ointment (Aclovate®)
Desonide	0.05% cream (DesOwen®)
	0.05% cream (Tridesilon®)
Fluocinolone acetonide	0.01% cream/solution (Synalar®)

Adapted from Del Rosso J, Friedlander SF. Corticosteroids: options in the era of steroid-sparing therapy. J Am Acad Dermatol. 2005;53:S50–8; with permission.

Topical doxepin (Sinequan®, Zonalon®) has been shown to be effective in modulating pruritus because of its antihistamine activity. Risks of sedation and development of allergic contact dermatitis limits its use (6).

Systemic Therapies

Particularly recalcitrant AD or flares of otherwise well-controlled disease may require systemic agents for management.

Systemic CS control the pruritus and inflammation of AD. However, discontinuation often leads to a rebound flare. Chronic use is not recommended because of serious adverse effects, including Cushing syndrome, increased risk of cutaneous and systemic infections, hypopituitary-pituitary-adrenal axis suppression, glaucoma, cataracts, and osteoporosis (4).

Cyclosporine (Neoral®, Gengraf®, Sandimmune®) is a systemic calcineurin inhibitor, which suppresses T-cell activity. Cyclosporine may be associated with the development of hypertension, anemia, and renal or hepatic insufficiency. Complete blood count, electrolytes, including magnesium and phosphate, renal and hepatic function, and blood pressure should be monitored closely. Recombinant gamma interferon (Actimmune®) reduces inflammation and clinical symptoms by inhibiting the aberrant Th2 immune response of AD. Adverse effects, including neutropenia, hepatic transaminitis, and flu-like symptoms are common and limit its use. Efalizumab (Raptiva®), a monoclonal antibody to CD11, is effective in treating severe AD (7). Risks include serious infections, malignancies, thrombocytopenia, hemolytic anemia, and arthritis. Other systemic therapies that have demonstrated efficacy in AD include methotrexate (Trexall®, Rheumatrex®), azathioprine (Imuran®), and mycophenolate mofetil (CellCept ®) (4).

Sedating antihistamines are recommended for the sleep disruption that may be associated with pruritus, but these agents may have little impact on pruritus of AD (6). Sedating antihistamines include diphenhydramine (Benadryl®), chlorpheniramine (Chlor-Trimeton®), cyproheptadine (Periactin®), hydroxyzine (Atarax®), alimemazine (Vallergan®), and promethazine (Phenergan®).

Secondary Infections

Topical antibiotics, such as mupirocin (Bactroban®) and retapamulin (Altabax®), have limited utility except for application on very localized sites of infection. Management of more serious or widespread infections requires oral antibiotics to improve both the bacterial infection and the resulting AD flare (4). Cultures and susceptibility should guide antibiotic selection.

Phototherapy

Ultraviolet light (UV) reduces inflammation and pruritus through anti-proliferative and anti-inflammatory mechanisms. Several forms of phototherapy, including broadband UVB/UVA, Psoralen plus UVA (PUVA), narrowband

UVB (nb-UVB), and UVA1, are effective in the treatment of AD (6). Treatments are given 2 to 3 times per week. The most common side effects are redness and pain at exposed sites, similar to sunburn. Both melanoma and non-melanoma skin cancers may develop with long-term use.

Treatment of Atopic Dermatitis in Pregnancy

Pregnant or lactating women with AD can be managed with emollients, nb-UVB, and/or topical CS. TCI and super-potent topical CS should be used with caution (3). Methotrexate, mycophenolate mofetil, and azathioprine are contraindicated during pregnancy and lactation (see Table 9-6).

Treatment of nipple eczema includes emollients and low-to-mid-potency topical CS. Topical medications should be applied after breast-feeding and removed prior to subsequent feedings.

References

1. **Harrop J, Chinn S, Verlato G, et al.** Eczema, atopy and allergen exposure in adults: a population-based study. Clin Exp Allergy. 2007; 37:526–35.
2. **Boone SL BK, Paller AS, West DP.** Atopic DERMATITIS Update: Topical Calcineurin Inhibitors and Disease Management, in press 2008.
3. **Weatherhead S, Robson SC, Reynolds NJ.** Eczema in pregnancy. BMJ. 2007;335:152–4.
4. **Paller A.** Eczematous Eruptions in Childhood. In Hurwitz Clinical Pediatric Dermatology, 3rd ed, eds: Paller AS, Mancini AJ. Philadelphia: Elsevier Saunders. 2006. pp. 49–82.
5. **Whitaker-Worth DL, Carlone V, Susser WS, et al.** Dermatologic diseases of the breast and nipple. J Am Acad Dermatol. 2000;43 (5 Pt 1):733–51; quiz 52–4.
6. **Hanifin JM, Cooper KD, Ho VC, et al.** Guidelines of care for atopic dermatitis, developed in accordance with the American Academy of Dermatology (AAD)/American Academy of Dermatology Association Administrative Regulations for Evidence-Based Clinical Practice Guidelines. J Am Acad Dermatol. 2004;50:391–404.
7. **Takiguchi R, Tofte S, Simpson B, et al.** Efalizumab for severe atopic dermatitis: a pilot study in adults. J Am Acad Dermatol. 2007;56:222–7.
8. **Stevens SR, Hanifin JM, Hamilton T, et al.** Long-term effectiveness and safety of recombinant human interferon gamma therapy for atopic dermatitis despite unchanged serum IgE levels. Arch Dermatol. 1998;134:799–804.
9. **Grundmann-Kollmann M, Podda M, Ochsendorf F, et al.** Mycophenolate mofetil is effective in the treatment of atopic dermatitis. Arch Dermatol. 2001;137:870–3.
10. **Del Rosso J, Friedlander SF.** Corticosteroids: options in the era of steroid-sparing therapy. J Am Acad Dermatol. 2005;53:S50–8.

10

Gastrointestinal Disorders

A. Inflammatory Bowel Disease
Debra J. Helper, MD

B. Gallstone Disease
Raufu A. Lasisi, MD; Julia K. LeBlanc, MD

C. Peptic Ulcer Disease
Jonathan Benson, MD; Rakesh Vinayek, MD

D. Gastroesophageal Reflux Disease
Kenneth Berman, MD; Hala Fatima, MD; Rakesh Vinayek, MD

A. Inflammatory Bowel Disease

Debra J. Helper

KEY POINTS

* Inflammatory bowel disease (IBD) affects approximately 1 million Americans.
* Females and males are affected equally.
* Disease onset is typically during child-bearing years.
* Current treatments induce and maintain remission while limiting steroid use.
* Managing the pregnant patient requires special considerations.

Epidemiology

Idiopathic inflammatory bowel disease (IBD) is comprised of predominantly two conditions—ulcerative colitis (UC) and Crohn disease (CD). Indeterminate colitis (IC) is a term used for an idiopathic colitis that cannot be confidently determined to be either UC or CD. Both are relapsing and remitting disorders of the bowel causing gastrointestinal (GI) symptoms of diarrhea and abdominal pain, systemic symptoms such as fever and weight loss, sometimes associated with extraintestinal manifestations, including iritis, arthritis, skin lesions, and liver disease.

These conditions affect approximately 1 million Americans and have a prevalence and incidence that vary widely around the world. It is more common in people of northern European descent and Ashkenazi Jews, although the incidence in other parts of the world is increasing. Males and females are generally affected equally.

UC is an inflammation of the colon only, always involving the rectum and the colon in a continuous manner from the anus some distance proximally into the colon. Except in fulminant colitis, it involves the mucosa only, whereas CD is a transmural inflammation of the GI tract that can occur anywhere from mouth to anus. Most commonly, CD involves the terminal ileum and colon. Because of the transmural nature of the inflammation, CD is associated with complications such as stricture with obstruction, fistulae, and perforation with abscess.

Etiology and Pathogenesis

IBD is an immune dysfunctional disease with the T lymphocyte acting as the mediator for inflammation. While UC typically involves the TH2 pathway, CD involves TH1. The GI tract (among other areas) functions as an immunologic organ and acts as a barrier to the outside world,

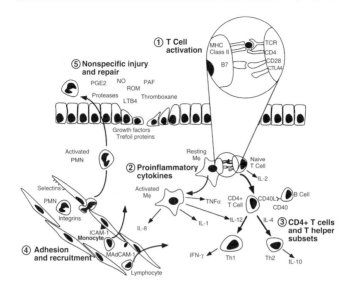

Figure 10-1 Mediators of inflammation and injury in IBD. Heavier curved lines indicate movement or differentiation of cells. TCR, T-cell receptor; PGE2, prostaglandin E2; NO, nitric oxide; PAF, platelet-activating factor; ROM, reactive oxygen metabolites; LTB4, leukotriene B4; MΦ, macrophage; PMN, polymorphonuclear cell; CD40L, CD40 ligand; ICAM-1, intercellular adhesion molecule-1; MAdCAM-1, mucosal addressin cellular adhesion molecule-1; IFN-γ, interferon-γ; TNF-α, tumor necrosis factor-α. (From Sands BE. Inflammatory Bowel Dis. New York: Lippincott-Raven Publishers. 1997;3:95–113; with permission.)

protecting an individual from various environmental antigens and pathogens. There are multiple sites of potential dysfunction, which can lead to inflammation and complications (Figure 10-1).

Although the cause of IBD is unknown, both genetic factors and environmental factors clearly play a role. Neither UC nor CD is inherited in a Mendelian fashion, and, in fact, only one member of a pair of monozygotic twins may be affected. Of the environmental factors known to affect IBD, cigarette smoking is an exacerbating factor in CD. NSAIDs and ASA may exacerbate either disease. Antibiotics, as well as infections, even those outside the GI tract, may be associated with flare-ups. Current theories of pathogenesis include lack of tolerance to luminal bacteria, as suggested by genetically altered animal models (1).

Clinical Manifestations

IBD may present with a variety of intestinal and non-intestinal symptoms. Classically, UC presents as bloody diarrhea, abdominal pain, weight loss, and fever. However, inflammation limited to the rectum (proctitis) may present as "constipation." CD typically presents as abdominal pain, with or without diarrhea, bloating, fever, and weight loss. Extraintestinal manifestations are more common with extensive colitis (UC or CD) and include eye inflammation (iritis, episcleritis, uveitis, conjunctivitis), arthritis/arthralgias, or skin lesions, such as erythema nodosum and pyoderma gangrenosum, and primary sclerosing cholangitis. Because of small bowel involvement by CD, other extraintestinal manifestations may be due to malabsorption and include growth failure with malnutrition, kidney stones (typically calcium oxalate), osteoporosis, and gallstones. Complications of extensive colitis include hemorrhage, toxic megacolon, development of dysplasia, and cancer. Additional complications of CD include obstruction, stricture, abscess, and fistulae (perianal, rectovaginal, enteroenteric, enterovesical, enterocutaneous).

The diagnosis of IBD is made based on symptoms, along with various diagnostic tests—most involving some imaging of the bowel. The diagnosis of UC is made in patients who present with bloody diarrhea when other causes are excluded (Box 10-1). Colonoscopy allows for visualization of the entire colon, as well as the terminal ileum, with biopsies to confirm the presence of a chronic colitis. Features of chronic colitis by biopsy include gland architecture distortion with basilar plasmacytosis. These are not unique to UC and can be seen in any chronic colitis. Therefore, it is important to exclude all other causes before making the diagnosis of UC. Endoscopically, the appearance of UC is that of continuous inflammation from the anus some distance proximally, typically with erythema, exudate, and erosions, but without discrete ulcers. CD involving only the colon may present as bloody or non-bloody diarrhea, with abdominal pain, and is suggested by the endoscopic appearance of discontinuous inflammation, aphthous ulcers, discrete ulcers, or cobblestoning. The presence of perianal disease, such as indurated skin tags, fissures, or fistulae, suggests the diagnosis of CD (Figure 10-2). Although the terminal ileum may be mildly erythematous in individuals with UC involving the whole colon (a condition known radiographically as backwash ileitis), aphthae, edema, or narrowing of the lumen suggests CD. Likewise, a finding of non-caseating granuloma by biopsy is diagnostic of CD.

Imaging of the small bowel is accomplished by radiographic methods, including dedicated small bowel follow-through or enteroclysis, with or without CT. Video capsule endoscopy is not recommended as an initial evaluation in patients with symptoms suggestive of obstruction. Double-balloon enteroscopy is a relatively new technique for direct endoscopic imaging of the small bowel, which may be useful in cases where suspicion of CD is high but other studies are negative, or if there is a need for biopsies or endoscopic treatment of a small bowel stricture. Abdominal and pelvic CT are used to evaluate for complications such as abscess, obstruction, or fistula.

Differential Diagnosis

In women, the prevalence of irritable bowel syndrome (IBS) is far greater than that of IBD. Because the symptoms of CD are very similar to those of IBS, patients with CD can remain misdiagnosed as having IBS for many years. There is no diagnostic test for IBS; it is a diagnosis of exclusion.

Box 10-1   Differential Diagnosis of Inflammatory Bowel Disease

Infections
Viral
- Acute self-limited colitis
- CMV
- Norovirus
- Adenovirus
- Astrovirus
- Herpes virus
- HIV

Bacterial
- *Shigella*
- *Salmonella*
- Shiga-toxin producing *E.Coli*
- *Campylobacter*
- *Yersinia*
- *Clostridium difficile*

Mycobacterial
- *M. tuberculosis*

Fungal
- Aspergillosis

Protozoal/Parasitic
- *Entamoeba histolytica*
- *Lymphogranuloma venereum*
- Cryptosporidiosis
- *Cyclospora*
- *Giardia*

Vascular
- Vasculitis
- Low-flow colonic ischemia
- Chronic mesenteric ischemia
- Radiation enteritis
- Cocaine abuse

Medications
- NSAIDs
- Gold
- Isotretinoin
- Colon cleansing prep
- High-dose pancreatic enzymes

Miscellaneous
- Graft versus host disease
- Diverticula-associated colitis
- Solitary rectal ulcer syndrome

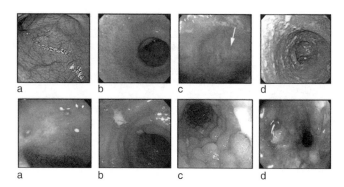

Figure 10-2a   Top Row (a) normal colon (b) mild ulcerative colitis (c) moderate ulcerative colitis, sharp line of demarcation at arrow and (d) severe ulcerative colitis. Bottom row (a) Crohn's colitis, aphthous ulcers (b) Crohn's colitis, discrete ulcers (c) Crohn's colitis, cobblestone pattern and (d) Crohn's colitis, inflammatory stricture.

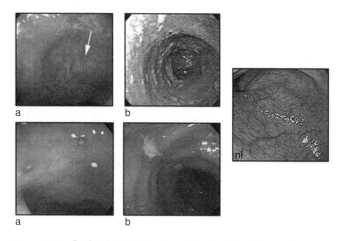

Figure 10-2b   Top Row (a) mild ulcerative colitis, sharp line of demarcation at arrow (b) moderately severe ulcerative colitis. Bottom row (a) Crohn's colitis, aphthous ulcers (b) Crohn's colitis, discrete ulcers.

It is unreasonably hazardous and expensive to exclude CD in everyone suspected of having IBS. Features that should prompt a search for IBD include the presence of alarm symptoms and signs such as blood in the stool, nocturnal diarrhea, weight loss, fever, anemia, or hypoalbuminemia. Suspicion should remain high for those with a family history of IBD or other autoimmune diseases and in patients with extraintestinal manifestations suggestive of IBD. Lack of response to therapy for IBS should be an indication to investigate further for IBD. Serologic markers for inflammation, such as

C-reactive protein and sedimentation rate, also may suggest the presence of IBD in a patient with symptoms otherwise typical of IBS.

Management

Medical treatment is directed at controlling inflammation (putting the disease into remission) and maintaining remission. Other goals of therapy are to close fistulae, treat complications, restore nutrition, and achieve a normal lifestyle. Surgical therapy is reserved for treatment of complications, such as abscesses, obstruction due to fixed stricture, medically refractory disease, or development of dysplasia or cancer.

The following agents are effective to induce remission in UC: 5-aminosalicylates (5-ASA or mesalamine); corticosteroids; the anti-TNF alpha monoclonal antibody infliximab (2); and cyclosporine A. There are a number of oral and topical 5-ASA agents available (Table 10-1). While topical 5-ASA is more effective than oral 5-ASA or steroids for active disease limited to the rectum and left side of the colon, no single oral agent is superior to any other for inducing or maintaining remission in UC (3).

Induction of remission may be accomplished in CD with 5-ASA agents released in the terminal ileum (Asacol and Pentasa), corticosteroids, and controlled-ileal release budesonide (for ileum and right colon only). Biologic agents, including infliximab, adalimumab (a humanized anti-TNF alpha monoclonal antibody), and an anti-alpha integrin monoclonal antibody, natalizumab, can induce remission. Traditional treatment has been "step-up," starting with a 5-ASA agent for mild to moderate disease and moving to steroids for moderate to severe disease, while reserving biologic agents for patients who fail to enter remission with conventional therapies. That concept is being challenged by a "top-down" strategy of earlier use of biologic agents. More data are needed to determine which patients with IBD might benefit most from either strategy. The American Gastrointestinal Association (AGA) has convened an expert panel to review the risks and benefits of biologic agents in IBD and to develop a consensus on the use of such agents (4).

Maintenance of remission in UC and CD is achieved by continuation of the agent that induced remission, with the exception of steroids. In the case of steroids, a maintenance agent should be introduced as soon as the steroid has been shown to be effective and tapering of the steroid has

Table 10-1 Distribution of 5-Aminosalicylic acid Compounds

Agent	Colon	Small bowel
Sulfasalazine	Yes	No
Olsalazine	Yes	No
Balsalazide	Yes	No
Mesalamine oral	Yes	Yes
Enemas	Rectum to splenic flexure	No
Suppositories	Rectum only	No

begun. Steroid-sparing maintenance agents include the purine analogs, aza-thioprine and 6-mercaptopurine (6-MP) (5), which have also been shown to close fistulae, and infliximab for both UC and CD. Additional steroid-sparing maintenance agents shown to be effective in CD include methotrex-ate (6), adalimumab, and natalizumab. Some patients with CD may benefit from longer-term therapy with lower dose (6 mg/d) budesonide (7).

5-ASA agents are usually quite safe, though they rarely may cause hemo-lytic anemia, nephritis, hepatitis, and worsened colitis. Allergic reactions to the sulfa-containing portion of sulfasalazine can be avoided by the use of a different 5-ASA compound. Less commonly, allergy is to the salicylate por-tion common to all of these agents. Corticosteroids produce side effects, including hypertension, mood swings, hypokalemia, hyperglycemia, weight gain, moon facies, striae, infection, bone demineralization, cataracts, and, rarely, aseptic necrosis. Steroids are not effective as a long-term treatment of either UC or CD. Budesonide has fewer steroid side effects over the short term but is not recommended as a long-term treatment at induction doses (9 mg/d). The anti-TNF biologic agents are potentially more toxic. Reactivation of tuberculosis (TB) can be a lethal effect of the anti-TNF agents; they are con-traindicated in those individuals with a high risk of TB. All patients receiv-ing these agents need to be screened for TB with PPD and chest x-ray, if necessary. Other infections, such as fungal, other mycobacterial, and bac-terial disease, may occur, especially as abscesses in patients with CD and perianal disease. Lupus-like reactions, demyelinating disease, worsening congestive heart failure, acute allergic reaction, delayed infusion reaction, and an increased risk of lymphoma have been associated with the use of anti-TNF agents. Natalizumab also increases the risk of infection and can induce acute allergic reactions. A rare, but devastating, infection with Jakob-Creutzfeld (JC) virus (progressive multifocal leukoencephalopathy, PML) was diagnosed in patients receiving natalizumab while on another immuno-suppressant. It should be used with caution and only as a monotherapy in CD. Azathioprine and 6-MP also increase the risk of infection, particularly viral. They can cause bone marrow suppression, pancreatitis, hepatitis, and lymphoma. Methotrexate increases the risk of infection, may cause hepatitis leading to cirrhosis, and has been associated with neuropathy and hyper-sensitivity pneumonitis. Cyclosporine increases the risk of infection and can cause nephropathy, tremor, paresthesias, seizures, hyperkalemia, hyperten-sion, and hypomagnesemia. Prophylactic antibiotics and antiviral agents are recommended while a patient is on high-dose cyclosporine.

Surgical therapy for UC involves removal of the entire colon and rectum, with either an end-ileostomy or an ileoanal pouch anastomo-sis (IAPA). This is performed in the case of failure of medical therapy or development of dysplasia or cancer of the colon. In CD, surgery may involve partial resections for failure of medical therapy, strictures or fis-tulae, stricturoplasty, incision and drainage, or perianal abscesses, and treatment of perianal fistulae. Total proctocolectomy with end-ileostomy may be necessary for extensive refractory colitis, with or without perianal disease, as well as for the development of dysplasia or cancer of the colon. IAPA is generally not an option for patients with CD colitis.

Issues of particular concern for women with IBD include fertility, pregnancy (8), and bone health. Fertility is generally normal in women with CD unless there has been extensive pelvic sepsis. It is also normal in women with UC who have not undergone an IAPA. The outcome of pregnancy is primarily determined by the health of the mother. It is better in women who remain in remission through the course of the pregnancy. Remaining in remission through the pregnancy is more likely in women who are in remission at the time of conception. When the disease is active, babies are more likely to be born prematurely and have low birth-weight. All of the therapies used to induce and maintain remission in IBD may be used in pregnancy, except for methotrexate. Azathioprine and 6-MP are considered Category D in pregnancy, and, although they have been used safely in pregnancy in IBD, their use must be individualized. Women with IBD should discuss the use of various therapies during conception and pregnancy with an IBD specialist and a high-risk obstetrical specialist. The mode of delivery should be determined according to usual obstetrical guidelines, although patients with active perianal disease may require Caesarean section.

The risk of cervical cancer is increased in women with IBD on immunosuppressive therapy, particularly azathioprine and 6-MP. Such individuals should be monitored closely and treated aggressively if cervical dysplasia develops.

Bone disease in IBD is worsened by smoking, malabsorption, decreased intake of calcium and vitamin D, hypogonadism, effect of steroids, and decreased physical activity. Clearly, those who smoke should be encouraged and given the tools to stop at every point of encounter. Calcium and vitamin D intake should be recommended, and, if this is not possible and if there is a suspicion of malabsorption, vitamin D levels should be measured, with replacement therapy as indicated. Physical exercise should be recommended, and disease activity and symptoms should be aggressively treated to allow for this. Bone density should be measured in all patients with IBD. Corticosteroids should be avoided in IBD patients with low bone density, but, if steroids are necessary, a bisphosphonate may be added early in the course of steroid therapy to avoid additional bone loss. The time of exposure to corticosteroids should be limited in all patients with IBD by the early addition of a steroid-sparing agent (9).

References

1. **Cho J, Weaver C.** The genetics of inflammatory bowel disease. Gastroenterology. 2007;133:1327–39.
2. **Rutgeerts P, Sandborn WJ, Feagan BG, et al.** Infliximab for induction and maintenance therapy for ulcerative colitis. N Engl J Med. 2005;353:2462–76.
3. **Hanauer SB.** Medical therapy for ulcerative colitis. In Kirsner JB (ed): Inflammatory Bowel Disease, 5th ed. Philadelphia: WB Saunders; 2000. pp. 529–56.
4. **Clark M, Colombel, JF, Feagan BG, et al.** American Gastroenterological Association consensus development conference on the use of biologics

in the treatment of inflammatory bowel disease, June 21–23, 2006. Gastroenterology. 2007;133:312–39.

5. **Present DH, Korelitz BI, Wisch N, et al.** Treatment of Crohn's disease with 6-mercaptopurine. A long-term, randomized, double-blind study. N Engl J Med. 1980;302:981–7.

6. **Feagan BG, Fedorak RN, Irvine EJ, et al.** A comparison of methotrexate with placebo for the maintenance of remission in Crohn's disease. North American Crohn's Study Group Investigators. N Engl J Med. 2000;342:1627–32.

7. **Hanauer S, Sandborn WJ, Persson A, et al.** Budesonide as maintenance treatment of Crohn's disease: a placebo-controlled trial. Aliment Pharmacol Ther. 2005;21:363–71.

8. **Kane S.** Inflammatory bowel disease in pregnancy. Gastroenterol Clin North Am. 2003;32:323–40.

9. **Lichtenstein GR, Sands BE, Pazianas M.** Prevention and treatment of osteoporosis in inflammatory bowel disease. Inflamm Bowel Dis. 2006;12:797–813.

B. Gallstone Disease

Raufu A. Lasisi and Julia K. LeBlanc

KEY POINTS

- The prevalence of gallstones in women in the U.S. between the age of 20 and 50 years ranges from 5–20%; among those over 50 years, the prevalence is 25–30%.
- Gallstones are twice as common in women as in men.
- Conditions associated with an increase in the prevalence of gallstones in women include family history of gallstones, pregnancy, use of hormonal contraceptives, and hormone replacement therapy.
- Cholecystectomy remains the gold standard of treatment.
- Prevention of gallstones is currently under investigation; however, reduction of obesity is recommended.

Epidemiology

There are more than 20 million individuals with gallstones in the U.S. (1). Among gastrointestinal disorders, gallstone disease is one of the most common diagnoses requiring hospitalization. Direct cost of gallstone disease in the U.S. in 1998 was approximately $5.8 billion (2). Eighty percent of all gallstones in Americans are composed of cholesterol, while pigment

stones account for the remaining 20%. While ultrasound is useful in identifying gallstones, it cannot differentiate between the types of stones.
Women are 2–3 times more likely to have gallstones than are men. The
prevalence of gallstones increases with age, since gallstones rarely dis-
solve spontaneously. In American women between the ages of 20 and 50
years, the prevalence ranges from 5–20% and increases to 25–30% among
those over 50 years. The prevalence among Mexican-American women is
26.7% (1). Most notably, the highest prevalence in the world exists among
Pima Indians (Native American) with a prevalence of 73% in women over
the age of 25 years (3). In other Native American groups in the U.S., up
to 30% of men and 64% of women have gallstone disease (4–6). Gallstone
disease in women of African or Asian descent ranges from 3–5% (7).

Most gallstones never cause symptoms; however, the prevalence of
symptomatic gallstone disease in women has been reported to range from
18–65% (8). Although the incidence is more difficult to assess, 1–3% of
women without a history of gallstones develop them during pregnancy (9).

Risk Factors

Risk factors for gallstones in women (Box 10-2) include diabetes, obesity, metabolic syndrome, hypertriglyceridemia and low HDL, ileal Crohn's
disease, and cirrhosis. In a large prospective study of obese women,
those with a body mass index (BMI) >45 kg/m^2 were 7 times more
likely to develop gallstones (10). Thus, reduction of obesity is thought to
decrease the chance of developing gallstones. On the other hand, rapid
weight loss is another risk factor for gallstones. Up to half of patients will
develop gallstones or biliary sludge (microlithiasis) within 6 months of
gastric bypass surgery. Formation is thought to be secondary to increased
cholesterol secretion during diet restriction. The prophylactic use of ursodeoxycholic acid has had some success in this population (11). It also has
been recommended that weight loss should not exceed 1.5 kg/week.

Box 10-2   Risk Factors for Cholesterol Gallstone Disease in Women

- Fecundity
- Increasing age
- Obesity
- Diets: high refined carbohydrate, low fiber, high cholesterol
- Hypertriglyceridemia and low HDL cholesterol
- Pregnancy
- Hormones: estrogen replacement therapy, oral/non-oral contraceptives
- Sedentary life-style
- Rapid weight loss
- Drugs: octreotide, ceftriaxone, fibrates
- Insulin resistance during pregnancy
- Ileal Crohn disease
- Cirrhosis

Medications have been linked to the formation of gallstones (12). Fibrate drugs are a risk factor for developing gallstones, since their use may result in supersaturation of cholesterol and subsequent cholesterol gallstone precipitation. Ceftriaxone causes gallstones by precipitating out of bile as it forms complexes with calcium. Octreotide contributes to gallstone formation by inhibiting gall bladder motility.

During pregnancy, bile is more lithogenic, probably because of the effects of increased estrogen, which results in increased cholesterol secretion and supersaturation of bile (13). In addition, it has been observed that progesterone contributes to stasis of the gall bladder by modulating extracellular calcium entry.

Clinical Presentation

Patients with symptomatic gallstone disease usually present with biliary colic. Biliary colic is a sharp and constant severe pain that results from increased pressure in the gall bladder and may occur in the setting of gall bladder or cystic duct outlet obstruction. It is typically located in the right upper quadrant or mid-abdominal region or in the chest, and it usually occurs 1–2 hours after eating. The pain may radiate to the back and may last 1–24 hours. In women, the pain may be described as a sensation akin to tight undergarments around the upper abdomen. The pain is occasionally unrelated to meals and often is associated with nausea and vomiting. No factors have been found to relieve the pain, and it is not exacerbated by movement. In the setting of right upper quadrant pain, fever, and jaundice (Charcot's triad), one should suspect acute cholecystitis. Patients also may present with other complications of gallstone disease, such as biliary acute pancreatitis, choledocholithiasis (bile duct stones), chronic cholecystitis, gangrene, perforation, cholecystoenteric fistula involving the small bowel, gallstone ileus, or emphysematous cholecystitis. The abdominal examination is often unremarkable. In the setting of acute cholecystitis, however, the patient may experience right upper quadrant tenderness from the ultrasound probe during transabdominal ultrasound of the gallbladder (Murphy's sign) (14).

Diagnosis

Various tests are used to diagnose gallstone disease (Table 10-2). Laboratory studies that may be helpful in identifying complications of gallstone disease, such as acute pancreatitis, acute cholecystitis, and choledocholithiasis, include white blood cell count and differential, amylase, lipase, AST (aspartate aminotransferase), ALT (alanine aminotransferase), total bilirubin, fractionated bilirubin, alkaline phosphatase, and GGT (gamma glutamyltransferase). Because ALT is found almost exclusively in the liver, it is a better indicator of hepatobiliary injury than is AST, which also is found in cardiac, skeletal, kidney, and brain tissue. In the setting of choledocholithiasis, an elevated AST is usually the earliest abnormality detected and is typically elevated less than five-fold. Alkaline phosphatase is made by bile duct epithelial cells and is elevated in biliary obstruction. In this setting, an elevated alkaline phosphatase can be

Table 10-2   Tests Used in Gall Bladder Disease

Test	Considerations
Transabdominal Ultrasound	Most frequent first test
	Less useful in detecting stones <3 mm
	Useful in detecting pericholecystic fluid
MRI/MRCP	Expensive
	Useful in detecting choledocholithiasis >5 mm
Endoscopic ultrasound (EUS)	Requires conscious sedation
	Useful in detecting choledocholithiasis <5 mm
	Not widely available
Computed tomography (CT)	Useful in detecting acute pancreatitis
	Not used for diagnosing gallstones
Cholescintigraphy (HIDA)	Used in diagnosing acute cholecystitis

observed without elevations of total bilirubin. Since alkaline phosphatase also is made by liver, bone, and the intestinal tract, GGT elevation is more sensitive than alkaline phosphatase in biliary obstruction.

Transabdominal ultrasound has a specificity of 99%; however, gallstones <3 mm may not be detected. Ultrasound also is useful in detecting pericholecystic fluid, which occurs in the setting of inflammation. Magnetic resonance cholangiopancreatography (MRCP) and endoscopic ultrasound (EUS) are useful in detecting choledocholithiasis (bile duct stones) (15). Computed tomography (CT) and EUS should be requested if pancreatitis due to choledocholithiasis is suspected (16). Cholescintigraphy (hepatobiliary iminodiacetic acid, or HIDA) is valuable in the diagnosis of acute cholecystitis, since it can be used to assess cystic duct patency. The specificity of the HIDA scan in acute cholecystitis is 90%. Elevation of liver function tests also support the diagnosis of biliary obstruction. Up to 10% of patients with acute cholecystitis are acalculous (17).

Management

Management of symptomatic gallstones involves cholecystectomy. Biliary colic is treated by mitigating the underlying cause, which may include removal of common bile duct stones and treatment of related complications or infection. The pain medication of choice is meperidine, because it does little to increase the pressure of the sphincter of Oddi (18). The method of gallstone removal varies based on patient comorbidities related to surgery. For patients who are good surgical candidates, laparoscopic cholecystectomy is recommended. It is associated with early oral intake, a shorter length of stay in hospital, and a shorter recovery time. Compared to open cholecystectomy, however, there is no difference in mortality, complications, or operative time.

In 10% of laparoscopic cholecystectomy cases, the procedure is converted to an open cholecystectomy (19). Laparoscopic cholecystectomy may be associated with common bile duct injury, such as laceration or stricture formation, and 15% of the patients will develop frank diarrhea postoperatively (20). The risk of developing right-sided colon cancer has been reported to increase 10 years after cholecystectomy (21). The pathophysiology for this observation remains unclear but may be related to continuous exposure of the colon to biliary acids and fat. In patients who are unable to undergo surgery because of comorbidities, bile acid therapy with ursodeoxycholic acid or chenodeoxychoic acid may be a reasonable alternative. However, up to 40% of patients will develop gallstones again within 5 years (22). Bile acid therapy and external shockwave lithotripsy also have resulted in significant recurrence rates (23). Endoscopic retrograde cholangiopancreatography (ERCP) with biliary sphincterotomy is another alternative in patients who cannot undergo surgery, since a sphincterotomy of up to 1 cm in size can be made.

References

1. **Everhart JE, Khare M, Hill M, et al.** Prevalence and ethnic differences in gallbladder disease in the United States. Gastroenterology. 1999;117:632–9.
2. **Sandler RS, Everhart JE, Donowitz M, et al.** The burden of selected digestive diseases in the United States. Gastroenterology. 2002;122:1500–11.
3. **Sampliner RE, Bennett PH, Comess LJ, et al.** Gallbladder disease in Pima Indians. Demonstration of high prevalence and early onset by cholecystography. N Engl J Med. 1970;283:1358.
4. **Thistle JL, Eckhart KL Jr, Nensel RE, et al.** Prevalence of gallbladder disease among Chippewa Indians. Mayo Clin Proc. 1971;46:603.
5. **Williams CN, Johnston JL, Weldon KLM.** Prevalence of gallstones and gallbladder disease in Canadian Micmac Indian women. Can Med Assoc J. 1977;117:758.
6. **Everhart JE, Yeh F, Lee ET, et al.** Prevalence of gallbladder disease in American Indian populations: Findings from the Strong Heart Study. Hepatology. 2002;35:1507.
7. **Kratzer W, Mason RA, Kachele V.** Prevalence of gallstones in sonographic surverys worldwide. J Clin Ultrasound. 1999;27:1–7.
8. **Diehl AK.** Symptoms of gallstone disease. Bailliere's Clinical Gastroenterology. Nov 1992;6:643–4.
9. **Valdivieso V, Covarrubias C, Siegel F, et al.** Pregnancy and cholelithiasis: pathogenesis and natural course of gallstones diagnosed in early puerperium. Hepatology. 1993;1–4.
10. **Stampfer MJ, Maclure KM, Colditz GA, et al.** Risk of symptomatic gallstones in women with severe obesity. Am J Clin Nut. 1992;55:652–8.
11. **Shiffman ML, Kaplan GD, Brinkman-Kaplan V, et al.** Prophylaxis against gallstone formation with ursodeoxycholic acid in patients in very-low-calorie diet program. Ann Intern Med. 1995;122:899.
12. Anonymous. Gallbladder disease as a side effect of drugs influencing lipid metabolism. Experience in the Coronary Drug Project. N Engl J Med. 1977;296:1185.
13. **Van Bodegraven AA, Bohmer CJ, Manoliu RA, et al.** Gallbladder contents and fasting gallbladder volumes during and after pregnancy. Scand J Gastroenterol. 1998;33:993.

14. **Adedeji OA, McAdam WA.** Murphy's sign, acute cholecystitis and elderly people. J R Coll Surg. Edinb. Apr 1996;41:88.

15. **Ledro-Cano L.** Suspected choledocholithiasis: endoscopic ultrasound or magnetic resonance cholangio-pancreatography? A systematic review. Eur J Gastroenterol Hepatol. 2007;19:1007–11.

16. **Chak A, Hawes RH, Cooper GS, et al.** Prospective assessment of the utility of EUS in the evaluation of gallstone pancreatitis. Gastrointest Endosc. 1999;49:599.

17. **Barie PS, Fischer E.** Acute acalculous cholecystitis. J Am Coll Surg. 1995;180:232.

18. **Elta GH, Barnett JL.** Meperidine need not be proscribed during sphincter of Oddi manometry. Gastrointest Endosc. 1994;40:7.

19. **Livingston EH, Rege RV.** A nationalwide study of conversion from laparoscopic to open cholecystectomy. Am J Surg. 2004;188:205–11.

20. **Bernard HR, Hartman TW.** Complications after laparoscopic cholecystectomy. Am J Surg. 1993;165:533.

21. **Ekbom A, Yuen J, Adami HO, et al.** Cholecystectomy and colorectal cancer. Gastroenterology. Jul 1993;105:286–8.

22. **Hood KA, Ruppin DC, Dowling RH.** The British-Belgian Gallstone Study Group. Gallstone recurrence and its prevention: the British-Belgian Gallstone Study Group's posts-dissolution trial. Gut. 1993;34:1277–88.

23. **Sackmann M, Niller H, Klueppelberg U, et al.** Gallstone recurrence after shock wave therapy. Gastroenterology. 1994;106:225–30.

C. Peptic Ulcer Disease

Jonathan Benson and Rakesh Vinayek

KEY POINTS

- Ten percent of Americans are affected by peptic ulcer disease (PUD), costing $10 billion annually.
- *Helicobacter pylori* (*H. pylori*) and non-steroidal anti-inflammatory drugs (NSAIDs) are the most significant risk factors for peptic ulcers.
- Patients using chronic NSAIDs and patients with peptic ulceration who cannot stop NSAIDs may require long-term acid-suppression therapy or misoprostol.
- Correlation of symptoms to PUD found on endoscopy (the gold standard for peptic ulcer diagnosis) is weak.
- PUD found in pregnancy should be treated with lansoprazole (a proton pump inhibitor) or H2 receptor antagonists.
- Of those with dyspepsia, only 10% have peptic ulcers.

Peptic ulcers are defined as defects in the gastrointestinal mucosa that occur as a result of gastric acid and pepsin. They are most commonly located in the stomach and duodenum, where concentrations of acid are highest. Less commonly, they occur in the lower esophagus, the distal duodenum, the jejunum (as in unopposed hypersecretory states such as Zollinger-Ellison syndrome), in hiatal hernias (Cameron ulcers), or in ectopic gastric mucosa (e.g., Meckel's diverticulum) (1,2). Anti-secretory medications, in conjunction with the discovery that infection with *H. pylori* and use of NSAIDs are strong risk factors for peptic ulcer disease (PUD), have allowed significant advances in prevention, management, healing, and limiting recurrence of peptic ulcers (3).

Epidemiology

Although the incidence of peptic ulcers in Western countries has declined over the last 3 decades, possibly as a result of the increasing use of proton pump inhibitors and decreasing rates of *H. pylori* infection, approximately 10% of all Americans are still affected. Approximately 500 000 persons develop peptic ulcer disease in the U.S. each year. In 70% of patients, it occurs between the ages of 25 and 64 years. The annual direct and indirect health care costs of the disease are estimated at about $10 billion (2). The worldwide ulcer prevalence differs, with duodenal ulcers dominating in Western populations and gastric ulcers being more frequent in Asia, especially in Japan. Interestingly, hospitalizations for ulcer complications have increased in the elderly population in the past few decades. This is likely due to increased use of NSAIDs and age-related decline in prostaglandin levels in elderly persons (1). *H. pylori* infection and NSAIDs are independent risk factors for peptic ulcer disease (PUD) that have additive or synergistic effects on adverse gastrointestinal outcomes. Other factors, such as cigarette smoking, oral bisphosphonates, immunosuppressive medications, potassium supplements, and psychological stress, all have been suggested as contributors to the development of PUD (4,5).

Etiology

As noted above, *H. pylori* infection and the use of NSAIDs are the predominant causes of PUD in the U.S., accounting for approximately 50% and 25% of cases, respectively (6). Uncommon causes include hyper-secretory states, such as gastrinoma, antral G-cell hyperplasia, retained antrum syndrome, idiopathic hyper-secretory duodenal ulcers, systemic mastocytosis, and basophilic leukemia. Crohn's disease and viral infections such as *Herpes simplex* virus type-1 and cytomegalovirus also cause gastroduodenal ulcerations. Critical illnesses, surgery, cirrhosis, chronic renal failure, or hypoperfusion may result in gastroduodenal erosions or ulcers (stress ulcers) (7).

Helicobacter pylori

The isolation of *H. pylori* in the early 1980s was one of the most exciting advances in the history of PUD, and it has dramatically changed the management of peptic ulcers. Eradication of *H. pylori* infection is now the mainstay of treatment for PUD and has resulted in very high ulcer healing rates. Recurrence rates have dropped dramatically, especially for individuals with duodenal ulcers. Although *H. pylori* is present in the gastroduodenal mucosa in most patients with duodenal ulcers, only a minority (10–15%) of patients with *H. pylori* infection develop PUD (8).

H. pylori is a gram-negative spiral-shaped bacterium containing 4–6 unipolar flagellae. It produces urease and mucolytic proteases that help the bacterium survive the hostile environment of the stomach. Urease is responsible for the resistance of *H. pylori* to acid. *H. pylori* organisms may be found in otherwise healthy persons (1). In developing countries, the infection is acquired in childhood. In developed countries, such as the U.S., the prevalence may vary depending on the ethnic group and socioeconomic status (*H. pylori* prevalence is inversely related to socioeconomic status) (4). Currently, the specific mode of transmission (fecal–oral, oral–oral, or gastric–oral) is not well understood, although there is evidence that the organism is transmitted from person to person (9).

H. pylori evades attack by the host immune system and causes chronic, indolent inflammation via several mechanisms. *H. pylori* can damage the mucosal defense system by reducing the thickness of the mucus gel layer, diminishing mucosal blood flow, and interacting with the gastric epithelium throughout all stages of the infection. The presence of an outer inflammatory protein and a functional cytotoxin-associated gene, *Cag*A, increases virulence and ulcerogenic potential by interfering with gastric epithelial cell-signaling pathways, thereby regulating cellular responses and possibly contributing to apical junction barrier disruption, interleukin-8 secretion, and phenotypic changes to gastric epithelial cells. *H. pylori* infection also can increase gastric acid secretion by producing various antigens, virulence factors, and soluble mediators. *H. pylori* induces inflammation, which increases parietal cell mass and, therefore, the capacity to secrete acid. The presence of bacteria in the antrum leads to a loss of D cells, which release somatostatin, and allows the antral G cells to release gastrin without inhibition. This, in turn, leads to increased gastric acid secretion and ulcer formation (10). Patients with *H. pylori* infection have increased resting and meal-stimulated gastrin levels and decreased gastric mucus production and duodenal mucosal bicarbonate secretion, all of which favor ulcer formation. Eradication of *H. pylori* greatly reduces the incidence of ulcer recurrence from 67% to 6% in patients with duodenal ulcers and from 59% to 4% in patients with gastric ulcers (11).

Non-Steroidal Anti-inflammatory Drugs

Despite their well-accepted anti-inflammatory and analgesic benefits, NSAID use is probably the most common cause of gastrointestinal mucosal injury in developed countries. NSAIDs, including aspirin, significantly increase the risk of adverse gastrointestinal events, particularly those related to gastric and/or duodenal mucosal injury, erosions, ulcers, and ulcer complications, especially bleeding (12). The clinician needs to have a high index of suspicion, since 30–50% of patients may not even report using these drugs, many of which are available in over-the-counter preparations. NSAIDs disrupt the mucosal defense mechanism by both topical and systemic effects. Topical effects of NSAIDs cause direct injury to the gastric epithelium. Systemically, by inhibiting the cyclooxygenase enzymes, NSAIDs inhibit the formation of prostaglandins and their protective cyclooxygenase-2-mediated effects. This leads to a decrease in mucus and bicarbonate production, mucosal blood flow, and epithelial cell proliferation, which in turn leads to increased hydrogen ion back-diffusion and mucosal injury. Prostaglandin inhibition also results in alterations in the tight intercellular junctions and trapping of neutrophils within the capillaries. The neutrophils release cytokines, increasing the inflammatory reaction (13). Coexisting *H. pylori* infection increases the likelihood and intensity of NSAID-induced damage (14).

Duodenal ulcers occur in approximately 10% of persons taking NSAIDs long-term. Risk factors associated with ulcer formation and gastrointestinal bleeding include: age above 60 years; personal history of PUD; past history of gastrointestinal hemorrhage; ingestion of more than one NSAID concurrently; taking anticoagulants with NSAIDs; and comorbid conditions, primarily cardiovascular disease. NSAIDs are responsible for approximately half of perforated ulcers, which occur most commonly in older patients who are taking aspirin or other NSAIDs for cardiovascular disease or arthropathy. Attempts have been made to avoid gastrointestinal ulceration through the use of newer agents that preferentially inhibit the cyclooxygenase (COX)-2 isoform (15). Although these agents are less ulcerogenic, and the risk of ulcers among those taking these drugs appears to be about 3–5%, the potential gastroduodenal-sparing effects of these drugs are lost when they are used along with aspirin. Prophylactic therapy with high-dose H-2 receptor antagonists or proton pump inhibitors (PPIs) may be as effective as misoprostol (Cytotec) in preventing gastroduodenal ulceration caused by NSAIDs (16).

Clinical Features or Presentation

The clinical features of PUD range from silent ulceration presenting with upper gastrointestinal tract hemorrhage or perforation to the classical symptoms of dyspepsia and epigastric pain. The classical symptoms traditionally ascribed to a duodenal ulcer are gnawing or burning epigastric pain, occurring 2–5 hours after meals or on an empty stomach, and nocturnal pain relieved by food intake, antacids, or anti-secretory agents (2). These symptoms occur in only 50% of patients with duodenal ulcers. Pain related to gastric ulcers is often associated with onset shortly after a meal but may be difficult to distinguish by history from duodenal ulceration. Pain does not define an ulcer, however, and the absence of pain does not preclude the diagnosis, especially in the elderly, who can present with "silent ulcer" complications. No specific symptom helps to differentiate between *H. pylori*-associated or NSAID-associated ulcers, but a careful history can identify surreptitious NSAID users and an appropriate *H. pylori* test can detect infected individuals. Less common symptoms include nausea, vomiting, cramping pain, indigestion, heartburn, intolerance to fatty foods, and anorexia (although 20% of patients may describe weight gain or increased appetite) (6). Weight loss precipitated by fear of food intake is characteristic of gastric ulcers. In a Scandinavian study (17), symptoms of anxiety, depression, and neurasthenia were seen significantly more commonly among female patients with chronic PUD when compared to a control group of women without PUD.

Psychosocial Issues

Psychosocial factors, such as stress, remain controversial in the development of PUD. Up to 20% of patients with PUD have no clear risk factors. Stress is well-described as being associated with dyspeptic symptoms, but convincing evidence is lacking to suggest that stress has a causal relationship to peptic ulceration. This may be partly due to the decrease in original investigations into the "stress-acid theory" that took place after the discovery of other dominant risk factors for PUD (5). Still, historical medical databases (6) suggest that during times of extreme stress, such as air-raids during World War II, earthquakes, etc., the incidence of perforated peptic ulcers increases transiently. At present, however, no study has definitively shown an association of emotional stress with peptic ulcer formation.

Pregnancy and Contraception

Dyspeptic symptoms are common during pregnancy, and often empiric PPI therapy is initiated. Ulcer symptoms are milder and may improve during pregnancy. Vomiting, when it occurs, is often nocturnal or postprandial and worse during the third trimester. Multiple trials have evaluated PPI therapy in pregnancy, and there appears to be no increased risk of malformations, low birth-weight, or number of preterm deliveries while taking PPIs prior to or during pregnancy in most large studies (18–20). Limited evidence in an animal study suggested that omeprazole may be associated with birth defects (21); because of this, PPIs remain second-line after H2-receptor antagonists (ranitidine and famotidine are category B) during pregnancy. If a PPI is necessary, lansoprazole is recommended (category B). If *H. pylori* is diagnosed during pregnancy, treatment may be delayed until after delivery (21–23).

The use of any medication while taking oral contraceptives raises concern for decreasing the effectiveness of contraception if bioavailability is affected. The effects of lansoprazole, a PPI, on the bioavailability of ethinyloestradiol and levonorgestrel were investigated, and no effect on bioavailability was found, indicating that effectiveness of contraception is not hampered by taking these medications together (24).

Diagnosis

Since the symptoms and signs of PUD are not specific and may overlap with other gastrointestinal conditions, diagnosis on the basis of medical history and physical examination alone is difficult. The diagnosis is usually based on the results of esophagogastroduodenoscopy (EGD) or an upper gastrointestinal tract radiographic study. The findings of these two tests correlate in 80–90% of the cases. EGD is the preferred method for evaluating suspected duodenal ulcer disease, because the upper gastrointestinal radiographic study is less sensitive and not as effective in detecting small ulcers (1). Furthermore, EGD allows biopsies of the antrum for *H. pylori*, biopsies of gastric ulcers to differentiate benign from malignant ulcers, and evaluation of infectious, infiltrative, or granulomatous causes of ulcers. The patient also should be evaluated for alarm symptoms (Box 10-3) (3). Anemia, hematemesis, melena, or heme-positive stools suggest bleeding; vomiting suggests gastric ulcer or obstruction secondary to pyloric stenosis; anorexia or weight loss suggest cancer; persistent abdominal pain radiating to the back suggests penetration (continuation of the ulcer into adjacent organs, such as liver or pancreas); and severe, spreading, upper abdominal pain suggests perforation. The decision regarding when to perform endoscopy for symptoms of upper abdominal pain may be aided by the American Gastroenterological Association (AGA) position statement regarding approach to dyspepsia symptoms (25). Those patients <55 years of age should be tested for *H. pylori* and treated with triple therapy if positive (in populations in which *H. pylori* prevalence is >10%), since *H. pylori* "test-and-treat" is more cost-effective than EGD in this group of patients. Triple therapy is defined as an acid-suppressing medication (usually a PPI) and two antibiotics (Table 10-3). Patients >55 years and those with alarm symptoms should be referred for prompt EGD (25). Figure 10-3 outlines an approach to dyspeptic symptoms.

Box 10-3   Alarm Signs

- Bleeding
- Anemia
- Early satiety
- Unexplained weight loss
- Progressive dysphagia
- Odynophagia
- Persistent vomiting
- Family history of GI malignancy
- Personal history of GI malignancy

Dyspeptic symptoms with alarm signs should be evaluated with EGD.

From Sleisenger MH, Fordtran JS (eds): Gastrointestinal Disease: Pathophysiology, Diagnosis, and Management, 8th ed. Copyright Elsevier 2006; with permission.

Table 10-3   Treatment for PUD Based on ACG Guidelines

Treatment modality	First line therapy	Eradication rate (%)
H. pylori negative	PPI therapy	80–100 at 4 wk
	H2 receptor inhibitor therapy	70–80 at 4 wk
H. pylori positive	Amoxicillin 1 g bid, clarithromycin 500 mg bid, and PPI for 10–14 d	70–85
H. pylori positive with PCN allergy	Clarithromycin 500 mg bid, metronidazole 500 mg bid, and PPI for 10–14 d	70–85
	Metronidazole 250 mg bid, tetracycline 500 mg qid, bismuth 525 mg qid, for 14 d, and H2 receptor antagonist (or PPI) for 28 d	75–90
H. pylori positive salvage for persistent infection (avoid antibiotics taken previously)	Metronidazole 250 mg bid, tetracycline 500 mg qid, bismuth 525 mg qid, for 14 d and H2 receptor antagonist (or PPI) for 28 d	68
	Levofloxacin 500 mg qd, amoxicillin 1 g bid, PPI	87

From Chey WD, Wong BCY. Practice Parameters Committee of the American College of Gastroenterology guideline on the management of Helicobacter pylori infection. American Journal of Gastroenterology. 2007;102:1808–25; with permission.

Diagnostic testing for *H. pylori* has become essential in the diagnosis and management of PUD. Tests that require samples of gastric mucosa include histological examination for evidence of chronic active gastritis with the presence of *H. pylori* culture and polymerase chain reaction (PCR) of gastric biopsy specimens. The mucosal biopsy specimen can be tested for urease with the urease test, called the "CLO (Campylobacter-like organism) test." It is imperative to be aware that recent therapy with PPIs or antibiotics or a recent gastrointestinal tract hemorrhage can produce false-negative results (26).

Non-endoscopic tests include the ^{13}C-urea or ^{14}C-urea breath test (UBT), serology (IgG antibody), or an *H. pylori* stool antigen test. The serological tests are as sensitive and specific as a biopsy and are very useful in the initial diagnosis of *H. pylori* infection. For patients in whom EGD is unnecessary or contraindicated, serologic tests are quick, inexpensive, and accurate. However, they are less helpful in confirming cure after treatment because a marked loss of titers may take 6–12 months after therapy. The *H. pylori* stool assay appears to be highly accurate. It is a noninvasive, simple, and cost-effective test that is used to diagnose *H. pylori* infection in symptomatic adults and to monitor response to therapy. The UBT is accurate but can be false-negative if the patient used antibiotics or PPIs recently. The UBT is the test of choice (where available) to confirm eradication of *H. pylori*. This should

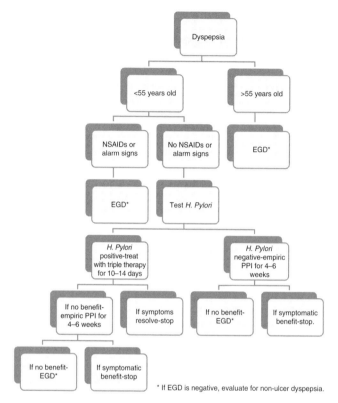

Figure 10-3   Algorithm for evaluating dyspepsia.

be performed 4 weeks after treatment with antibiotics or discontinuation of PPIs (27).

Management of Peptic Ulcer Disease

The treatment of PUD has changed remarkably with the discovery of the role of *H. pylori* in peptic ulcers. The recurrence of PUD has decreased from approximately 90% at 1 year to 1–2% after eradication of the organism. It is imperative that *H. pylori* initially be considered as the cause of ulcer disease in all patients. If the *H. pylori* testing is negative, alternative explanations such as NSAIDs or hyper-secretory states should be considered. The treatment of PUD should include eradication of *H. pylori* in patients with this infection (8).

Standard treatment for *H. pylori* is amoxicillin 1 g po bid for 14 days, clarithromycin 500 mg po bid for 14 days, and a PPI (such as esomeprazole 40 mg bid) for 14 days. For penicillin-allergic patients, amoxicillin may be substituted by metronidazole 500 mg po bid for 14 days. If *H. pylori* testing is negative or if symptoms persist after completed *H. pylori* therapy, empiric treatment with a PPI for 6–8 weeks is recommended (27). EGD is recommended if the symptoms persist after 8 weeks. Repeat EGD with biopsy is recommended to confirm healing of gastric ulcers and to rule out malignancy. Refractory peptic ulcer disease (i.e., disease that fails to heal after 8–12 weeks of therapy) may be caused by persistent or resistant *H. pylori* infection, continued NSAID use, giant ulcers requiring longer healing time, cancer, tolerance of/or resistance to medications, or hyper-secretory states (5). Medications, particularly NSAIDs, should be discontinued if possible, and patients should be strongly encouraged to discontinue alcohol and smoking (25). If NSAIDs cannot be discontinued, a PPI may be taken for the duration of the NSAID use, both to heal the ulcer and to prevent ulcer recurrence.

Administration of an H-2 blocker or PPI for 4 weeks induces healing in most duodenal ulcers. However, PPI therapy provides superior acid suppression, healing rates, and symptom relief, and is recommended as initial therapy for most patients. A recent systematic review of randomized controlled trials (28) showed that PPIs healed duodenal ulcers in >95% of patients at 4 weeks and gastric ulcers in 80–90% of patients at 4 weeks. Therefore, there is little reason to prescribe PPIs for longer than 4 weeks for duodenal ulcers unless the ulcers are large, fibrosed, or unresponsive to initial treatment (2). Table 10-3 shows a comparison of PUD healing rates and *H. pylori* regimens.

Complications

Approximately 25% of patients with PUD have serious complications, such as hemorrhage, perforation, or gastric outlet obstruction. Silent ulcers and complications are more common in older patients and in patients taking NSAIDs. The incidence of serious complications among persons in the general population who do not take NSAIDs is extremely low (13).

Bleeding

Upper gastrointestinal bleeding occurs in 15–20% of patients with PUD. It is the most common cause of death and the most common indication for surgery in the disease. In older patients, 20% of bleeding results from asymptomatic ulcers. Patients may present with hematemesis, melena, fatigue caused by anemia, orthostasis, or syncope. In a stable patient, potentially ulcerogenic medications should be discontinued. A PPI should be administered intravenously; this reduces transfusion requirements needed for surgery and duration of hospitalization, although it does not reduce mortality. Once the patient is resuscitated with fluids and/or packed red blood cells, EGD should be performed to identify characteristics that may suggest a high rate of bleeding recurrence (e.g., ulcer >1 cm, visible vessel, or actively bleeding vessel). EGD also permits treatment of the bleeding site with appropriate therapeutic modalities, including thermocoagulation, hemoclips, and injection of epinephrine (29).

Oral PPI therapy should be initiated as soon as patients resume oral intake. Patients should be tested for *H. pylori* infection and should receive eradication therapy if results are positive. Treatment of *H. pylori* infection is more effective than anti-secretory therapy without eradication of *H. pylori* for preventing recurrent bleeding. If continued administration of aspirin or other NSAIDs is required, concurrent administration of misoprostol or a PPI should be considered. Patients with malignant-appearing or non-healing gastric ulcers should be biopsied to rule out cancer (30).

Angiographic embolization of bleeding vessels or surgery is indicated if a patient's vital signs or laboratory results suggest continued or recurrent bleeding. Surgical options include gastroduodenotomy and oversewing of the blood vessel with or without vagotomy and drainage in duodenal ulcers, and excision of the ulcer with vagotomy and drainage or partial gastrectomy in bleeding gastric ulcers (6,29).

Perforation

Perforation occurs in approximately 2–12% of peptic ulcers. It usually involves the anterior wall of the duodenum, but may less commonly be a complication of antral or lesser curve gastric ulcers. Peritonitis, caused by perforation (evidenced by clinical peritonitis on exam or finding of free air on abdominal imaging), is a surgical emergency. Initial resuscitation should include large volumes of crystalloids, nasogastric suction, and administration of intravenous broad-spectrum antibiotics. This may be followed by emergency laparotomy and placement of an omental patch in patients with a perforated duodenal ulcer. In otherwise healthy patients with chronic ulcer and minimal peritoneal contamination, a concurrent definitive, anti-ulcer procedure (e.g., vagotomy and drainage, highly selective vagotomy) may be considered (6). Perforated gastric ulcers are treated with an omental patch, wedge resection of the ulcer, or a partial gastrectomy with re-anastomosis (2). Coexisting *H. pylori* infection should be eradicated to reduce recurrence and minimize the need for long-term anti-secretory therapy and further surgical intervention. In older patients, the mortality rates from perforation may be as high as 30–50% (31).

Gastric Outlet Obstruction

Fewer than 8 % of cases of gastric outlet obstruction are caused by PUD. Chronic or recurrent ulcers in the distal stomach, pyloric channel, or proximal duodenum can cause obstructive symptoms via edema, spasm, fibrosis, and scarring. Obstructive symptoms include early satiety, vomiting, and persistent bloating after meals. Weight loss, dehydration, and hypochloremic, hypokalemic metabolic alkalosis may result. Malignancy, a more common cause of obstruction (responsible for over 50% of cases), should be ruled out (32). EGD or gastroduodenography is recommended for the determination of the site, cause, and degree of obstruction. Obstruction resulting from acute inflammation or edema responds well to nasogastric decompression, administration of intravenous antisecretory agents, and eradication of *H. pylori*. Prokinetic medications should be avoided. Endoscopic pyloric balloon dilatation or surgery (vagotomy and pyloroplasty, antrectomy, or gastroenterostomy) are options for the relief of chronic obstruction (2).

Prevention

Primary prevention of peptic ulcers in the absence of risk factors is not a clinically practical or cost-effective approach to care. As noted above, *H. pylori* infection and NSAID use are the most significant risk factors for PUD. A meta-analysis evaluated the role of testing and treating *H. pylori* in patients requiring chronic NSAIDs prior to ulcer development and showed that *H. pylori* eradication was particularly effective for patients who were previously NSAID-naive. However, this approach was still less effective than PPI therapy (30). Smoking cessation or avoidance should be recommended for all patients because of adverse cardiovascular, pulmonary, and malignancy risks; the association of PUD and cigarette smoking provides another reason to support cessation (18). Smoking impairs ulcer healing and may be related to decrease in mucosal blood flow and direct injury by increasing production of free radicals, promoting secretion of vasopressin, and secretion of endothelin by the gastric mucosa. Smoking also affects the mucosal protective mechanisms, such as inhibiting gastric mucous secretion, gastric prostaglandin generation, duodenal mucosal bicarbonate secretion, and pancreatic bicarbonate secretion (33). Selective COX-2 inhibitors showed promise in reducing adverse GI events. Unfortunately, celecoxib, and other Cox-2 inhibitors were associated with unfavorable cardiovascular events in 3 large studies, though the trials were not designed to examine cardiovascular events (8,34). Prior to choosing a COX-2 inhibitor over an NSAID/PPI combination, careful discussion with the patient and evaluation of cardiovascular risk factors should be considered (16).

Overview

While symptoms of upper abdominal pain are common, the likelihood that dyspeptic symptoms are due to PUD is as low as 10%. With symptoms for PUD being neither sensitive nor specific, a directed approach to diagnosis is needed, as outlined above. Careful history, particularly regarding NSAID use and smoking, as well as consideration of *H. pylori* testing, age, and "alarm signs," can aid in stratifying the risk of underlying peptic ulceration (35). Once a diagnosis of PUD is made, treatment with acid suppression and/or removal of risk factors should be instituted.

References

1. **Chan FKL, Leung WK.** Peptic-ulcer disease. [see comment]. Lancet. 2002;360:933–41.
2. **Ramakrishnan K, Salinas RC.** Peptic ulcer disease. American Family Physician. 2007;76:1005–12.

3. **Meurer LN.** Treatment of peptic ulcer disease and nonulcer dyspepsia. Journal of Family Practice. 2001; 50:614–9.

4. **Jones MP.** The role of psychosocial factors in peptic ulcer disease: beyond *Helicobacter pylori* and NSAIDs. Journal of Psychosomatic Research. 2006;60:407–12.

5. **Levenstein S.** Stress and peptic ulcer: life beyond Helicobacter. BMJ. 1998;316:538–41.

6. **Harbison SP, Dempsey DT.** Peptic ulcer disease. Current Problems in Surgery. 2005;42:346–454.

7. **Kurata JH, Nogawa AN.** Meta-analysis of risk factors for peptic ulcer. Nonsteroidal antiinflammatory drugs, *Helicobacter pylori*, and smoking. Journal of Clinical Gastroenterology. 1997;24:2–17.

8. **Louw JA.** Peptic ulcer disease. Current Opinion in Gastroenterology. 2006;22:607–11.

9. **Konturek SJ, et al.** *Helicobacter pylori* and its involvement in gastritis and peptic ulcer formation. Journal of Physiology & Pharmacology. 2006;57:29–50.

10. **Dzierzanowska-Fangrat K, Dzierzanowska D.** *Helicobacter pylori*: microbiology and interactions with gastrointestinal microflora. Journal of Physiology & Pharmacology. 2006;57:5–14.

11. **Dzieniszewski J, Jarosz M.** Guidelines in the medical treatment of *Helicobacter pylori* infection. Journal of Physiology & Pharmacology. 2006;57:143–54.

12. **Fennerty MB.** NSAID-related gastrointestinal injury. Evidence-based approach to a preventable complication. Postgraduate Medicine. 110:87–8, 2001.

13. **Lanza FL.** A guideline for the treatment and prevention of NSAID-induced ulcers. Members of the Ad Hoc Committee on Practice Parameters of the American College of Gastroenterology. American Journal of Gastroenterology. 1998;93:2037–46.

14. **Sung J, et al.** Non-steroidal anti-inflammatory drug toxicity in the upper gastrointestinal tract. Journal of Gastroenterology & Hepatology. 2000;15:G58–68.

15. **Goldstein JL, et al.** A multicenter, randomized, double-blind, active-comparator, placebo-controlled, parallel-group comparison of the incidence of endoscopic gastric and duodenal ulcer rates with valdecoxib or naproxen in healthy subjects aged 65 to 75 years. Clinical Therapeutics. 2006;28:340–51.

16. **Strand V.** Are COX-2 inhibitors preferable to non-selective non-steroidal anti-inflammatory drugs in patients with risk of cardiovascular events taking low-dose aspirin? Lancet. 2008;370:2138–51.

17. **Sjodin I, Svedlund J.** Psychological aspects of non-ulcer dyspepsia: a psychosomatic view focusing on a comparison between the irritable bowel syndrome and peptic ulcer disease. Scandinavian Journal of Gastroenterology—Supplement. 1985;109:51–8.

18. **Garbis H, et al.** Pregnancy outcome after exposure to ranitidine and other H2-blockers. A collaborative study of the European Network of Teratology Information Services. Reproductive Toxicology. 2005;19:453–8.

19. **Lalkin A, et al.** The safety of omeprazole during pregnancy: a multicenter prospective controlled study. American Journal of Obstetrics & Gynecology. 1998;179:727–30.

20. **Nikfar S, et al.** Use of proton pump inhibitors during pregnancy and rates of major malformations: a meta-analysis. Digestive Diseases & Sciences. 2002;47:1526-9.

21. **Mahadevan U, Kane S.** American gastroenterological association institute technical review on the use of gastrointestinal medications in pregnancy. Gastroenterology. 2006;131:283-311.

22. **Richter JE.** Gastroesophageal reflux disease during pregnancy. Gastroenterology Clinics of North America. 2003;32:235-61.

23. **Richter JE.** Review article: the management of heartburn in pregnancy. Alimentary Pharmacology & Therapeutics. 2005;22:749-57.

24. **Fuchs W, Sennewald R, Klotz U.** Lansoprazole does not affect the bioavailability of oral contraceptives. British Journal of Clinical Pharmacology. 1994;38:376-80.

25. **Talley NJ, et al.** AGA technical review: evaluation of dyspepsia. American Gastroenterological Association. Gastroenterology. 1998;114:582-95.

26. **Gisbert JP, Abraira V.** Accuracy of Helicobacter pylori diagnostic tests in patients with bleeding peptic ulcer: a systematic review and meta-analysis. American Journal of Gastroenterology. 2006;101:848-63.

27. **Chey WD, Wong BCY.** Practice Parameters Committee of the American College of Gastroenterology guideline on the management of *Helicobacter pylori* infection. American Journal of Gastroenterology. 2007;102:1808-25.

28. **Ford AC, et al.** Eradication therapy in Helicobacter pylori positive peptic ulcer disease: systematic review and economic analysis. American Journal of Gastroenterology. 2004;99:1833-55.

29. **Adler DG, et al.** ASGE guideline: The role of endoscopy in acute non-variceal upper-GI hemorrhage. [erratum appears in Gastrointest Endosc. 2005 Feb;61:356. Note: Quereshi, Waqar A [corrected to Qureshi, Waqar A]]. Gastrointestinal Endoscopy. 2004;60:497-504.

30. **Vergara M, et al.** Meta-analysis: role of *Helicobacter pylori* eradication in the prevention of peptic ulcer in NSAID users. Alimentary Pharmacology & Therapeutics. 2005;21:1411-18.

31. **Yeomans ND.** Management of peptic ulcer disease not related to Helicobacter. Journal of Gastroenterology & Hepatology. 2002; 17:488-94.

32. **Shone DN, et al.** Malignancy is the most common cause of gastric outlet obstruction in the era of H2 blockers. [see comment] American Journal of Gastroenterology. 1995;90:1769-70.

33. **Eastwood GL.** Is smoking still important in the pathogenesis of peptic ulcer disease? Journal of Clinical Gastroenterology. 1997;25: S1-7.

34. **Bresalier RS, et al.** The Editor's round: cyclooxygenase-2 inhibitors and cardiovascular risk. American Journal of Cardiology. 2005;96: 1589-604.

35. Feldman: **Sleisenger & Fordtran's** Gastrointestinal and Liver Disease, 8th ed. Philadelphia: Saunders, 2006

D. Gastroesophageal Reflux Disease

Kenneth Berman, Hala Fatima, and Rakesh Vinayek

KEY POINTS

- Gastroesophageal reflux disease (GERD) is a common disease that affects quality of life and leads to substantial health care and productivity costs.
- Obesity and obstructive sleep apnea are risk factors for reflux disease.
- Severity of symptoms does not correlate well with severity of esophageal damage.
- Major complications of GERD are peptic strictures, Barrett's esophagus, adenocarcinoma, chest pain, asthma, dental erosions, and cough.
- Differential diagnosis for esophagitis includes GERD/NERD (most common), pill esophagitis, infectious esophagitis, and eosinophilic esophagitis.
- In the absence of alarm symptoms, empiric diagnosis and treatment with life-style changes and PPI therapy are appropriate.
- Patients refractory to PPI therapy typically do not respond well to anti-reflux surgery.
- Reflux is common in pregnancy and should be treated in step-up fashion as pharmacological data is limited.

Background

GERD is a common digestive disorder characterized by reflux of gastric contents into the esophagus, leading to troublesome symptoms or complications. The Montreal definition (1) expanded the category of GERD to include complications of esophagitis and extra-esophageal symptoms with or without established evidence on the correlation with GERD. Symptomatic patients lacking evidence of mucosal breaks are termed NERD (non-erosive reflux disease) (2) or endoscopic negative reflux disease (ENRD) and comprise about 50% of patients with reflux symptoms. The spectrum of disease extends from NERD/ENRD to erosive reflux disease (ERD) with varying degree of erosive esophagitis on endoscopy and complicated reflux disease characterized by nocturnal breakthrough, extra-esophageal manifestations, esophageal strictures, Barrett's esophagus, and adenocarcinoma. While the typical symptoms of GERD are heartburn and regurgitation, many patients present with cough, asthma, hoarseness, and chest pain. Given the nature of the disorder, GERD has been shown to affect quality of life and work productivity (3) and also has been shown to be associated with substantial costs, both as a result of health care costs (4) and loss of productivity (5).

Epidemiology

The prevalence of GERD in the Western world is approximately 10–20% (1,6). There is growing evidence to suggest that the prevalence of GERD-related symptomatology is rising worldwide. In the U.S., there is approximately a 4% increase per year in prevalence of weekly GERD symptoms on the average, with similar trends reported in South America, Asia, and Europe. The data from the U.S. Ambulatory Medical Care Survey clearly show that there is an increasing proportion of visits for GERD in primary care settings, with a 46% increase in GERD-related visits in the last 3 years, and most GERD-related patients were women (7). In addition, incidence of Barrett's esophagus and adenocarcinoma are rising (8). GERD has been identified as the 5th most common GI complaint seen at outpatient visits.

Pathophysiology

Multiple mechanisms for reflux exist, including gastric function abnormalities, dysfunction of the anti-reflux barrier, autonomic nervous dysfunction, and abnormal esophageal transit. Transient lower esophageal sphincter relaxations (TLESRs) are thought to be the most common mechanism. TLESRs are stimulated by gastric distension and are the physiologic mechanism for belching. However, not all TLESRs result in gastroesophageal reflux. It has been suggested that mechanical events related to the TLESR (i.e., duration, magnitude of relaxation, pressure gradient across the lower esophageal sphincter (LES) could be the factors that determine the occurrence and type of reflux during TLESRs. GERD may be associated with disturbances of the autonomic nervous system, which can be revealed as an alteration in heart rate variability studies. The diaphragm assists the sphincter by applying external pressure at the LES. Hiatal hernias contribute to reflux via loss of external pressure on the LES, thereby decreasing competence. Additionally, fatty foods, alcohol, caffeine, and other drugs will decrease LES tone. Obesity is a risk factor for GERD in men and women. Jacobson demonstrated that women with a BMI >25 have a 2–3-fold increased risk of reflux symptoms. The association with BMI is thought to be related to mechanical changes as well as hormonal features of adiposity (9). Finally, obstructive sleep apnea (OSA) is a risk factor for GERD; approximately 60–70% of patients with OSA suffer from GERD.

Clinical Features

The hallmark symptom of GERD is heartburn, which is described as retrosternal burning discomfort, usually experienced postprandially. It is typically worse with certain foods, such as spicy or acidic foods, caffeine, chocolate, fatty foods, and alcohol. Other less common symptoms are sour taste in the mouth, nausea, hematemesis, and globus sensation. Some patients, particularly the elderly, may be asymptomatic. Moreover, the degree of esophageal damage does not correlate well with the severity of symptoms. Men and women seem to have similar symptoms from GERD and appear to have generally similar patterns of endoscopic severity of GERD, but women are less likely to have Barrett's esophagus. The severity of symptoms in women is significantly greater than in men and may contribute to earlier disease recognition and different disease management. Men and women have similar LES function, esophageal motility, gastric emptying, and gastric acid secretion. Differences in symptom sensitivity and thresholds for discomfort may account for this (10). Complications of GERD include peptic stricture, Barrett's esophagus, and adenocarcinoma.

GERD may be associated with multiple extra-esophageal symptoms. GERD may mimic cardiac chest pain and may lead to asthma due to bronchospasm from gastric acid aspiration. Other manifestations are chronic cough, laryngitis, laryngeal cancer, obstructive sleep apnea, and dental erosions.

Differential Diagnosis

Reflux esophagitis is the most common type of esophagitis. Other common types of esophagitis can often be separated by history. Medication or pill esophagitis typically has a more acute presentation and is most frequently seen with tetracycline antibiotics (particularly doxycycline), anti-inflammatory medications, ferrous sulfate, potassium chloride, and bisphosphonates. In regard to bisphosphonates, early reports suggested increased incidence of esophagitis with alendronate; however, further studies with alendronate and other bisphosphonates have not indicated this. When taken appropriately (i.e., before a meal, with 8 oz. of water and maintenance of upright posture for 30 minutes) the risk of esophagitis with bisphosphonate therapy appears to be quite low. Odynophagia and dysphagia suggest infectious esophagitis, such as herpes, cytomegalovirus, and Candida esophagitis. Diagnosis of infectious esophagitis is made endoscopically with biopsies. Eosinophilic esophagitis (EE) tends to be more common in young men, presenting with dysphagia, food impaction, and heartburn. This is often mistakenly diagnosed as GERD. Half of these patients have asthma, and significant numbers of these patients have food allergies. A trial of PPI is recommended even when a diagnosis of EE is established before contemplating topical and systemic steroids. Functional dyspepsia often can manifest with reflux-like symptoms. About 30–50% of patients with NERD have heartburn symptoms despite having normal esophageal acid exposure. These patients are referred to as having functional heartburn, the pathophysiology of which may be related to hypersensitivity to physiologic degrees of acid reflux, *H. pylori* infection, and psychosocial factors.

Diagnosis

According to the American College of Gastroenterology, empiric treatment, including life-style modifications, is sufficient to diagnose patients with uncomplicated GERD (6). Postprandial heartburn symptoms that are worse with bending over or lying down and that improve with antacids in combination with endoscopic changes are 97% specific for GERD (11). In the absence of alarm symptoms (see below), a trial of PPI therapy is recommended as a therapeutic and diagnostic step. PPIs prove more cost-effective compared to H2RA (H2 receptor antagonists) in empiric treatment, producing higher efficacy, decreased office visits, decreased need for endoscopy, and better quality of life (12). However, because of the additional cost of PPIs, a trial of H2RA therapy may be reasonable in patients with milder symptoms. If symptoms do not improve, further testing is warranted. It is important to note that symptoms do not predict the degree of esophagitis or complications (13).

Endoscopy at presentation should be considered in the circumstances listed in Box 10-4.

While endoscopy is the preferred modality to evaluate symptoms of complicated GERD, at least 50% of symptomatic patients have normal endoscopy and are classified as NERD (1). However, this does not correlate with the severity of symptoms or ease of control with medications.

Findings of reflux esophagitis on endoscopy diagnose GERD with a specificity of 90–95% (15). Endoscopy also allows collection of specimens for pathology and microbiology. Biopsies and/or brush cytology should be obtained in immunocompromised hosts, if irregular or deep ulceration or mass is present, if the proximal esophagus is involved, or if a malignant-appearing stricture is seen.

Box 10-4　Alarm Signs and Symptoms

1. Screen for Barrett's esophagus (BE) in chronic GERD (>5 y) in Caucasian males, >50 y of age, with a family history of BE and/or adenocarcinoma of the esophagus
2. Lack of response to empiric therapy
3. Persistent vomiting
4. Alarm symptoms: anorexia, weight loss (>5%), dysphagia, odynophagia, bleeding/iron deficiency anemia. Patients with alarm symptoms are more likely to have peptic strictures, esophagitis, or esophageal cancer
5. Patients requiring continuous acid suppression and those experiencing symptom recurrence upon withdrawal of successful medical therapy
6. Extra-esophageal symptoms: coughing, hoarseness
7. Imaging study showing mass, stricture, or ulcer
8. Preoperative evaluation for anti-reflux surgery
9. Recurrence of symptoms after anti-reflux procedures
10. Placement of wireless esophageal pH monitoring device (14)

In patients without mucosal damage noted during endoscopy, ambulatory reflux monitoring may be helpful to confirm a diagnosis of GERD. Newer methods of monitoring allow for evaluation of esophageal pH by using a radio-telemetry capsule without the discomfort of a nasoesophageal tube. Ambulatory reflux monitoring is best utilized in a patient who is failing acid suppression therapy to determine whether the failure is in the management of reflux or in the diagnosis. In refractory cases, impedance and manometry measurements may assist the management and diagnosis. Manometry provides preoperative measurement of esophageal peristalsis and lower esophageal sphincter functions prior to Nissen's fundoplication. Additionally, it is a valuable diagnostic tool in identifying patients with various esophageal motility disorders. Multi-channel impedance monitoring is a new technique that allows detection of all reflux episodes, and its combination with pH allows the characterization of such episodes as acid or non-acid. Adding impedance to pH monitoring improves the diagnostic yield and allows better symptom analysis than pH monitoring alone. The persistence of symptoms in patients on PPI therapy either are not associated with reflux (30–50% of the cases) or might be associated with non-acid reflux in 20–30% of cases.

Although the role of acid reflux in the pathogenesis of GERD is established, bile also has been implicated in the pathophysiology of GERD. Most patients with esophagitis have a variable combination of acid and duodeno-gastroesophageal reflux (DGER) containing bile. Using 24-hour pH-bilitec monitoring, we now have the ability to identify patients with mixed acid and bile reflux, which has been associated with severe mucosal injury and the greatest deterioration of esophageal function.

Medical Treatment

Given the high percentage of NERD and absence of correlation of symptoms with the degree of esophageal damage, patients with symptoms of uncomplicated GERD can be managed with an initial trial of empirical therapy, including life-style modifications (6). These include decreasing fat intake, smoking cessation, and avoiding foods that lower LES pressure (chocolate, alcohol, peppermint, coffee, carbonated beverages, and citrus juices). Head of bed elevation (especially with nocturnal or laryngeal symptoms) and avoidance of late meals may provide additional benefit. Obesity has been found to be a risk factor for GERD, erosive esophagitis, and esophageal adenocarcinoma (16). Therefore, weight loss should be strongly encouraged.

Many patients will have already tried over-the-counter treatment by the time they present for medical attention. Antacids are often a first choice among patients, presumably because they are inexpensive, provide quick relief, and are relatively safe. Antacids directly neutralize gastric pH, providing rapid relief. In general, however, antacids only will be sufficient in milder cases of GERD. H2RA are particularly useful when taken before a meal or exacerbating activity, such as exercise. They provide symptom relief in about 30 minutes, but, unlike antacids, last about 10 hours. Potency of H2RAs and antacids is similar.

Proton pump inhibitors (PPIs) are currently the most effective agents available for the treatment of GERD and have become the mainstay of treatment. PPIs have been shown to provide more complete symptom resolution and more rapid healing of esophagitis when compared to H2RAs (17). PPIs are very effective in providing symptom relief in patients with erosive esophagitis; there is 10–15% discordance between symptom resolution and mucosal healing. The various PPIs are of similar efficacy, with meta-analysis studies failing to demonstrate significant differences among them at standard doses (17). Nevertheless, some patients may respond better to one PPI than to another. The proportion of NERD patients responding to a standard PPI dose is about 20–30% lower than those with erosive esophagitis (18). Daily dosing should be taken 30 minutes before a meal. A small percentage of patients respond better to twice-daily dosing. For patients with persistent nighttime breakthrough symptoms despite twice-daily PPI therapy, the addition of an H2RA before bedtime has been shown to be superior to a third dose of PPI or placebo; however, tachyphylaxis to H2RA develops within a week of therapy (19).

Maintenance Therapy

Since GERD is a chronic disease, maintenance therapy is typically used to control symptoms and prevent complications. The people who are appropriate for long-term maintenance therapy are most patients with severe erosive esophagitis, patients with nocturnal/extraesophageal symptoms of GERD, and patients with complications of GERD (esophageal ulcer, stricture, and Barrett's esophagus). PPIs at a standard dose are more effective than H2RAs at maintaining symptomatic and endoscopic remission of esophagitis (20). Long-term treatment of reflux does prevent peptic esophageal strictures; however, Barrett's esophagus does not appear to improve with chronic acid suppression.

Patients appropriate for "on-demand" therapy with H2RAs or PPIs include those with symptomatic NERD and some patients with low-grade erosive esophagitis. The patients' compliance with long-term therapy is an issue in GERD, with non-compliance seen in 30–74% of patients.

In general, PPI therapy is safe. Headache, diarrhea, and abdominal pain are the most common adverse events reported, in the range of 3–5% of patients. Development of chronic atrophic gastritis is a theoretical issue with long-term therapy, especially if *H. pylori* is present. However, since the risk is small, *H. pylori* should not be checked routinely in these patients.

The risk of pneumonia attributable to PPI use is slight (21). There also is an increased risk of *C. difficile* diarrhea secondary to PPI use (22). PPI therapy also has been associated with B12 deficiency, presumably due to achlorhydria, and B12 levels should be checked periodically in patients on long-term therapy. A dose- and duration-dependent risk of hip fracture has been demonstrated with long-term PPI use (23), likely due to decreased calcium absorption from acid suppression, as well as inhibition of osteoclastic proton pumps.

Role of Endoscopy

Endoscopy allows therapeutic maneuvers, like esophageal dilation for strictures and endoscopic mucosal resection or photodynamic therapy for dysplastic Barrett's esophagus. In case of erosive esophagitis, follow-up endoscopy is indicated if symptoms fail to respond to therapy, additional biopsies are needed to clarify diagnosis, or if esophageal ulceration is present. Endoscopy also may have a role in ruling out Barrett's esophagus once mucosal healing has been achieved (24).

Endoluminal therapy of GERD is evolving. This includes delivery of radiofrequency energy to the gastroesophageal junction and suture plication of the proximal fundic folds. Data on efficacy, safety, and economics are lacking, and at present there are no definite indications for their use (25).

Surgical Treatment

Surgery is an option for reflux treatment in patients who respond well to PPI therapy but cannot or prefer not to take medications on a long-term basis and for patients with aspiration symptoms due to significant volume reflux. Patients refractory to PPI therapy typically do not respond well to anti-reflux surgery and often have alternative etiologies for symptoms. Laparoscopic Nissen fundoplication, the most commonly performed anti-reflux surgical procedure, has a <1% mortality rate, but dysphagia, bloating, and increased flatus are common. Early studies comparing surgery to medical therapy showed benefit for surgery; however, this has not been so in the era of PPIs. The response to surgery is lower in NERD patients compared with those suffering from erosive esophagitis.

Reflux Disease during Pregnancy

Heartburn occurs in 30–50% of pregnant women (26). Incidence is the same across all 3 trimesters (27). Most women who develop heartburn during pregnancy have resolution after delivery. The mechanism seems to be related to a progesterone- and estrogen-dependent failure of LES pressure to increase with increasing abdominal compression. Endoscopy has been determined to be a safe diagnostic tool in pregnancy. As with non-pregnant patients, treatment starts with life-style modification. Antacids are commonly used. Sucralfate, a non-absorbable, locally acting inhibitor of pepsin activity, has been shown to control symptoms in over 80% of pregnant women. For patients not responding to the above treatment, H2RAs and PPIs may be used. All H2RAs carry an FDA category B rating during pregnancy; however, ranitidine is the only member in this class with documented efficacy in pregnancy. Of the

5 PPIs, omeprazole carries an FDA class C rating, while the others are rated as class B. Omeprazole has teratogenicity in rats and case reports of birth defects in humans; however, prospective studies have not demonstrated this. Animal studies have not shown teratogenicity with the other PPIs. The safest approach, however, would be to reserve PPIs for patients who have failed to respond to H2RAs.

References

1. **Vakil N, van Zanten SV, Kahrilas P, et al.** [The Montreal definition and classification of gastroesophageal reflux disease: a global, evidence-based consensus paper]. Z Gastroenterol. 2007;45:1125-40.
2. **Fass R, Fennerty MB, Vakil N, et al.** Nonerosive reflux disease–current concepts and dilemmas. American Journal of Gastroenterology. 2001; 96:303-14.
3. **Wahlqvist P, Brook RA, Campbell SM, et al.** Objective measurement of work absence and on-the-job productivity: a case-control study of US employees with and without gastroesophageal reflux disease. J Occup Environ Med. 2008;50:25-31.
4. **Willich SN, Nocon M, Kulig M, et al.** Cost-of-disease analysis in patients with gastro-oesophageal reflux disease and Barrett's mucosa. Aliment Pharmacol Ther. 2006;23:371-6.
5. **Brook RA, Wahlqvist P, Kleinman NL, et al.** Cost of gastro-oesophageal reflux disease to the employer: a perspective from the United States. Aliment Pharmacol Ther. 2007;26:889-98.
6. **DeVault KR, Castell DO, American College of G, et al.** Updated guidelines for the diagnosis and treatment of gastroesophageal reflux disease. American Journal of Gastroenterology. 2005;100:190-200.
7. **Niemcryk SJ, Joshua-Gotlib S, Levine DS, et al.** Outpatient experience of patients with GERD in the United States: analysis of the 1998-2001 National Ambulatory Medical Care Survey. Dig Dis Sci. 2005;50:1904-8.
8. **Gibbs JF, Rajput A, Chadha KS, et al.** The changing profile of esophageal cancer presentation and its implication for diagnosis. J Natl Med Assoc. 2007;99:620-6.
9. **Jacobson BC, Somers SC, Fuchs CS, et al.** Body-mass index and symptoms of gastroesophageal reflux in women. N Engl J Med. 2006; 354:2340-8.
10. **Lin M, Gerson Lauren, Lascar R, et al.** Features of gastroesophageal reflux disease in women. Am J Gastroenterology. 2004;99:1442-7.
11. **Tefera L, Fein M, Ritter MP, et al.** Can the combination of symptoms and endoscopy confirm the presence of gastroesophageal reflux disease? Am Surg. 1997;63:933-6.
12. **Gerson L, Robbins A, Garber A, et al.** A cost-effectiveness analysis of prescribing strategies in the management of gastroesophageal reflux disease. Am J Gastroenterology. 2000;95:2:395-407.
13. **Avidan B, Sonnenberg A, Schnell TG, et al.** There are no reliable symptoms for erosive oesophagitis and Barrett's oesophagus: endoscopic diagnosis is still essential. Alimentary Pharmacology & Therapeutics. 2002;16:735-42.

14. **Chotiprashidi P, Liu J, Carpenter S, et al.** ASGE technology status evaluation report: wireless esophageal pH monitoring system. Gastrointestinal Endoscopy. 2005;62:485–7.

15. **Moayyedi P, Talley NJ, Moayyedi P, et al.** Gastro-oesophageal reflux disease. [see comment]. Lancet. 2006;367:2086–100.

16. **Hampel H, Abraham NS, El-Serag HB, et al.** Meta-analysis: obesity and the risk for gastroesophageal reflux disease and its complications. Ann Intern Med. 2005;143:199–211.

17. **Vakil N, Fennerty MB.** Systematic review: direct comparative trials of the efficacy of proton pump inhibitors in the management of gastro-oesophageal reflux disease and peptic ulcer disease. Aliment Pharmacol Ther. 2003;18:559–68.

18. **Dean BB, Gano AD, Jr., Knight K, et al.** Effectiveness of proton pump inhibitors in nonerosive reflux disease. [see comment]. Clinical Gastroenterology & Hepatology. 2004;2:656–64.

19. **Fackler WK, Ours TM, Vaezi MF, et al.** Long-term effect of H2RA therapy on nocturnal gastric acid breakthrough. [see comment]. Gastroenterology. 2002;122:625–32.

20. **Ip S, Bonis P, Tatsioni A, et al.** Comparative effectiveness of management strategies for gastroesophageal reflux disease. Evidence Report/Technology Assessment No. 1. (Prepared by Tufts-New England Medical Center. Evidence-based Practice Center under Contract No. 290-02-0022.) Rockville, MD: Agency for Healthcare Research and Quality. Available at: www.effectivehealthcareahrqgov/reports/finalcfm December 2005.

21. **Laheij RJ, Sturkenboom MC, Hassing RJ, et al.** Risk of community-acquired pneumonia and use of gastric acid-suppressive drugs. [see comment]. JAMA. 2004;292:1955–60.

22. **Leonard J, Marshall JK, Moayyedi P, et al.** Systematic review of the risk of enteric infection in patients taking acid suppression. American Journal of Gastroenterology. 2007;102:2047–56; quiz 57.

23. **Yang YX, Lewis JD, Epstein S, et al.** Long-term proton pump inhibitor therapy and risk of hip fracture. [see comment]. JAMA. 2006;296:2947–53.

24. **Hanna S, Rastogi A, Weston AP, et al.** Detection of Barrett's esophagus after endoscopic healing of erosive esophagitis. [see comment]. American Journal of Gastroenterology. 2006;101:1416–20.

25. **Falk GW, Fennerty MB, Rothstein RI, et al.** AGA Institute technical review on the use of endoscopic therapy for gastroesophageal reflux disease. Gastroenterology. 2006;131:1315–36.

26. **Richter JE.** Gastroesophageal reflux disease during pregnancy. Gastroenterology Clinics of North America. 2003;32:235–61.

27. **Rey E, Rodriguez-Artalejo F, Herraiz MA, et al.** Gastroesophageal reflux symptoms during and after pregnancy: a longitudinal study. Am J Gastroenterol. 2007;102:2395–400.

11

Endocrine Disorders

A. Diabetes

Melissa K. Cavaghan

KEY POINTS

- ◆ Diabetes is occurring in epidemic proportions.
- ◆ The majority of diabetes care occurs in the primary care setting.
- ◆ The key to reducing complications of diabetes is aggressive control of hyperglycemia, hypertension, and hypercholesterolemia.
- ◆ Women of child-bearing potential need preconception counseling and tight glycemic control during pregnancy.

Epidemiology

The worldwide epidemic of diabetes is one of the most serious health care issues of this century. A near *doubling* of the incidence of the disease is projected between the years 2000 and 2030, with approximately 30 million cases in the U.S. alone (1). This staggering increase, predominantly in type 2 diabetes, is attributable to increasing obesity and physical inactivity. Furthermore, type 2 diabetes, previously rare in the pediatric population, is now commonplace. For unclear reasons, the incidence of autoimmune type 1 diabetes also is increasing worldwide.

Diabetes is a major cause of preventable blindness, limb loss, end-stage renal disease, and premature death from cardiovascular and cerebrovascular causes. Since diabetic patients vastly overwhelm the availability of diabetes specialists, it is essential that primary care physicians be familiar with screening, prevention, and comprehensive care of diabetes and its complications.

Clinical Features

Symptoms of significant hyperglycemia include polyuria, polydipsia, weight loss, blurry vision, and fatigue. Prompt diagnosis and aggressive treatment is essential in this setting. However, once symptoms are evident, it is estimated that diabetes and its complications have been present for many years. Therefore, systematic screening for diabetes is of paramount importance.

Diabetic complications are usually asymptomatic until late in their development. Sudden asymmetric vision impairment may indicate infarction, embolism, or hemorrhage, and warrants immediate ophthalmologic evaluation. Symptoms of diabetic neuropathy vary widely, and up to 50% of patients are asymptomatic. The typical "stocking-glove" pattern of combined sensorimotor neuropathy, with or without paresthesia and dysesthesia, is the most common presentation of peripheral neuropathy. Early recognition is important to allow the exclusion of treatable non-diabetic neuropathies (e.g., hypothyroidism, vitamin B12 deficiency); compression neuropathies (e.g., carpal tunnel syndrome), cranial, and peripheral mononeuropathies also occur. Autonomic neuropathy may manifest as supine hypertension, orthostatic hypotension, exercise intolerance, and gustatory sweating. Gastroparesis can manifest with any combination of nausea, vomiting, constipation, and diarrhea. Individuals with less obvious symptoms may have unpredictable glucose control.

Less common diabetic complications include arthropathies (i.e., Charcot arthropathy), dermopathies, and diabetic muscle infarction. Ischemic heart disease in diabetic patients is more likely to be silent because of cardiac autonomic neuropathy. In addition, diabetes erases the "female advantage": diabetic women develop heart disease at ages equivalent to men.

Diagnosis and Differential Diagnosis

Diabetes. Physicians should be familiar both with the categories of glucose tolerance (Table 11-1) and with the subcategories of diabetes (Box 11-1) used to describe the underlying physiology with as much specificity as possible. The importance of differentiating type 1 from type 2 diabetes arises from the need to recognize the risk for life-threatening diabetic ketoacidosis (DKA), which occurs when insulin is withheld from a patient with type 1 diabetes. The traditional simple clinical paradigms (type 1 diabetes is a disease of children; type 2 diabetes is a disease of overweight adults) should be abandoned. For instance, type 1 diabetes diagnosed during adulthood may progress slowly and appear to be type 2 diabetes at the time of diagnosis. Antibodies to glutamic acid decarboxylase (GAD) are usually positive in these patients. Conversely, type

Table 11-1   Criteria for the Categorization of Glucose Intolerance in Nonpregnant Adults

---

DIABETES is diagnosed with ONE of the following:
* Non-stressed plasma glucose ≥126 mg/dL (7 mmol/L) on 2 occasions
* Random glucose ≥200 mg/dL (11.1 mmol/L) accompanied by symptoms consistent with hyperglycemia (polyuria, polydipsia, weight loss)
* 2-h glucose ≥200 mg/dL after 75 g of oral glucose during an OGTT performed in the morning after an overnight fast

PRE-DIABETES is diagnosed with ONE of the following:

Impaired Fasting Glucose

Fasting plasma glucose ≥100 mg/dL (5.6 mmol/L) but <125 mg/dL

Impaired Glucose Tolerance

2-hour glucose ≥140 mg/dL (7.8 mmol/L) but <200 mg/dL after 75 g of glucose during an OGTT

From Standards of Medical Care in Diabetes—2008. Diabetes Care. 2008;31:S12–54. (Updated each January at www.diabetes.org); with permission.

Box 11-1   Classification of Type of Diabetes (American Diabetes Association)

- Type 1 diabetes—loss of insulin secretion from beta cell destruction, usually resulting in complete or near complete loss of insulin
- Type 2 diabetes—relative insulin deficiency on a background of increased demand for insulin (i.e. insulin resistance)
- Other specific subtypes (secondary to steroid treatment, cystic fibrosis, specific genetic mutations)
- Gestational diabetes

From Standards of Medical Care in Diabetes—2008. Diabetes Care. 2008;31:S12–54. (Updated each January at www.diabetes.org); with permission.

---

2 diabetes now frequently occurs in children because of the increasing incidence of obesity. Finally, patients with type 1 diabetes also may have obesity and the metabolic syndrome.

Risk factors indicating the need for testing for pre-diabetes and type 2 diabetes are listed in Box 11-2. There are no screening recommendations for type 1 diabetes. The fasting glucose is recommended for screening because of its ease of use, but it is less sensitive than the 75-gram oral glucose tolerance test (OGTT). Hemoglobin A1C (HbA1C) is not reliable for screening. Patients who become hyperglycemic during an acute illness may or may not be diabetic and should have glucose levels reassessed in the absence of illness.

Box 11-2   Recommendations for Testing for Pre-Diabetes and Diabetes

Overweight adults (BMI ≥25 kg/m²) with at least one additional risk factor:
- Physical inactivity
- First-degree relative with diabetes
- High risk ethnicity (African-American, Latino, Native American, Asian American, Pacific Islander)
- Women with a history of GDM* or baby >9 lb
- Hypertension (≥140/90 mmHg or current therapy for hypertension)
- HDL <35 mg/dL
- Triglycerides >250 mg/dL
- Polycystic ovary syndrome
- History of pre-diabetes
- Clinical suggestion of insulin resistance (severe obesity or acanthosis nigricans)

Age ≥45 y regardless of other risk factors
Repeat testing every 3 y unless risk factors increase
*GDM = gestational diabetes mellitus

From Standards of Medical Care in Diabetes—2008. Diabetes Care. 2008;31:S12–54. (Updated each January at www.diabetes.org); with permission.

Gestational diabetes mellitus (GDM) refers to diabetes diagnosed during pregnancy. Women at highest risk (extreme obesity, history of GDM or large infant, glycosuria, polycystic ovary syndrome [PCOS], and strong family history of diabetes) should be assessed for diabetes at the first prenatal visit using criteria for non-pregnant adults (2). Otherwise, OGTT testing is performed between weeks 24 and 28, using the criteria shown in Box 11-3. Only women who meet all of the low-risk criteria (age <25, normal pre-pregnancy weight, low-risk ethnic group, absent family history of diabetes, absent personal history of abnormal glucose tolerance, absent history of poor obstetrical outcome, inclusive) do not require testing (2).

Complications of diabetes. Diabetic **nephropathy** is the leading cause of end-stage renal disease (ESRD). Early stages are marked by persistent microalbuminuria (30–299 mg/24 hours or spot microalbumin/creatinine ratio of 30–299). Macroalbuminuria (≥300 mg/24 hours) frequently progresses to ESRD. Spot measurements must be confirmed, since false-positive results occur in the setting of infection, significant hypertension or hyperglycemia, or recent exercise. Deterioration of glomerular filtration rate (GFR) may or may not parallel the progression of albuminuria, so estimates of GFR must be made concurrently to detect early kidney dysfunction. Non-diabetic nephropathy should be suspected if the decline in GFR has been rapid, in the absence of other significant microvascular complications, or if there is an active urine sediment (2). Diabetic **retinopathy** is diagnosed by the presence of microaneurysms, exudates, or hemorrhages on funduscopic examination and is more common in patients with nephropathy and hypertension (2). Peripheral **neuropathy** is diagnosed clinically by testing for pinprick sensation, vibration (with a 128-Hz tuning fork), the ankle reflex, and light touch with a standard 10-gram monofilament. Gastroparesis is evaluated by a gastric emptying study during normoglycemia. Cardiovascular autonomic neuropathy is indicated by resting tachycardia or orthostatic hypotension (2).

Box 11-3   Criteria for the Diagnosis of Gestational Diabetes Mellitus

GDM is diagnosed when two or more glucoses are abnormal during the 100-g OGTT, performed in the morning, after an 8-h overnight fast.
- Fasting ≥95 mg/dL (5.3 mmol/L)
- 1 h ≥180 mg/dL (10 mmol/L)
- 2 h ≥155 mg/dL (8.6 mmol/L)
- 3 h ≥140 mg/dL (7.8 mmol/L)

This test can be performed with or without the 50-g screening test performed on a previous day. Patients with glucose <140 mg/dL (7.8 mmol/L) after 50 g of oral glucose can avoid the 3-h test.

From Standards of Medical Care in Diabetes—2008. Diabetes Care. 2008;31:S12–54. (Updated each January at www.diabetes.org); with permission.

Prevention and Clinical Care

Prevention of diabetes. Up to 70% of individuals with pre-diabetes will eventually develop diabetes. Several large diabetes prevention trials have demonstrated that progression to diabetes can be reduced by approximately 60% by either significant life-style modification (30 minutes of moderate activity on most days and a goal weight loss of 5–10%) or thiazolidinedione therapy. Treatment with metformin, acarbose, or orlistat reduces diabetes by 20–30% (2,3).

Treatment of pre-diabetes. Current recommendations include life-style modification, consideration of metformin for individuals at higher risk, and annual laboratory monitoring for diabetes (2,3). Metformin is most effective in individuals under age 60 and with body mass index (BMI) ≥35 kg/m^2 (4).

The risk for cardiovascular events is increased in patients with pre-diabetes, independent of the components of the metabolic syndrome (e.g., low HDL, hypertension) which also are frequently present. Although prevention of diabetes itself will substantially reduce cardiovascular risk, optimal treatment of hypertension and dyslipidemia also must be a priority in this population (3).

Treatment of diabetes. A comprehensive clinical assessment of the patient with diabetes should include nutritional and life-style evaluation, review of home glucose monitoring, assessment of hypoglycemia and awareness of hypoglycemia, BMI, blood pressure measurement, thyroid and foot examinations, and laboratory measurement of HbA1C. Retinal and peripheral neurologic examination, fasting lipid panel, liver function, urine albumin/creatinine ratio, and serum creatinine with calculated GFR are recommended at least annually. Thyroid-stimulating hormone (TSH) is recommended every 1–2 years for patients with type 1 diabetes and in women over age 50 years or patients with dyslipidemia (2). All patients require comprehensive diabetes education and instruction on medical nutrition therapy from a nurse educator and registered dietician at the time of diagnosis and periodically thereafter. Referral to mental health services, dentistry, nephrology, cardiology, and podiatry also may be necessary. Annual influenza vaccination and pneumococcal vaccination are recommended (2).

Self-monitoring of blood glucose (SMBG) should be carried out 3 or more times per day while treatment regimens are changing and in patients using multiple daily injections of insulin or insulin pump therapy. Monitoring postprandial glucose may help guide therapy when preprandial glucoses are near target but HbA1C is >7%. More frequent monitoring is needed in patients with frequent hypoglycemia or hypoglycemia unawareness and in pregnant women. HbA1C should be measured (preferably at the point-of-care) at least semi-annually in patients meeting glycemic goals and quarterly in patients with changing therapy or who are not at glycemic targets.

Life-style modification is a mainstay of diabetes care, aiming for weight maintenance or weight loss, as needed, and regular physical activity, as tolerated, to improve insulin resistance and improve cardiovascular risk. Clinical judgment should guide whether cardiac stress testing ought to be performed prior to initiating an exercise program. The hypoglycemic effects of exercise can be avoided by pre-exercise carbohydrate ingestion. Specific nutritional goals include restriction of saturated fat, minimization or elimination of *trans* fat, high fiber, and whole grain intake, patient familiarity with carbohydrate serving size and consistency in carbohydrate intake, and restriction of alcohol intake to 1 drink daily for women and 2 for men. No specific single diet plan is endorsed (2).

Goals of therapy. Tight glycemic control aimed at near normalization of blood sugars (Table 11-2) has been shown in major trials involving large groups of patients with both type 1 and type 2 diabetes to reduce complications (5–8). Less stringent glycemic goals can be considered in children and in patients with short life expectancies, serious comorbidities, or severe hypoglycemia.

Therapy for type 1 diabetes. The landmark Diabetes Control and Complications Trial (DCCT) clearly showed that patients with type 1 diabetes had improved glycemic and microvascular outcomes as a result of intensive therapy: 3 or more injections per day or insulin pump therapy (5). Fifteen years later, the availability of insulin analogs which mimic physiologic insulin secretion patterns makes intensive therapy easier to implement with less risk of the hypoglycemia seen in the DCCT. (See Figure 11-1 for the onset and duration of action of various insulin preparations.) Ideal therapy is a combination of basal insulin (glargine once or twice daily or detemir twice daily, dosed morning, evening, or both) and pre-meal analog insulin dosed immediately before eating.

Table 11-2   Treatment Goals in Patients with Diabetes Mellitus

GLUCOSE	Nonpregnant adults[2]		Pregnancy[9]
	ADA	ACE/AACE	
H bA1C	<7.0%*	≤6.5%	
Fasting	70–130 mg/dL	<110 mg/dL	≤95 mg/dL
1-h postmeal	N/A	N/A	≤140 mg/dL
2-h postmeal	<180 mg/dL	<140 mg/dL	≤120 mg/dL
BLOOD PRESSURE <130/80 mm Hg			
CHOLESTEROL LDL <100 mg/dL, optional goal of <70 mg/dL when CVD is present HDL >40 mg/dL in men, >50 mg/dL in women TRIGLYCERIDES <150 MG/DL			

ADA = American Diabetes Association, ACE = American College of Endocrinology, AACE = American Association of Clinical Endocrinologists
*<7% is a general goal. For an individual, the goal is "as close to normal (<6%) as possible without significant hypoglycemia."[2]

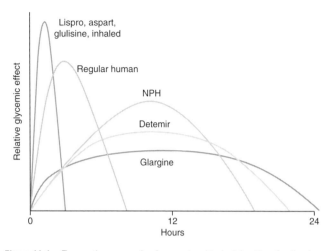

Figure 11-1   Time-action curves showing onset and typical duration of action for individual insulin preparations. Premixed insulins are not shown. (Reprinted from McMahan G, Dluhy R. N Engl J Med. 2007;357:1759–61; with permission.)

(NPH insulin is less costly but is usually needed 3–4 times per day to adequately provide basal insulin needs.) Total daily requirements are typically between 0.5–0.8 U/kg/day, with half as basal insulin and half as pre-meal insulin. Pre-meal insulin can be prescribed in fixed doses along with fixed, consistent carbohydrate intake, or can be flexibly adjusted by the patient for varying carbohydrate intake using formulas (e.g., 1 unit for 15 grams carbohydrate). Supplemental insulin is added to pre-meal insulin when the pre-meal blood sugar is elevated. The "Rule of 1800" (credited to Dr. Paul Davidson, Atlanta, GA) predicts that 1 unit of supplemental analog insulin will reduce blood sugar by an amount equal to 1800 ÷ (patient's total daily insulin dose, all insulins combined). When using regular insulin as pre-meal insulin, 1500 is substituted for 1800. Continuous subcutaneous insulin pump therapy offers advantages for many patients and is increasingly utilized, usually requiring referral to a comprehensive diabetes clinic. Pramlintide, a novel injectable therapy, may be used as an adjunct to meal-time insulin with expected benefits of improved postprandial hyperglycemia and possible mild weight loss.

Episodes of hypoglycemia (usually <70 mg/dL) may significantly limit optimal glycemic control and may require that glycemic goals be raised. Avoidance of beta blockers, which impair autonomic responses to hypoglycemia, is helpful, when possible. Two weeks of strict avoidance of hypoglycemia may also improve hypoglycemic awareness. Continuing education about balancing insulin and carbohydrate intake, correct treatment of hypoglycemia, anticipating the effects of exercise, and the importance of frequent blood sugar monitoring is essential. Patients also need "sick day rules" when diabetes worsens temporarily as a result of intercurrent illness, steroid use, or significant psychological stress. Access to a diabetes treatment team is essential during these episodes to either successfully manage illness at home or determine if hospitalization is needed to treat or avoid dehydration or diabetic ketoacidosis (DKA).

Therapy for type 2 diabetes. When initial anti-hyperglycemic therapy is selected, the starting HbA1C should guide whether oral therapy, alone or in combination, or insulin is appropriate (10,11). Each medication used at maximum doses will likely reduce HbA1C by approximately 1–1.5% (less for nateglinide and alpha glucosidase inhibitors). Larger effects may be seen when the starting HbA1C is high (i.e., above 9%). Agents that do not cause hypoglycemia are preferred when HbA1C is close to goal. When sulfonylurea or insulin is used, hypoglycemia risk increases, and more attention must be paid to consistency in carbohydrate intake. Initial combination therapy with two agents is synergistic and is appropriate for many patients. Initial HbA1C levels above 9.5–10% or significant hyperglycemia (fasting >250, random >300 mg/dL) should prompt consideration of immediate insulin therapy, even if oral agents are later considered for maintenance (10,11).

Multiple anti-hyperglycemic agents are available, both oral and injectable, with different and complimentary mechanisms of action and side effect profiles (Table 11-3). Metformin is universally recommended, when not contraindicated, as first-line therapy because of its safety record, low cost, lack of hypoglycemia, and possible associated mild weight loss. Because of frequent GI side effects, initial doses are low and are gradually increased over 2–3 weeks. When additional therapy is needed, no data indicate superiority of one agent over another with respect to long-term outcomes. Clinicians must choose therapy based on tolerability, cost, and nonglycemic effects. All of the oral medications may be used as monotherapy or in combination with other agents, although not every possible combination is FDA-approved. Exenatide may be used in combination with 1 or 2 oral agents. Basal insulin administered at night is usually added after failure of combination oral agents at a dose of 0.2 units/kg (or 10 units) and is then titrated rapidly until fasting glucose is at goal. Once fasting glucoses reach goal, if HbA1C is still elevated, prandial insulin should be added and most oral agents sequentially withdrawn for the sake of regimen simplicity and cost savings. The intensive insulin regimens described above for type 1 diabetes are also appropriate for insulin-requiring type 2 diabetes, although usual doses exceed 1 unit/kg/day. When pre-mixed insulins are used (combination of short- and long-acting insulins, such as lispro 75/25), 2/3 of the dose is typically given before breakfast and 1/3 before the evening meal. Strict attention to timing of injections and meal times is needed (10).

Despite many effective therapies for hyperglycemia, the progressive nature of type 2 diabetes with gradual loss of insulin secretion is not altered by treatment as we know it. Adequacy of therapy must be

Table 11-3   Non-Insulin Medications for Type 2 Diabetes

Medication class	Mechanism of action	Common side effects	Rare but serious toxicities	Precautions	Dosing
Biguanide (metformin)	Inhibits hepatic glucose output	GI distress, diarrhea	Lactic acidosis	Renal or hepatic insufficiency, heavy alcohol use, heart failure, acidosis	Oral, 1–3 times daily
Thiazolidinediones (pioglitazone, rosiglitazone)	Decrease insulin resistance	Edema, weight gain	Heart failure, fractures in women; rosiglitazone may increase MI rate	Heart failure	Oral, once daily
Secretagogues (glimepiride, glyburide, glipizide, repaglinide, nateglinide)*	Stimulate insulin secretion	Hypoglycemia, weight gain		Renal or hepatic insufficiency, particularly for longer acting agents	Oral, 1–3 times daily
DPP4 Inhibitor† (sitagliptin)	Prolongs incretin concentrations	None		Dose reduction in renal insufficiency	Oral, once daily
Alpha glucosidase inhibitors (acarbose, miglitol)	Inhibit intestinal absorption of carbohydrate	GI distress		Gastrointestinal disease	Oral, 1–3 times daily with meals
GLP-1 agonist (exenatide)	Increases insulin secretion, decreases glucagon secretion, delays gastric emptying	Nausea, weight loss, vomiting	Pancreatitis	Severe gastrointestinal disease, ESRD	SQ, twice daily
Pramlintide‡	Decreases glucagon secretion, delays gastric emptying	Nausea, weight loss, vomiting		Severe gastrointestinal disease	SQ, thrice daily, with insulin

*listed in order of duration of action, longest to shortest

†DPP4, dipeptidyl peptidase 4

‡Pramlintide is approved for use together with insulin in both type 1 and type 2 diabetes

continually assessed; patients should be counseled to expect periodic intensification of therapy, including eventual insulin treatment, as a normal part of diabetes (10). The most common error made in the care of diabetic patients is failure to intensify therapy when treatment goals are not being met.

Reducing complications. The ultimate goal of reducing long-term complications of diabetes requires aggressive treatment of nonglycemic risk factors (hypertension, dyslipidemia) which are major contributors to both microvascular and macrovascular complications.

Initial pharmacologic therapy for **hypertension** includes an angiotensin converting enzyme (ACE) inhibitor or angiotensin II receptor blocker (ARB), with a diuretic added if needed. Most diabetic patients will require combination therapy to achieve blood pressure goals (see Table 11-2). No specific anti-hypertensive therapy is contraindicated in patients with diabetes, although high doses of beta blockers may impair hypoglycemic awareness and have mild adverse metabolic effects (2).

Treatment recommendations for **lipid management** include the lifestyle changes recommended above and statin therapy for patients over age 40 years with one other risk factor for cardiovascular disease (CVD), regardless of baseline lipid values. Low density lipoprotein (LDL) is the primary target, supported by overwhelming clinical evidence. Ezetimibe or binding resins (cholesevelam, cholestyramine) may be added to lower LDL further, but cholestyramine may raise triglycerides and interfere with absorption of other medications. Triglycerides and high density lipoprotein (HDL) are secondary targets and frequently require the addition of fenofibrate, gemfibrozil, or niacin. The risk of rhabdomyolysis and transaminitis is increased when statins and fibrates are used concurrently; prudent monitoring is advised. Rhabdomyolysis occurs more often with higher statin doses and in renal insufficiency. Smoking cessation may raise HDL and is recommended for all diabetic patients. Current recommendations apply to all diabetic individuals, although the weight of the evidence arises from studies in type 2 diabetes (2).

Anti-platelet therapy (aspirin 81–325 mg daily, others) is recommended unless contraindicated for those with a history of CVD or who are over age 40 years with traditional cardiac risk factors or albuminuria (2).

Testing for coronary disease should be prompted by typical or atypical cardiac symptoms or an abnormal electrocardiogram. Although the incidence of silent ischemia in diabetic patients is high, screening asymptomatic individuals remains controversial. Screening for peripheral arterial disease with an ankle–brachial index may be considered in asymptomatic patients.

Treating microvascular disease. ACE inhibitors or ARBs are recommended to slow the progression of diabetic **nephropathy** if albuminuria, hypertension, or renal insufficiency is present. Creatinine and potassium are measured, particularly after initiation of therapy. Blood pressure and albuminuria are monitored to judge the effectiveness of therapy. Protein restriction may be considered for early (0.8–1.0 g/kg body wt/day) or later (0.8 g/kg/day) stages of nephropathy (2). Care of diabetic **retinopathy** includes careful ophthalmologic observation with laser photocoagulation and other therapies when necessary (2). For diabetic **neuropathy,** tight glycemic control is the only measure shown to prevent or slow disease progression. Treatment is supportive. Pregabalin (slowly titrated to 100 mg tid) and duloxetine (60–120 mg/day) are FDA-approved medications for painful diabetic neuropathy, but other agents are also commonly used (tricyclic antidepressants and anticonvulsants). Since peripheral neuropathy predicts a higher risk of foot ulcers, patients should be instructed on regular foot inspection, foot hygiene, supportive footwear, and possible podiatric referral. Foot examination should assess sensation, skin integrity, calluses, nail pathology, and bony deformity. For autonomic neuropathy, resting tachycardia is cautiously treated with beta blockade if tolerated. Gastroparesis may improve with pro-kinetic agents (2).

Preconception care of diabetes. Unfortunately, nearly two-thirds of diabetic pregnancies are unplanned. All women and adolescents of childbearing potential should receive regular counseling about the risks of malformations and the importance of contraception. No contraceptive method is specifically contraindicated in women with diabetes. Pregnancy should be delayed until the HbA1C is as close to 6.0% as possible without hypoglycemia, since the increased risk of congenital malformations is present at the time of conception in women whose HbA1C is >1% above the normal range. Diabetic complications, including coronary artery disease, may be already present, so a comprehensive assessment should be undertaken. Pregnancy in women with untreated coronary artery disease is associated with a high mortality rate. Retinopathy may accelerate unpredictably during pregnancy, and preconception ophthalmologic consultation is essential. The risk of hypertensive disease during pregnancy is increased in women with urinary protein >190 mg/24 hours, and intrauterine growth retardation is more common when urinary protein is >400 mg/24 hours. Hypothyroidism is more common in women with type 1 diabetes; TSH should be checked prior to pregnancy or as soon as pregnancy is confirmed (2,9,12).

Treatment of diabetes during pregnancy. Insulin is the only approved therapy for diabetes during pregnancy. Metformin and acarbose are not recommended but are category B (no evidence of risk). More stringent pregnancy glycemic treatment goals are shown in see Table 11-2. Glucose records are reviewed frequently (many clinicians review weekly). Patients are seen and HbA1C is measured monthly. Insulin needs may decrease in early pregnancy, increasing the risk for hypoglycemia, and hypoglycemic unawareness may occur for the first time. Later pregnancy is characterized by insulin resistance and increasing insulin needs, which may occur dramatically and quickly at times. Hyperglycemia during pregnancy increases the risk of fetal macrosomia, respiratory distress, perinatal death, maternal hypertension, and Caesarean section.

The risk for worsening retinopathy continues throughout pregnancy and for several months after delivery. Preexisting nephropathy may worsen during pregnancy but is usually transient. However, women with creatinine clearance <50 ml/min frequently have permanent worsening of renal function. ACE inhibitors, ARBs, and statins are contraindicated during pregnancy (2,9,12).

References

1. **Wild S, Roglic G, Green A, et al.** Global prevalence of diabetes: estimates for the year 2000 and projections for 2030. Diabetes Care. 2004;27:1047–53.

2. Standards of Medical Care in Diabetes—2008. Diabetes Care. 2008;31: S12–54. (Updated each January at www.diabetes.org)

3. **Nathan DM, Davidson JM, DeFronzo RA, et al.** Impaired fasting glucose and impaired glucose tolerance: implications for care. Diabetes Care. 2007;30:753–9.

4. **Knowler WC, Barrett-Conner E, Fowler SE, the Diabetes Prevention Program Research Group, et al.** Reduction in the incidence of type 2 diabetes with lifestyle intervention or metformin. N Engl J Med. 2002;346:393–403.

5. DCCT: The effect of intensive treatment of diabetes on the development and progression of long-term complications in insulin-dependent diabetes mellitus. The Diabetes Control and Complications Trail Research group. N Engl J Med. 1993;329:381–9.

6. **Nathan DM, Cleary PA, Backlund JY, et al.** Intensive diabetes treatment and cardiovascular disease in patients with type 1 diabetes. N Engl J Med. 2005;353:2643–53.

7. UKPDS: Effect of intensive blood-glucose control with sulphonylureas or insulin compared with conventional treatment and risk of complications in patients with type 2 diabetes (UKPDS 33). UK Prospective Diabetes Study (UKPDS) Group. Lancet. 1998;352:837–53.

8. UKPDS: Effect of intensive blood-glucose control with metformin on complications in overweight patients with type 2 diabetes (UKPDS 34). UK Prospective Diabetes Study (UKPDS) Group. Lancet. 1998;352:854–65.

9. **Metzger BE, Coustan DR.** Summary and recommendations of the Fourth International Workshop-Conference on Gestational Diabetes Mellitus. The Organizing Committee. Diabetes Care. 1998;21: B161–7.

10. **Nathan DM, Buse JB, Davidson MB, et al.** Management of hyperglycemia in type 2 diabetes: A consensus algorithm for the initiation and adjustment of therapy. A consensus statement from the American Diabetes Association and the European Association for the study of diabetes. Diabetes Care. 2006;29:1963–72.

11. ACE/AACE Diabetes Road Map Task Force. Road maps to achieve glycemic control in type 2 diabetes mellitus. Endocrine Practice. 2007;13:261–8.

12. American Diabetes Association: Preconception care of women with diabetes (Position Statement). Diabetes Care. 2004;27:S76–8.

B. Thyroid Disease

Melissa K. Cavaghan

KEY POINTS

◆ Thyroid disease disproportionately affects women.

◆ Thyroid-stimulating hormone (TSH) is the appropriate screening test for disorders of thyroid function.

◆ Levothyroxine is the preferred therapy for hypothyroidism, aiming for a TSH of 1–2 mU/L.

◆ Management of hyperthyroidism depends on etiology and includes medical therapy, radioactive iodine (RAI), and surgery.

◆ Thyroid nodules should be systematically evaluated for hyperfunction or malignancy.

◆ Thyroid disease during and after pregnancy is common, poses risks to the baby and mother, and must be carefully managed.

Epidemiology

Disorders of thyroid function are congenital (rare) or acquired. Most acquired hypothyroidism is either surgical or autoimmune. The incidence of autoimmune thyroid disease increases with age, is higher in patients with a personal or family history of autoimmune disease, and disproportionately affects women at a ratio of 7–10:1. Non-autoimmune hypothyroidism is more common in areas of iodine deficiency. Hyperthyroidism is most commonly due to autoimmunity (i.e., Graves' disease), followed by nodular disease and thyroiditis. Elevated and low levels of TSH are seen in 2.5% of pregnancies and 0.1–0.4% of pregnancies, respectively. Postpartum thyroiditis occurs in up to 15% of women (1,2).

Nodular thyroid disease is more common in women, and its frequency increases with age, exposure to ionizing radiation, and iodine deficiency. Approximately 10% of thyroid nodules are cancers. Most of these have an excellent prognosis with appropriate treatment (3).

Clinical Features

Autoimmune thyroid disease—general comments. The symptoms of thyroid disease are variable and nonspecific. Patients may have only a few, or even no, symptoms. Autoimmune thyroid disease also is occasionally a component of a polyglandular autoimmune syndrome, which includes adrenal insufficiency, type 1 diabetes, vitiligo, pernicious anemia, and hypogonadism, so additional symptoms may be present.

Hypothyroidism (Box 11-4). Women often report heavier and/or less frequent menstruation and may experience infertility and more frequent miscarriages. The disease not uncommonly presents in reproductive-age women as a result of postpartum thyroiditis. The time course of symptoms is usually gradual (weeks to months). On physical examination, patients may have a small, smooth, firm goiter (variable), dry skin, coarse hair, brittle nails, and delay in the relaxation phase of the ankle deep tendon reflex. Diastolic blood pressure may be elevated. More severe signs include bradycardia, edema, pleural and pericardial effusions, and hoarseness.

Causes of hypothyroidism are listed in Box 11-5. It is frequently detected asymptomatically on screening laboratory testing. Rare cases of central (pituitary) hypothyroidism may present with symptoms of deficiency of adrenal or reproductive hormones (e.g., fatigue, anorexia, weight loss, and amenorrhea) (1).

Hyperthyroidism (Box 11-6). Women report more frequent but lighter menstrual flow and may have amenorrhea. The hyperthyroidism of postpartum thyroiditis may interfere with lactation and may precipitate or exacerbate postpartum mood disorders. These cases present 2-10 months after pregnancy, miscarriage, or pregnancy termination, recur frequently after subsequent pregnancies, and may result in permanent hypothyroidism. Graves' disease also may present or recur in the postpartum state as a result of immune reconstitution.

Hyperthyroidism has multiple etiologies (Box 11-7). Typical physical findings in patients with overt disease include tachycardia, wide pulse pressure, warm, sweaty, smooth skin, widened palpebral fissures (i.e., the thyroid "stare"), agitation, fine tremor, and brisk deep tendon reflexes. Older patients may present with "apathetic hyperthyroidism," characterized by fatigue, weight loss, dizziness, and failure to thrive. A small or minimally enlarged smooth, soft gland may indicate painless (silent, lymphocytic) thyroiditis. These patients typically present in their 3rd-6th decade. A tender gland indicates the less common subacute thyroiditis. The presence of multiple thyroid nodules suggests

---

Box 11-4   Symptoms of Hypothyroidism

- Fatigue
- Weakness
- Modest weight gain
- Cold intolerance
- Hair loss
- Difficulty with concentration, memory
- Depressed mood
- Dry skin
- Constipation, anorexia
- Menorrhagia, lengthened menstrual cyclicity, amenorrhea

Box 11-5   Causes of Hypothyroidism

Primary
- Autoimmune thyroiditis (Hashimoto's disease)
- Thyroiditis (silent, postpartum, subacute)
- Thyroid surgery
- Radioactive iodine
- External radiation (late effect)
- Iodine deficiency (more common outside the U.S.)
- Iodine excess (temporary, often due to iodinated contrast)
- Infiltrative disorders
- Drugs (amiodarone, lithium, interferon alfa, interleukin-2, ribavirin, tyrosine kinase inhibitors)
- Congenital

Central
- Pituitary tumors (including hemorrhage, infarction)
- Aneurysms
- Surgery
- Head trauma
- Infiltrative and infectious diseases
- Lymphocytic hypophysitis (*i.e.*, postpartum)
- Congenital

Adapted from Devdhar MD, Ousman YH, Burman KD. Hypothyroidism. Endocrinol Metab Clin N Am. 2007;36:595–615; with permission from Elsevier.

Box 11-6   Symptoms of Hyperthyroidism

- Fatigue
- Weight loss
- Muscle weakness
- Increased heart rate/palpitations/arrhythmia
- Heat intolerance
- Hair loss
- Insomnia, anxiety, restlessness, irritability, tremor
- Appetite increase or decrease
- Nausea, vomiting, hyperdefecation
- Increased sweating
- Decreased menstrual cyclicity, shorter periods, amenorrhea

---

toxic multi-nodular goiter as the cause. A single prominent nodule with atrophy of the surrounding tissue indicates an autonomously function-ing nodule. Graves' disease typically causes a very firm, diffusely enlarged thyroid, although mild cases may present with only a minimally enlarged gland. A thyroid bruit may be present. Graves' disease is also suggested

---

Box 11-7   Causes of Hyperthyroidism

Primary
- Graves' disease
- Toxic multinodular goiter
- Toxic single nodule
- Thyroiditis (silent, subacute, postpartum)

Secondary
- Iatrogenic/exogenous
- hCG-mediated hyperthyroidism
- Drug-induced (amiodarone)
- Iodine (in underlying toxic multinodular goiter, indolent Graves' disease)
- TSH-producing tumor (rare)
- Metastatic functional thyroid cancer (rare)
- Struma ovarii (rare)

Adapted from Nayak B, Hodak SP. Hyperthyroidism. Endocrinol Metab Clin N Am. 2007;36:617–56; with permission from Elsevier.

---

by the presence of other autoimmune diseases or thyroid ophthalmopathy: conjunctival irritation, swelling/inflammation of extraocular muscle insertion sites, and proptosis. Less commonly, ophthalmoplegia (restriction of lateral and/or upward gaze) or blurry vision is present; rarely, pretibial myxedema, the often red, raised, indurated lesion in the lateral tibial area, is seen (4).

Thyroid nodules/goiter. Most nodules are asymptomatic, but patients may report pressure during swallowing. Larger nodules also may significantly impact breathing. Pain, when present, may radiate to the ears. Multiple thyroid nodules present as a slowly expanding goiter, sometimes leading to locally compressive symptoms. Voice change, rapid growth, and progressive local symptoms are unusual and suggest malignancy.

Benign thyroid nodules are mobile with swallowing; very firm, non-mobile nodules or the presence of cervical lymphadenopathy suggests malignancy. Hyperthyroidism will accompany single thyroid nodules about 5% of the time. Patients with multi-nodular goiters are usually euthyroid at presentation. Hyperthyroidism develops slowly in approximately 25% of these cases, usually after the age of 50 years. Symptoms are typically mild or absent. Less commonly, an enlarged thyroid may contain no nodules. If hypothyroidism is not present, this is referred to as simple goiter (3).

Diagnosis and Differential Diagnosis

Laboratory evaluation of thyroid function. Laboratory evaluation should be performed in "steady-state" when possible. Because the half-life of thyroid hormone is 6–7 days, levels change very slowly. The pituitary response (TSH) also changes slowly. "Steady-state" refers to

5–6 weeks of a stable clinical condition or thyroid hormone dosing without changes in interfering medications or conditions (e.g., pregnancy, acute illness). In the vast majority of cases, the TSH response to prevailing thyroid levels should be relied upon to indicate a person's thyroid status. Except in cases of acute illness, known pituitary disease, or resolving hyperthyroidism (see "Pitfalls" below), assessment with TSH is highly reliable. If thyroxine levels are measured, the free hormone should be ordered (i.e., free T4, free thyroid index, and others) instead of total levels, which are subject to laboratory artifacts causing misleading results. Measuring T3 (triiodothyronine) levels in addition to T4 is useful in hyperthyroidism, because of the possibility of T3-predominant Graves' or nodular hyperthyroidism. There is no need to assess T3 levels in hypothyroidism.

TSH varies inversely with serum thyroid levels. TSH <0.05 mU/L indicates hyperthyroidism; TSH >8–10 mU/L indicates hypothyroidism. Free hormone levels are then measured to document the severity of disease. However, pituitary secretion of TSH is highly sensitive to peripheral thyroid levels and will be abnormal with only a small (~5%) change in serum thyroxine concentrations. In these mild cases, previously referred to as "subclinical" disease, TSH is abnormal (between 0.05 and 0.4 mU/L or between 4 and 10 mU/L, respectively), while T4 levels are still normal. Because thyroid status may fluctuate, treatment should not be initiated until these mild abnormalities in TSH are confirmed after 6–12 weeks (1,4).

Ninety percent of patients with autoimmune thyroid disease will have antibodies to thyroid peroxidase (a.k.a., anti-microsomal antibodies). If TSH is normal, the presence of antibodies does not indicate disease but rather the risk for developing future disease. Thyroid-stimulating immunoglobulin is the pathogenic antibody in Graves' disease and is used in the evaluation of pregnant women with hyperthyroidism where nuclear thyroid scanning is contraindicated. It also is measured in late pregnancy in all women with current or past Graves' disease to predict both the likelihood of fetal Graves' disease and, in untreated patients, postpartum thyrotoxicosis (2,4). Thyroglobulin and anti-thyroglobulin antibodies have no role in the evaluation of routine thyroid disease.

Hypothyroid patients also may have increased low-density lipoprotein (LDL), triglycerides, homocysteine, creatine kinase (CK), and prolactin. Hyponatremia is seen in more severe cases. Laboratory abnormalities associated with hyperthyroidism include increased transaminases and alkaline phosphatase, leukocytosis, hyperglycemia, and hypercalcemia. Anemia may accompany both hypo- and hyperthyroidism (1,4).

Pitfalls in the Interpretation of Thyroid Function Tests

Resolving hyperthyroidism. Patients with hyperthyroidism often have prolonged suppression of pituitary secretion of TSH. Free T4 and T3 levels must be followed until the TSH is in the normal range for at least 3 months.

Non-thyroid illness. Patients with significant illness (usually hospitalized patients) or malnutrition (including eating disorders) may have an inappropriately low TSH and, over time, a higher likelihood of low T4 and T3 as well. These laboratory abnormalities correct spontaneously when the underlying disease resolves and rarely represent actual thyroid disease.

Resistance to thyroid hormone. This is a rare inherited disorder of impaired thyroid hormone action characterized by a compensatory increase in thyroid hormone levels. TSH is usually normal and should be relied upon to indicate euthyroidism.

Abnormalities in thyroid binding. Thyroid hormone is highly protein-bound. Abnormal or low binding can be inherited or acquired. High levels of binding proteins also may be inherited or acquired (e.g., pregnant women, estrogen use, acute liver disease). In these cases, it is particularly important to rely upon free hormone measurements.

Thyroid function tests during pregnancy. Thyroid-binding globulin increases during pregnancy due to higher estrogen levels, which elevate total T4 and total T3 concentrations. In addition, the rise of hCG (human chorionic gonadotrophin) during early pregnancy stimulates the TSH receptor, causing a mild increase in T4 and T3 with a concomitant decrease in TSH in approximately 15% of women. These laboratory findings are present in 30–50% of women with hyperemesis gravidarum. Although it may be difficult clinically to differentiate true hyperthyroidism from the typical thyroid laboratory abnormalities of pregnancy, the latter resolve spontaneously by approximately 20 weeks (2,4).

Functional and anatomic evaluation of the thyroid. [123]I and ^{131}I scanning differentiates the cause of hyperthyroidism: an increased 24-hour uptake of the iodine tracer is seen in Graves' disease, toxic multinodular goiter, and toxic single nodule; a low uptake indicates thyroiditis. There is no role for thyroid nuclear scanning in the diagnosis of hypothyroidism (4).

Clinical evaluation of thyroid nodules. Nodules must be evaluated for the possibility of hyperfunction or malignancy (Figure 11-2). Initial evaluation includes a review of local and systemic symptoms, history of neck radiation, family history of possible thyroid disease or multiple endocrine neoplasia type 2, and a thorough examination of the thyroid and cervical lymph nodes. TSH is measured; a low value suggests a hyperfunctioning nodule. Hyperfunctioning nodules are rarely malignant and do not require biopsy. These autonomous nodules are confirmed as "hot" by thyroid nuclear scanning. The majority (~95%) of nodules, however, are not hot. Thus, when the TSH is normal, the thyroid nuclear scan is omitted. These nodules must be further evaluated by neck ultrasound to precisely measure nodule size and characterize high-risk ultrasound features (e.g., irregular borders, hypoechogenicity, fine calcifications, increased nodule vascularity, and cervical lymphadenopathy). Neck CT or MRI is useful only in evaluating airway impingement or substernal extension. In particular, infused neck CT should be avoided since the iodine content of the contrast agent will prevent the diagnostic or therapeutic use of RAI for several months.

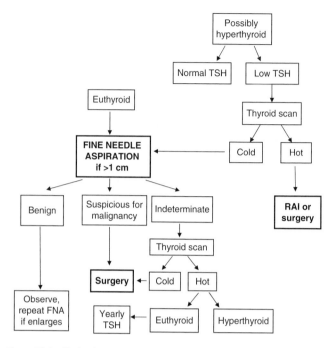

Figure 11-2   Evaluation and management of thyroid nodules.

Fine needle aspiration (FNA) is indicated for nodules >1–1.5 cm and for smaller nodules with high-risk ultrasound characteristics, even when multiple nodules are present. FNA should be performed under ultrasound guidance by physicians experienced in nodule evaluation. Results of FNAs typically fall into 1 of 4 categories: 1) non-diagnostic, or insufficient sample (must be repeated); 2) benign colloid nodule; 3) suspicious for papillary thyroid carcinoma; and 4) indeterminate. Indeterminate samples are problematic; ambiguous wording on reports may include "no evidence of malignancy" or "favor benign" (3).

Prevention and Clinical Care

Adequate iodine intake is essential for prevention of goitrous hypothyroidism and is especially important during pregnancy. Screening for thyroid disease is important in certain high-risk populations, such as the elderly, pregnant women, and patients with other autoimmune diseases.

Hypothyroidism (Box 11-8). Levothyroxine (T4) is the preferred treatment for overt hypothyroidism because its long half-life results in stable,

Box 11-8 Treatment of Hypothyroidism

Initiate treatment
- TSH >8–10 mU/L × 2 measurements without symptoms
- TSH <10 × 2 measurements with symptoms of hypothyroidism

Consider treatment
- TSH 4–10 × 2 measurements with positive microsomal antibodies

Observe
Positive microsomal antibodies, TSH <4

Thyroxine dosing
- Nonpregnant healthy patients: 1–1.6 mcg/kg/d
- Pregnant patients: 1 mcg/kg/d for mild disease, 2 mcg/kg/d for overt disease
- Cardiac disease: 25–50 mcg starting dose

Monitoring
- TSH every 6 wk until at goal of 1–2 mU/L

Interfering substances/medications
- Avoid co-administration with iron, calcium, soy
- Dose adjustment with oral estrogens, SSRIs, acid blockers, others

Adapted from Beshay VE, Beshay JE, Halvorson LM. Pituitary tumors: diagnosis, management, and implications for reproduction. Seminars in Reproductive Medicine. 2007;25:388–401; with permission.

physiologic levels of both T4 and T3, and TSH is normalized. The average dose is 1.6 mcg/kg/day on an empty stomach, specifically avoiding calcium, iron, and soy supplements within several hours of the dose. Initial doses of 25–50 mcg are recommended in patients with heart disease. The occasional missed dose should be added to the following day's dose, except in patients with heart disease. The target goal for TSH is 1–2 mU/L. Only small adjustments (~3–5%) in the weekly dose of T4 are needed to lower the TSH from the upper range of normal to the goal range of 1–2 mU/L and may require splitting pills or different doses on different days of the week. TSH should be measured no sooner than after 5 weeks of stable therapy. Oral estrogens, SSRIs (selective serotonin reuptake inhibitors), antidepressants, and acid blockers may increase thyroid hormone requirements. Attention must be paid when these medicines are started or stopped.

Whether to treat patients whose TSH is at or just above the upper limit of normal remains controversial. Treatment of asymptomatic patients with minimally elevated TSH is optional, keeping in mind that these patients progress to overt hypothyroidism at a rate of 4–18% per year (1).

Fertility/pregnancy/lactation. Thyroid disease can affect fertility and maintenance of pregnancy and should be optimally treated prior to attempting pregnancy. Women taking thyroid hormone should have a TSH drawn 6–8 weeks after stopping oral contraceptives. Some data suggest that women with positive anti-microsomal antibodies can lower their elevated risk for miscarriage by taking thyroid supplementation (1). Normal levels of maternal thyroid hormone are crucial for normal fetal neurologic development; since thyroid requirements may increase as early as the fourth week of pregnancy, TSH levels must be checked early and followed closely throughout pregnancy. When overt hypothyroidism is diagnosed during pregnancy, the starting dose of levothyroxine is 2 mcg/kg/day. Thyroid hormone doses return to pre-pregnancy requirements immediately after parturition. Failure to reduce the dose may interfere with lactation (2).

Hyperthyroidism (Box 11-9). The treatment of hyperthyroidism varies depending on the etiology. Graves' disease does not remit spontaneously and must be treated with anti-thyroid drugs, RAI (radioactive iodine), or surgery. Medical therapy is chosen to prepare a patient for RAI or

---

Box 11-9   Treatment of Hyperthyroidism

Medical therapy
- Beta blockade for symptom control until euthyroid
- Methimazole starting dose 10–30 mg/d OR
- Propylthiouracil starting dose 100–400 mg/d, divided
- Monitor T4 and T3 every 6 wk until euthyroid, then monitor TSH

Indications for medical therapy
- Induction of remission in Graves' disease
- Patient preference
- Pregnancy, lactation

Radioactive iodine
- Pre-treat with medical antithyroid therapy until euthyroid by T4/T3 levels in vulnerable patients
- Discontinue antithyroid therapy 5 d before radioactive iodine

Indications for radioactive iodine
- Definitive therapy for Graves' disease, toxic multinodular goiter, toxic single adenoma
- Intolerance to medical antithyroid therapy

Surgery
- Pre-treat with medical antithyroid therapy until euthyroid by T4/T3 levels in all patients

Indications for surgery
- Graves' ophthalmopathy
- Definitive therapy in patients ineligible for radioactive iodine
- Failure of radioactive iodine therapy
- Large compressive goiters
- Goiter where malignant potential is uncertain

surgery (to reduce operative risk) or to attempt to induce a remission. Methimazole is preferred in non-pregnant adults because it can be dosed once a day, enhancing compliance. Propylthiouracil (PTU) is preferred in pregnancy and lactation because of its demonstrated safety, and in thyroid storm because it reduces T4 to T3 conversion. Beta-blockers are added until symptomatic tachycardia resolves. The TSH is unreliable after significant hyperthyroidism, so T4 and T3 levels must be monitored and kept in the normal range. Side effects of anti-thyroid therapy include allergy and dysgeusia. Hepatotoxicity and leukopenia are infrequent and usually reversible. Vasculitic reactions are rare. RAI and surgery are definitive treatments and will render the patient hypothyroid. RAI is contraindicated in pregnant or lactating women. It also should be avoided in patients with Graves' ophthalmopathy and, possibly, in smokers, in whom there is a higher risk of worsening or new ophthalmopathy after such treatment.

Nodular hyperthyroidism often is asymptomatic and progresses slowly, making the timing of intervention less obvious than when overt disease is present. It is prudent to measure TSH for 6–12 months in mild cases to ensure that treatment is needed. Methimazole and PTU are effective, but definitive therapy with RAI or surgery is preferred. Non-functioning nodules, which also may be present, must be evaluated for possible malignancy before a decision about treatment is made.

Hyperthyroidism from thyroiditis resolves spontaneously within 3–6 months but may be followed by transient or permanent hypothyroidism. These patients should be monitored for 6–12 months. Hyperthyroidism caused by an iodine load (e.g., iodinated contrast) usually resolves in 4–6 weeks. Amiodarone-induced hyperthyroidism is more persistent and difficult to treat.

Hyperthyroidism increases the risk for atrial arrhythmias (especially in patients >65 years of age) and bone loss. Even patients with only mild suppression of TSH should be considered for treatment of their thyroid disease in order to lower these risks. Calcium and vitamin D supplementation is encouraged, and bone mineral density measurement should be considered (4).

Fertility/pregnancy/lactation. Hyperthyroidism in pregnancy should be managed by experienced clinicians to ensure that overtreatment does not occur. If hyperthyroidism persists or recurs postpartum, propylthiouracil (PTU) is the preferred agent because of its lower concentration in breast milk. Under-treatment may interfere with lactation (2).

Benign thyroid nodules. Sub-centimeter nodules or larger nodules proven benign by FNA should be measured again by ultrasound after 6 months and then at less frequent intervals if stable. Enlarging nodules require repeat FNA. Suppressive therapy with T4 is ineffective. If local symptoms are progressive, surgery may be needed.

Multi-nodular goiter. Benign hyperthyroid goiters are treated with RAI or surgery; bulky goiters causing significant local symptoms may require surgery.

Indeterminate and malignant thyroid nodules. Nodules of indeterminate cytology carry a 20% risk of malignancy and require hemi-thyroidectomy for definitive pathology. Malignant nodules require complete thyroidectomy. Thyroid surgery should be performed by a surgeon with sufficient experience to minimize complications and ensure that the appropriate surgical management is performed, particularly in the case of thyroid cancers. Most thyroid cancers require thyroid remnant ablation with RAI and long-term follow-up by endocrinologists (3).

References

1. **Devdhar MD, Ousman YH, Burman KD.** Hypothyroidism. Endocrinol Metab Clin N Am. 2007;36:595–615.
2. **LeBeau SO, Mandel SJ.** Thyroid disorders during pregnancy. Endocrinol Metab Clin N Am. 2006;35:117–36.
3. **Gharib H, Papini E.** Thyroid nodules: clinical importance, assessment, and treatment. Endocrinol Metab Clin N Am. 2007;36:707–25.
4. **Nayak B, Hodak SP.** Hyperthyroidism. Endocrinol Metab Clin N Am. 2007;36:617–56.

C. Polycystic Ovary Syndrome and Hirsutism

Rebecca A. Austin

KEY POINTS

- Polycystic ovarian syndrome (PCOS) is a clinical syndrome that includes menstrual irregularities and hyperandrogenism.
- To diagnose PCOS, other causes of irregular menses and hyperandrogenism should be excluded.
- The prevalence of PCOS is about 5% in women of child-bearing years, making it the most common endocrinopathy in women.
- PCOS is the most common cause of anovulatory infertility.
- Women with PCOS are at high risk of insulin resistance, metabolic syndrome, and type 2 diabetes.
- Hirsutism, abnormal growth of terminal hair, affects 5–10% of all women.
- Hirsutism can be a sign of PCOS, a normal variant, or a harbinger of other endocrine abnormalities.

Epidemiology

The prevalence of PCOS is 3–10% in women of reproductive age, making it the most common reproductive and metabolic disorder in women in this age group (1). PCOS is a major contributor to anovulatory infertility, which prevents pregnancy in approximately 10–25% of infertile couples (2). The underlying pathology of PCOS is unclear, but the leading hypothesis is that primary insulin resistance causes abnormal ovarian androgen secretion, which, in turn, causes anovulation and the signs of hyperandrogenism (elevated serum androgens) associated with PCOS (1).

Clinical Features

Symptoms of PCOS include oligomenorrhea, amenorrhea, or dysfunctional uterine bleeding, usually beginning at menarche. Other common symptoms are infertility, obesity, which may occur in 40–50% of patients, acne, and hirsutism (3). Many women with PCOS also have some outward signs of hyperandrogenism, including hirsutism (abnormal growth of dark, terminal hair), acne, and acanthosis nigricans (1). Obesity is another common feature of PCOS and can contribute to the insulin resistance seen in many of the patients. Skin tags and sleep apnea are uncommon symptoms associated with PCOS (4).

Diagnosis and Differential Diagnosis

The revised Rotterdam diagnostic criteria for PCOS are the most commonly used. To be diagnosed with PCOS, a woman must meet 2 out of the following 3 criteria (5):

1. Oligomenorrhea or amenorrhea;
2. Clinical and/or biochemical evidence of hyperandrogenism;
3. Presence of polycystic ovaries and exclusion of other hormonal disorders with similar clinical features, such as congenital adrenal hyperplasia (CAH), hyperprolactinemia, adrenal or ovarian adenomas, hyperthecosis, and Cushing's syndrome.

Tests of insulin resistance are not necessary to make the diagnosis of PCOS, but all obese women who have PCOS should be screened for insulin resistance and type 2 diabetes (5). Many women with PCOS have elevated fasting insulin levels and abnormal glucose tolerance tests (6). Up to 25% of all women have multiple ovarian cysts on ultrasound, so an abnormal ultrasound is not necessarily a sign of PCOS (1). However, in a woman with other clinical criteria of PCOS, an abnormal ultrasound is supportive of the diagnosis (4). The classic description of ovarian cysts on ultrasound includes 12 or more follicles, often on the periphery of the ovary (5).

Practical Diagnosis of PCOS

In practice, the diagnosis of PCOS includes the clinical syndrome of irregular menses and hyperandrogenism, after other similar disorders have been excluded. Either ultrasound findings of polycystic ovaries or an elevated testosterone level should be used to help confirm the diagnosis. PCOS is thus a clinical diagnosis, a diagnosis of exclusion, and ultra-sonographic and laboratory testing are used secondarily for confirmation or to rule out competing diagnoses (3).

Laboratory testing is used to confirm the diagnosis of PCOS, exclude other causes of hyperandrogenism, and screen for the common associated metabolic disturbances that can accompany PCOS. In women who have a clear diagnosis of PCOS and no worrisome physical findings, laboratory testing for testosterone and DHEA-S is not required, but is commonly done to confirm the diagnosis. If, however, a woman shows signs of virilization (voice changes, clitoromegaly, receding hairline, etc.) or if the diagnosis is unclear, laboratory testing is indicated to exclude an androgen-secreting tumor as the cause of her hyperandrogenism.

In women with either oligomenorrhea or amenorrhea, pregnancy testing is the first step in diagnosis. If the subject is not pregnant, laboratory testing should include thyroid stimulating hormone (TSH) and prolactin levels to exclude 2 common causes of anovulation. Subsequently, follicle-stimulating hormone (FSH) and a luteinizing hormone (LH) levels should be obtained (5). An elevated FSH level signifies premature ovarian failure. In women with PCOS, LH is often elevated and, if not elevated, the ratio of LH to FSH is greater than 3:1. Testing to exclude other causes of hyperandrogenism should include free testosterone, dehydroepiandrosterone-sulfate (DHEA-S), and, possibly, a 17-hydroxyprogesterone level (17-OHP) (1). Serum free testosterone is generally elevated in patients with PCOS but may suggest an androgen-secreting tumor if the level is over 200 ng/dL. DHEA-sulfate, similarly, may be somewhat elevated but should not be markedly so. Levels of 7000 mcg/dL or greater may suggest an adrenal tumor. 17-OHP should be obtained if there is a suspicion of congenital adrenal hyperplasia due to 21-hydroxylase deficiency. A 17-OHP value of <3 ng/dL during the follicular phase excludes this entity (1) (Table 11-4).

Prevention and Clinical Care

PCOS is associated with an increased risk of metabolic syndrome (MS) (for more information, see Section E), insulin resistance, obesity, and type 2 diabetes. Therefore, the American College of Obstetricians and Gynecologists recommends (7):

Level A Evidence: (supported by high quality randomized controlled trials)
- All women with PCOS should be screened for glucose intolerance with a 2-hour glucose tolerance test (GTT).
- Women should be screened for hyperlipidemia with a fasting lipid profile.

Table 11-4   Differential Diagnosis of PCOS

Diagnosis	Signs	Testing
Ovarian hyperthecosis	• Severe hirsutism • Clitoromegaly and temporal balding • Marked insulin resistance • Acanthosis nigricans	Pelvic ultrasound shows enlarged, thickened stroma (pathologically, luteinized theca cells with dense fibroblasts)
Congenital adrenal hyperplasia (adult onset)	• Clitoromegaly • Regular menses • Short stature • Familial pattern (autosomal recessive)	Elevated 17-hydroxy-progesterone level
Cushing's syndrome	• Moonlike facies • Buffalo hump • Abdominal striae • Hypertension • Osteoporosis • Muscle wasting	Increased urinary free cortisol, failure of dexamethasone suppression, no polycystic findings in ovaries
Androgen-producing tumors of ovary or adrenal gland	• Rapid onset of hirsutism • Male body habitus • Clitoromegaly • Acne • Menses variable	Elevated androgens Pelvic, abdominal, or retroperitoneal mass

From Hunter MH, Sterrett JJ. Polycystic ovarian syndrome: it's not just infertility. American Family Physician. 2000;62:1079–88,90. Chang R, Jeffrey A. A practical approach to the diagnosis of polycystic ovarian syndrome. American Journal of Obstetrics and Gynecology. 2004;191:713–7; with permission.

Level B Evidence: (supported by systematic reviews or high quality case control studies)

• Improved insulin sensitivity (via weight loss, metformin, and/or thiazolidenediones) may improve risk factors for diabetes and cardiovascular disease.

Treatment of Symptoms

Symptomatic treatment in women with PCOS involves correcting their anovulation and treating unwanted signs of hyperandrogenism (mostly hirsutism). Treatment of amenorrhea in patients not desiring fertility commonly includes oral contraceptive pills (OCPs) (7). All OCPs increase sex hormone-binding globulin (SHBG) production in the liver. This increased level of SHBG binds more free testosterone, thereby helping to decrease signs of hyperandrogenism, as well as regulating the menstrual cycle. Many practitioners recommend using OCPs with low androgenic progestins. Progesterone alone may be used to induce withdrawal bleeding cyclically and regulate menses in women who do not need contraception (7).

Non-pharmacologic treatment of infertility includes weight reduction. Weight reduction of as little as 5% improves insulin sensitivity and can increase ovulation and rates of fertility in up to 75% of women with PCOS (2). All overweight women with PCOS should be counseled on eating a healthy diet and performing regular exercise.

Medications for infertility resulting from anovulation include clomiphene citrate (which induces ovulation) and metformin. Metformin works by decreasing insulin resistance to increase ovulation and fertility, compared with placebo, and improves ovulatory pattern (8). Studies comparing metformin with clomiphene show variable results in pregnancy rates, and metformin added to clomiphene does not improve rates of ovulation (9). Metformin also may reduce the risk of spontaneous abortion and should be continued in a successful pregnancy through the first trimester. Metformin is recommended only for women with PCOS who have insulin resistance (10). Clomiphene citrate is the first-line treatment for induction of ovulation in women with PCOS and infertility (10).

Thiazolidinediones (TZDs) increase the chances of ovulation and insulin sensitivity but are classified as FDA pregnancy category C (see appendix for FDA pregnancy categories), rather than B, and, therefore, have not been evaluated as much studied or recommended (4).

Clomiphene citrate has been studied in patients with PCOS, as well as in other patients with ovulation difficulties. Ovarian size is followed via ultrasound during clomiphene therapy (2).

Hirsutism

Clinical Presentation

Hirsutism, or abnormal growth of coarse, dark hair in areas normally free from such hair, occurs in 5–10% of all women and is a common symptom of PCOS. It may occur with or without virilization. Normal amounts of hair growth in women vary depending on ethnicity. Hirsutism is caused by high androgen levels (from ovaries or adrenals) or by increased sensitivity to normal androgen levels and their actions on hair follicles (11). Women may report abnormal facial or body hair that causes distress.

The physical examination of a woman with hirsutism begins with an evaluation of the degree of hair growth at 11 specific sites on the body: upper lip, chin, chest, upper and lower abdomen, thigh, upper and lower back, upper arm, forearm, and upper and lower leg (11). Documentation of hair growth can aid in assessing future treatment. Evaluation for any signs of virilization (clitoromegaly, increased muscle mass, deepening voice, infrequent menses, or frontotemporal balding) is also important to exclude malignant causes of hyperandrogenism (11). A rapid onset of symptoms or progression of hair growth can signify an androgen-secreting tumor. Idiopathic hirsutism, PCOS, and Congenital adrenal hyperplasia (CAH) more typically present at puberty with slow, progressive hair growth (11). Less common physical findings, which may be helpful, include palpable ovarian tumors, acanthosis nigricans (which can be a clue to insulin resistance), and the moon facies, buffalo hump, and abdominal striae of Cushing's syndrome (11).

Differential Diagnosis

In women who have hirsutism with virilization, the differential diagnosis includes PCOS, hyperthecosis, HAIR-AN (hyperandrogenism, insulin resistance, acanthosis nigricans), tumors, CAH, and Cushing's syndrome. In women who have hirsutism without virilization, the differential diagnosis includes PCOS, racial, familial, physiologic causes (puberty, pregnancy, and menopause), hypothyroidism, acromegaly, Hurler's syndrome, porphyria, hamartomas, drugs, and central nervous system lesions (12).

Laboratory Testing

Initial laboratory testing should focus on evaluation of hyperandrogenism and should include DHEA-S and total or free testosterone (11). If hirsutism has an onset at puberty, a 17-OH progesterone level should be obtained to evaluate for CAH (11).

Treatment of Hirsutism

The treatments for hirsutism are shown in Tables 11-5 and 11-6.

Table 11-5 Pharmacotherapy for Treatment of Hirsutism

Therapy	Comments
OCPs	Reduce free testosterone by increasing SHBG; consider use of low androgenic progestin
Spironolactone	Androgen receptor blocker
Vaniqua (eflornithine HCL topical cream)	Improvement may be seen in 4–8 wk; hair will return to normal growth rate 8 wk after cessation
Glucocorticoids	Treatment for a year, then should be discontinued. Best for hirsutism of short duration

From Hunter MH, Carek PJ. Evaluation and treatment of women with hirsutism. American Family Physician. 2003;67:2565–72. Habif TP, editor. Clinical Dermatology 4th Edition, 2004. Mosby, Elsevier, Amsterdam, The Netherlands; with permission.

Table 11-6   Cosmetic Therapy for Treatment of Hirsutism

Shaving	Does not increase number or thickness of hairs	Shave with the grain to avoid folliculitis
Waxing and plucking	Removes hair at root	May last up to 6 wk
Bleaching	Helpful for light-skinned patients	Skin irritation may occur
Depilatories	Break down hair shaft; remove some hair below skin level	May last longer than shaving, but may cause irritation
Electrolysis	Permanent follicular destruction with electrical probe	Expensive, painful, slow; may cause hypertrophic scars
Lasers	Multiple types; some better for dark vs. light skin	Expensive, can cause erythema, multiple treatments needed

From Hunter MH, Carek PJ. Evaluation and treatment of women with hirsutism. American Family Physician. 2003;67:2565–72. Habif TP, editor. Clinical Dermatology 4th Edition, 2004. Mosby, Elsevier, Amsterdam, The Netherlands; with permission.

References

1. **Hunter MH, Sterrett JJ.** Polycystic ovarian syndrome: it's not just infertility. American Family Physician. 2000;62:1079–88, 90.
2. **Katz VL, editor.** Comprehensive Gynecology 2007; 5th edition. Elsevier, Amsterdam, Netherlands.
3. **Chang R, Jeffrey A.** A practical approach to the diagnosis of polycystic ovarian syndrome. American Journal of Obstetrics and Gynecology. 2004;191:713–7.
4. **Futterweit W.** Polycystic ovarian syndrome: a common reproductive and metabolic disorder necessitates early recognition and treatment. Primary Care: Clinics in Office Practice. 2007;34:761–89.
5. Rotterdam ESHRE/ASRM-sponsored PCOS consensus working group. Revised 2003 consensus on diagnostic criteria and long term health risks related to PCOS. Fertility and Sterility. 2004;81:19–25.
6. **Hoffman LK, Ehrmann DA.** Cardiometabolic features of polycystic ovarian syndrome. National Clinical Practice of Endocrinology and Metabolism. 2008;4:215–22.
7. American College of Obstetricians and Gynecologists. Clinical guidelines on diagnosis and treatment of polycystic ovarian syndrome. Obstetrics and Gynecology. 2002:100: 1389–402.
8. **Lord JM, flight IH, Normal RJ.** Metformin in polycystic ovarian syndrome: a systematic review and meta-analysis. BMJ. 2003;327:951–3.
9. **Moll E, et al.** Effect of clomiphene citrate plus metformin and clomiphene citrate and placebo on induction of ovulation in women with newly diagnosed polycystic ovarian syndrome: randomized double blind clinical trial. BMJ. 2006;332:1485.

10. Thessaloniki ESHRE/ASRM-sponsored polycystic ovarian syndrome consensus working group. Consensus on infertility treatment related to polycystic ovarian syndrome. Human Reproduction. 2008;23:462–77.
11. **Hunter MH, Carek PJ.** Evaluation and treatment of women with hirsutism. American Family Physician. 2003;67:2565–72.
12. **Habif TP, editor.** Clinical Dermatology, 4th Edition, 2004. Mosby, Elsevier, Amsterdam, The Netherlands.

D. Pituitary Disorders

Sarina B. Schrager

KEY POINTS

- Pituitary disorders in women have multiple reproductive consequences, most commonly abnormal menses and infertility.
- Pituitary tumors account for 15% of all intracranial tumors and are predominantly benign.
- Hypopituitarism is associated with increased mortality.
- Prolactinomas are the most common hormonally active tumors of the pituitary gland.
- TSH-secreting adenomas can be difficult to diagnose and usually present with normal to high TSH levels and elevated T3 and T4 levels.
- Women with gonadotropin deficiency from hypopituitarism should be given estrogen/progestin supplementation until menopause.

Epidemiology

The pituitary gland is an endocrine gland the size of a pea located at the base of the skull. The pituitary gland produces many hormones, several of which have a direct effect on women's reproductive functioning. Pituitary hormones include prolactin, growth hormone (GH), adrenocorticotropic hormone (ACTH), thyroid-stimulating hormone (TSH), anti-diuretic hormone (ADH), luteinizing hormone (LH), and follicle stimulating hormone (FSH). Prolactin, TSH, LH, and FSH have the most impact on women's reproductive health and will be the focus of this section.

The most frequent cause of pituitary disorders is tumors. Pituitary tumors are the most commonly occurring intracranial neoplasms, accounting for up to 15% of all intracranial tumors (1). The vast majority

Table 11-7   Causes of Pituitary Insufficiency

Brain Damage	Tumors	Infection	Infarction	Miscellaneous
Brain injury	Pituitary	Abscess	Sheehan's	Lymphocytic
Subarachnoid	adenomas	Hypophysitis	syndrome	hypophysitis
hemorrhage	Metastatic	Meningitis	Apoplexia	Hemachromatosis
Neurosurgery	tumors	Encephalitis		Granulomatous
Radiation	Primary brain			disease
CVA	tumors			Perinatal damage
				Idiopathic

Adapted from Schneider HJ, Aimaretti G, Kreitschmann-Andermahr I, et al. Hypopituitarism. Lancet. 2007;369:1461–70; with permission.

of pituitary tumors are benign, but they can cause morbidity by creating hypersecretion of certain hormones. Pituitary tumors can also cause a mass effect by their growth, which can, in turn, cause other hormones normally produced by the pituitary gland to be decreased. Additionally, the mass effect may affect other nearby structures (e.g., the optic nerve). Prolactinoma is the most common hormonally active pituitary tumor (1).

Hypopituitarism is the other common disorder that affects the pituitary gland. It is also known as pituitary insufficiency and can include a deficiency of some or all of the hormones normally produced by the pituitary gland. Hypopituitarism is usually a lifelong disorder and is associated with increased mortality (2). People can have symptoms related to decreased production of one or several of the normally produced pituitary hormones. Pituitary insufficiency can be caused by many different factors, including tumors, infections, trauma, and autoimmune disorders (2) (Table 11-7).

Clinical Features

Although deficiency and hypersecretion of all of the pituitary hormones can cause morbidity and mortality, prolactin, TSH, and the gonadotropins (LH and FSH) are the most clinically relevant in women.

Prolactin

Low prolactin levels can be caused by pituitary insufficiency. The clinical implications of low prolactin levels are mostly seen in postpartum women with inability to breastfeed. Elevated prolactin levels are much more common and can cause infertility, breast tenderness, and galactorrhea. Elevated prolactin levels can be caused by pituitary adenomas as well as multiple other disorders. (Table 11-8)

Prolactin-secreting pituitary adenomas, or prolactinomas, can be classified by size as either microadenomas or macroadenomas. Clinical presentation of these tumors can include signs and symptoms of

Table 11-8   Causes of Hyperprolactinemia

Medications	Central Tumors	Physiologic	Other
Antipsychotics (dopamine receptor blockers) SSRIs Tricyclic antidepressants Verapamil Alpha methyl dopa	Prolactinomas Other pituitary adenomas Hypothalamic lesions Empty sella syndrome	Pregnancy Breast stimulation (i.e. nipple piercing) Breastfeeding	Chest wall trauma Primary hypo- thyroidism Renal failure (decreased clearance)

Adapted from Beshay VE, Beshay JE, Halvorson LM. Pituitary tumors: diagnosis, management, and implications for reproduction. Seminars in Reproductive Medicine. 2007;25:388–401; with permission.

hyperprolactinemia or symptoms of visual field deficits caused by growth of the tumor and compression of the optic nerve (macroadenomas).

Treatment of hyperprolactinemia is mostly medical with the dopamine receptor agonists bromocriptine or cabergolide. In most cases of microadenomas, this treatment is sufficient to bring prolactin levels down low enough to resolve symptoms. In some cases, when macroadenomas do not shrink while on medication, surgical removal is indicated. Studies have shown that cabergolide has improved response rates over bromocriptine with fewer side effects. However, since it has not been available for as long as bromocriptine, it is not as commonly used in pregnancy. There is a theoretical possibility of tumor growth due to the estrogen stimulation of pregnancy, but studies have shown that in women with microadenomas, pregnancy has little effect on the tumor size (3). However, in women with macroadenomas, the increased levels of estrogen during pregnancy can cause significant tumor enlargement in pregnancy (4).

Thyroid-Stimulating Hormone

Thyrotropin-secreting pituitary adenomas are the least common type of pituitary tumors and account for 1–2% of these tumors (1). They are a very rare cause of hyperthyroidism (5). Women commonly present with signs of hyperthyroidism but often have a normal TSH level in the context of elevated T3 and T4 levels. The diagnosis of these lesions may be difficult but should include an MRI and possibly a thyroid-releasing hormone (TRH) stimulation test. Distinguishing central hyperthyroidism from Graves' disease can be a challenge, but women with TSH-secreting tumors do not have antibodies associated with autoimmune thyroiditis. Because the diagnosis is difficult, most of the time these tumors are not discovered until they become macroadenomas (6). Treatment is usually surgical, though medical administration of somatomedin can sometimes control symptoms.

Hyperthyroidism from these tumors can cause oligomenorrhea, amenorrhea, and infertility in women. Hyperthyroidism itself also can cause increased conversion of androgens to estrogen (1).

Central hypothyroidism from pituitary insufficiency is similar to peripheral hypothyroidism and is diagnosed with elevated TSH levels with low levels of free T4. Hypothyroidism also can cause reproductive abnormalities predominantly associated with ovulatory disorders. Women with hypothyroidism can have amenorrhea, oligomenorrhea, and subsequent infertility. Treatment of central hypothyroidism consists mainly of thyroid hormone replacement therapy.

Gonadotropins (Follicle Stimulating Hormone and Luteinizing Hormone)

Gonadotropin-secreting pituitary adenomas (gonadotropinomas) are fairly uncommon. These tumors usually secrete FSH but rarely at high levels (1). Consequently, women with gonadotropinomas rarely exhibit symptoms of gonadotropin excess and, instead, present with less specific signs of hypopituitarism (due to the undersecretion of other hormones) or hyperprolactinemia. Macroadenomas can cause compression of adjacent structures and present as headaches or visual field disturbances. Diagnosis of these lesions may be difficult and involve an MRI in addition to hormone assays.

Gonadotropinomas can cause anovulation with consequent amenorrhea and infertility. The treatment of these tumors is usually surgical.

Deficiency of LH and FSH from hypopituitarism usually presents with menstrual irregularities such as oligomenorrhea and amenorrhea. Laboratory evaluation shows low LH and FSH levels signaling secondary hypogonadism (2). Treatment in premenopausal women is with estrogen/progestin-containing contraceptives or hormone replacement therapy until menopause. In women who wish to become pregnant, injectable synthetic FSH can be administered.

References

1. **Beshay VE, Beshay JE, Halvorson LM.** Pituitary tumors: diagnosis, management, and implications for reproduction. Seminars in Reproductive Medicine. 2007;25:388–401.
2. **Schneider HJ, Aimaretti G, Kreitschmann-Andermahr I, et al.** Hypopituitarism. Lancet. 2007;369:1461–70.
3. **Christin-Maitre S, Delemer B, Touraine P, et al.** Prolactinoma and estrogens: pregnancy, contraception, and hormonal replacement therapy. Annals of Endocrinology. 2007;68:106–12.
4. **Molitch ME.** Pituitary disorders during pregnancy. Endocrinology and Metabolism Clinics of North America. 2006;35:99–116.
5. **Beck-Peccoz P, Brucker-Davis F, Persani L, et al.** Thyrotropin-secreting pituitary tumors. Endocrinology Review. 1996;17:610–38.
6. **Foppiani L, Del Monte P, Ruelle A, et al.** TSH-secreting adenomas: rare pituitary tumors with multifaceted clinical and biological features. Journal of Endocrinologic Investigation. 2007;30:603–9.

E. Metabolic Syndrome: A Clustering of Cardiometabolic Risk Factors

Michael J. Waddell and Rattan Juneja

KEY POINTS

- Metabolic syndrome is an increasing problem worldwide, potentially reaching pandemic proportions.
- A unifying definition of metabolic syndrome is difficult to come by, since different organizations have not used the same criteria to describe the condition.
- In broad terms, metabolic syndrome encompasses a clustering of factors contributing to cardiac risk.
- Central obesity and insulin resistance are thought to be key underlying factors in its pathophysiology, with waist circumference being a clinical surrogate for its presence.
- The overall goal of management is to reduce cardiac risk; therefore, treatment is targeted at management of the underlying cardiovascular risk factors.

Definitions

The concept of metabolic syndrome emerged decades ago when a correlation between obesity, the risk of diabetes, and coronary artery disease became apparent. Gerald Reaven first described "Syndrome X" in 1988 to encompass a cluster of abnormalities involving glycemic control, hypertension, and dyslipidemia (1). This syndrome has since been referred to by many different names, including the insulin resistance syndrome and, more recently, the metabolic syndrome.

It is important to note that metabolic syndrome is not a discrete entity but a clustering of attributes that predispose to cardiac and metabolic risk. Hence, the term cardiometabolic syndrome also is used to describe the condition. Although insulin resistance and abdominal obesity appear to be central to its occurrence, no single pathogenic mechanism for its development has been clearly identified. This has led to different organizations developing their own interpretations of what constitutes the metabolic syndrome (Table 11-9). The first formal definition was proposed in 1998 by the World Health Organization (WHO) and centered on the presence of insulin resistance, as measured in a laboratory using an insulin clamp (2). The European Group for the Study of Insulin Resistance released its modifications to the WHO definition in 1999,

Table 11-9 Criteria Proposed for the Diagnosis of Metabolic Syndrome

Clinical Measure	WHO (1998)	EGIR	ATP III (2001)	AACE (2003)	IDF (2005)
Insulin resistance	IGT, IFG, DM2, or lowered insulin sensitivity* **plus any 2 of the following**	Plasma insulin >75th percentile **plus any of the following**	None, but **any 3 of the following 5 features**	IGT or IFG **plus any of the following based on clinical judgment**	None
Body weight	Men: waist to hip ratio >0.90 Women: waist to hip ratio >0.85 And/or BMI >30	WC ≥94 cm in men or ≥80 cm in women	WC ≥102 cm in men or ≥88 cm in women[†]	BMI ≥25	Increased WC (population specific)[#] **plus any 2 of the following**
Lipid	TG ≥150 and/or HDL ≤35 in men or ≤39 in women	TG ≥150 and/or HDL ≤39 in men or women	TG ≥150 HDL <40 in men or <50 in women	TG ≥150 and HDL <40 in men or <50 in women	TG ≥150 or on TG Rx HDL <40 in men or <50 in women or on HDL Rx
Blood pressure	≥140/90 or on hypertension Rx	≥140/90 or on hypertension Rx	≥135/85	≥135/85	≥135 systolic or ≥85 diastolic or on hypertension Rx
Glucose	IGT, IFG, or DM2	IGT or IFG but not diabetes	>110 mg/dL (includes diabetes)[‡]	IGT or IFG but not diabetes	≥100 mg/dL (includes diabetes)
Other	Microalbuminuria			Other features of insulin resistance[§]	

DM2 indicates type 2 diabetes; WC indicates waist circumference; BMI body mass index; TG triglycerides

*Insulin sensitivity measured under hyperinsulinemic euglycemic conditions, glucose uptake below lowest quartile for background population under investigation.

†Some male patients can develop multiple metabolic risk factors when the WC is only marginally increased (94–102 cm). Such patients should benefit from changes in lifestyle habits.

‡The 2001 definition identified fasting plasma glucose ≥110 as elevated. This was modified in 2004 to be ≥100 in accordance with the ADA's updated definition of IFG.

§Includes family history of type 2 diabetes, polycystic ovarian syndrome, sedentary lifestyle, advancing age, and ethnic groups susceptible to type 2 diabetes.

‖WC ≥94 cm in Europid men and ≥80 cm in Europid women. WC ≥90 cm in Chinese/South Asian men and ≥80 cm in Chinese/South Asian women. WC ≥85 cm in Japanese men and ≥90 cm in Japanese women.

In 2005, the American Heart Association/National Heart, Lung, and Blood Institute issued a statement of guidance on metabolic syndrome. The criteria are essentially the same as the ATP III with the addition of "drug treatment" as a positive for any of the components.

From Grundy SM, Cleeman JI, et al. Diagnosis and management of metabolic syndrome: an American Heart Association/National Heart, Lung, and Blood Institution Scientific Statement. Circulation. 2005;112:2735–52. Grundy SM, Brewer B, Cleeman JI et al. Definition of metabolic syndrome. Circulation. 2004;109:433–8.Simonson GD, Kendall DM. Diagnosis of insulin resistance and associated syndromes: the spectrum from metabolic syndrome to type 2 diabetes. Coronary Artery Disease. 2005;16:465–72; with permission.

again focusing on insulin resistance (2). In 2001, perhaps the most well-known and utilized definition of metabolic syndrome was proposed by the National Cholesterol Education Program (NCEP) Adult Treatment Panel III (commonly referred to as ATP III criteria) (3). This definition was designed for simplicity of use in the clinical setting. It requires any 3 of the following: abdominal obesity, as determined by waist circumference; elevated triglycerides; reduced HDL; elevated blood pressure; and elevated fasting glucose (impaired fasting glucose [IFG] or type 2 diabetes) to make a diagnosis. In 2003, the American Association of Clinical Endocrinologists (AACE) released another set of criteria based on the ATP III definition but now including insulin resistance, as determined by clinical surrogates (see Table 11-9). In 2005, the International Diabetes Foundation (IDF) published yet another modification of the ATP III criteria, this time lowering the threshold for abdominal obesity and separating it by ethnicity (2).

Given these disparate descriptions, it is obvious that a single, straightforward definition of metabolic syndrome does not exist. However, the presence of metabolic syndrome does point to one fact: an elevated cardiovascular risk. Therefore, one could surmise that for patients at a high risk for cardiovascular disease, the healthcare provider must screen for individual risk factors. For uniformity throughout this chapter, the term metabolic syndrome will be used to encompass all of the above descriptions.

Epidemiology

Metabolic syndrome is a growing problem, both in the U.S. and around the world, reaching pandemic proportions. As grows the girth of a nation, so does the number of patients with this condition. The overall prevalence among U.S. adults is about 23%, or 47 million people, and it increases with age (4). Data from NHANES III showed a prevalence of 7% in the 20–29-year-old age group, 20% in those 40–49 years, 44% in the 60–69-year range, and 42% in those >70 years (5). Among ethnic groups in the U.S., the highest rates of metabolic syndrome are seen in Latinos, followed by non-Latino Whites and African Americans. This may be secondary to the higher prevalence of obesity in Latinos and, likewise, the lower frequency of dyslipidemia in African Americans (4).

Females have a lower prevalence of metabolic syndrome than males, at least up to the age of 65 years (6). After this, due to the relative estrogen-deficient state of menopause, an android pattern of fat distribution (an increase in visceral fat) in females leads to an increased prevalence of the syndrome (see clinical features below) (6,7). Females with a history of gestational diabetes mellitus have a 3-fold increased risk (7), and high-carbohydrate intake and physical inactivity increase the risk in both sexes. Additionally, childhood obesity, with its prolonged insulin resistance, has been postulated to lead to hypertension and dys-lipidemia as the child ages (4).

Clinical Features

Given the plethora of definitions, metabolic syndrome is probably best described as a clustering of cardiac and metabolic risk factors. These factors include hypertension, abdominal obesity, dyslipidemia, and an insulin-resistant state. A pro-inflammatory and pro-thrombotic milieu are thought to coexist, probably due to obesity's association with an increase in adipokines and a decrease in adiponectin (see Pathophysiology). Taken together, these factors interact to cause an increase in atherogenesis and, thus, an increased risk of morbidity and mortality from cardiovascular disease (5).

The underlying metabolic derangements in this syndrome are thought to originate from insulin resistance and/or central obesity. The uni-fying pathophysiological attribute for all of the risk factors in meta-bolic syndrome is probably insulin resistance. Clinically, however, insulin resistance is difficult to quantify (8); therefore, measures of obesity, body mass, and central adiposity have been postulated to be reasonable surrogates. Abdominal obesity by ATP III criteria is a waist circumference >102 cm (or 40 inches) in men and >88 cm (or 35 inches) in women of Caucasian descent. With obesity, the location of the adipose tissue becomes extremely important. Visceral or intra-abdominal adiposity makes patients much more susceptible to meta-bolic syndrome than does subcutaneous fat (6). Phenotypically, this presents as an "apple"-shaped body habitus, compared to a "pear" shape (Figure 11-3). Men tend to carry more intra-abdominal fat (and, thus, are "apple"-shaped), while women are generally "pear"-shaped. But women who have an "apple"-shaped habitus have higher rates of insulin resistance and metabolic syndrome than women of the same weight who have a "pear"-shaped habitus. Measuring the waist circum-ference at the level of the iliac crest (see Figure 11-3) is the most easily obtainable clinical marker for abdominal obesity and, thus, indirectly for insulin resistance (8).

Other clinical conditions that are linked with metabolic syndrome include fatty liver, asthma, cholesterol gallstones, sleep apnea, and polycystic ovarian syndrome (PCOS) (3). There is also speculation that metabolic syndrome may be related to an increase in breast cancer risk (9) and recurrence, modulated through changes in adipokines (see Pathophysiology).

Pathophysiology

Pathophysiologically, metabolic syndrome is believed to be related to a complex series of interactions involving intra-abdominal obesity and insulin resistance (Figure 11-4).

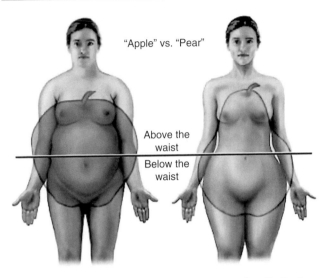

Figure 11-3   Apple vs. pear shaped body habitus. (From http://graphics8.nytimes.com/images/2007/08/01/health/adam/19265.jpg)

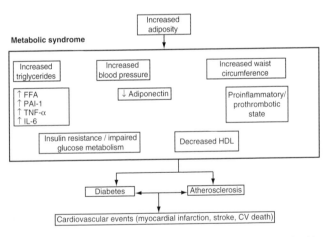

Figure 11-4   The metabolic storm of metabolic syndrome and cardiovascular risk.

Abdominal Obesity and Disorders of Adipose Tissue

In general, an increase in intra-abdominal obesity is considered harmful. It is now established that adipose tissue is an endocrine organ that produces adipokines, such as interleukin-6 (IL-6), tumor necrosis factor-α (TNF-α), and plasminogen activator inhibitor-1 (PAI-1). Changes in the levels of these adipokines can induce insulin resistance, inflammation, dyslipidemia, hypercoagulability, and endothelial dysfunction (5). In addition, adipose tissue also produces adiponectin. Unlike adipokines, adiponectin improves insulin sensitivity and has anti-diabetic and anti-atherosclerotic properties. An increase in intra-abdominal obesity is associated with a paradoxical decrease in the levels of adiponectin, thus contributing to the worsening of insulin resistance and atherosclerosis (10). This decrease in adiponectin is postulated to be secondary to antagonistic effects of the increased levels of the adipokine, TNF-α. An increase in intra-abdominal obesity leads to increased mobilization of non-esterified fatty acids. These fatty acids overload liver metabolism and lead to ectopic fat deposition causing fatty liver and non-alcoholic fatty liver disease (NFLD) (10).

Insulin Resistance/Dyslipidemia

Insulin resistance can best be thought of as a failure of insulin to perform its physiological activities to the extent expected. The roles of insulin resistance, obesity, and liver metabolism are intertwined through a series of metabolic pathways. Insulin resistance leads to increased mobilization of free fatty acids as a result of an increase in lipolysis. These free fatty acids, when oxidized in the muscles, result in decreased glucose utilization, thus elevating blood glucose levels. In addition, as these free fatty acids flow into the liver, they get packaged into very low-density lipoprotein (VLDL) particles, elevating triglycerides. Through the enzyme cholesteryl ester transferase protein (CETP), high density lipoprotein (HDL) transfers its lipid into VLDL, resulting in the classic low-HDL and high-triglyceride lipid abnormalities seen in metabolic syndrome (7). Insulin resistance is postulated to cause an increase in adrenergic tone and fluid retention, thus contributing to hypertension, another hallmark of the syndrome (5).

In pathophysiologic terms, therefore, this syndrome could be considered to be the result of a "metabolic storm": increased intra-abdominal obesity interacting with insulin resistance, generating adipokines, and suppressing the protective adiponectin, all of which ultimately culminates in an increased cardiovascular risk.

Clinical Management

In the absence of a unifying definition, or even the existence of a specific condition, clinical management can best be done by treating individual cardiac and metabolic risk factors that predispose to cardiovascular risk. This strategy is often referred to as cardiometabolic risk reduction (11). For instance, if a patient has diabetes or known cardiovascular disease, aggressive management of all risk factors is the standard of care, regardless of an actual diagnosis of metabolic syndrome. On the other hand, a diagnosis of metabolic syndrome in the absence of established diabetes or cardiovascular disease does carry with it an increased risk of developing either or both of these conditions. Therefore, the goals of management would really depend on the clinical circumstance.

The cornerstone of management involves life-style changes designed to achieve weight loss (and thus a decrease in intra-abdominal fat). Weight loss can improve all components of this syndrome. A reasonable goal would be to strive for a 7–10% weight loss over 6–12 months (2). Weight loss should be encouraged via increased physical activity, a healthier diet, and a decrease in caloric intake. In the Diabetes Prevention Program, an NIH-funded study of pre-diabetes patients (12), exercising just 30 minutes a day, 5 days a week, reduced the risk of developing diabetes by 58%.

Drugs for weight loss have had minimal long-term success due to lack of compliance and/or side effects. Sibutramine (Meridia), a neuronal serotonin reuptake inhibitor, suppresses appetite via inhibition of serotonin and norepinephrine reuptake, resulting in weight loss (3.5–7.8 kg) and improvement in lipids and glycemic control. However, the norepinephrine effect can lead to hypertension (13,14). Orlistat (Xenical or Alli) works as an intestinal lipase inhibitor that prevents absorption of fat. However, the modest weight loss of 1.5–6 kg achieved is limited by diarrhea from the malabsorption of fats, thus decreasing its acceptability by patients (12,13). A novel agent, Rimonabant, works as an endocannabinoid receptor antagonist and has shown promise in treating obesity, dyslipidemia, insulin resistance, and glycemic control. The cannabinoid receptor, CB1, present in the brain, is involved in central regulation of food intake. Endocannabinoids (cannabinoid produced in the body in response to neural signals) stimulate appetite by binding to these receptors. Rimonabant, by competitively binding to the CB1 receptor, inhibits endocannabinoid binding, thus suppressing appetite and facilitating weight loss (13,14). However, reports of increase in depressive symptoms with this medication have limited its use, and further trials are needed before this drug can come to market in the U.S. Bariatric surgery might be an option, especially for those with a BMI >40 kg/m^2, or BMI >35 kg/m^2 with significant comorbidities, such as diabetes, heart disease, or severe sleep apnea.

Along with weight loss, management should consist of appropriate therapies directed at the other components of metabolic syndrome that contribute to cardiovascular risk, such as hypertension and dyslipidemia, in keeping with established guidelines for targets to be achieved for each individual condition (Table 11-10).

In summary, perhaps the greatest clinical value in considering a diagnosis of metabolic syndrome is to "raise a red flag" for cardiometabolic risk. Making a diagnosis would facilitate the incorporation not only of life-style changes on the part of the patient but also aggressive treatment of individual components of the syndrome with appropriate pharmacotherapy by the physician.

Table 11-10   Management of Metabolic Syndrome. The Cornerstone Is Weight Loss and Lifestyle Changes. Treatment of Individual Components Is Warranted if Needed (Based on Cardiovascular Risk Level)

Component	Possible therapies
Abdominal obesity	Lifestyle changes, bariatric surgery, anti-obesity agents
Hypertension	Antihypertensive agents
↑ Glucose	Antidiabetic agents
↑ Triglycerides	Lipid modifiers
↓ HDL cholesterol	Lipid modifiers
↑ LDL cholesterol	Lipid modifiers
Insulin resistance	Insulin sensitizers
↑ Thrombotic state	Antiplatelet agents

While we wait for further research and management breakthroughs, we can significantly impact the lives of millions of patients who have this syndrome by prompting healthier life-styles with better food choices and exercise.

References

1. **Reaven GM**. Banting Lecture 1988, Role of insulin resistance in human disease. Diabetes. 1988;37:1595-607.

2. **Grundy SM, Cleeman JI, et al.** Diagnosis and management of metabolic syndrome: an American Heart Association/National Heart, Lung, and Blood Institution Scientific Statement. Circulation. 2005;112:2735-52.

3. **Grundy SM, Brewer B, Cleeman JI, et al.** Definition of metabolic syndrome. Circulation. 2004;109:433-8.

4. **Kolovou GD, Anagnostopoulou KK, Salpea KD, et al.** The prevalence of metabolic syndrome in various populations. The American Journal of Medical Sciences. 2007;333:362-71.

5. **Fulop T, Tessier D, Carpenter A.** The metabolic syndrome. Pathologie Biologie. 2006;54:375-86.

6. **Mitrakou A.** Women's health and the metabolic syndrome. Annals New York Academy of Sciences. 2006;1092:33-48.

7. **Schneider JG, Tompkins C, Blumenthal RS, et al.** The metabolic syndrome in women. Cardiology in Review. 2006;14:286-91.

8. **Simonson GD, Kendall DM.** Diagnosis of insulin resistance and associated syndromes: the spectrum from metabolic syndrome to type 2 diabetes. Coronary Artery Disease. 2005;16:465-72.

9. **Reaven GM**. Chapter 28 syndrome X insulin resistance, hyperinsulinemia, and coronary heart disease. Endotext.com, February 16, 2005.

10. **Despres JP, Lemieux I.** Abdominal obesity and metabolic syndrome. Nature. 2006;444:881-7.

11. **Grundy SM.** Metabolic syndrome: a multiplex cardiovascular risk factor. The Journal of Clinical Endocrinology and Metabolism. 2007;92:399-404.

12. Diabetes Prevention Program, http://www.niddk.nih.gov/patient/dpp/ dpp.htm, accessed 11/13/08.
13. **Molavi B, Rasouli N, Kern PA.** The prevention and treatment of metabolic syndrome and high-risk obesity. Current Opinion in Cardiology. 2006;21:479–85.
14. **Fujioka K.** Metabolic syndrome treatment strategies. Pharmacotherapy. 2006;26:222S–6S.

F. Osteoporosis

James Edmondson

KEY POINTS

- Osteoporosis is the most common bone disease, affecting approximately 45 million people in the U.S. and nearly 50% of those over the age of 80 years.
- Osteoporosis affects both men and women, but almost 80% of patients with osteoporosis are women.
- High-risk groups for osteoporosis are those who are treated with chronical glucocorticoid therapy.
- Treating osteoporosis reduces the risk of fractures of the spine, hip, and long bones.
- Not all subjects with low bone density have osteoporosis. Vitamin D deficiency and hyperparathyroid states must be excluded.
- Calcium is required during the entirety of life, and primary care physicians should counsel all women annually about appropriate amounts of calcium and vitamin D intake.

Epidemiology

Forty-five million men and women have abnormally low bone density, 10 million of whom have osteoporosis and 35 million of whom have low bone density, which is also called osteopenia. By age 80 years, >50% of women and men have bone density values in the osteoporotic range. Osteoporosis is the most important risk factor for fracture, but the other predictors of fracture are advanced age and prior fractures. The 3 most common osteoporotic fractures in women are fractures of the spine, wrist, and hip. Hip fracture is a common reason for nursing home placement and has a 25% one-year mortality.

Clinical Presentation

Before a fracture occurs, osteoporosis is asymptomatic, and a bone density measurement must be performed in order to make the diagnosis (1-3). Bone density studies should be performed in women at age 65 years, or at 60 years if there is a high risk for osteoporosis, including postmenopausal women, women with primary hyperparathyroidism, and those who will be receiving glucocorticoid therapy in doses >5 mg/d of prednisone or its equivalent for 3 months or more (4). Amenorrhea in younger women is also a concern for bone loss. Primary care physicians should focus on women in high-risk groups, including those with eating disorders and women receiving depomedroxyprogesterone acetate for contraception. Women in these groups should have a bone mineral density test and increase their calcium intake to 1500 mg daily with at least 800 IU/day of vitamin D.

Diagnosis and Differential Diagnosis

Prior to fracture, the diagnosis of osteoporosis requires measurement of bone density. Dual energy x-ray absorptiometry (DXA) is the most accurate diagnostic tool for establishing a diagnosis of osteoporosis because of its general availability, its use in clinical fracture trials of osteoporosis pharmacotherapy, and the low dose of radiation to which the patient is exposed. Serial measurements of bone mineral density (BMD) must be performed using the same BMD equipment in order to determine if an individual's bone density has changed. The diagnosis of osteoporosis by DXA requires that a T score more negative than −2.5 be present in the spine, hip, or wrist. T score is the bone density value in standard deviation units of young adult women aged 22-29 years (i.e., those who are at peak bone mass). Z score, by contrast, is the age-adjusted bone density in standard deviation units. In the presence of an osteoporotic fracture, a T score less negative than −2.5 may be used to make a clinical diagnosis of osteoporosis. Severe osteoporosis is considered present when a T score of −2.5 or more negative is present together with an osteoporotic fracture. The World Health Organization is currently working on tools for estimating absolute 10-year fracture risk, but these methods are still not ready for routine use.

Not all women with T scores more negative than −2.5 have osteoporosis, since other bone diseases also may produce low bone density. Other common metabolic bone diseases from which osteoporosis must be differentiated include osteomalacia and primary hyperparathyroidism. Uncommonly, other disorders may be confused with osteoporosis. These conditions include Cushing's syndrome, multiple myeloma, and hyperthyroidism. Helpful laboratory studies include measurement of serum total calcium, inorganic phosphorus, creatinine, intact parathyroid hormone (PTH), alkaline phosphatase, and 25-hydroxy-vitamin D. When a less common disease is being considered, dexamethasone suppression testing, thyroid-stimulating hormone (TSH), and serum protein electro-phoretic studies are useful (5).

In the future, instead of providing a T score, bone densitometry meas-urements will generate an absolute fracture risk based on bone mineral density, age, prior fracture history, and other fracture risk predictors.

Clinical Care

General osteoporosis treatment measures include assuring an adequate calcium intake of approximately 1500 mg per day in women. Calcium supplementation is better absorbed with food and in divided doses. Proton pump inhibitor (PPI) therapy may interfere with gut calcium absorption and also is known to increase the risk of hip fracture in the elderly. In women using PPIs, calcium intake of >1500 mg/day is needed (6,7).

Vitamin D supplementation also is needed as a general measure in the treatment of osteoporosis. Among the elderly, vitamin D insuf-ficiency is common, and supplementation in doses exceeding 800 IU per day may be required based upon measurement of the 25-hydroxy-vitamin D blood level (8,9). A 25-hydroxy-vitamin D blood level should be measured in women who will be actively treated for osteoporosis. Physical activity reduces the frequency of falling and should be employed in the general treatment of individuals with osteoporosis. Walking for 30 minutes daily provides an appropriate way of increasing physical activity and potentially provides addition vitamin D availability.

Pharmacotherapy of osteoporosis involves administering either an agent that reduces bone resorption or an anabolic agent (Table 11-11). All of the available osteoporosis treatment options reduce the risk of fracture at one or more of the common osteoporotic sites by nearly 50% or more. Selection of the appropriate agent should be based on patient-specific criteria, including age, gender, sites of lowest bone density, prior

Table 11-11 Properties of Osteoporosis OP Pharmacotherapy

	Bisphosphonates	Raloxifene	Calcitonin	Teriparatide
Class of agent	Resorption inhibitor	Resorption inhibitor	Resorption inhibitor	Anabolic
Administration	Oral/IV	Oral	Intranasal	Subcutaneous
Vertebral fractures	√	√	√	√
Hip fractures	√			
Peripheral fractures	√			
Male OP	√			√
GIOP*	√			
Cost ($/mo)	90	96	120	860
Black box warnings		DVT, Stroke		Osteosarcoma

GIOP = glucocorticoid-induced OP

fracture history, the presence of comorbidities, including esophageal disease, and the presence of primary or secondary hyperparathyroidism. There are no uniformly accepted durations of active therapy for osteoporosis, except for teriparatide, which should not be given for more than 18–24 months. BMD should be measured about every 24 months when a woman is being treated for osteoporosis. Concomitant therapy with 2 or more osteoporosis agents is rarely necessary, since benefit based on better fracture reduction has not been established, and the cost of therapy and the potential for adverse events are higher. The optimal duration of osteoporosis therapy has not been determined, but many women who are actively treated for osteoporosis discontinue therapy within a few months. Osteoporosis therapy which can be administered at infrequent intervals has become available and offers the advantage of enhanced patient adherence.

References

1. **Favus MJ (ed).** Primer on the Metabolic Bone Diseases and Disorders of Mineral Metabolism. Philadelphia: Lippincott Williams & Wilkins. 2003.
2. **Gass M, Dawson-Hughes B.** Preventing osteoporosis-related fractures: an overview. Am J Med. 2006 Apr;119:S3–11.
3. **Moreira Kulak CA, Schussheim DH, McMahon DJ, et al.** Osteoporosis and low bone mass in premenopausal and perimenopausal women. Endocrin Prac. 2000 Jul–Aug;6:336–7.
4. **Lewiecki EM.** Update on bone density testing. Curr Osteoporos Rep. 2005 Dec;3:136–42.
5. Report of the Surgeon General's Workshop on Osteoporosis and Bone Health December 12–13, 2002, Washington, D.C.
6. National Osteoporosis Foundation. Physician's Guide to Prevention and Treatment of Osteoporosis. Washington, DC: National Osteoporosis Foundation;2003.
7. **Yang, Yu-Xiao, Lewis James D, Epstein, Solomon, et al.** Long-term proton pump inhibitor therapy and risk of hip fracture. JAMA. 2006;296:2947–53.
8. **Zadshir A, Tareen N, Pan D, et al.** The prevalence of hypovitaminosis D among US adults: data from the NHANES III. Ethn Dis., 2005 Autumn;15: S5–97,S101.
9. **Dawson-Hughes B, Harris SS, Krall EA, et al.** Effect of calcium and vitamin D supplementation on bone density in men and women 65 years of age or older. N Engl J Med. 1997;337:670–6 [PMID: 9278463].

12

Women's Role in Society

A. Intimate Partner Violence: How Can Healthcare Providers Make a Difference?

DaWana Stubbs

KEY POINTS

- Intimate partner violence (IPV) affects everyone.
- It is not the fault of the victim.
- Power and control are the key components of IPV.
- Healthcare providers should routinely screen all of their female patients for IPV.
- Healthcare providers can make a difference.
- Success is asking about the problem.

Epidemiology

IPV (also called domestic violence, DV) is a public health epidemic affecting people of all ages, races, religions, and socioeconomic levels, and both sexes. However, >95% of IPV involves women being abused by men (1). Research suggests that IPV is the greatest single cause of serious injury to women in the U.S.: IPV is responsible for more injuries than rape, motor vehicle accidents, and muggings combined (2). Abused women are at increased risk of problems with pregnancy and childbirth, depression and anxiety, substance abuse, and chronic medical illnesses (1,3,4). Subsequently, these women have higher rates of health care use as compared to their non-abused counterparts (1,4). Unfortunately, women are not the only victims of IPV. IPV may occur in as many as 1 of every 4 U.S. families (3). Annual estimates reveal that 3.3 million U.S. children are exposed to IPV (4), which places them at risk for injury, either deliberately or incidentally (1). Furthermore, children exposed to IPV have an increased risk of suicide, substance abuse, poor school performance, violent and aggressive behavior, and chronic somatic disorders (1,4).

The Problem

IPV can be defined as the establishment of control and fear in a relationship through violence and other forms of abuse. Violence may not occur often or constantly but remains a hidden and constant terrorizing factor (2,5). The use of violence is a **choice** made by the batterer. It is *not* the fault of or due to any behavior of the victim. In fact, IPV is *not* caused by any of the following: stress, alcohol or drugs, mental or physical illness, financial problems, or poverty (5).

IPV can occur in several forms, including emotional, verbal, financial, sexual, and physical abuse. Emotional abuse can include trickery, dishonesty, lying to others about the victim, and being jealous. Verbal abuse can include yelling, insults, derogatory comments, and sexual comments. Financial abuse may include making victims ask for money and preventing them from getting or keeping a job or from keeping the money they earn. Sexual abuse can be the most difficult for women to discuss and may include rape, unwanted sexual contact, rude comments, and not listening to "no." The most notable form is physical abuse, which usually escalates in both frequency and severity and may be fatal. Physical abuse includes a wide range of actions, including destroying property, blocking one's path, being overly aggressive or insistent, spitting, slapping, pulling hair, pushing, punching, kicking, choking, throwing things, using weapons, punching walls, and breaking things in sight of the other person (6).

All of the above actions are used by batterers to gain and maintain control over their partners. One important aspect that must be understood regarding IPV is that power and control are its driving forces. This theory is illustrated by the Power and Control Wheel, shown in Figure 12-1. This was developed by the Domestic Abuse Intervention Project in Duluth, Minnesota. The wheel shows the relationship of physical and sexual abuse to other forms of abuse. It places power and control at the center or in the hub of the wheel. The spokes symbolize the different behaviors used by batterers to exert their control. The wheel is held together by the rim of physical and sexual abuse (2,5).

Screening for Intimate Partner Violence

The American College of Physicians, as well as several other professional organizations, recommends routine screening for IPV. Punukollu (7) cites studies that provide evidence that screening is beneficial at detecting IPV and increasing referrals to appropriate resources, which results in improved quality of life and fewer violence-related injuries. For example, a qualitative study conducted by Nicolaidis (8) revealed that screening enables a woman to recognize a problem even if she is not ready for help at that time. Additionally, it indicated that battered women rated validating their experience, emphasizing their worth as a human being, and listening in a non-judgmental manner, as highly desirable behaviors in their physicians (8). Healthcare providers have a unique opportunity, if not a responsibility, to intervene on behalf of their patients in abusive relationships (3,9). Providers need not be experts on the dynamics of IPV; yet, they can make a difference simply by identifying pertinent historical and physical findings, asking the right questions, documenting their findings, assessing patient safety, and making the appropriate referrals (1,10,11).

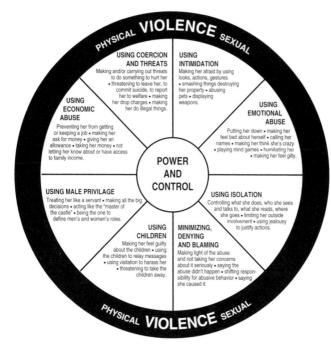

Figure 12-1   Power and control wheel. Developed by the Domestic Abuse Intervention Project in Duluth, Minnesota; with permission.

Patient Presentation: Red Flags

The common physical injuries and medical findings suggestive of abuse include, but are not limited to, the following (1,10,11):

- Somatic disorders
- Depression
- Anxiety
- Chronic pain syndromes
- Story and injury inconsistencies
- Injuries to face, torso, breast, abdomen (central distribution)
- Defensive injuries to the forearms
- Injuries in different stages of healing
- Any type of injury caused by sexual assault
- Delay in seeking treatment

Inquiry

The most important part of screening is to maintain the patient's confidentially. Therefore, any discussion of IPV should be done in private.

The partner or anyone else close to the patient should not be present during the screening process (10).

Framing statements should be used to open the discussion of IPV. These statements help to destigmatize the issue and produce a feeling of not being singled out. An example may be: "I ask all of my patients about their relationships and family so I can understand them better and be available to discuss any problems that they may be experiencing" (10).

Once the door has been opened, and based on the initial discussion, providers may ask either indirect or direct questions. Indirect questions remain fairly general but allow for a deeper inquiry into possible abuse. An example may be: "Every couple fights—what are fights or disagreements like in your home? Do they ever become physical?" Direct questions should be used if indirect questioning, physical examination, or other observation raises any suspicion of current abuse. For example, such questions might include: "Has your partner or ex-partner ever hit or hurt you?" or "Has your partner or ex-partner ever threatened to hurt you or someone close to you?"(10). Recent studies show that abused women prefer and appreciate their physician asking direct questions (12) and openly discussing any clinical suspicion of abuse (8).

Interestingly, recent work from Canada has indicated that women there prefer self-administered screening tools to provider inquiries (13). Whether these data will be generalizable to the U.S. remains to be seen.

Documentation

If screening reveals abuse, it should be documented, just as any other medical problem. Your documentation may be helpful to your patient in both criminal and civil court proceedings. Documentation can occur in 3 forms: as a written description, freehand or printed sketches, and photos.

The written description should be framed in neutral and non-judgmental language that outlines the chronology of the event(s) in the patient's words and describes the physical findings (10). It is very important that the handwritten documentation be **legible**. Avoid phrases or words that sound either belittling or blaming and give the impression of disbelief, such as: *"Is that all?," "just claims," and "only"* (11). The written description should include answers to the following questions (11):

- Who injured you?
- How is the batterer related to you?
- How many times has this happened before?
- When was the last episode? What's the worst episode you can remember?
- Were any children at home during the abuse? If so, were they injured?

Freehand or printed sketches can be used as an adjunct to the written narrative. The physician/provider should record all new or old injuries, showing their location, size, depth, and appearance (1). Additionally, record any areas that the patient reports to be tender, as bruising may appear later. Any photos of injuries should be documented and linked to the sketch.

Photographs provide additional information and should be obtained only with the patient's consent. Photographs should be obtained with color film, using either a ruler or other standardized object in the photo to clarify the size of the wound or bruise. Photos should be taken from different angles before medical treatment is given, and at least one should include the patient's face. All photos should be labeled with the name of the patient and photographer, location of injury, and date (10).

Safety

The final step in screening is an assessment of the patient's safety. Both the patient's immediate and long-term safety should be explored. This can be accomplished by inquiry about the frequency and severity of the abuse, the presence of weapons, threats of homicide or suicide, and the patient's own comfort with returning home (1,14).

The following are examples of safety plans, which are available from the Family Violence Prevention Fund (www.endabuse.org).

When Victim Cohabits with Perpetrator
- Identify who victim can call in a crisis
- Work out signal with children or neighbor to call for help
- Identify where she will go
- Develop escape routes from the home
- If possible, remove weapons from the home
- Identify locations/rooms to avoid
- Place important documents, extra clothing, money, and keys in safe location

Eviction of Perpetrator
- Change locks on doors and windows
- If possible, install security system
- Teach children to call the police or family and friends if they are kidnapped by the perpetrator
- Alert school and childcare provider of situation
- In rural areas, cover mailbox with bright colored paper
- Obtain an order of protection

Leaving the Perpetrator
- Identify how and when it is most safe for her to leave
- Determine what she and others can do so that the perpetrator will not find her
- Ensure she knows the numbers of local shelters
- Plan for how she will travel to ensure her safety
- Identify who she can and cannot tell about leaving

Referral

IPV is a complex problem, and, therefore, the healthcare provider is not expected to work on it alone. IPV requires coordinated efforts of the healthcare provider and various social service agencies. Providers should have available phone numbers of local IPV agencies, including shelters, legal services, counseling, and support groups. Below (see Resources) is a list of national organizations that can assist healthcare providers in finding out what is available in their communities.

Conclusion

As healthcare providers, we have been trained to find solutions to our patient's problems. We can prescribe medications and recommend procedures to "fix" whatever ails them and usually judge our success based on their improvement. However, IPV does not fit into the usual medical paradigm. In the case of IPV, the patient has become the expert. Only she can decide what is best, whether that is to leave or to stay. On average, women will leave an abusive partner 7 times before leaving for good, and women are at the greatest risk for injury and death when they do leave (11). Providers must understand that, in the case of IPV, they cannot and should not make decisions for their patient but rather they can assist her in reviewing available options and then determining which option is most applicable to her situation. Therefore, the goal of any healthcare provider should be the following (1,8,11,12,14):

- Ask routinely about abuse
- Display compassion and concern
- Behave non-judgmentally
- Document the abuse
- Assess safety
- Review options and make appropriate referrals
- Be patient (will take more than one visit to resolve problems)

Women have routinely reported that a good patient-provider relationship is an important element in breaking the cycle of violence and in the recovery process (1,11,12,14).

Success should be measured by asking about the problem not by finding the solution!

Resources

National Domestic Violence Hotline:
Phone: 1-800-799-SAFE (7233)
Website: www.ndvh.org

National Coalition against Domestic Violence:
Phone: (303) 839-1852
Website: www.ncadv.org

Family Violence Prevention Fund:
Websites: 1. www.fvpf.org
2. www.endabuse.org

References

1. **Eisenstat SA, Bancroft L.** Domestic violence.[see comment]. New England Journal of Medicine. 1999 Sep 16;341:886–92.
2. Domestic Violence Handbook. http://www.domesticviolence.org/. Accessed January 7, 2008.
3. **Alpert EJ.** Domestic violence and clinical medicine: learning from our patients and from our fears. Journal of General Internal Medicine. 2002 Feb;17:162–3.
4. **Zuckerman B, Augustyn M, Groves BM, et al.** Silent victims revisited: the special case of domestic violence. Pediatrics. Sep 1995;96:511–3.
5. **Silliman B.** Domestic Violence Thrives in Silence. http://www.ccsd.ca/pubs/2004/nowhere/nowhere_to_turn.pdf. Accessed January 7, 2008.
6. American Medical Association Diagnostic and Treatment Guidelines on Domestic Violence.[erratum appears in Arch Fam Med 1992 Nov;1:287]. Archives of Family Medicine. 1992 Sep;1:39–47.
7. **Punukollu M.** Domestic violence: screening made practical. Journal of Family Practice. 2003 Jul;52:537–43.
8. **Nicolaidis C.** The voices of survivors' documentary: Using patient narrative to educate physicians about domestic violence. Journal of General Internal Medicine. 2002;17:117–24.
9. **Coker AL.** Preventing intimate partner violence: how we will rise to this challenge.[comment]. American Journal of Preventive Medicine. 2006 Jun;30:528–9.
10. **Alpert EJ, Albright CL.** Domestic violence: screening and documentation. Hippocrates. 2000 Mar:39–43.
11. **Berlinger JS.** Answers to your questions about domestic violence. "Why don't you just leave him?" Nursing. 1998 April;28:34–9.
12. **Fogarty CT, Burge S, McCord EC.** Communicating with patients about intimate partner violence: screening and interviewing approaches. Family Medicine. 2002 May;34:369–75.
13. **MacMillan HL, Wathen CN, Jamieson E, et al**. Approach to screening for intimate partner violence in health care settings: A randomized trial. JAMA. 2006;296:530–6.
14. **Alpert EJ, Albright CL.** Domestic Violence: Risk Assessment and Safety Planning. Hippocrates. 2000 April:33–6.

B. Eating Disorders

Theresa Rohr-Kirchgraber and Mary Rouse

KEY POINTS

◆ Eating disorders (ED), such as anorexia nervosa (AN) and bulimia nervosa (BN), affect more than 11 million Americans, >90% of whom are female.

◆ Millions more have a variant of an ED.

◆ The mortality rate for patients with ED may be as much as 12 times that of the general population.

◆ Early recognition and treatment are critical.

◆ Primary care providers must become comfortable with the screening, identification, initiation of treatment, and the care of the patient after recovery.

Epidemiology

While EDs are more common in women, men comprise as much as 15% of the cases of AN and 40% of binge eating disorders (BED) (1). More common in young women, an ED can occur in those over the age of 40 years and is now increasingly recognized in younger children as well (1). It is estimated that up to 3% of *all* young women have an ED, with perhaps twice that number having a variant of disordered eating (1). For many, the patterns of disordered eating may go on for years before a diagnosis is made.

An ED is believed to be caused by a combination of genetic, cultural, psychological, and neurochemical factors (2). It is more prevalent in industrialized societies and crosses socioeconomic classes, races, and cultures. It is seen more frequently in those who participate in activities that promote thinness, such as figure skating, ballet, wrestling, dance, modeling, and running. Young women with type 1 diabetes seem to have a higher incidence of AN (3).

Eating disorders CAN be treated and early intervention is essential. About 50% of those diagnosed with an ED make a full recovery, and 30% have at least a partial recovery. First, though, physicians must be aware of the possibility of an ED and screen screen for it and, since 50% of EDs are undiagnosed (4).

Definition

There are 3 major recognized eating disorders: anorexia nervosa, bulimia nervosa, and eating disorder not otherwise specified (EDNOS) (5). Binge eating disorder currently is a category within EDNOS. Other EDs are being studied and proposed, such as purging disorder, which encompasses those patients who do not binge but consistently purge regular meals and are of relatively normal weight.

DSM-IV-TR Criteria (5)

Anorexia Nervosa (AN): Purging and Non-Purging

- Refusal to maintain body weight (BW) at or above a minimally normal weight for age and height (*e.g.*, weight loss leading to maintenance of BW <85% of that expected or failure to make expected weight gain during a period of growth, leading to BW <85% of that expected).
- Intense fear of gaining weight or becoming fat, even though underweight.
- Disturbance in the way in which BW or shape is experienced, undue influence of BW or shape on self-evaluation, or denial of the seriousness of the current low BW.
- In post-menarchal females, amenorrhea (i.e., the absence of at least 3 consecutive menstrual cycles).
- Restricting type: The person does not engage in any binge eating or purging behaviors.
- Purging type: The person regularly engages in binge eating or purging behaviors while still fulfilling the other criteria for AN.

Bulimia Nervosa (BN)

- Repeated episodes of bingeing, eating a larger than normal amount in a discrete period of time, with a sense of lack of control.
- Purging, typically by self-induced vomiting, abuse of laxatives, diet pills, diuretics, excessive exercise, or fasting.
- Bingeing and purging must occur at least twice weekly for 3 months.
- Extreme concern with body weight and shape.
- The disturbance does not occur during periods of AN.

Eating Disorder Not Otherwise Specified

- Some, but not all, signs/symptoms of AN or BN.
- Binge eating disorder—excessive eating with feelings of guilt and shame.
- Female athlete triad—disordered eating, amenorrhea, and osteoporosis.

Characteristics

It is not unusual for the patient to come to the attention of medical personnel because of the concern of parents and friends. Often, the patient may not recognize the problem or insist that it does not exist (6). Some are so adept at hiding their lack of proper nutrition or bingeing and purging behaviors, that it can go unrecognized for years. Food can get shoved around on a plate; a fork can be raised and lowered towards the mouth, while the meal gets deposited into napkins, the floor, or folds of clothing, never making it to the designated target, the stomach. Bingeing can occur away from the home with all the evidence thrown away, or when one is home alone, often with the food replaced before the family returns. Frequent trips to the bathroom within minutes of a meal may be the opportunity to purge.

Patients may become very proficient at cooking but refuse to eat in the presence of others, claiming that they just ate, they will eat on the way to school, or they ate so much while they were cooking that they just do not have any more room. Frequently, because of the stress and anxiety the patient has about food, social activities that include food will be avoided. Parents or friends may bring the patient to the physician, worried about the withdrawn behavior, worsening grades/work patterns, abnormal food restrictions, compulsive exercising, significant weight loss, or amenorrhea, while the patient may not express any complaints (6). Alternatively, the patient may present with symptoms such as abdominal pain, fatigue, uncontrolled vomiting, or lightheadedness, with no report of ED behaviors.

Some of the psychological characteristics of EDs are included in Box 12-1 (6).

Diagnosis/Assessment

Screening tools, such as SCOFF (4) (Box 12-2) and the Eating Attitudes Test (EAT) (7), do help in identifying patients with ED. We have found that

---

Box 12-1   Psychological Characteristics of EDS

For anorexia
 1. Fear of growing up
 2. Inability to separate from the family
 3. Need to please or be liked
 4. Perfectionism
 5. Need to control
 6. Need for attention
 7. Lack of self-esteem
 8. High family expectations
 9. Parental dieting
10. Family discord
11. Temperament—often described as the "perfect child"
12. Teasing about weight and body shape
For bulimia
13. Difficult regulating mood
14. More impulsive—sometimes will be involved in shoplifting, substance abuse, etc.
15. Sexual abuse
16. Family dysfunction

---

starting with the following simple questions is an easy method of opening the dialogue about the role food plays in the patient's daily life (8):

- Are you comfortable with your current body/weight?
- What have you done to change your body shape or weight in the last year?

The review of systems should include questions regarding:

- Menstrual history
- Fainting, fatigue, and overall weakness
- Hair loss
- Depression and anxiety screening
- Sleep habits
- Caffeine intake
- Bowel movements

Studies to order if considering the diagnosis of an ED include (1,3):

Laboratory Studies

- Complete blood count with differential
- Complete metabolic panel, including liver functions, sodium, potassium, chloride, bicarbonate, blood urea nitrogen, creatinine, glucose
- Calcium, magnesium, phosphate
- Pregnancy test
- Pre-albumin (may be normal in severe AN)
- Carotene level
- Amylase
- Thyroid-stimulating hormone (TSH), thyroxine (T4)
- Urinalysis
- Erythrocyte sedimentation rate
- Urine drug screen

X-Rays

- DXA scan for bone density

Other

- EKG

Examination

The physical exam in an ED patient has some special characteristics. The height of the patient should be measured at the initial visit (and at least every few months in a growing child) (9). It is this height that is used to calculate the BMI, not the patient's self-reported height. The weight should be taken in the exam room while the patient is wearing only a hospital gown and standing on the scale backwards so she cannot see the result. Orthostatic blood pressure and pulse should be obtained at each visit (9). A thorough exam of the skin for evidence of self-harm should be conducted, especially at the initial visit. This might include cutting, burns to the skin, recent scars, and bruising, and should be discussed and documented (6).

The exam in AN may note evidence of malnutrition such as those listed in Box 12-3 (1). Box 12-4 lists items that may be included in the exam in BN (1):

Data Results (2):

Box 12-3   Key Exam Findings in AN

- BMI <18.5
- Skin pale dry and yellow (hypercarotenemia)
- Muscle wasting
- Bony protuberances
- Thin and brittle hair
- Acrocyanosis (cold and blue extremities)
- Lanugo (soft, fine coat of hair that forms on the arms and other body parts)
- Hypothermia
- Hypotension
- Bradycardia
- Orthostasis
- Breast atrophy
- Systolic heart murmur (usually due to mitral valve prolapse, MVP)
- Scaphoid abdomen
- Stool palpable in the left lower quadrant
- Pretibial edema

Box 12-4   Key Exam Findings in BN

- Normal weight, but can be under- or overweight
- Bilateral painless parotid enlargement
- Loss of tooth enamel
- Calluses on the dorsum of the hand (Russell's sign)

Anorexia Nervosa

- Exam can be normal
- Leukopenia
- Thrombocytopenia
- Anemia
- Hypoglycemia
- Electrolyte abnormalities (hypokalemia, hyponatremia, hypophos-phatemia)
- Elevated liver function tests (LFTs)
- Hypercarotenenemia
- Decreased hormones (T3, LH, FSH, estradiol, testosterone)

Bulimia Nervosa

- Exam can be normal
- Electrolyte disturbances (hypokalemia, hyperamylasemia)

Differential Diagnosis (10)

Gastrointestinal disorders: Inflammatory bowel disease, celiac disease, Crohn disease

Endocrine disorders: Hyper/hypothyroidism, diabetes mellitus, panhypopi-tuitarism, Addison's disease

Infections: AIDS, intestinal parasitosis, tuberculosis

Malignancy: Occult carcinoma, lymphoma

Psychiatric disorder: Depression, schizophrenia, conversion disorder

Complications

ED can affect any organ system, causing acute and long-term effects. Constipation, rectal prolapse, delayed gastric emptying, decreased intestinal motility, hematemesis, Mallory-Weiss tears, and gastric dilation and rupture can be noted in the gastrointestinal (GI) tract. Cardiac effects include cardiomyopathy, arrhythmia, decreased left ventricular mass, mitral valve prolapse, hypotension, and bradycardia. The reproductive system can be affected, leading to problems with infertility, low birthweight babies, and insufficient weight gain during pregnancy. Reversible cortical atrophy, peripheral neuropathy, and ventricular enlargement have been noted in the neurological system, which may result in permanent cognitive problems and changes in behavior (1). Dental caries, cheilosis, enlargement of the parotid gland, and submandibular adenopathy are noted in the oromaxillary system (9). Multiple endocrine abnormalities, including the electrolyte disturbances noted above, osteoporosis, delay in puberty, amenorrhea, lipid abnormalities, hypercortisolism, low testosterone and estradiol levels, and hypothyroidism may be seen (9).

Treatment

Although an ED is classified as a psychological illness, as demonstrated with a DSM-IV-TR classification, it is important for the primary provider to recognize his/her unique ability to intercede–first as the diagnostician, then as a leader of the treatment team. A team approach is the most useful method for treating an ED and usually includes a generalist physician, psychiatrist, psychologist or master's level therapist, and a registered dietician. All should be comfortable dealing with EDs and working as a team. Involving the parents is essential in treating younger patients, and engaging family and friends can be helpful in all age groups (2).

After the initial evaluation, the physician must determine whether the patient is medically stable for continued outpatient therapy. A patient may be considered for hospitalization for reasons listed in Box 12-5 (3).

If stable for outpatient therapy, the physician monitors the patient frequently for medical problems, including frequent visits for weight and blood pressure/heart rate checks. Depending on the patient, these visits may need to occur twice weekly and progress to monthly over time. A mental health professional works with the patient to recognize dysfunctional thoughts and maladaptive behaviors and to re-establish healthy relationships. Formal dietary counseling helps the patient to better understand her body's need for food, to determine how best to achieve the weight goal in AN, and to help the patient with BN know that a balanced adequate diet will both help control binges and allow weight to be maintained in a healthy range (1).

Some patients may be restricted from physical activity until a target weight is achieved. Medications may be helpful, especially in BN or EDNOS, where there is a greater association of depression and anxiety. An anxiolytic or an atypical anti-psychotic, such as olanzapine, may have a role in AN, if the patient has severe anxiety related to eating (1). Fluoxetine, which has shown some benefit in BN and EDNOS, has not demonstrated significant benefit in anorexic patients (1). Trials of Topiramate or Ondansetron for BN also have had some success in controlling bingeing, although further studies are needed (6). A proton pump inhibitor can help prevent further esophageal damage in BN (11), while a multivitamin is helpful in replacing those nutrients that are lacking until nutritional rehabilitation is complete.

Box 12-5   Consideration for Hospitalization

- Weight 25–30% below ideal that
- Rapid and severe weight loss is refractory to outpatient therapy
- Marked symptomatic hypotension or syncope
- Pulse <35–40 beats/min
- Arrhythmias
- Severe electrolyte abnormalities
- Suicidality

Conclusion

ED encompasses a range of disordered eating from severe restriction to binge eating and purging behaviors. The patient may not be diagnosed for many years and may present with other somatic complaints. It is not unusual for multiple medical tests to have been performed prior to the diagnosis in order to investigate the somatic symptoms. Screening all patients for ED will help to increase awareness, encourage discussions on healthy eating, promote understanding, and provide earlier intervention for this disease.

Resources

Academy for Eating Disorders http://www.aedweb.org/

The Anna Westin Foundation http://www.annawestinfoundation.org

Eating Disorders Coalition for Research. Policy & Action (EDC) http://www.eatingdisorderscoalition.org

National Eating Disorders Association (NEDA) http://www.nationaleatingdisorders.org

Eating Attitudes Test http://www.psychcentral.com/quizzes/eat.htm http

References

1. **Becker AE, Grinspoon SK, Klibanski A, et al.** Eating disorders. N England J Med. 1999;340:1092–98.

2. **Yager J, Andersen AE.** Anorexia nervosa. N England J Med. 2005;353:1481–88.

3. **Mehler PS.** Diagnosis and care of patients with anorexia nervosa in primary care settings. Ann of Internal Medicine. 2001;134:1048–59.

4. **Morgan JF, Reid F, Lacey JH.** The SCOFF questionnaire: Assessment of a new screening tool for eating disorders. BMJ. 1999;319:1467–68.

5. **Wilfley DE, Bishop ME, Wilson GT, et al.** Classification of eating disorders: Toward DSM-V. International Journal of Eating Disorders. 2007;40:S123–29.

6. **Herzog DB, Franko DL.** Unlocking the Mysteries of Eating Disorders: A Life-Saving Guide to Your Child's Treatment and Recovery. New York, McGraw-Hill 2008.

7. **Garner DM, Olmsted MP, Bohr Y, et al.** The eating attitudes test: psychometric features and clinical correlates. Psychological Medicine. 1982 Nov;12:871–78.

8. **Rouse M and the Division of Adolescent Medicine.** Guidelines for the Care of the Adolescent Patient: Indiana University School of Medicine. Unpublished.

9. American Academy of Pediatrics: Committee on Adolescence. Identifying and Treating Eating Disorders, Pediatrics. 2003;111:204–11.

10. Ferri: Ferri's Clinical Advisor 2008, 1st edition 2008 Mosby.

11. **Eiro M, Katoh T, Watanabe T**. Use of a proton-pump inhibitor for metabolic disturbances associated with anorexia nervosa. N Engl J Med. 2002;346:140.

C. Balancing Life Roles

Heather L. Paladine

KEY POINTS

♦ Both men and women may experience stress from work–family conflict and role overload; however, it is a particularly significant problem for women.

♦ Women continue to spend more time on home and family responsibilities than do men.

♦ Role overload can lead to increased rates of anxiety and depression in women.

♦ Supportive work environments, rewarding work, and separation of work and family life can help to reduce work–family conflict.

♦ Flexible work arrangement can help alleviate some work–family conflict.

Epidemiology

In the 21st century, women have many different roles to fill. They are likely to work outside the home, as well as to have responsibilities to children, partners, and/or elderly relatives. They also have limited time for self-care, exercise, and relaxation. Although all of these roles can be rewarding, multiple life roles may lead to contradictory demands on a woman's time. Stress related to these conflicting pressures can result in poor health, work absenteeism, and mental health concerns.

Both men and women may experience conflict from these demands on their time. The 2002 National Study of the Changing Workforce found that 43% of all employees (both men and women) with families described some or a lot of interference between their jobs and family life (1). However, some conflicts are unique to, or more significant for, women. Both sexes have increased time pressures related to work and family, while gender discrimination and balancing work with pregnancy/childbirth affect only women. Seventy-eight percent of married salaried workers or wage-earners live in dual-career households (1). Between 1977 and 2002 the number of hours per week that a dual-earning couple works has increased from 81 to 91. In addition, the amount of time spent with children has increased from 5 to 6 hours a day. Consequently, parents have less time to spend on themselves. Working women on average have 0.9 hours to themselves per day (down from 1.6 hours in 1977) compared to 1.3 hours a day that fathers spend on themselves (down from 2.1 hours in 1977) (1).

Work Issues

Although women are responsible for most of the duties in the home, their hours spent working in the home have decreased over the past few decades while men's hours have increased (2). Over the past 30 years, women's weekly hours of housework have decreased from 30 to 17.5, and men's weekly hours increased from 4.9 to 10 (2). Even so, mothers in a family with children perform 60% of household tasks and often take on more of the "emotional burden" of the family (3). In general, in families with children, fathers work longer hours in paid employment and earn more money. Over 50% of men in dual-earning families earn >$75 000 compared to only 14% of women (3). Women tend to have lower job satisfaction, likely because of the probability of performing part-time work at lower paying jobs (3). An average women will earn $37 000 annually, compared to men earning $53 000 (1).

Women also bear a greater responsibility for child care than do men (3). Even when non-family members care for children, the responsibility for arranging child care usually is borne by the woman (3). Women are also more likely to be the ones to care for children when they are sick and cannot attend child care or school (i.e., women are more likely to miss days of work because of the need to stay home in such circumstances) (3).

Women are more likely to work part-time than men, but the gap in hours is closing. The average work hours for women are 42 per week, compared with 49 hours per week for men (1). However, work hours for both men and women have increased over the past 20 years (1). As working hours have lengthened, they also have become more irregular, and employees may have to work during hours that were previously devoted to family time, such as evenings or weekends. Finally, both women and men in the U.S. spend longer hours at work than people in other developed countries.

Given this complex situation, women may feel pressured by multiple responsibilities. Work-family conflict occurs when the stress or time demands of one role interfere with participation in the other life role. In a 2001 survey of employees (women and men) in Canada, 88% reported moderate to high levels of role overload, i.e., the feeling that they have too much to do in a given amount of time (4). Most of the role overload comes from work pressures intruding into family life, rather than the opposite (4). For example, women are more likely to bring work home with them than to have family responsibilities interfere with work time. People with high levels of role overload are more likely to report work absenteeism, job stress, and poor health; therefore, role overload and work-life conflict are of increasing concern to employers (5). A study of 155 women who worked full-time found that role overload was negatively correlated with psychological health, job satisfaction, and leisure satisfaction (5).

The single strongest predictor of work-life conflict is whether an organization's culture is supportive of family responsibilities. Employer policies can go a long way toward mitigating or worsening role overload. For example, employers who value long hours spent at work or who pressure employees to choose between work and family responsibilities have employees with higher levels of role overload. Flexible time policies at work can help to relieve work-life conflict, but it is important to keep work and home separated as much as possible. Flexible work arrangements lead to more job satisfaction, increased employee loyalty, and better employee retention (1).

Flexible work arrangements (FWA), such as flexible work hours or part-time work, result in less work pressure (6). However, written or unwritten policies may make it difficult for women to take advantage of flexible work hours (7). Women's career advancement and income may also suffer if they work fewer hours or use flexible time for family responsibilities (7). Part-time employees may not be eligible for health insurance and other benefits. Women are more likely than men to want to work in flexible work situations, especially if they have young children (8). In 1997, over 26% of all women who worked full-time participated in some type of FWA (9).

FWA have been divided into flex-time and flex-space (8). Flex-time is a means by which employees may be flexible with their work hours, and flex-space is where employees may telecommute from home or other locations not at the work site. Several issues have arisen concerning these alternate work arrangements, including less "face time" at work, not feeling like a part of the team, resentment by traditional full-time workers and "boundary" issues. Women set up limits or boundaries between the different aspects of their life. When women work at home, these lines can be blurred (8). Women working at home may be tempted to take a break to complete tasks involved in taking care of children or the house. In addition, if a person is telecommuting from home, but needs to be sitting at the computer all day, she is not truly flexible (8). A meta-analysis of the effect of FWA on work-family conflict indicated that family-friendly work environments and spousal support were the most effective in decreasing work-family conflict (7). Additionally, flex-time seems to be more effective than flex-space in decreasing work-family conflicts (8).

Factors that increase job satisfaction, such as feeling that the job is meaningful or that there are opportunities for advancement, are associated with lower levels of work-life conflict (10). A study from the Netherlands found that work-role explained an excess of depression and anxiety in women. In this study, women had poorer quality of work, less job control, and lower salaries, all of which contributed to psychological distress. In women, employment had a less favorable effect on mental health compared to men (10).

Clinical Implications

Primary care providers often see women suffering from stress-related conditions, including depression and anxiety. Counseling about life balance may play a role in managing these conditions. Strategies for work–life balance of successful executives who were focused equally on work and family include: setting strict boundaries between work and family time,

> **Box 12-6** Tips for Patients
>
> 1. Get enough sleep
> 2. Exercise regularly
> 3. Eat a healthy diet
> 4. Limit caffeine and alcohol
> 5. Take some time for yourself on a regular basis
> 6. Ask for help when you need it
> 7. Negotiate with your family about spreading out the workload
> 8. Maintain relationships and support networks
> 9. Look for a job that may provide some flexibility
> 10. Negotiate with your supervisor for some flexibility in either time or space

being fully present when at home or at work, taking time for themselves to rest and pursue other interests, and focusing on their priorities in life (11).

Some commonsense tips for patients are listed in Box 12-6.

Conclusion

Achieving a balance between work and family life can be difficult. Focusing on self-care, life priorities, and working with employers to promote family-friendly work environments may help women negotiate this complex arena.

References

1. **Bond JT, Thompson C, Galinsky E, et al.** Highlights of the national study of the changing workforce: executive summary. Family and Work Institute, 2002. Available at http:www.familiesandwork.org.
2. **Bianchi SM, Milkie MA, Sayer LC, et al.** Is anyone doing the housework? Trends in the gender division of household labor. Social Forces. 2000;79:191–228.
3. **Schneider B, Waite LJ.** eds. Being Together, Working Apart: Dual career families and the work-life balance (2005). Cambridge, UK: Cambridge University Press.
4. **Duxbury L, Higgins C.** Work-life conflict in Canada in the new millennium—a status report. Accessed at: http://www.phac-aspc.gc.ca/publicat/work-travail/pdf/rprt_2_e.pdf, January 3, 2008.
5. **Pearson QM.** Role overload, job satisfaction, leisure satisfaction and psychological health among employed women. Journal of Counseling and Development. 2008; 86:57–63.
6. **Russell H, O'Connell PJ, McGinnity F.** The impact of flexible working arrangements on work-life conflict and work pressure in Ireland. Working Papers 189, Economic and Social Research Institute (ESRI).
7. **Mesmer-Magnus JR, Viswesvaran C.** How family friendly work environments affect work/family conflict: a meta-analyis. Journal of Labor Research. 2006;27:555–74.

8. **Shockley KM, Allen TD.** When flexibility helps: Another look at the availability of flexible work arrangements and work-family conflict. Journal of Vocational Behavior. 2007;71:479–93.

9. **Beers TM.** Flexible scheduling and shift work: replacing the 9 to 5 work day? Monthly Labor Review. 2000;113(6) (http://www.bls.gov/opub/mlr/2000/06/contents.htm)

10. **Praisier I, et al.** Work and family roles and the association with depression and anxiety disorders: differences between men and women. Journal of Affective disorders. 2008;105:63–72.

11. **Galinsky E.** Dual-centric: a new concept of work-life. Data from the leaders in the global economy study. Available at www.familiesandwork.org.

D. Access to Health Care for Uninsured Women

Tammy Quall

KEY POINTS

- Women without health insurance in the U.S. tend to be young; single, working part-time, self-employed, unemployed, poor or near poor, have less than a high school diploma, and/or are not U.S. citizens.
- Uninsured women are the least likely to have a regular provider of primary care, more likely to be diagnosed in advanced disease states, and less likely to receive treatment.
- Resources for uninsured women include the Medicaid program, Federally Qualified Community Health Centers, and Free Clinics.
- Medical homes decrease barriers in access and increase quality of care for uninsured women.
- Characteristics of an effective medical home include a regular provider or place of care, the ability to contact a provider easily by phone, the ability to get care or advice on weekends or evenings, and office visits that are organized and on schedule.

Uninsured Women: Who Are They?

While uninsured women range significantly in age and backgrounds, as a group they share certain socioeconomic characteristics. Women without health insurance in the U.S. tend to be young, single, working part-time, self-employed, unemployed, poor or near poor, have less than a high school diploma, and/or are not U.S. citizens (1).

Over 20% of women from 18 to 34 years of age are uninsured (2). Thirty-five percent of women who are unmarried and living with a partner are uninsured, as are 20% of women who are divorced (2). While 1 in 10 women who works full-time is uninsured, 26% of self-employed women are without any coverage (2).

Women who report poor health are more likely to be uninsured than women who report good to excellent health. One fifth (22%) of women under 65 years who report fair or poor health are without some form of health coverage (2).

Women with the lowest incomes are the most likely to be uninsured. Those with incomes <100% of the Federal Poverty Level (FPL) are >6 times as likely to be uninsured than women with incomes >300% of the FPL (2). One hundred percent of the federal poverty threshold in 2007 was $17 170 for a family of 3 (Figure 12-2).

There is significant variation among states in the number of women without health insurance. The 2 ends of the spectrum are Texas, with the highest rate of uninsured women at 28.1%, and Minnesota, with the lowest rate at 9.1% (3). In addition, racial disparities exist in health insurance coverage for women. Hispanic and Native American women are >2.5 times as likely to be uninsured as white women (3) (Figure 12-3).

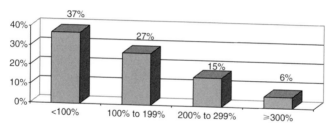

Figure 12-2   Uninsured women by poverty level; women 18 to 64 years. (From Henry J. Kaiser Family Foundation. Women and Health Care: A National Profile. Key Findings from the Kaiser Women's Health Survey, July 2005; with permission.)

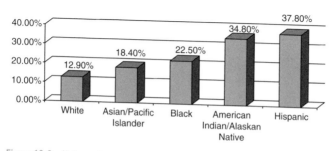

Figure 12-3   Uninsured women by race and ethnicity. (From Data source: National Women's Law Center. Making the Grade on Women's Health: A National and State-by-State Report Card 2007; with permission.)

Uninsured Women and Their Health Care Issues

According to the 2004 Kaiser Women's Heath Survey, women without insurance consistently fare worse on multiple measures of access to care: "Uninsured women are the least likely to have had a provider visit in the past year (67%), compared to women with either private (90%) or public insurance-Medicaid (88%) and Medicare (93%). Two-thirds of uninsured women (67%) report delayed/forgone care due to costs, 4 times as high as women with private coverage or Medicare." (2) Almost 40% of uninsured women do not have a regular provider of primary care (4), and uninsured women consistently report lower rates of preventive screening tests (2). (Figure 12-4)

Uninsured, low-income women are more likely to experience a broader range of chronic health problems than insured women with higher incomes, and, once over the age of 45 years, they are at much greater risk for chronic disease (2). Latinas, one of the racial/ethnic groups at highest risk for diabetes, for instance, report the greatest restrictions in access, care provided, and perception of health and impairment (4) (Figure 12-5).

Uninsured adults with chronic disease often do not receive the care they need to manage their health conditions (5). The Institute of

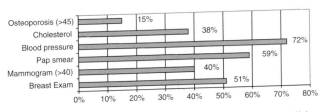

Figure 12-4   Uninsured women's prevention screening rates. (From Henry J. Kaiser Family Foundation. Women and Health Care: A National Profile. Key Findings from the Kaiser Women's Health Survey. July 2005; with permission.)

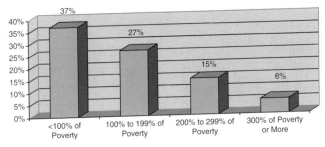

Figure 12-5   Rates of chronic disease in low income women over age 45. (From Kaiser Family Foundation. Women and Health Care: A National Profile. Key Findings from the Kaiser Women's Health Survey, July 2005; with permission.)

Medicine's Committee on the Consequences of Uninsurance examined treatment and outcomes for 5 chronic diseases (diabetes, cardiovascular disease, end-stage renal disease, HIV infection, and mental illness) and found that "uninsured patients have consistently worse clinical outcomes than insured patients" (5).

Uninsured women also are diagnosed at more advanced disease states (6). According to the Kaiser Foundation Report, *Sicker and Poorer: The Consequences of Being Uninsured*, "having health insurance reduces mortality rates for the uninsured by 10 to 15 percent" (6).

Almost 20% of uninsured women report unmet needs for medical or surgical services, almost 8% for prescription drugs, and >23% report the need for dental care (4). Research has found that low-income, uninsured primary care patients report that their most common chronic health problems are headaches, chronic back problems, arthritis, and mood disorders (7). In addition, chronic pain and mental illness are likely to co-occur in patients.

The needs of uninsured women can be overwhelming in a healthcare delivery system that focuses on efficiency and limits time that providers spend with their patients. In addition, primary care providers are often not adequately trained in areas that allow them to address significant psychosocial and mental health needs (7).

Resources for Uninsured Women

Medicaid: Medicaid is a health care coverage program that is funded by both state and federal dollars. It provides coverage for over 20 million low-income women (8). Women comprise 69% of the adults who are enrolled in the program and receive a wide range of services, including reproductive, chronic disease, prevention, and long-term services (8).

In order to be eligible for Medicaid, a woman must fit into a certain "group," such as being pregnant, age 65 years or older, mother of a child under 18, or having a disability (8). In addition, women must meet income criteria that vary from state to state. Generally, income thresholds are very low. The extremes of the spectrum of income eligibility levels for pregnant women range from 133% of the Federal Poverty Level (FPL) in 8 states to 275% in Minnesota, and for working parents levels range from 18% of FPL in Arkansas to 275% in Minnesota (8). Some states might have their own name for the Medicaid program, such as "Medi-Cal" in California.

Low-income seniors and disabled women who qualify for Supplemental Security Income (SSI) can receive full Medicaid benefits (8). SSI is a federal income supplement program for aged, blind, and disabled people, who have little or no income. It provides a small, monthly cash subsidy to eligible beneficiaries to meet basic needs.

As of 2007, 26 states have made family planning services available to women who otherwise do not meet the categorical and income requirements for Medicaid (8). These women are covered under Medicaid for family planning and related prevention services only. In addition, all states have adopted a program that extends Medicaid coverage to pay for cancer treatment for uninsured women who do not meet a categorical requirement but do meet the income requirements for Medicaid (8). In addition, these women must have been diagnosed with breast or cervical cancer through a federal CDC screening program (8).

Women with Medicaid utilize primary care in a manner similar to women with private insurance coverage (8). One long-standing issue for Medicaid is the limited participation by private physicians, particularly specialty providers (8). Women on Medicaid consistently report barriers to accessing specialty care.

The Center for Medicare and Medicaid Services web site provides further information on Medicaid coverage and services (http://www.cms.hhs.gov/home/medicaid.asp).

Federally Qualified Community Health Centers: The U.S. Health Resources and Services Administration's (HRSA) Bureau of Primary Health Care administers the program for Federally Qualified Health Centers (FQHC). There are 4 types of FQHC programs: Community Health Centers, Migrant Health Centers, Healthcare for the Homeless Programs, and Public Housing Primary Care Programs that address the healthcare needs of underserved populations. FQHCs serve 13 million people in both rural and urban settings at over 4000 sites in the U.S.

FQHCs must locate in or serve a high need community and provide comprehensive primary care services, as well as supportive services such as translation and transportation. In addition, they must make services available to all residents of the service area, with fees adjusted based on the ability to pay. Of those served by FQHCs, >90% have incomes <200% of the FPL, and >60% are members of racial and ethnic minorities. Many FQHCs also provide dental and mental health services and focus on caring for chronic disease. The above and additional information on FQHCs can be found at the HRSA Web site (http://bphc.hrsa.gov/about/). The following Web site provides information on how to find FQHC clinical sites throughout the country: http://ask.hrsa.gov/pc/.

Free Clinics: Free Clinics bring together volunteer healthcare professionals and other community volunteers to provide free or low-cost healthcare to low-income people. Free Clinics can provide medical, dental, pharmaceutical, and/or mental health services to uninsured people at little or no cost. Each Free Clinic is unique in the services it provides, types of providers, and hours of operations. These clinics are generally funded at the local level with minimal government support (http://www.freeclinics.us/).

Implications for the Primary Care Visit

In spite of efforts of some states to expand Medicaid coverage, many women continue to be uninsured. The concept of the "medical home" has been proposed as a model for delivering high-quality healthcare to the entire population. According to The Commonwealth Fund 2006 Health Care Quality Survey, "when adults have health insurance coverage and a medical home, racial and ethnic disparities in access and quality are reduced or even eliminated" (9).

The survey found that the following characteristics of a medical home contribute to the quality of care that is capable of reducing health disparities (9):

- A regular provider or place of care
- Ability to easily contact a provider by phone
- Ability to get care or advice on weekends or evenings
- Office visits that are organized and on schedule

Medical homes increase the likelihood of patients receiving routine preventive screenings. Again, according to The Commonwealth Fund Survey, "rates of cholesterol, breast cancer, and prostate screening are higher among adults who receive patient reminders. Even among the uninsured, having a medical home affects whether patients receive preventive care reminders. Two-thirds of both insured and uninsured adults with medical homes receive preventive care reminders, compared with half of insured and uninsured adults without medical homes." (9)

The survey suggests that by creating a "medical home" for uninsured women, providers can improve their health outcomes (9). However, achieving the above characteristics of a primary care home can be more complicated when addressing the socioeconomic issues that many uninsured women face.

Lessons learned by FQHCs from the National Health Disparities Collaboratives (HDC) can provide insight into caring for an underserved, uninsured population. The HDCs were created nationally to modify primary care practice to improve health outcomes for low-income patients and to address health disparities (10). HDCs largely focus on chronic disease and prevention interventions. Some of the tools utilized in the HDCs include use of clinical registries and evidenced-based clinical guidelines, patient self-management resources and protocols, health education resources, and outreach and nutrition services (10) (www. healthdisparities.net/hdc/html/home.aspx).

In addition, many FQHCs and other providers of care to at-risk populations utilize support services, such as social, translation, and case management services, that have demonstrated improved access and outcomes in working with this population. To the extent possible that these resources can be obtained, they can help address the many barriers that are associated with at-risk socioeconomic characteristics.

References

1. **Freeman, G, Lethbridge-Cejku, M.** Access to health care among Hispanic or Latino women: United States, 2000–2002. Advance Data. 2006;(368):1–25.
2. Henry J. Kaiser Family Foundation. Women and health care: a national profile. Key findings from the Kaiser Women's Health Survey. Henry J. Kaiser Family Foundation, July 2005.

3. National Women's Law Center. Making the grade on women's health: a national and state-by-state report card 2007. National Women's Law Center, 2007.
4. **Almeida R, Dubay L, Ko G.** Access to care and use of health services by low-income women. Health Care Financing Review. 2001;22:27–47.
5. Committee on the Consequences of Uninsurance. Care without coverage: too little, too late. Institute of Medicine of the National Academies. May2002.
6. Henry J. Kaiser Family Foundation. Sicker and poorer: The consequences of being uninsured. Henry J. Kaiser Family Foundation. February 2003.
7. **Mauksch LB, Katon WJ, Russo J, et al.** The content of a low-income, uninsured primary care population: including the patient agenda. Journal of the American Board of Family Practice. 2003Jul–Aug;16: 278–89.
8. Henry J. Kaiser Family Foundation. Issue brief: an update on Women's Health Policy, Medicaid's Role for Women. Henry J. Kaiser Family Foundation. October2007.
9. **Beal A, Doty M, Hernandez S, et al.** Closing the divide: How medical homes promote equity in health care: results from the Commonwealth Fund 2006 Health Care Quality Survey. The Commonwealth Fund. June2007.
10. Association of States and Territorial Health Officials. Issue brief: Improving health outcomes through coordination: The Health Disparities Collaboratives. Association of States and Territorial Health Officials. 2006.

E. Disparities in Health for Vulnerable Women: Women in Prison and Immigrant Women

Nancy Pandhi, Rosalilia Mendoza, and Kala R. Kluender

KEY POINTS

- Poverty and stress are significant risk factors for poor health.
- Creative approaches are required to support vulnerable women's ability to self-manage chronic disease.
- It is critical to screen for depression and abuse in vulnerable populations.
- Maternal and neonatal complications are prevalent in immigrant populations.
- Immigrant women experience multiple stressors before and after migration.
- Incarceration facilities vary in level of medical services provided.

> ♦ Compared to the general population, the female incarcerated population has higher rates of HIV/AIDS, tuberculosis, hepatitis C, abnormal Pap smears, and psychiatric illness.
> ♦ Women who are incarcerated should be screened for chronic conditions and provided with reproductive counseling.

In 2006, U.S. Census data indicated that 5.6 million women aged 18 years and above had incomes below the federal poverty level (FPL). In that year, women earned 77 cents to every dollar earned by men (1). Women are vulnerable to poor health from the compounding effects of poverty and stress. This chapter will outline the influence of these risks on health and then focus in more detail on 2 specific groups of vulnerable women: immigrants and those who are incarcerated.

Aside from the obvious difficulties imposed by limited access to health care, vulnerable women may have difficulty adhering to medical recommendations because of multiple competing time demands and restricted opportunities for self-care. Chronic conditions, such as diabetes, obesity, and cardiovascular disease, are prevalent in this population and necessitate creative solutions for self-management support. Poor living conditions (e.g., inadequate housing, high neighborhood poverty concentrations, and environmental contaminants) and difficult working conditions with minimal autonomy (e.g., domestic work sales) also create demands on health.

Low-income women are at significant risk for depression, particularly due to chronic stressors and uncontrollable life events (2). Other mental health concerns in this population include post-traumatic stress disorder, often due to physical or sexual trauma, and anxiety disorders.

Immigrant Women

Immigrants are the largest and most rapidly growing population in the U.S. In 2003, approximately 11.7% of the U.S. population consisted of foreign-born individuals from Latin America (53.3%), Asia (25.0%), Europe (13.7%), and other regions (8.0%) (3).

Studies have shown that length of residency in the U.S. impacts health in several ways for diverse immigrant subpopulations (4). Among these different and heterogeneous populations, immigrant women's health disparities are illustrated in comparison to non-Native American U.S.-born or White women's health. For instance, from 1991 to 1997, foreign-born Black, Latino (Hispanic), and Asian women experienced more pregnancy-related deaths and higher pregnancy mortality rates than non-Native American U.S.-born women (5). U.S.-born Latino and Asian immigrant women are twice as likely to die from pregnancy-related complications as are non-Latino, U.S.-born White women (6). In addition, Latino immigrant women have a higher risk of delivering premature and low-birth-weight infants than their White counterparts (5).

Cancer rates are disproportionately high among certain immigrant populations: for example, Chinese and Japanese immigrant women have higher rates of colon cancer than Asian women born in the U.S. In addition, Haitian-born Black women and Black women in the U.S. experience higher rates of cervical cancer than Black women from English-speaking Caribbean countries (5). Interestingly, both immigrant groups have a lower rate of breast cancer than American-born Black women (5).

Immigrant women experience stressors that affect their health prior to migrating and after arriving in the U.S. Women have reported suffering some degree of trauma from the upheaval in their lives prior to emigrating, hardships in refugee camps, and/or witnessing family members being injured or killed (7). After migrating from their native country, social stressors that impact immigrant women's health include finding employment, loss of social status, loneliness and social isolation, and language barriers (7). Furthermore, immigrant women experience cultural and gender-related stressors that impact their well-being and may manifest as a change in eating patterns, crying, sadness and depression, headaches, rashes, and poor health in general (7).

Since immigrant women constitute a rapidly growing segment of the U.S. population, it is important for primary care providers to increase their awareness of these individuals, who represent multiple different cultures, in order to provide better health services. Providers should attempt to: 1) increase their knowledge and understanding of immigrant women's conceptualizations and health beliefs, based on their countries of origin (7); and 2) gain knowledge and promote research about harmful and protective factors that influence immigrant women's health, in the context of time, generation, and geography or regional communities (5).

Incarcerated Women

The number of women facing the "quadruple burden" of their gender, race/ethnicity, socioeconomic status, and criminal conviction is growing (8). Between 1990 and 2002, the female prison population increased 118%, and the number of female inmates continues to grow at a higher rate than that of males. Most likely incarcerated for non-violent drug or property offenses, women in correctional facilities are disproportionately African American. Indeed, data from 1999 reveal that African American women were incarcerated 7 times more frequently than White women and twice as often as Latino women (8). The median age of female prisoners in federal facilities is 36 years, while it is 33 at the state level and 31 in local institutions. Nearly 75% of women in jail (locally operated institutions for temporary confinement of individuals awaiting sentencing/transfer or serving a sentence up to 1 year in length) and 50% of those in prison (state and federal facilities that house convicted offenders with sentences of over 1 year) were unemployed at the time of their arrest (8). Histories of abuse are common among these women: 44–60% of incarcerated women report physical or sexual assault at some point in their lives (8).

Undoubtedly, common factors of poverty, drug use, homelessness, and traumatic relationships influence the health status of incarcerated women. Correctional facilities are required to provide health services, although their quality and availability fluctuate considerably among jails and prisons (8).

Reproductive health is of particular concern among incarcerated women, because they are often of child-bearing age, and many new inmates have vaginal or sexually transmitted infections (STIs) (9). Five to ten percent of women who enter correctional facilities are already pregnant, and over three-quarters of newly incarcerated women have abnormal Pap smears. In addition, the female inmate population has a high prevalence of other infectious diseases, such as HIV/AIDS, tuberculosis, and hepatitis C. Psychiatric disorders also occur at higher rates among incarcerated women compared to the general female population (8).

In a primary healthcare encounter, it is important to consider the complex psychosocial situation of women in or recently released from correctional facilities. Women who are or have been incarcerated are likely to face issues of poverty and, therefore, have restricted access to health insurance and regular healthcare providers. After release, women may lose access to medication coverage. A thorough medical history at intake should strive to identify ongoing and/or communicable illnesses. Screening and treatment for chronic conditions, such as cancer, asthma, and diabetes—as prevalent in these women as in the general population—may not have been available in their correctional facility and/or may have been interrupted by their release. Women with incarceration experiences will likely need reproductive counseling, as well as routine gynecological care, as strong links exist among drug use, commercial sex work, and STIs. Sensitivity to the economic desperation that might drive women to maintain violent relationships, prostitution, and drug use is necessary, as well as awareness of mental illnesses. In addition, the emotional strain experienced by women who are separated from their children and other family members while they are incarcerated should not be overlooked, since up to two-thirds of female inmates have children under the age of 18 years (8).

Women generally do not serve life sentences in correctional facilities and eventually re-enter society, with or without support services. Since their unique situations before, during, and after incarceration make them particularly vulnerable to poor health, the improvement of their well-being will ultimately translate to improved family and community health as well.

References

1. **DeNavas-Walt C, Proctor BD, Smith J.** Income, poverty, and health insurance coverage in the United States: 2006. In Current Population Reports. Washington, D.C., U.S: Census Bureau; 2007. pp. 60–233.
2. **Belle D, Doucet J.** Poverty, inequality and discrimination as sources of depression among U.S. women. Psychology of Women Quarterly. 2003;27:101–13.
3. **Larsen L.** The Foreign-born population in the United States: 2003. In Current Population Reports. Washington, D.C., U.S: Census Bureau; 2004. pp. 20–551.

4. National Center for Health Statistics. Examples of uses of data from NCHS. Hyattsville: MD; 2007.
5. **Williams DR.** Racial/ethnic variations in women's health: The social embeddedness of health. American Journal of Public Health. 2002;92:588-97.
6. U.S. Department of Health and Human Services. Safe motherhood: Finding one voice. Health Matters for Women. Atlanta: Centers for Disease Control and Prevention; 2002.
7. **Meadows LM, Thurston WE, Melton C.** Immigrant women's health. Social Science and Medicine. 2001;52:1451-8.
8. **Arriola KJ, Braithwaite RL, Newkirk CF.** An overview of incarcerated women's health. In Braithwaite RL, Arriola KJ, Newkirk CF (eds): Health issues among incarcerated women. New Brunswick: Rutgers; 2006. pp. 3-17.
9. **De Groot AS, Maddow R.** HIV/AIDS Infection among incarcerated women. In Braithwaite RL, Arriola KJ, Newkirk CF (eds): Health issues among incarcerated women. New Brunswick: Rutgers; 2006. pp. 237-47.

F. Racial Disparities

Sarina B. Schrager

KEY POINTS

- After controlling for socioeconomic factors, striking disparities still exist between women of color and Caucasian women.
- African American women have a lower incidence of breast cancer but a higher mortality than Caucasian women.
- Latinas have the highest rate of cervical cancer, followed by African American women.
- African American women with heart disease are 30% less likely to have bypass surgery than are Caucasian women.
- African American women account for over half of the newly diagnosed HIV/AIDS cases in the U.S. each year.
- African American women have a rate of gonorrhea infection that is 24 times as high as Caucasian women.
- African American women have higher preterm birth and infant mortality rates than women in all other groups.

Disparities in health reflect different outcomes or risk factors. "Racial disparities" is a term that describes differential health outcomes based on race or ethnicity. Attention to differences in health outcomes among women of different races or ethnicities has increased over the last 10 years. Differences can be due to social issues, like access to care, availability of health insurance, or socioeconomic status. African American women and Latinas together comprise almost a quarter of the total population of adult women in the U.S., making this a very important topic (1).

Women of color are much more likely to be uninsured than Caucasian women, which can affect access to screening tests and adequate treatment. Thirty-seven percent of Latinas and 20% of African American women are uninsured, as compared to 16% of Caucasian women (2). Furthermore, half of all Latinas experienced a period without insurance over a one-year time-frame (2). Women of color also are more likely than their white counterparts to have low incomes (2). Thirty-three percent of African Americans in the U.S. live in poverty, compared to 29% of Latinos and 11.6% of Caucasians (3). Many barriers exist to receiving and accessing health care, over and above availability of health insurance, including cost of co-pays, difficulty finding childcare, and lack of transportation. All of these factors are more prevalent among women of color (2). Even after controlling for many of these socioeconomic factors, striking disparities exist between Caucasian women and women of color (4).

Overall health status is poorer among women of color. A fifth of African American women (20%) rate their health status as fair or poor, compared to Latinas (29%) and Caucasian women (13%) (2). Life expectancy is lower for some women of color compared to Caucasian women (Non-Hispanic Black women, 74.3 years; Latinas 82.2 years; and White, Non-Hispanic women 80 years) (5). This chapter will review health disparities among women for some common health conditions.

Cancer

Breast cancer is the most common cancer among women of all races and ethnicities (6). It is the leading cause of cancer death among Latinas and the second among Caucasian, African American, Asian/ Pacific Islander, and Native American/Alaskan Native women (6). The incidence of breast cancer is higher in Caucasian women, yet mortality among African American women is greater (7). Controlling for treatment, mammogram screening, tumor characteristics at diagnosis, and comorbidities reduced but did not eradicate the mortality difference (8). Premenopausal African American women tend to have the highest incidence of aggressive cancers (7). Only 72% of African American women are alive 5 years after a breast cancer diagnosis compared to >87% of Caucasian women (5). Breast cancer mortality has been decreasing annually for Caucasian women but not for African Americans (5).

The overall rates of mammogram screening are not significantly different among the races (2). However, almost 30% of women over 50 of all races had not received a screening mammogram within the past

2 years (2). In addition, 32% of Latinas did not have a clinical breast exam during the past year, as compared to only 20% of Caucasians (2). Lack of insurance, poor access to primary care, and both cultural and language barriers are important reasons for why Latinas, Native Americans, and some Asian Americans do not get regular breast cancer screening (9). In addition, the interval between an abnormal screening test and a diagnostic procedure is longer for women of color than it is for Caucasian women (10).

Cervical cancer is a largely preventable cancer because of widespread Pap smear screening. Incidence rates of invasive cervical cancer are higher in both Latinas and African American women than in Caucasians (11). The incidence of cervical cancer per 100,000 women in the US is 8.9 for Caucasian women, 13.5 for African American women, 14.8 for Latinas, and 8.9 for Asian/Pacific Islander women. African American women have lower survival rates from cervical cancer, which may be explained mostly by socioeconomic factors, such as poverty and lack of access to health care (12). Vietnamese women have a 5-fold higher incidence of cervical cancer than Caucasians (9). This disparity may be in part because Asian American women get Pap smears at a rate much lower than Caucasians, African Americans, or Latinas (5).

Cardiovascular Disease

Heart disease is the leading cause of death for women of all races, except Asian/Pacific Islanders (5). In the latter group, heart disease is second to cancer as a cause of death (5). Mortality rates cardiovascular and cerebrovascular disease are also higher for women of color. African American women had death rates from heart disease that were 2.1 times greater than Latinas and 1.4 times higher than Caucasians, according to 1995 data (13). Much of the differential in mortality from heart disease among races can be accounted for by a different prevalence of risk factors. Fifty-seven percent of African American women between 45 and 64 years have hypertension, as compared to only 28% of Caucasian women in the same age group (2). Nearly 60% of Native American/ Alaskan Native women had at least one risk factor for heart disease (5). Native American/Alaskan Native women have a higher prevalence of smoking than all other groups (5). In addition, the rates of obesity are higher in African American women and Latinas compared to Caucasian women (5).

In addition to the difference in prevalence of risk factors among groups, women of color do not get as aggressive care for their cardiovascular (CV) disease as do Caucasian women. African American women are less likely to be referred for angiograms (5), and they are also 13% less likely to have angioplasty and >30% less likely to get bypass surgery than Caucasian women (10).

African American women have higher death rates from strokes compared to other groups as well (Table 12-1).

Table 12-1   Death Rates for Stroke per 100 000 U.S. Women

African American	78.1
Latina	36.3
Asian/Pacific Islander	48.2
American Indian/Alaskan Native	38.5
Caucasian	59.6

From Clark A, Fong C, Romans M. Health disparities among US women of color: an overview. Washington, D.C.: The Jacobs Institute of Women's Health;2002. Available at www.jiwh.org; with permission.

Diabetes

Both prevalence of diabetes mellitus and death from diabetic conse-quences are higher in women of color. Prevalence of diabetes is highest among the Native American/Alaskan Native population, followed by African Americans, Caucasians, and Latinas (14). The rate among Native American/Alaskan Native women is almost 3 times the overall rate in the U.S. (15). In addition, Japanese Americans, Filipino Americans, Chinese Americans, and Korean Americans all have higher rates of diabetes than the general population (15). The difference in prevalence is especially striking in older women. Thirty-two percent of African American women between 60 and 74 years and >25% of Latinas >50 years have diabetes (5). These rates are double those of Caucasian women of similar ages (5). Latinas have a higher prevalence of diabetes than do non-Latino whites. Within the Latino population, diabetes rates vary, with the highest occur-ring in women from Puerto Rico and those who live in the Southwestern U.S., and the lowest rates in women of Cuban ancestry (15).

The complication and mortality rates from diabetes are also quite different among races. African American women are more than twice as likely to develop renal disease from their diabetes as are Caucasian women (15). In addition, rates of proteinuria and of diabetes-induced blindness are higher in all women of color (15). The diabetes-related mortality rate per 100 000 for African Americans (both men and women) is 49.2, compared to 23.0 for Caucasians and 21.5 for other races (3).

Infections

The most striking disparity in infectious diseases is the differential preva-lence of HIV infection between women of color and Caucasian women. Between 2001 and 2005, African American women made up 58.9% of all the new HIV/AIDS diagnoses among injection drug users and 69.5% of all new diagnoses among people with heterosexual transmis-sion (16). During that same time period, regionally, African American women made up 71.5% of all new HIV/AIDS diagnoses in the South, 64% in the Northeast, and 63.5% in the Midwest (16). Among both men and women, the annual AIDS case rate per 100 000 was 7.2 among Caucasians, 68.6 among African Americans, and 23.3 among Latinos (3).

Table 12-2 New HIV/AIDS Diagnoses in Women between 2001 and 2005 (% of total)

Caucasian	African American	Latina	Asian/Pacific Islander	American Indian/ Alaskan Native
16.3	67.2	14.5	0.7	0.6

From Update to racial/ethnic disparities in diagnoses of HIV/AIDS—33 states, 2001–5. MMWR. 2007;56:189–93; with permission.

Table 12-3 Number of Cases of STIs per 100 000 U.S. Men and Women*

	African American	Caucasian	American Indian/ Alaskan Native	Asian/Pacific Islander
Chlamydia	805.9	90.2	512.1	108.0
Gonorrhea	570.4	24.2	96.1	18.3
Syphilis	9.4	1.1	2.3	0.8

*Data missing for Hispanic population
From Racial disparities in nationally notifiable diseases in the United States, 2002. MMWR. 2005;54:9–11; with permission.

Table 12-2 shows new HIV/AIDS diagnoses among women that occurred between 2001–2005 by race.

The rates of other sexually transmitted infections (STIs) are also higher in people of color (Table 12-3).

Maternal and Child Health

Racial disparities exist throughout the continuum of maternal and child health, from rates of preterm labor to infant mortality. African American women are less likely to receive early prenatal care than Caucasian women, which may be explained at least in part by socioeconomic factors (18). This decreased access to care may promote adverse outcomes. African American women are much more likely to have a preterm infant than are all other women (19) (Table 12-4).

In addition, the infant mortality rate is significantly higher among African American babies compared to the national average (14.1 vs. 6.9 per 1000 live births) (20). It is likely that a large percentage of this disparity is related to the higher rates of preterm deliveries. Other socioeconomic factors that may affect adverse pregnancy outcomes are poverty, lack of insurance, and stress from racism. A sample of over 10 000 African American and Latino women on Medicaid compared pregnancy outcomes between the two groups. African American women had higher rates of preterm births and stillbirths after controlling for socioeconomic factors, suggesting that poverty itself does not account for all of the disparity (21). Racism or perceived racism has been found to be a predictor of preterm birth in African American women as well (22).

Table 12-4 Preterm Birth Rates by Maternal Race/Ethnicity, 2002–2004*

Latina	Caucasian	African American	Native American	Asian
11.8	11.3	17.8	13.4	10.4

* All race categories exclude Hispanics
From Peristats, data on perinatal outcome. March of Dimes, available at www.marchofdimes. com/peristats. National Center for Health Statistics, final natality data. Retrieved February 4th, 2008, from www.marchofdimes.com/peristats; with permission.

Other Conditions

The prevalence of lupus is 3 times higher in African American than in Caucasian women (23). The disease is also more common in Latinas, Asian women, and Native American women (23). Women of color may experience a more severe course of the disease as well, getting symptoms at an earlier age and having more severe end-organ involvement (23). In addition, African American women have higher death rates from lupus than do Caucasian women (23). Arthritis is also more common in African American women than in Latinas and Caucasian women (40% prevalence compared to 33% and 32%, respectively) (2). Osteoporosis, however, is more common in Caucasian women and Latinas than in African American women (2). There is no significant racial difference in diagnosis of anxiety or depression (2).

Conclusion

Significant racial disparities exist in many areas of women's health. Many of these differences may be explained by socioeconomic factors. Primary care providers need to be vigilant in their care of women of color, taking into account the barriers to care that they may experience.

References

1. Racial and ethnic disparities in women's health. ACOG Committee Opinion. Obstetrics and Gynecology. 2005;106:889–93.
2. Racial and ethnic disparities in women's health coverage and access to care, findings from the 2001 Kaiser Women's Health Survey. Available at www.kff.org.
3. Key health and health care indicators by race/ethnicity and state. Kaiser Family Foundation, Available at statehealthfacts.org.
4. **Sudano JJ, Baker DW.** Explaining US racial/ethnic disparities in health declines and mortality in late middle age: the roles of socioeconomic status, health behaviors, and health insurance. Social Science and Medicine. 2006;62:909–22.
5. **Clark A, Fong C, Romans M.** Health disparities among US women of color: an overview. Washington, D.C.: The Jacobs Institute of Women's Health; 2002. Available at www.jiwh.org.
6. Statistics about health disparities in cancer among women, available at www.cdc.gov/cancer/healthdisparities/women.htm.

7. **Karliner LS, Kerlikowske K.** Ethnic disparities in breast cancer. Women's Health. 2007;3:679–88.

8. **Curtis E, Quale C, Haggstrom D, et al.** Racial and ethnic disparities in breast cancer survival: how much is explained by screening, tumor severity, biology, treatment, comorbidities, and demographics. Cancer. 2008;112:171–80.

9. Office of minority health and health disparities. Eliminate disparities in cancer screening and management. Available at, www.cdc.gov/omhd/AMH/factsheets/cancer.htm

10. AHRQ, Addressing racial and ethnic disparities in health care: fact sheet. Available at, http://www.ahrq.gov/research/disparit.htm

11. **Saraiya M, Ahmed F, Krisnan S, et al.** Cervical cancer incidence in a pre-vaccine era in the United States, 1998–2002. Obstetrics and Gynecology. 2007;109:360–70.

12. **Movva S, Noone AM, Banerjee M, et al.** Racial differences in cervical cancer survival in the Detroit metropolitan area. Cancer. 2008;112:1264–71.

13. **Casper ML, Barnett E, Halverson JA, et al.** Women and Heart Disease: an Atlas of Racial and Ethnic Disparities in Mortality, Second edition. Morgantown, WV: Office for Social Environment and Health Research, West Virginia University, 2000. Available at http://www.cdc.gov/dhdsp/library/maps/cvatlas_womens/womens_download.htm

14. National Center for Chronic Disease Prevention and Health Promotion. National diabetes fact sheet. Available at www.cdc.gov/diabetes/pubs/estimates.htm

15. AHRQ, Diabetes disparities among racial and ethnic minorities: fact sheet. Available at www.ahrq.gov/research/diabdisp.htm

16. Update to racial/ethnic disparities in diagnoses of HIV/AIDS—33 states, 2001–5. MMWR. 2007;56:189–93.

17. Racial disparities in nationally notifiable diseases in the United States, 2002. MMWR. 2005;54:9–11.

18. **Harper MA, Block SM.** Editorial, Racial disparities in obstetrical care. Journal of Perinatology. 2006;26:73.

19. Peristats, data on perinatal outcome. March of Dimes, available at www.marchofdimes.com/peristats.

20. Office of Minority Health and Health Disparities, Eliminate disparities in infant mortality. Available at www.cdc.gov/omhd/AMH/factsheets/infant.htm.

21. **Brown HL, Chireau MV, Jallah Y, et al.** The "Hispanic paradox": and investigation of racial disparity in pregnancy outcomes at a tertiary care medical center. American Journal of Obstetrics and Gynecology. 2007;197:1–7.

22. **Dominguez TP, Dunkel-Schetter C, Glynn LM, et al.** Racial differences in birth outcomes: the role of general, pregnancy, and racism stress. Health Psychology. 2008;27:194–203.

23. Office of Minortiy Health and Health Disparities, Eliminate disparities in lupus. Available at, www.cdc.gov/omhd/AMH/factsheets/lupus.htm

Part II

Life Cycle Structure

13

Adolescent Women

A. Menstrual Disorders in the Adolescent Patient

Mollie L. Kane

KEY POINTS

- Most adolescent females will experience some menstrual difficulties, ranging from excessive or irregular menstrual bleeding to amenorrhea, dysmenorrhea, or premenstrual syndrome.
- Many irregular menstrual patterns that adolescent females experience are normal variations due to lack of maturation of the hypothalamic–pituitary–ovarian axis. However, menstrual irregularities also can be a sign of important underlying disease.
- Adolescent females typically experience anovulatory cycles for an average of 18 months after menarche. These cycles are of variable length and duration, with varying amounts of blood flow.
- Excessive menstrual bleeding or dysfunctional uterine bleeding in adolescents is most commonly due to anovulation. However, anovulation is a diagnosis of exclusion, and other conditions such as bleeding disorders must be excluded.
- Amenorrhea is a common complaint in adolescent females. There are numerous causes of amenorrhea. Many causes are benign, but pregnancy and pathology always must be excluded.

Adolescent females experience a wide variety of menstrual patterns, ranging from regular, monthly menses, to non-pathologic variations, to disorders reflecting serious underlying pathology. Regardless of the cause, irregular menstrual bleeding patterns are often the cause of anxiety for the adolescent patient and her family. The clinical visit for a menstrual complaint provides the opportunity for important patient education and, at times, the early diagnosis of medical problems.

Most adolescent girls experience some menstrual difficulties, and many of them seek medical care for their concerns. Menstrual complaints in adolescent girls include amenorrhea, dysmenorrhea, premenstrual syndrome, and excessive or irregular uterine bleeding. Polycystic ovarian syndrome (PCOS) is also a common cause of menstrual irregularities.

Many adolescents feel sensitive or embarrassed discussing issues related to their menstrual cycles. For some, menstrual disorders are secondary to disordered eating, sexually transmitted infections, trauma, or other conditions. Therefore, for almost all adolescents presenting with menstrual complaints, at least part of the history should be obtained without parents or others in the room. Confidentiality laws should be respected when pregnancy related issues or sexually transmitted diseases are involved.

Normal and Anovulatory Menstrual Cycles

Young adolescents often present with a complaint of skipping menstrual periods or having periods close together. They may be concerned that some of their periods have heavy flow while others are light. These irregularities are usually caused by physiologic anovulatory menstrual cycles and require reassurance of the patient that her system is normal.

The normal, ovulatory, menstrual cycle is 28 days, +/− 7 days, in length, with an average duration of 4 days +/− 2 days. Normal blood loss is 20–80 mL per cycle, although the amount of bleeding can be difficult to assess clinically (1). These ovulatory menstrual cycles require a mature hypothalamic–pituitary axis.

It is normal for cycles to be anovulatory for an average of 18 months post-menarche while the hypothalamic–pituitary axis matures. Anovulatory cycles may be of variable length and duration. The amount of blood loss is generally normal, although prolonged, heavy bleeding can occur. While ovulatory cycles are often associated with premenstrual symptoms, dysmenorrhea, breast tenderness, cervical mucous changes, *mittleschmertz* (mid-cycle cramping with ovulation) and biphasic temperature changes, these findings are absent in anovulatory cycles. Other common causes of anovulatory cycles in this age group include thyroid and prolactin abnormalities, eating disorders, and physiologic stress due to excessive exercise.

Menorrhagia (Excessive Menstrual Bleeding)

Menorrhagia (excessive blood flow) may be due to prolonged duration of menses or excess volume of flow (>80 mL/cycle). Menorrhagia is quite common in adolescent patients and is caused by anovulatory cycles about 95% of the time (2). This lack of ovulation may be due to immaturity of the hypothalamic–pituitary axis, as described above, or to hypothalamic–pituitary dysfunction caused by stress, weight loss, chronic disease, disordered eating, or excessive exercise.

A smaller group of adolescents have excessive vaginal bleeding caused by pathologic conditions. These include complications of pregnancy, benign or malignant cervical or uterine lesions, complications of sexually transmitted infections, exogenous hormone use, polycystic ovarian syndrome, other androgen excess disorders, hyperprolactinemia, other endocrine disorders, trauma, foreign bodies, systemic disease such as systemic lupus erythematosus or liver disease, and systemic bleeding disorders.

Menorrhagia beginning at menarche is a strong indicator for a bleeding disorder, since between 5% and 24% of women with menorrhagia have an undiagnosed bleeding disorder (3). In women presenting with menorrhagia at menarche, the rate is probably even higher. Any patient with menorrhagia who has a history of heavy bleeding since menarche, family history of bleeding disorder or easy bleeding, excessive bleeding postpartum or after spontaneous or therapeutic abortion or surgery should have a work-up for bleeding disorder. Patients without any of these risk factors who are refractory to medical treatment of menorrhagia also should be evaluated. The most common bleeding disorders responsible for menorrhagia are Von Willebrand's Disease and disorders of platelet function. Other coagulation factor deficiencies are rare causes of menorrhagia.

The evaluation of menorrhagia should include a thorough history and physical examination and assessment of hemodynamic stability. The history should be directed toward menstrual history, sexual history, history of trauma, and medication use. Compliance with any hormonal contraceptives, symptoms such as easy bleeding, gingival bleeding, or epistaxis, and endocrine history such as hirsutism, galactorrhea, or thyroid symptoms should be reviewed. The physical exam should focus on endocrine abnormalities, Tanner stage, signs of pregnancy, or anatomic sources for the bleeding. In the very young patient (or in any patient) who has never been sexually active, an internal speculum exam is not generally needed. External genital exam is useful to look for Tanner stage and signs of hyperandrogenism. An internal digital exam may be helpful to rule out the presence of a foreign body. If an internal speculum exam becomes necessary, general anesthesia can be considered.

Laboratory studies always should include a pregnancy test and a CBC with smear and platelets. Thyroid stimulating hormone (TSH) and prolactin levels should be tested in cases of abnormal bleeding. In patients who are sexually active, testing should be performed for sexually transmitted infections.

When work-up for a bleeding disorder is indicated, studies to consider include PT, PTT, factor VIII, Von Willebrand factor antigen, Von Willebrand functional assay, collagen-binding assay, or ristocetin cofactor. Platelet dysfunction can be studied via platelet aggregometry and platelet function assay. If PT or PTT are abnormal, additional studies of coagulation factors and coagulation inhibitors may be indicated. Ideally, the bleeding disorder evaluation should be performed before oral contraceptives are started, since the latter may mask the diagnosis of Von Willebrand's disease by increasing levels of factor VIII. Aspirin and non-steroidal anti-inflammatory drugs also complicate the diagnosis of bleeding disorders.

Initial treatment should be aimed at stabilizing the patient and controlling bleeding (4,5). When bleeding is mild, with a hematocrit >33%, iron supplementation should be provided. Oral contraceptives may also be used to decrease bleeding. For moderate bleeding, with hematocrit or 27–33%, oral contraceptives should be administered together with iron supplements.

For patients with a contraindication to estrogen therapy, bleeding can be controlled with oral progesterone. High-dose oral progesterone also may stop the bleeding. These patients can then be continued on progestin-only OCPs (3).

If bleeding is severe (i.e., hematocrit <27% or signs of orthostasis), the patient should be admitted to the hospital for type and screen, IV fluids, and transfusion if appropriate. Intravenous estrogen should be started at 25 mg every 4–6 hours up to 4 doses. In some cases, oral contraceptives administered 4 times a day will control bleeding in place of intravenous medication. Many of these patients will need surgical intervention to stop the bleeding (3).

Amenorrhea

Amenorrhea, or lack of menstrual periods, is a very common presenting complaint for adolescents. While many causes of amenorrhea are benign, it can be the first sign of a serious underlying medical problem. In the adolescent patient, pregnancy always should be considered first as the possible cause of amenorrhea.

Amenorrhea can be primary or secondary. Primary amenorrhea is traditionally defined as having no menarche by age 16 in the presence of normal secondary sexual characteristics, or the absence of secondary sexual characteristics by age 14. However, 98% of females have menarche by age 15. Based on this statistic, it is practical to begin the evaluation for primary amenorrhea at age 15 (6,7). Similarly, 95% of girls will have developed secondary sexual characteristics by age 13, and it is reasonable to begin a work-up at age 13 if secondary sexual characteristics remain absent (5,8).

Normal female puberty usually occurs over an average of 4 years, with a normal range of 1–8 years. Tanner staging is a method that can be used to ensure that puberty is progressing normally. In 1962, Tanner and Marshall published a study of 420 British adolescent male and female patients who had been followed throughout puberty to determine normal rates of development (9,10). Female puberty starts with thelarche (breast budding) at a normal age range of 8–13 years. This should be followed by pubarche (first appearance of pubic hair) within an average of 6 months later. However, a number of normal females will experience pubarche as the first sign of puberty. Peak height velocity (growth spurt) appears next, followed by menarche.

All adolescent females should progress in a predictable pattern from Tanner stage 1 through Tanner stage 4. Not all females will progress to Tanner stage 5. This is normal and also varies by ethnic group. Menarche usually occurs when girls are at Tanner stage 4 for both breast and pubic hair development and should occur at 2.3 +/- 1.1 years after the beginning of Tanner stage 2 for breast development. Tanner staging for females is reviewed in Tables 13-1 and 13-2.

Menarche requires an intact central nervous system with normal hypothalamic–pituitary function, normal end organs with gonadal responsiveness, and an intact outflow tract (11). If any of these components are absent, primary amenorrhea will occur. Primary amenorrhea is quite rare and occurs in <1% of females. The most common causes of primary amenorrhea include: pregnancy: chromosomal abnormalities such as Turner's syndrome or Sawyer's syndrome; hypothalamic hypogonadism, which may be functional or caused by lesions or diseases of the hypothalamus, pituitary, or other endocrine organs; congenital absence of the uterus, cervix, or vagina; transverse vaginal septum; and imperforate hymen. Common causes of primary amenorrhea are explained

Table 13-1   Tanner Stages of Female Breast Development

Tanner Stage	Description	Age (in years)
Stage 1	Prepubertal, no breast tissue	
Stage 2	Breast bud present with diameter less than diameter of areola	8.0–13.0
Stage 3	Diameter of breast bed greater than diameter of areola	9.8–14.6
Stage 4	Areola mounded above the plane of the breast	11.4–15.0
Stage 5	Adult breast development	11.6–16.4

From Marshall WA, Tanner JM. Variations in pattern of pubertal changes in girls. Arch Dis Child. 1969;44:291–303. Sanfilippo JS, Hertweck SP. 2002. Physiology of menstruation and menstrual disorders. In S.B. Friedman, M.M., Fisher, S.K. Schonberg, & E.M. Alderman (Eds.), Comprehensive adolescent health care (2nd edition, pp. 1011–15). St. Louis, MO: Mosby; with permission.

Table 13-2   Tanner Stages for Female Pubic Hair Development

Tanner Stage	Description	Age (in years)
Stage 1	Prepubertal, no pubic hair	
Stage 2	Pubic hair just visible on mons or labia	8.0–12.8
Stage 3	Pubic hair clearly visible on mons	9.8–14.6
Stage 4	Pubic hair confined to suprapubic region	12.5–16.5
Stage 5	Pubic hair present on medial thighs	11.6–16.0

From Marshall WA, Tanner JM. Variations in pattern of pubertal changes in girls. Arch Dis Child. 1969;44:291–303. Sanfilippo JS, Hertweck SP. 2002. Physiology of menstruation and menstrual disorders. In S.B. Friedman, M.M., Fisher, S.K. Schonberg, & E.M. Alderman (Eds.), Comprehensive adolescent health care (2nd edition, pp. 1011–15). St. Louis, MO: Mosby; with permission.

in Table 13-3. There are numerous other very rare causes of primary amenorrhea, such as cyanotic heart disease, other severe chronic diseases (such as severe liver or kidney disease), testicular feminization, or congenital adrenal hyperplasia. In addition, any condition that causes secondary amenorrhea can also present at menarche as primary amenorrhea.

Secondary amenorrhea is defined as the absence of menstrual cycles for 3–6 months. Recent evidence supports initiating a work-up for secondary amenorrhea if no menses has occurred for 90 days (5). The most common cause of secondary amenorrhea in adolescents is dysfunction of the hypothalamic–pituitary–ovarian axis. Non-pathologic causes include anovulation, due to immaturity of the hypothalamic–pituitary axis, and chronic hypothalamic anovulation.

Other causes of secondary amenorrhea include pregnancy, use of some hormonal contraceptives, post-contraceptive amenorrhea, uterine adhesions (Asherman's syndrome), thyroid disease, and hyperandrogenism, as seen in polycystic ovarian syndrome. Ovarian failure leads to

Table 13-3   Causes of Primary Amenorrhea

Hypogonatropic Hypogonadism (Absence of Secondary Sex Characteristics)	Mullerian Agenesis	Androgen Insensitivity Syndrome	Congenital Outflow Obstruction	Hypergonadotropic Hypogonadism
Excessive exercise Excessive weight loss or malnutrition Hypothalamic or pituitary destruction Kallman syndrome Anorexia or bulimia Constitutional delay of growth or puberty Depression	Congenital absence of uterus and vagina Causes 15% of all primary amenorrhea	Normal breast development, no pubic hair Previously known as testicular feminization X-linked recessive disorder that causes a failure of normal development of external genitalia of genetic males (46 XY) Girl has lower vagina, but not upper or uterus or ovaries	Imperforate hymen Transverse vaginal septum	Absence of secondary sex characteristics Karyotype XO—Turner's syndrome Karyotype XX— premature ovarian failure

Adapted from Master-Hunter T, Heiman DL. Amenorrhea: Evaluation and treatment, Am Fam Physician. 2006;73:1374–82,1387; with permission.

secondary amenorrhea and may be idiopathic, autoimmune, or karyotypic, but this is very uncommon in adolescents.

Following a history and physical, the evaluation of secondary amenorrhea should always include a pregnancy test, followed by a prolactin level and TSH level.

Treatment of both primary and secondary amenorrhea depends on the specific cause. However, estrogen replacement should be considered in all cases (except when the cause of amenorrhea is pregnancy). Supplementation with calcium 1500 mg per day and vitamin D 400–800 IU per day should be given to minimize loss of bone density caused by a hypoestrogenic state. Most patients with secondary amenorrhea, as well as dysfunctional uterine bleeding, will ovulate at times. Patients need to be made aware that they are at risk for pregnancy, even when menses are absent or irregular.

Adolescent girls with amenorrhea or dysfunctional uterine bleeding are at increased risk for long-term health complications. Most of these patients have low levels of circulating estrogens, increasing their risk for loss of bone mineral density. Such loss has been shown to be significant by age 20 in many patients (12). While estrogen levels are low, in some patients they are unopposed by progesterone. In these cases, there is an increased risk of endometrial hyperplasia, which can lead to endometrial carcinoma. There also may be a negative effect on lipoprotein profiles (13). Many clinicians provide estrogen and progesterone supplementation, often in the form of OCPs, in hopes of preventing these complications. Others monitor patients with bone mineral density screening studies and lipid panels.

Dysmenorrhea

Dysmenorrhea is the presence of lower abdominal cramping associated with menses. It occurs in up to 90% of adolescent girls and is severe in about 15%. It is the leading cause of recurrent short-term school absences in teenage girls in the U.S. (14). Primary dysmenorrhea begins with the onset of ovulatory menstrual periods. It becomes less severe with age and after pregnancy. Discomfort may begin several hours before bleeding starts, typically peaks in 24 hours, and usually resolves by 48–72 hours after the onset of bleeding. Lower abdominal discomfort may be accompanied by low back pain, upper leg pain, headache, nausea, vomiting, malaise, and gastrointestinal distress.

Secondary dysmenorrhea is menstrual pain that is secondary to uterine lesions and is rare in adolescents. Many types of uterine pathology can cause secondary dysmenorrhea, such as endometriosis, cervical stenosis, or uterine fibroids. In young women, sexually transmitted infections, pelvic inflammatory disease, and complications of pregnancy should be considered first as possible causes of secondary amenorrhea. Symptoms of secondary dysmenorrhea do not generally follow the predictable pattern of symptoms seen in primary dysmenorrhea.

The diagnosis of dysmenorrhea is made by history and physical exam. In primary dysmenorrhea, an internal pelvic exam is not required for those patients who are not yet sexually active. However, pelvic exam and sexually transmitted disease testing are indicated in those patients who are sexually active. If dysmenorrhea is very severe or remains problematic despite treatment, ultrasound or laparoscopy may be considered to look for pathology such as endometriosis.

Many adolescents are very distressed by their dysmenorrhea and need to be reassured that it is normal and common. In addition to reassurance, treatment of primary dysmenorrhea includes increased time for sleep, regular exercise, and applications of heat. Nonsteroidal anti-inflammatory agents can be used. These are most effective if they are started before the dysmenorrhea begins and taken at regular intervals until 48 hours into the menstrual period. When these measures are not effective, or when the teen desires contraception, hormonal contraceptives can be used to suppress ovulation.

In the past, breast exam and pelvic exam with Pap smear were often considered prerequisites for prescribing oral contraceptives. This is no longer the case, since requiring these exams may prevent many teens from choosing to get treatment or contraception that they need. The decision to use oral contraceptives should include a review of any contraindications and a blood pressure check. Prescription of hormonal contraceptives should not be contingent upon performance of a pelvic exam and pap smear (15).

Premenstrual Syndrome

There are very few studies of premenstrual syndrome in a specifically adolescent population. It is thought that PMS occurs in adolescents in about the same rates as it does in older women and involves the same constellation of symptoms. When possible, adolescents with PMS should be treated with reassurance and conservative measures. However, treatments used in adults can be used safely and effectively in adolescent populations as well.

References

1. **Spellacy WN.** Abnormal bleeding. Clin Obstet Gynecol. 1983; 26:702–9.
2. **Rimsza ME.** Dysfunctional uterine bleeding. Pediatrics in Review. 2002;23:227–33.
3. **Strickland JL.** Management of abnormal bleeding in adolescents. Mo Med. 2004;101:38–41.
4. **Greenfield TP, Blythe MJ**, Menstrual disorders in adolescents. D.E. D.R. H.D. Essential Adolescent Medicine 2006. New York: McGraw-Hill Medical Publishers. pp. 591–612.
5. **Greydanus DE.** Breast and gynecologic disorders. A.D.D.E. Adolescent medicine 3rd edition. 1997Stamford, CT: Appleton & Lange. pp. 520–65.
6. National Center of Health Statistics. Age at Menarche: United States. Rockville (MD): MCHS: 1973. Available at http://wwwcdc.gov/nchs/data/series/sr_11/sr11_133.pdf. Retrieved January, 2008.

7. Menstruation in girls and adolescents: using the menstrual cycle as a vital sign. ACOG Committee Opinion No. 349. American Academy of Pediatrics; American College of Obstetricians and Gynecologists. Obstet Gynecol. 2006;108:1323–8.

8. **Reindollar RH, Byrd JR, McDonough PG**. Delayed sexual development: a study of 252 patients. Am J Obstet Gynecol. 1981;140:371–80.

9. **Tanner JM.** Growth at Adolescence, ed 2, Springfield, IL, 1962, Charles C Thomas.

10. **Marshall WA, Tanner JM.** Variations in pattern of pubertal changes in girls. Arch Dis Child. 1969;44:291–303.

11. **Sanfilippo JS, Hertweck SP.** 2002. Physiology of menstruation and menstrual disorders. In S.B. Friedman, M.M., Fisher, S.K. Schonberg, and E.M. Alderman (Eds.), Comprehensive Adolescent Health Care. 2nd edition St. Louis, MO: Mosby. pp. 1011–5.

12. **Park KH, Song CH.** Bone mineral density in premenopausal anovulatory women. J Obstet Gynaecol. 1995 Feb;21:89–97.

13. **Schachter M, Shoham Z.** Amenorrhea during the reproductive years–is it safe? Fertil Steril. 1994 Jul;62:1–16.

14. **French L.** Dysmenorrhea. Am Fam Physician. 2005;71:285–91.

15. Revised oral contraceptive labeling: FDA approves recommendation allowing delay of pelvic exam. Contracept Rep. 1993 Nov;4:4–7.

B. Teenage Pregnancy Planning

Marissa Harris and Marji Gold

KEY POINTS

- Health care providers play a valuable role in assisting adolescents with family planning.
- Contraceptive counseling should provide accurate information in a confidential manner.
- Teens have the right to privacy, but can elect to involve parent/s in such discussions.
- Providers can be helpful in facilitating discussions with teens and their families.
- The availability of many different contraceptive methods allows the adolescent to select the most appropriate method based on ease, privacy, cost and comfort.
- Close follow-up with the adolescent is recommended to reinforce safe-sex options and address satisfaction or discomfort with the chosen contraceptive method.

Epidemiology

Healthcare providers can play an important role in helping sexually active teens prevent unintended pregnancy. For the first time in 15 years, the rate of teen births in the U.S. increased from 40.5 live births/1000 females aged 15–19 years in 2005 to 41.9 births/1000 in 2006 (1). During the decade prior to 2006, the incidence of pregnancies in women aged 15–19 years had been steadily decreasing. Teen pregnancy rates in the U.S. remain higher than that of most industrialized nations (2). Eight hundred thirty-one thousand American between the ages of 15–19 years became pregnant in 2005 (3). In addition, there are significant racial differences in teen pregnancy rates: Latinas have a 35% risk of becoming pregnant between the ages of 15–19 compared with 27% for non-Hispanic blacks and 12% for non-Hispanic whites (4).

Adolescent pregnancy and child-bearing are associated with academic failure, high-risk pregnancies, and adverse clinical outcomes, including low birth-weight and elevated infant mortality rates (5). There may be socioeconomic consequences of early pregnancy as well, such as disruption of high school education, and financial difficulty in some teen mothers. This may not be as evident in those with supportive communities and families (5) (Box 13-1).

Although widely prevalent, sexuality education in high schools is highly variable. Comprehensive programs highlight abstinence as an effective means of protection, along with balanced education regarding other contraceptive methods. Abstinence-only programs, which have increased in number due to government funding, teach that abstinence is the only acceptable option for pregnancy and sexually transmitted infection (STI) prevention and often do not provide accurate information about STIs and contraceptive methods. Adolescents are instructed to delay initiation of sex until marriage, and other contraceptive methods are characterized as "ineffective." Recent data show that such programs are not effective at delaying teenage sexual contact (2,6). Most

---

Box 13-1 Youth Risk Behavior Facts

- 46.8% of high school students have had sexual intercourse
- 62.8% of sexually active high school students used a condom the last time they engaged in sexual intercourse
- 23.3% of high school teens consumed alcohol or drugs before their last sexual encounter
- 7.5% of all students have ever been physically forced to have sex
- 17.6% of sexually active students used birth control pills for pregnancy prevention during the last sexual intercourse

From Youth Risk Behavior Surveillance-United States 2005. Morbidity and Mortality Weekly Report. 2006;55:1–108; with permission.

adolescents do not remain abstinent and, without appropriate education, are more likely to have unprotected intercourse with subsequent vulnerability to STIs and unintended pregnancy. Primary care providers play a vital role in addressing this gap in the reproductive health education of adolescents.

Contraceptive Counseling

Every adolescent's visit to the primary care provider's office is an opportunity to reiterate pregnancy planning and STI prevention strategies. Many teens present to the office only for administrative examinations for school, sports, or work. These may be the only opportunities to address effective risk-reduction strategies while promoting healthy sexual relationships for teens.

Primary care physicians should have a focused approach to both address and advocate for teenage family planning. At the onset of adolescence, providers should establish themselves as trustworthy confidantes with whom teens can feel comfortable. Visits should include a complete sexual health history with inquiry about current relationship status, sexual activity, sexual orientation, and the extent of intimate physical contact. Discussion of sexual behavior and interest in pregnancy allows providers to connect with both male and female teenage patients, forming an alliance to protect the well-being of their sexual and reproductive health.

Clinicians should approach the adolescent patient in a nonjudgmental manner. Confidentiality should be established early in the relationship and explained to both the patient and the parent. The healthcare provider should explain that any information obtained during a visit with an adolescent can be shared with family members only if the adolescent patient permits it. This clear statement of confidentiality provides teens a safe environment and encourages their autonomy as young adults. The patient should be counseled and examined without the parent present in the room, unless the teen prefers otherwise (Box 13-2).

Eliciting sensitive information from the adolescent patient can be difficult. While the teen may be uncomfortable with the seemingly intrusive interview, he or she may be encouraged to discuss their sexual history if the provider introduces a clinical concern that is commonly shared by other teenagers. Peers often have great social influence/impact on

---

Box 13-2   Take Home Points

- Counseling with the adolescent should be safe, confidential, and free of judgment.
- Providers should take the opportunity to address contraception and sexual behaviors at every encounter.
- The counseling session should be concrete with role-play if necessary to aid the patient in selecting the most appropriate contraceptive method.

teens, so a provider can normalize the experience by asking about them. For instance, the conversation can begin with, "It's really common for teens to think about sex. Do your friends talk about this? Do you have any questions?" or "Many young women have felt afraid to say no to sex because they might lose their boyfriends. Have you ever felt this way?" Referring to a third person during questions is a technique that often encourages teens to open up.

The sexual history should screen for previous sexual experience and pleasure, as well as coercion, rape, and a history of other sexual abuse. In addition, primary care providers should inquire about sexual risk-taking behaviors, such as sex without condoms, intercourse while intoxicated or after illicit drug use, and multiple partners, in a non-threatening manner. The role of the provider in the contraceptive counseling session is to facilitate the selection of the appropriate method by the patient through the provision of factual information and concrete instructions for use. Psychosocial and cultural factors also may be relevant to contraceptive choice. The explanation of each method should include risks, benefits, and alternatives in language that is understandable to the patient. Box 13-3 contains useful teen sexual and reproductive health resources.

Many states in the country allow adolescents to receive reproductive health care without parental consent. Providers should familiarize themselves with the laws pertinent to their state. Consideration also should be given to the adolescent's insurance status. Although the visit is confidential, many teens face the potential for unintended disclosure when contraceptive services appear on the explanation of benefits addressed to the parent. This type of scenario should be anticipated and presented to the teen patient as a potential outcome should a prescription for birth control be dispensed using parental insurance.

Initiating Contraception

The male adolescent is commonly overlooked in contraceptive counseling. Providers should discuss pregnancy prevention with all male teens who have sexual relationships. As part of discussions about sexuality, the male patient can learn to effectively communicate with female sexual partners. The male patient also can benefit from factual education

---

Box 13-3   Internet Resources for Teens and Providers

- National Campaign to Prevent Teen and Unplanned Pregnancy www.teenpregnancy.org
- National Youth Behavior Risk Survey www.cdc.gov/yrbss
- Teen Wire www.teenwire.com
- The Pleasure Project www.thepleasureproject.org
- Advocates for Youth www.advocatesforyouth.org
- The Alan Guttmacher Institute www.guttmacher.org

about birth control and dual protection methods; he should especially be informed about accessibility and appropriate use of emergency contraception. An added benefit of counseling male teens to use condoms is protection from STIs and HIV.

For young women, a pelvic examination is not required to initiate any contraceptive method. Cervical cancer screening should commence 3 years after the onset of sexual activity or at age 21. The CDC recommends routine screening of adolescents for gonorrhea and chlamydia. Such testing can now be performed with a urine sample, thus allowing delay of pelvic examination until appropriate. For hormonal contraception, a blood pressure measurement should be performed. The HPV vaccination should also be administered to all teens if they have not already received it, regardless of their sexual history.

The teen years represent a developmental bridge between childhood and adulthood. The ability to adequately process abstract concepts may be present in the mature or older teen; it is difficult to assess developmental maturity solely based on age. Some teens may be ill-equipped to anticipate those scenarios that may derail their contraceptive use; it is the responsibility of the provider to work with every adolescent initiating contraception to create a plan for effective use. This may be mediated by the discussion of each contraceptive method, including concrete, provocative questions and instructions. Teens are more equipped to apply logic when such concrete situations are provided. For example, the provider should ask questions such as *"How would you remind yourself to take your birth control pill while staying with a friend for the weekend?"* and *"If you did not want your parent to know you were taking the pill, would you be able to hide it successfully?"* Such questions enable the adolescent to plan for the future through imagined role-play. Box 13-4 contains other helpful questions to facilitate the selection of the appropriate contraceptive method. Through the interactive process, the teen patient is allowed to autonomously make the appropriate choice, given individual social and cultural circumstances, but with the advantage of the provider's experience and expertise.

Box 13-4   Useful Questions for Screening the Adolescent for Contraceptive Method

---

- Would it be a problem for you if your friends or family found your birth control?
- It can be difficult to remember to take a pill everyday. Would it be easier if you placed it next to your toothbrush? (Is it safe to do that in your house?)
- Some young women feel uncomfortable touching their vagina or private parts to place the ring. Do you think this would apply to you?
- The shot can make your cycle very unpredictable and you may stop getting your period. How would you feel about this? Would it be a problem if your parent noticed this?
- Sometimes sex can be unplanned. If you had sex without protection would you be able to quickly get the "morning after" pill?

Contraceptive Methods

Detailed information regarding contraceptive methods and eligibility criteria are described in Chapter 4D and are not reiterated here. Instead this chapter will focus on contraceptive issues with particular relevance to adolescents.

1. Condoms

Condoms are mechanical barriers, which offer dual protection from STIs and pregnancy, and should be recommended for all sexually active patients. Male condoms are quite accessible and convenient at a low cost, making them a valuable method for teens. Female condoms are not as widely used due to comfort, but can also be an effective method for teens.

The YRBS found an overall increase in male condom usage from 46.2% to 56.2% between 1991 and 2005 (3). With perfect use, the male condom's failure rate is 2%, and is 15% with typical use (7).

The female condom is also an effective barrier method. Its failure rate is 5% with perfect use and 21% with typical use (7). It should not be used with the male condom concurrently, since the two devices may become adherent and displaced. Teens may find the female condom cumbersome, since it can be both bulky and noisy.

Since condoms require the cooperation of both partners, the provider should emphasize the need for active participation and communication. The provider can be helpful in allowing the adolescent patient to practice communicating in potentially awkward scenarios.

2. Oral Contraceptives

Oral contraceptive pills (OCPs) are the most widely prescribed method of reversible contraception. Forty-four percent of adolescents employing contraception use the pill (2). OCPs are quite effective; however, daily administration may be difficult for some adolescents. In particular, progestin-only pills require administration at the same time each day, making them very impractical for many teens. OCPs have additional benefits for teens with menorrhagia, dysmenorrhea, and dysfunctional uterine bleeding. With use of OCPs, women experience decreased menstrual and anovulatory bleeding. Most OCPs also offer improvement in acne.

Providers should stress the importance of the consistent use of OCPs. Providers can offer simple suggestions such as cell phone alarms to discreetly remind the patient to take her pill daily. For the adolescent wishing to use a daily method, back-up methods such as condoms and emergency contraception should be reviewed in case of missed pills.

3. Hormonal Transdermal Patch

Hormonal methods that do not require daily administration can be appealing to many adolescents. The teen needs to remember to change the patch once a week; cell phone alarms may be useful here, as well as with the OCPs. The patch may be visible to family members and partners;

so young women can be instructed to place the patch in areas that are less commonly visible.

4. Vaginal Contraceptive Ring

The vaginal ring is a hormonal contraceptive that requires attention only twice a month. It offers privacy and simplicity. The ring is inserted in the vagina and removed after 21 days, followed by a 7-day ring-free interval before inserting a new one. The adolescent patient should be assessed for her comfort level in touching her genitalia before prescribing the ring. In some situations, her hesitation may be allayed by practicing ring placement and removal in the office.

5. Injectable Hormonal Contraception

Depot medroxyprogesterone acetate (DMPA) is a long-acting progesterone, which is administered intramuscularly by a health care provider at 11–13-week intervals. It is highly effective, with a perfect use failure rate of 0.3% after 1 year and typical use failure of 3% (2,7). DMPA is a viable contraceptive method for adolescents, since it is private and does not require daily or weekly administration. However, regular office visits are required. Teens should be assessed for feasibility of follow-up in the context of missing school and potential disclosure through insurance explanation of benefits sent to the parent.

The most common side effect of DMPA is menstrual irregularity leading to complete amenorrhea in 50% of users after the first year. Teens may find this a problem, especially if their mothers or other family members monitor their menstrual cycle. Patients considering this method must be adequately counseled about unpredictable uterine bleeding. Upon discontinuation of this method, there may be a 9–18-month delay before menstrual regularity resumes, which teens also may find problematic. Other possible effects include weight gain, headaches, and acne, which may be troubling issues for teens and should be discussed with the patient during counseling.

Concern has been raised regarding the effect of DMPA on bone mineral density (BMD), particularly among adolescents who have not yet achieved peak bone density. Several studies have found that DMPA use is associated with a decrease in BMD (8). In 2004, the FDA issued a warning discouraging the use of DMPA beyond 2 years unless other long-term contraceptive alternatives were not feasible (9). However, BMD is quickly restored in women aged 14–18 upon discontinuation of DMPA, and both the World Health Organization and the Society of Adolescent Medicine have released statements discouraging the restriction on the use of DMPA, stating that the benefits in teens outweighed the long-term risk of fracture (8,9).

6. Intrauterine Contraception

Intrauterine devices are the most widely used reversible contraceptive method in the world. Their use in the U.S. has been limited by fears and concerns about infertility, particularly in nulliparous women. The two intrauterine devices available in the U.S. are the Copper T 380A

(Paragard™) and the Levonorgestrel-IUS (Mirena™). This highly efficacious method is advantageous for teens who desire long-term reversible protection. The Copper T 380A is approved for use for 10 years, while the LNG-IUS may be used for 5 years. Adolescents who have difficulty adhering to daily or weekly regimens, or who need to keep their contraceptive method secret, may find intrauterine contraception an attractive choice.

Clinician fears about an association between intrauterine contraception and the risk of pelvic inflammatory disease (PID) and subsequent infertility have led to decreased use of IUDs in adolescents. These concerns were based upon flawed studies conducted in the 1970s where nulliparity was confounded by high-risk sexual behavior and STIs (10). The WHO recommends that intrauterine contraception should not be inserted in individuals with active PID, current purulent cervicitis, or gonorrhea or chlamydia infections (10). Still, the overall risks of PID and infertility with intrauterine contraception are low, making it a good option for adolescents.

7. Emergency Contraception

Since sex is often unplanned and spontaneous, adolescents should be informed about emergency contraception (EC). Plan B is a 2-pill progestin regimen that can be used up to 120 hours after an unprotected sexual encounter. A copper IUD also can be inserted up to 120 hours after unprotected sex for women who wish to continue using the method.

Plan B was recently made available to adult women without a prescription; however, women below the age of 18 require prescriptions. Because EC efficacy decreases with treatment delay, it is important for providers to review its correct use with the adolescent patient and prescribe prescriptions at every visit. The Plan B regimen, usually given at a 12-hour interval, is equally effective when both pills are administered simultaneously. Thus, through advanced counseling and prescription, there is a decreased likelihood for treatment failure.

Adolescents should be reassured that there is no teratogenicity associated with Plan B and that it will not affect an established pregnancy. It is important to review the mechanism of EC with each teen patient to avoid confusion with mifepristone (RU-486), an abortifacient. Plan B is generally well-tolerated; common side effects include nausea, vomiting, and dizziness.

8. Abstinence

Abstinence includes the delay of sexual initiation, as well as avoiding future sex after sexual experience has commenced, until marriage or adulthood. As previously mentioned, abstinence counseling must be provided with comprehensive sexual risk reduction strategies.

References

1. Teen birth rate rises for the first time in 15 years. News Release, National Center for Health Statistics December 5 2007; www.cdc.gov/nchs/pressroom/07newsreleases/teenbirth.htm.

2. Committee on Adolescence Policy Statement. Contraception and Adolescents. Pediatrics. 2007;120:1135–48.

3. Youth Risk Behavior Surveillance-United States 2005. Morbidity and Mortality Weekly Report. 2006;55;1–108.

4. **Abma J, Martinez G, Mosher W, et al.** Teenagers in the United States: Sexual activity, contraceptive use, and childbearing, 2002. Vital Health Statistics. 2004;23:1–48.

5. **As-Sanie S, Gantt A, Rosenthal M.** Pregnancy prevention in adolescents. Am Fam Phys. 2004;70:1517–24.

6. **Santelli J, Ott M.** Abstinence-only education policies and programs: A position paper of the Society of Adolescent Medicine. J Adol Health. 2006;38: 83–7.

7. **Hatcher R, Trussel J, Stewart F, et al.** Contraceptive Technology. 18th Ed, New York: Ardent Media; 2004.

8. Department of Reproductive Health and research. WHO statement on hormonal contraception and bone health. Contraception. 2006;73:443–4.

9. Society for Adolescent Medicine. Depot medroxyprogesterone acetate and bone mineral density in adolescents—The Black Box warning: a position paper of the Society of Adolescent Medicine. J Adolesc Health. 2006;39:296–301.

10. WHO medical eligibility criteria for contraceptive use, 3rd Ed., Geneva, World Health Organization, 2004, www.who.int/reproductive-health/publications/mec/mec.pdf

C. Screening Adolescents for Sexually Transmitted Infections

Mollie L. Kane

KEY POINTS

- Adolescents are at disproportionately high risk for sexually transmitted infections (STIs,) with about 9 millions new STIs diagnosed each year in 15–24 year olds.
- Often, those adolescents who are most in need of STI screening are least likely to seek care.
- Clinicians can help adolescents overcome some barriers to care by offering STI screening at a variety of types of visits, such as sports physicals and acute care visits.
- Some adolescents may be more likely to seek care for STIs if they understand confidentiality laws.
- Screening recommendations vary for each type of STI.

Background

STIs disproportionately affect adolescent patients, compared to adults, in the U.S. Of the estimated 19 million new STIs that occur in the U.S. each year, almost half occur in 15–24 year olds (1). Half of all new HIV infections also occur in this age group. In fact, by age 25 one half of sexually active Americans will have acquired a STI. The actual number of STIs in American teenagers may be even higher, since teens are one of the groups least likely to seek STI diagnosis and treatment (2).

Both behavioral and biological factors cause increased risk for STIs among adolescents. Because adolescence is a time of risk-taking, the initiation of sexual activity often begins during this period. Risk-taking with drugs and alcohol also increases the chance of high-risk sexual behaviors. Biological factors relate to the maturation of the female genital tract. The single layer columnar cells of the exocervix found during adolescence may be more susceptible to infection than the multilayer squamous cells that replace them as puberty progresses. Once an adolescent has an STI, it can cause inflammation of the cervix, which then increases susceptibility to additional infections.

STIs are preventable, treatable, and often curable. However, without early diagnosis and treatment, many STIs may have long-term medical consequences. It has been estimated that the lifetime medical costs of STIs acquired by Americans between the ages of 15 and 24 in the year 2000 alone totaled at least $6.5 billion (3). Improved prevention and screening could decrease physical and emotional suffering as well as economic costs.

Screening

Each clinician's approach to screening for STIs will have an important impact on his/her patient population, as well as on the public's health. The clinician must feel comfortable speaking with his/her adolescent patients about sexual activity and STIs. S/he must be able to make the patient feel at ease during the clinical visit in order to optimize chances that the patient will seek ongoing care.

Adolescents may experience many barriers to seeking care regarding sexual health. These include lack of medical insurance or ability to pay, inability to seek help from parents or trusted adults in getting care, fear that parents will be billed for care, embarrassment or lack of self-confidence, lack of knowledge about the medical system, transportation problems, and fear of broken confidentiality.

Clinicians can help to overcome some of these barriers with regular counseling and education at every opportunity. Each teen should be assessed for risk and, when possible, offered appropriate screening and immunizations, at least annually and more often if indicated by history. Many patients who would not seek STI-related care can be assessed and screened during sports physicals, well child visits, sick visits, or visits for emergency contraception. All adolescent patients should be educated about the symptoms of STIs, the asymptomatic nature of many infections, and the short- and long-term consequences of infection that can be prevented with screening and treatment. When appropriate, sexual partners should be identified, and the clinician should do everything possible to ensure that partners also receive care, although confidentiality must still be respected.

In the U.S., all states allow for confidential care of adolescents regarding STI and HIV diagnosis and treatment. While the details of the laws may vary from state to state, at minimum, adolescents may consent to their own STI-related care, and providers are permitted to provide that confidential care within the parameters of the laws of their state. Many medical professional organizations, including the American Medical Association, The American College of Obstetrics and Gynecology, the American Academy of Pediatrics, and the American Association of Family Physicians support the right of teenagers to receive confidential care for the diagnosis and treatment of STIs, while encouraging parental involvement whenever possible (4-7).

Most adolescents and many clinicians are not aware of confidentiality laws. However, adolescents are much more likely to seek the care that they need when they know that confidentiality is an option. The clinician should have effective office policies in place to educate patients about their rights, to make patients feel at ease, and to maintain confidentiality if needed. This must extend to how the patient will receive results after the appointment and how the patient will get billed.

Clinicians and their patients also must be aware that state laws may stipulate a variety of circumstances where confidentiality cannot be maintained. At minimum, these include instances where a reportable disease is diagnosed, or where the life or health of the patient or another individual may be at risk.

Table 13-4   Recommendations for STI Screening in Adolescents

Chlamydia	Routine screening for asymptomatic women aged 24 years and younger
	Insufficient evidence to recommend for or against screening in asymptomatic males
Gonorrhea	Routine screening for high risk females of all ages
	Insufficient evidence to recommend for or against screening in asymptomatic males
Genital Herpes	Routine screening in asymptomatic males and females is not recommended.
Human Papillomavirus	Routine screening in asymptomatic males and females is not recommended; however, cervical cytology should be performed as recommended to prevent complications of HPV disease.
Syphilis	Routine screening for high risk males and females
HIV	Universal screening for all males and females aged 13–64

Screening for Chlamydia Infections in Adolescents

Chlamydia is the most common bacterial STI in women in the U.S. and is more common in adolescents than in older women. Young age is the most significant risk factor for Chlamydia in the U.S. Seventy to ninety percent of women with Chlamydia are asymptomatic. However, Chlamydia can cause significant complications in women, including pelvic inflammatory disease (PID), ectopic pregnancy, infertility, and chronic pelvic pain. Men with non-gonococcal urethritis and acute epididymitis from Chlamydia infections may develop complications like infertility or chronic prostatitis. Asymptomatic women of age 24 and younger who have been sexually active should be screened at least annually to reduce the risk of PID and other complications of infection. Repeat screening should be considered at shorter intervals if new exposures may have occurred or if the patient becomes symptomatic. There is insufficient evidence to recommend for or against routine screening of adolescent males for Chlamydia, because most morbidity occurs in women. However, testing and treating adolescent males will decrease infections in females (8). Sexual partners who may have been exposed should be tested and treated or treated presumptively. Rates of re-infection with Chlamydia following treatment are high. Therefore, repeat testing about 12 weeks after treatment is generally recommended (9).

Endocervical swabs in females and urethral swabs in males have been the traditional modalities for Chlamydia screening. These samples can be cultured with very high sensitivity and 100% specificity. In sexual assault examinations, cultures are preferable. Endocervical and urethral swabs also can be tested via direct fluorescent antibody or enzyme immunoassay studies. Sensitivity is >70%, with specificities of 97–99% (10).

Urine samples may now be used for screening in place of swabs. Urine collection is generally preferred by adolescent patients. While sensitivity and specificity are slightly reduced, a much larger population of adolescents will consent to screening, thereby increasing the rate of diagnosis. Urine samples can be tested by ligase chain reaction, polymerase chain reaction, strand-displacement amplification, or transcription-mediated amplification.

Screening tests should be used for asymptomatic patients but are not a substitute for full pelvic examinations in cases of suspected infection. In these cases, a more complete exam is needed to look for evidence of other STIs and to rule out PID or other complications.

Screening for Gonorrhea Infection in Adolescents

The prevalence of gonorrhea in adolescents has increased in recent years. Women with asymptomatic gonorrhea infection are at risk for PID, ectopic pregnancy, and chronic pelvic pain. Annual screening for gonorrhea is recommended for asymptomatic high-risk females of all ages. In general, sexually active adolescents can be considered high-risk and should be screened. However, prevalence rates vary widely based on geographic location. Clinicians may wish to take into account prevalence rates in their communities when deciding whether to offer screening to all adolescent females. When universal screening is not done, screening should be targeted toward those adolescent patients with risk factors, including a history of STIs, new or multiple sexual partners, inconsistent condom use, sex work, and drug use. Adolescent patients presenting to STI clinics or juvenile detention facilities are generally also at higher risk. There is insufficient evidence to recommend for or against routine screening of adolescent males without symptoms, because most males with gonorrhea do have symptoms (11). Gonorrhea is a nationally reportable infection, and all positive tests must be reported to local health departments or other sites designated by each state.

The ideal interval between screening tests for gonorrhea has not been determined and must be decided on an individual basis. After treatment for gonorrhea, a repeat test in about 12 weeks is recommended to rule out re-infection.

Culture of endocervical swabs in females and urethral swabs in men provides 100% specificity and 62–93% sensitivity when suitable transport conditions can be arranged. Nucleic acid amplification tests may be used on urine specimens, endocervical or urethral swabs, or blind vaginal swabs. Nucleic acid probes have sensitivity ranging from 54% to 100%, with almost 100% specificity. Nucleic acid amplification testing of urine samples allows screening without pelvic examination, potentially allowing for more widespread screening of high-risk patients. It does not require special transport conditions, swabs can be stored up to 7 days without refrigeration, and a single specimen can be used for both gonorrhea and Chlamydia screening. However, sensitivity is lower (11).

Screening for Genital Herpes Infection in Adolescents

Routine screening for genital herpes infections in asymptomatic adolescents is not recommended. While risks of screening are low, there is no evidence that diagnosing asymptomatic individuals can improve outcomes. Genital herpes infections may be diagnosed by history and physical exam when symptoms are classical, but "atypical" presentations are more common. In cases where there is uncertainty, direct tests for virus by culture or PCR or type-specific serological testing may be helpful.

Screening for Human Papillomavirus Infection in Adolescents

Currently, screening directly for human papillomavirus (HPV) is not recommended. HPV is extremely common in adolescent women, and many cases regress on their own. However, screening cervical cytology should be performed in adolescent females according to current guidelines to rule out precancerous or cancerous lesions of the cervix caused by HPV infection. HPV typing may be performed as needed for individuals with abnormalities found on Pap smear. Widespread use of the HPV vaccine will be the most effective method to prevent HPV infection and its complications.

Screening for Syphilis Infection in Adolescents

Screening for syphilis should be based on risk factors regardless of the patient's age or gender. There are no adolescent-specific screening recommendations. Populations at increased risk for syphilis infection include men who have sex with men and engage in high-risk sexual behavior, commercial sex workers, persons who exchange sex for drugs, and persons in adult correctional facilities. Patients who have had an STI may be engaging in higher risk behaviors. Whether to screen them for syphilis must be decided on a case by case basis. Ideal intervals for re-screening have not been determined.

Initial screening is done using non-treponemal tests, either the Venereal Disease Research Laboratory (VDRL) or the Rapid Plasmin Reagin (RPR). Confirmatory testing is required with a fluorescent treponemal antibody absorbed (FTA-ABS) or *T. pallidum* particle agglutination (TP-PA). Sensitivity of the non-treponemal tests is >78%, with specificity of at least 85%. The FTS-ABS has a sensitivity of at least 84% and specificity of 96% (12).

Screening for Human Immunodeficiency Virus in Adolescents

The Centers for Disease Control and Prevention (CDC) recommends that all individuals between the ages of 13 and 64 be screened for HIV regardless of risk factors (13). Ideal intervals for re-screening have not been determined and must be assessed on an individual basis. HIV testing is generally done via the repeatedly reactive enzyme immunoassay, followed by confirmatory Western blot or immunofluorescent assay. These tests together have a sensitivity and specificity of >99%. Rapid HIV testing is also available with sensitivity and specificity of 96–100%. The test can be performed at the point of care with results available in 10–30 minutes (14). Rapid testing is an especially attractive option for many adolescent patients who worry about confidentiality issues when receiving results. Adolescents also may be more likely to choose to get tested if they know their results will be available right away.

References

1. **Weinstock H, Berman S, Cates W. Jr.** Sexually Transmitted diseases in American youth: incidence and prevalence estimates, 2000. Perspectives on Sexual and Reproductive Health. 2004;36:6–10.
2. **Cates JR, Herndon NL, Schulz SL, et al.** Our Voices, Our Lives, Our Futures: Youth and Sexually Transmitted Diseases. 2004; Chapel Hill, NC: School of Journalism and Mass Communication, University of North Carolina at Chapel Hill.
3. **Chesson JW, Blandford JM, Fift TL, et al.** The estimated direct medical cost of sexually transmitted diseases among American Youth, 2000. Perspectives on Sexual and Reproductive Health. 2004;36:11–9.

4. **Kane ML, Rosen DS.** Sexually transmitted infections in adolescents: practical issues in the office setting. Adolesc Med Clinics. 2004;15:409–21.

5. **Workowski KA, Berman SM.** Sexually transmitted diseases treatment guidelines, 2006. MMWR Recomm Rep. 2006;55:1.

6. ACOG Committee Opinion #301: Sexually transmitted diseases in adolescents. Obstet Gynecol. 2004;104:891.

7. American Academy of Pediatrics. Recommendations for preventative pediatric health care. Pediatrics. 2000;105:645.

8. United States Preventive Services Task Force. Screening for Sexually Transmitted Infection, at http://www.ahrq.gov/clinic/uspstf/usps.htm, accessed January 20, 2008.

9. **Fortenberry JD, Brizendine EJ, Katz BP, et al.** Subsequent sexually transmitted infections among adolescent women with genital infection due to *Chlamydia trachomatis, Neisseria gonorrhoeae*, or *Trichomonis vaginalis*. Sex Transm Dis. 1999;26:26.

10. **Rager KM, Biro FM.** Techniques of testing for sexually transmitted diseases. Curr Women's Health Rep. 2001;1:111–5.

11. U.S. Preventive Services Task Force. Screening for Gonorrhea: Recommendation Statement. AHRQ Publication No. 05-0579-A, May 2005. Agency for Healthcare Research and Quality, Rockville, MD. http://www.ahrq.gov/clinic/uspst05/gonorrhea/gonrs.htm, accessed January, 2008.

12. U.S. Preventive Services Task Force. Screening for Syphilis Infection: Recommendation Statement. July 2004. Agency for Healthcare Research and Quality, Rockville, MD. http://www.ahrq.gov/clinic/3rduspstf/syphilis/syphilrs.htm, accessed January, 2008

13. **Branson BM, Handsfield JJ, Lampre MA, et al.** Revised recommendations for HIV testing of adults, adolescents, and pregnant women in health-care settings. MMWR Recomm Rep. 2006;55:1.

14. U.S. Preventive Services Task Force. Screening for HIV: Recommendation Statement. Issued July 2005, amended April 2, 2007. AHRQ Publication No. 07-0597-EF-2. Agency for Healthcare Research and Quality, Rockville, MD. http://www.ahrq.gov/clinic/uspstf05/hiv/hivrs.htm, accessed January, 2008.

14

Reproductive Age Women

A. Pap Smear Screening

Heather L. Paladine and Julie Howard

KEY POINTS

- Women should begin having Pap tests within 3 years of becoming sexually active, or at age 21, whichever comes first.
- Sexually active teens and women in their twenties require yearly screening.
- Women over the age of 30 years with previous normal Pap smears can be screened every 3 years unless they are high risk.
- Women who have had a hysterectomy for benign causes do not need Pap tests.
- Women over 65 years of age, with previous normal Pap smears do not need Pap tests.
- Human papillomavirus (HPV) testing is a useful adjunct to cervical cytology.

Epidemiology

Cervical cancer is currently the third most common cancer in women in the world (1) and was formerly one of the most common types of cancer among women in the U.S. It's incidence has declined dramatically in the U.S. since the Pap test was introduced in 1955. In 2003, 11 800 women were diagnosed with cervical cancer in the U.S., and 3919 women died from cervical cancer, making it the 13th most common type of cancer in women and the 13th most common cause of cancer deaths in women. Annual expenditures to treat cervical cancer in the U.S. are approximately $2 billion (2).

Infection with high-risk subtypes of the HPV is the major risk factor for development of cervical cancer (3). It is estimated that 99.7% of cervical cancers contain HPV DNA (3). Fortunately, cervical cancer develops very slowly from precancerous lesions that can be detected and then treated.

Screening Recommendations

Women should begin having Pap tests within 3 years of the onset of sexual activity, or at age 21, whichever comes first (3). The frequency for primary cervical cancer screening has changed in the past few years. Women over the age of 30 years who are considered low-risk for cervical cancer and who have a history of normal screening require testing only every 3 years. "Low-risk" specifically means three consecutive normal Pap tests and the absence of an immunocompromised state (like HIV), DES exposure, or high risk sexual behavior. Women over 30 years of age also may opt testing for high-risk HPV (Subtypes 16, 18, 45 and 56) along with a Pap test as their primary screening. For sexually active teens and women in their twenties, annual screening is still the practice standard. For women of all ages with abnormal primary screening, the frequency of re-screening is dependent on their colposcopic findings and/or treatment.

Pap test screening can be stopped in women who have had a total hysterectomy for benign causes (3). Strong evidence supports the lack of benefit in this population, based on cost and the fact that vaginal dysplasia is much less common than cervical dysplasia. Women >65 years with previous normal screening tests can stop having Pap tests. Women with normal cervical cytology at 65 years are very unlikely to develop new abnormalities that will become clinically significant. However, if women over 65 begin sexual contact with a new partner, the clinician may consider restarting periodic pap tests due to potential for new infection with HPV.

Table 14-1   Recommendations for Frequency of Pap Tests

	USPSTF (3)	ACOG (10)	ACS (11)
Age to begin Pap tests	Within 3 y after beginning sexual activity or age 21, whichever comes first (A recommendation)	3 y after beginning sexual activity or age 21, whichever comes first (A recommendation)	3 y after beginning sexual activity or age 21, whichever comes first (strong evidence)
Age to stop Pap tests	Age 65, as long as the patient has had previous normal Pap tests (D recommendation)	Individualize (C recommendation)	Age 70, as long as the patient has had 3 previous normal Pap tests and no abnormal Paps within 10 y (strong evidence)
Frequency of Pap tests	At least every 3 y (A recommendation)	Yearly for women under age 30, every 2–3 y for women over 30 with previous normal Pap tests (A recommendation)	Yearly with conventional Pap tests or every 2 y with liquid-based Paps, can be every 2–3 y in women over 30 (strong evidence)
Pap tests after hysterectomy	Not recommended for benign disease (D recommendation)	Not recommended for benign disease (A recommendation)	Not recommended for benign disease (strong evidence)

Types of Pap Tests

Liquid-based Pap testing was introduced in 1996. Although it does reduce the false-negative rate of traditional (slide) Pap testing, it can also increase the false-positive rate. Cost of this test is also significantly higher than traditional Pap tests. There is not yet enough evidence to recommend liquid-based Pap testing as the standard for routine screening (4). It does have the advantage of allowing testing for high-risk HPV, gonorrhea, and Chlamydia infections using the same sample. Table 14-2 shows the comparison of the two methods for sensitivity and specificity at different thresholds of abnormal findings (5).

Performing the actual collection of cells for a Pap test is relatively simple, but there are some recommendations that should be followed. Specifically, menses should be avoided, and the woman should not douche, have sexual intercourse, use tampons, or apply any vaginal medications within 48 hours prior to testing. These factors do not necessarily preclude testing, but, if followed, they reduce false-negative results by minimizing obscuring material and inflammation. The use of lubrication for speculum insertion does not affect screening. In all cases, the cervix should be wiped with a cotton swab before collection of the sample (3).

The goal of Pap testing is to obtain a representative sample of cells from the cervix. When using conventional slide methods, an extended tip spatula swept across the ectocervix and a cytobrush tip placed inside the cervical os and rotated 360° provide the best sample with the highest yield of endocervical cells. Applying the fixative immediately and correctly, whether in spray or liquid form, is an important part of the procedure. If the fixative is not applied quickly enough, some of the cells may be obscured by drying artifacts making the slide more difficult to evaluate. The practitioner should familiarize her/himself with the proper application of slide fixative and have all supplies ready prior to performing the Pap smear (3).

Table 14-2   Conventional versus Liquid Pap Tests

	Sensitivity (%) (95% confidence interval)	Specficity (%) (95% confidence interval)
Conventional Pap tests		
HSIL or higher	55.2 (45.5–64.7)	96.7 (95.6–97.5)
LSIL or higher	75.6 (66.5–83.0)	81.2 (71.9–88.0)
ASCUS or higher	88.2 (80.2–93.2)	71.3 (58.3–81.6)
Liquid Pap tests		
HSIL or higher	57.1 (46.3–67.2)	97.0 (93.8–98.6)
LSIL or higher	79.1 (70.1–86.0)	78.8 (69.8–85.7)
ASCUS or higher	90.4 (82.5–95.0)	64.6 (50.1–76.8)

From Arbyn M, Bergeron C, Klinkhamer P, et al. Liquid compared with conventional cervical cytology: a systematic review and meta-analysis. Obstet Gynecol. 2008;111:167–77; with permission.

Liquid-based Pap tests suspend the cells in a liquid medium. The practitioner can use a plastic extended-tip spatula and an endocervical brush or a cervical broom to collect the sample in the same manner as above for this method, and each must be swirled vigorously in the vial 10 times.

Human papillomavirus Screening

Testing for high-risk strains of HPV is an important adjuvant to cervical cancer screening. It provides invaluable information for those women who have atypical squamous cells of undetermined significance (ASCUS) on Pap test. New evidence shows HPV testing, along with the Pap smear, can lead to earlier detection of high-grade cervical intraepithelial neoplasia (CIN) and cancers and, therefore, may become a standard screening method in high-risk women (6). Although HPV testing alone is not FDA-approved for primary cervical cancer screening, recent studies suggest that for detection of high-grade CIN, it is more sensitive and only slightly less specific than Pap testing alone (6). Women over 30 years of age who use HPV tests in place of Pap may have lower rates of CIN in the future. However, until there is more evidence, HPV testing is best used in combination with Pap test for women over 30 years or as additional testing in women with ASCUS on their initial Pap tests. Future studies, though, may transform cervical cancer screening (7–9).

References

1. U.S. Cancer Statistics Working Group. United States Cancer Statistics: 2004 Incidence and Mortality. Atlanta (GA): Department of Health and Human Services, Centers for Disease Control and Prevention, and National Cancer Institute; 2007.
2. **Brown ML, Lipscomb J, Snyder C.** The burden of illness of cancer: economic cost and quality of life. Annual Review of Public Health. 2001;22:91–113.
3. **Hartman KE, Hall SA, Nanda K, et al.** Screening for cervical cancer: systematic evidence review. Prepared for: U.S. Department of Health and Human Services Agency for Healthcare Research and Quality 2101 East Jefferson Street Rockville, MD 20852. 2002
4. **Davey E, Barratt A, Irwig L, et al.** Effect of study design and quality on unsatisfactory rates, cytology classifications, and accuracy in liquid-based versus conventional cervical cytology; a systematic review. Lancet. 2006;367;122–32.
5. **Arbyn M, Bergeron C, Klinkhamer P, et al.** Liquid compared with conventional cervical cytology: a systematic review and meta-analysis. Obstet Gynecol. 2008;111:167–77.
6. **Bulkmans NW, Berkhof J, Rozendaal L, et al.** Human papillomavirus DNA testing for the detection of cervical intraepithelial neoplasia grade 3 and cancer: a 5-year follow-up of a randomized controlled implementation trial. Lancet. 2007;370:1764–72.
7. **Koliopoulos G, Arbyn M, Martin-Hirsch P, et al.** Diagnostic accuracy of human papillomavirus testing in primary cervical screening; A systematic

review and meta-analysis of non-randomized studies. Gyn Onc. 2007;104:232–46.

8. **Mayrand MH, Duarte-Franco E, Rodriques I, et al.** For the Canadian Cervical Cancer Screening Trial Study Group. Human papillomavirus DNA versus Papanicolau screening tests for cervical cancer. N Engl J Med. 2007;357:1579–88.

9. **Nauder P, Ryd W, Tornberg S, et al.** Human papillomavirus and Papanicolaou tests to screen for cervical cancer. NEJM. 2007;357:1589–97.

10. American College of Obstetricians and Gynecologists (ACOG). Cervical cytology screening. Washington (DC): American College of Obstetricians and Gynecologists (ACOG); 2003 Aug. 11 p. (ACOG practice bulletin; no. 45).

11. **Saslow D, Runowicz CD, Solomon D, et al.** American Cancer Society guideline for the early detection of cervical neoplasia and cancer. CA Cancer J Clin. 2002 Nov–Dec;52:342–62.

B. Pregnancy Options Counseling: Choosing between Parenting, Adoption and Abortion

Marji Gold, Emily Jackson, and Tara B. Stein

KEY POINTS

- Unintended pregnancy is very common. All providers should be prepared to discuss the pregnancy test results with their patients and empower women to make the choice that is best for them.

- Providers should take the time to clarify their own personal values toward unintended pregnancy and identify what factors play into their own feelings.

- Every woman with an unintended pregnancy should be offered accurate information about her options for parenting, adoption, and abortion.

- Counseling should be patient-centered in order to elicit the woman's point of view. Effort should be made to remain non-judgmental and present all information in a neutral way.

- Support should be given to the patient's decision by offering treatment or an appropriate referral.

- All women should be screened for domestic violence.

Nearly half of all women will have at least one unintended pregnancy by the age of 45 (1). Many women will first present to their primary care physician for diagnosis or confirmation of their pregnancy, for information, support, and assistance regarding pregnancy options, or to initiate prenatal or abortion care. Providers should be able to offer options counseling to pregnant women who are unsure or undecided about how they would like to proceed. Options counseling provides the information necessary and support required for a woman to make an informed choice between the three pregnancy options: parenting; continuing the pregnancy and placing the child for adoption; and abortion. Primary care providers, who have the benefit of a preexisting relationship with a patient, are in a unique position to assess and counsel women who face this decision. However, any medical professional who cares for women has the opportunity to normalize the experience of an unplanned pregnancy within a patient's life and offer options counseling. Pediatricians, family physicians, internists, obstetrician/gynecologists, nurse practitioners, and midwives are some of the providers who will encounter patients with an unintended pregnancy, and they should be prepared to accurately and nonjudgmentally assist women and their families in making a decision.

Values Clarification

Before offering options counseling to patients, it is helpful for the clinician to clarify his/her own values and beliefs about the three options facing a pregnant woman. Personal experiences, life stage, family upbringing, religious beliefs, societal and cultural norms, and professional training all can influence one's values. Clinicians need to recognize their own values in order to provide unbiased care to women.

Although this is not a comprehensive exercise, Box 14-1 includes some helpful questions for clinicians to ask themselves to clarify their own values surrounding pregnancy options.

Box 14-1   Values Clarification*

- What similarities or differences exist between the values you presently hold about parenting, adoption, or abortion and those of your family?
- Do you think there is an ideal age for a woman to have her first child? Have your views changed about this since you were 18? Since you were 30? What influenced these changes?
- How comfortable or uncomfortable do you feel about discussing the following topics with your patients: Sexual abuse/assault? Sexually transmitted diseases? Drugs and alcohol? Unplanned pregnancies? Birth control options?
- Would gestational age of the fetus affect how you feel about a patient's decision to have an abortion? Does your feeling change with increasing gestational age?
- Under what circumstances would you feel comfortable with a woman's decision to have an abortion?

---

*Adapted from The Abortion Option: A Values Clarification Guide for Health Care Professionals. National Abortion Federation, 2005; with permission.

Options Counseling

Most counseling sessions consist of the following segments, which are further detailed below: delivering pregnancy test results in a neutral manner; providing accurate information about the three pregnancy options of parenting, terminating a pregnancy, or placing a child for adoption; eliciting from the patient how she feels about each of these options; supporting a woman's decision-making process; and initiating care for the patient in accordance with her wishes. Of course, during an options counseling session, it is the job of the provider to create a comfortable environment and to be aware of his/her own and the patient's, tone and body language. The clinician's goal must be to frame the discussion in a caring and nonjudgmental manner.

Giving Pregnancy Test Results

Given the widespread availability of accurate home pregnancy tests, many women will come to a physician's office already knowing that they are pregnant. In some offices, the patient may receive her pregnancy test results from a nurse or medical assistant before the session with her provider begins. If the clinician has the opportunity before the pregnancy test is performed, it is beneficial to ask the patient how she feels about the possibility of being pregnant. Providers can use this time to bring up all of the pregnancy options, establishing for the patient a safe environment in which she can discuss her opinions. Information gained from this brief conversation can guide the discussion later when the pregnancy test results are available.

When providing pregnancy test results to women, it is important to avoid any statements that may suggest your own values, such as "Congratulations, you are pregnant" or "I am sorry to inform you that your test was positive." Certain words to describe the pregnancy such as "baby" or "child" also should be avoided. Instead, give the patient her results in a neutral manner, for example, "Your pregnancy test is positive," and remain silent to give her a chance to react. Women have many different, and often competing, reactions when they find out that they are pregnant, and they may benefit from several quiet moments devoted to processing this information.

Eliciting the Patient's View

Many women have already considered their options and are quite clear about their choice. They have come to the physician to receive care or to get a referral to a provider who can provide the care they request. Other women may need the physician's help to assess their various options and come to a decision regarding how to proceed (2). Open-ended questions that explore what the pregnancy means to the patient, as well as the patient's current life circumstances and future goals, can assist both the provider and the patient in placing the current unplanned pregnancy into context and helping her decide on her choices (see Box 14-2 for examples).

Box 14-2   Options Counseling Quick Reference

Giving pregnancy test results

1. Your pregnancy test is positive.
2. Were you expecting this result?
3. Under what circumstances would you like to become pregnant?

Eliciting the patient's view

1. What are your thoughts about abortion/adoption/parenting?
2. What makes this a good or bad time for you to be pregnant?
3. Where do you see yourself in one year? Five years? How would continuing or not continuing your pregnancy at this time change or affect those goals?
4. What are the best and worst things that you think might happen if you choose to abort/adopt/parent?

Providing accurate information about the options

1. Having an early (first-trimester) abortion will not affect your ability to get pregnant in the future
2. Many medical providers do early (first-trimester) abortions in their office without general anesthesia. It is a safe, simple procedure that takes about 10 minutes. However, if you would like to be put to sleep for the procedure, this is an option.
3. An abortion does not cause the fetus pain.
4. Is there someone you know who might be interested in adopting your child and with whom you would feel comfortable about this situation? If not, there are services available to help you find an adoptive family.
5. You can choose to meet the adoptive family and/or stay in contact with them in the future.
6. During pregnancy, it is important to avoid exposure to alcohol, drugs or environmental toxins that can cause fetal abnormalities.
7. If you plan to continue your pregnancy, you should increase your folic acid intake to prevent neural tube defects. I can give you a prescription for a prenatal vitamin today.
8. Choosing to parent is a big responsibility and many women choose to attend prenatal or parenting classes to help them prepare for their decision.
9. Check out www.pregnancyoptions.info for more information on all your choices.

Supporting the patient's decision-making process

1. Although it can be helpful to discuss this matter with friends and family members, it is ultimately your right and responsibility to make the best decision for yourself.
2. Do you have someone with whom you can talk about this? What do you think she/he would say?
3. It can be a good parenting decision to decide not to parent.
4. Many women feel conflicting emotions when trying to make a decision like this and the right decision for you isn't necessarily an easy decision.
5. Whatever decision you make will be the right decision for you.

Many patients' concerns are unrelated to the pregnancy itself but instead revolve around social issues such as finances, housing, or partner involvement. In such cases, the provider is unlikely to be able to resolve these problems with the patient, but asking these questions is often very helpful to the woman (3). These questions will demonstrate the provider's interest in the woman as a whole person, and her responses may reveal the influences that are affecting her choices and her life situation.

Provide Accurate Information about the Options

Patients with an unintended pregnancy may present to their providers in order to get accurate information about their pregnancy options. As a medical provider, it is crucial to be knowledgeable about all of the patient's options, including parenting, adoption, and abortion. By asking women what they believe are the short- and long-term consequences of each pregnancy option, the clinician can uncover and address a woman's specific concerns. This section will address some basic facts about these topics.

Abortion

Twenty-four percent of all pregnancies in the U.S. end in abortion. For those with unintended pregnancies, 4 in 10 women will choose abortion (1). Common reasons for choosing abortion include current responsibilities to other children or family members, the cost of raising a child, interference with work or school, and problems with partners. In the first trimester, women can choose between a medication and procedural abortion. Both of these options have virtually no long-term risk of future problems, such as infertility, ectopic pregnancy, spontaneous abortion (miscarriage), or congenital malformation (birth defect), and little or no risk of subsequent preterm or low-birth-weight deliveries. This is true for women who have had one or multiple abortions. Additionally, a fetus does not develop the structures necessary to feel pain until the third trimester of pregnancy (after 24 weeks). Several recent studies have shown that it is unlikely that a fetus can feel pain before the third trimester of pregnancy (4). Some additional facts about abortion are included in Box 14-3.

Adoption

Adoption is the least common choice made by women with an unplanned pregnancy. Family members, such as grandparents, adopt most of the children who are adopted. Non-familial adoptions can either be "confidential," where the birth mother and adoptive family have no communication, or "open" where there is at least some communication between the families. Adoption agencies, attorneys, or private facilitators can coordinate the adoption process. Although there are some general legal guidelines surrounding adoption, adoption laws vary from state to state, and providers should be familiar with laws in their area (see Box 14-4 for further information).

Box 14-3   Abortion Facts*

- 2% of women aged 15–44 have an abortion each year.
- 52% of women who have abortions are younger than 25 y old; 33% are 20–24; 19% are <20.
- Over 60% of abortions occur in women who have had one or more children.
- 88% of all abortions take place within the first 12 wk of pregnancy.
- The risk of death associated with childbirth is about 12 times as high as that associated with abortion.
- In repeated studies since the early 1980s, leading experts have concluded that abortion does not pose a hazard to a woman's mental health.

*From Guttmacher Institute, Facts on induced abortion in the United States, In Brief, New York: Guttmacher Institute, 2008, http:/guttmacher.org/pubs/fb_induced_abortion. html; with permission.

Parenting

Women choosing to continue their pregnancy and parent will need to initiate prenatal care. The clinician also may want to offer referrals to social work or nutritional services, as appropriate.

Facilitating the Decision-Making Process

After ensuring that the patient has accurate and unbiased information about her pregnancy options, the provider has the opportunity to support the patient through her decision-making process. Open-ended questioning and active listening are effective means to allow the patient to express, in her own words, her feelings about the pregnancy, as well as the decision before her. Validating those emotions in a kind and caring manner helps convey to the patient that the provider is receptive to hearing what she has to say. The aim of the discussion is to help the

---

Box 14-4   Adoption Facts*

- In the 2000 U.S. census, adopted children account for approximately 2.5% of all children.
- Compared to women with unintended pregnancy who choose to parent, mothers who choose to place their child for adoption are more likely to finish school; are more likely to be employed; and are less likely to live in poverty.
- Children who are adopted have similar health, educational and social outcomes as those who are raised by their biological parents.
- Individual state laws can be found at: http:/www.infantadopt.org/re-statelaws. php.

*Adapted from NCFA's Adoption Factbook IV, National Council for Adoption; 2007; with permission.

woman to evaluate how her life would be impacted by continuing this pregnancy or by choosing abortion. For women who find it difficult to proceed with this exercise, it is helpful to normalize their feelings by use statements such as, "Many women that I have seen in this situation feel conflicted..." (see Box 14-2). This can help allay anxiety and reassure the patient that she is not alone in this experience.

Many important life decisions are accompanied by some degree of ambivalence. Decisions regarding an unplanned pregnancy are no different and often are affected by a patient's unique circumstances, including her personal religious beliefs, concerns about the morality of abortion, grief over the potential loss of the pregnancy or of a child placed for adoption, and expectations of family members and others. Although the goal of the options counseling session is to encourage the patient' to make a decision regarding how to proceed, the provider should feel comfortable suggesting that the patient take more time to consider her decision if she is unsure about what she would like to do. It is appropriate to offer more supportive counseling, provide the patient with written information, hotlines, or unbiased Web site addresses where she can seek further information, and invite the patient to return at a later date to continue the discussion.

It is useful to ask the patient whom she has told or plans to tell about the pregnancy and to elicit their reactions. The viewpoints of friends and family can exert a strong influence on a patient's decision-making process. If the patient has not already done so, the provider should encourage the identification of those individuals close to her who may or may not be able to offer support and assistance, regardless of her decision. Given the prevalence of violence against women in our society, it is also necessary to assess the patient's safety were she to disclose her pregnancy or her decision to friends and family (see the Special Populations section below for further information).

Support the Patient's Decision

Once the patient has reached her decision, it is the responsibility of the provider to treat or refer her appropriately. This may mean initiating prenatal care with a qualified provider, referring the patient to a social worker or adoption agency to discuss placement of a child, providing the patient with an in-office medication or procedural abortion, or helping the patient to make an appointment with a clinic or other provider offering abortion services. Physicians and other medical practitioners who do not provide abortion services are required to provide accurate information about abortions to patients and refer patients to a legitimate abortion provider if requested. Abortion laws vary from state to state (including waiting periods, parental notification, and gestational age limits), and providers should review the current laws in their own state to ensure timely access to services for their patients.

Whatever her decision, if the provider is not directly involved with the patient's care the provider should follow up with the patient to ensure that there has been a successful referral, if needed, and that the woman has the social support she needs. Those providers who have a preexisting relationship with the patient may continue to be an important source of support. All providers who offer options counseling can make what may be a stressful or confusing time easier by reassuring each woman that whatever decision she has made is the best one for her. It also may be helpful to state that the choice she makes today will be the best one for her, although it may be very different from one she would make at some other time.

Special Populations

While women of all ages may experience violence, studies indicate that women are at greatest risk of intimate partner violence (IPV) during their reproductive years. Women who are in abusive relationships may be less able to make decisions about contraception or protect themselves against pregnancy and sexually transmitted infections. The stress of coping with an unintended pregnancy may raise new emotions or put an already vulnerable woman at even more risk of abuse. Different studies have estimated the prevalence of violence during all pregnancies to be between 4% and 8% (5), with higher rates among women with unintended pregnancies. During an options counseling session, it is important to ask every woman if she feels safe at home right now, and if she can safely disclose her pregnancy and/or decision to parent, terminate, or place a child for adoption to her partner and/or family. It is also necessary to ensure that her final decision is her own and not made under duress from a partner or parent. Many other life circumstances might also affect a woman's choice, including immigration status, homelessness, or age (see Chapter 13B). It is crucial to remember that a woman's particular situation will heavily inform which decision is right for her at that time. If a social stressor is identified during the interview, it is appropriate to refer the patient to social work or other supportive services.

References

1. **Henshaw S.** Unintended pregnancy in the United States. Family Planning Perspectives. 1998;30:24-46.
2. **Singer J.** Options counseling: Techniques for caring for women with unintended pregnancies. Journal of Midwifery and Women's Health. 2004;49:235-42.
3. **Goodman S, Wolfe M, Hawkins M, et al.** Early Abortion Trainer's Workbook, 2nd Edition. UCSF Center for Reproductive Health Research and Policy: San Francisco, CA. 2007.
4. **Lee S, Ralston H, Drey E, et al.** Fetal pain: a systematic multidisciplinary review of the evidence. JAMA. 2005;294:947-54.
5. **Gazmararian J, et al.** Prevalence of violence against pregnant women. JAMA. 1996;275:1915-20.

15

Pregnancy and Postpartum

A. Chronic Medical Illness in Pregnancy
Anne-Marie Lozeau, MD, MS

B. Rashes in Pregnancy
Michael A. Umland, MD
Helen Luce, DO

C. Office Management of Miscarriage
Honor MacNaughton, MD
Linda W. Prine, MD

A. Chronic Medical Illness in Pregnancy

Anne-Marie Lozeau

KEY POINTS

- Women with mild chronic hypertension without superimposed preeclampsia have pregnancy outcomes similar to the general obstetrical population.

- Anti-hypertensive therapy has not been documented to improve maternal or neonatal outcomes in the setting of mild chronic hypertension. Blood pressure medications may be safely withheld if blood pressures remain <150 mm Hg systolic and 100 mm Hg diastolic.

- In the setting of severe chronic hypertension, anti-hypertensive therapy is necessary to reduce the acute risk of renal failure, stroke, and congestive heart failure in the mother.

- Women with severe asthma have the greatest risk for pregnancy complications.

- The goal of asthma treatment is prevention of hypoxic episodes in the mother in order to maintain adequate oxygenation of the fetus.

- Universal screening for thyroid dysfunction in pregnant women is not supported. Screening is appropriate in pregnant women with a history of thyroid disease, in women with hyperemesis gravidarum, or type I diabetes, women with autoimmune disorders, and in women with symptoms of thyroid disease.

- Untreated maternal hyperthyroidism increases the risk for preeclampsia, preterm delivery, heart failure, and low birth-weight. Untreated maternal hypothyroidism increases the risk of preeclampsia and inadequately treated maternal hypothyroidism increases the risk of low birth-weight infants.

- Pregestational diabetes is observed in 1% of all pregnancies. Perinatal outcomes are best when glucose control is achieved prior to conception and in the absence of maternal vascular disease.

- All antiepileptic drugs have been associated with an increased risk of fetal malformations.

Chronic medical conditions may complicate pregnancy. Increased maternal age in the U.S. has resulted in a higher incidence of pregnancy comorbidities due to more pregestational chronic disease. Advances in medical technology also have led to an increase in pregnancy comorbidities, because more women with severe illnesses of childhood are surviving to reproductive age. With proper medical care, women can enjoy a healthy pregnancy the majority of the time. This chapter will focus on the following pre-gestational chronic diseases that can complicate pregnancy: chronic hypertension, asthma, thyroid disease, pre-gestational diabetes, and epilepsy.

Chronic Hypertension and Pregnancy (i.e., hypertension that predates pregnancy)

Epidemiology

Chronic hypertension is present in approximately 1–5% of pregnant women who can be categorized as low- or high-risk based on the severity of their disease. Low-risk women have mild chronic hypertension without any end-organ involvement. Women with mild chronic hypertension have up to a 25% superimposed risk of preeclampsia (1–3). High-risk women (with some type of end-organ involvement) with severe chronic hypertension prior to pregnancy have a superimposed risk of preeclampsia ranging from 50 to 75%, intrauterine growth restriction (IUGR) of 25–40%, and abruption placentae of 10–20% (1). Perinatal mortality is increased 3–4-fold compared to the general obstetric population in these high-risk women. They also are at risk for maternal complications, such as hypertensive encephalopathy, retinopathy, cerebral hemorrhage, acute renal failure, and pulmonary edema (2). These women should receive aggressive anti-hypertensive therapy.

Clinical Features or Presentation

Women of childbearing age with chronic hypertension often have stage I or II hypertension, with systolic blood pressures in the 140–179 mm Hg range and diastolic pressures ranging from 90–109 mm Hg without signs of organ damage, these women are considered low-risk during pregnancy (2,3). Women with a history of perinatal loss, organ damage such as left ventricular dysfunction, retinopathy, microvascular disease, stroke, or with systolic blood pressures 180 mm Hg or greater or diastolic blood pressures 110 mm Hg or greater have severe hypertension and are considered high-risk during pregnancy (2).

Diagnosis and Differential Diagnosis

Hypertension in pregnancy is defined by a systolic blood pressure of at least 140 mm Hg or diastolic blood pressure of at least 90 mm Hg on two or more occasions, at least 4 hours apart (2). The National Heart, Lung and Blood Institute Working Group on high blood pressure in pregnancy identified chronic pregestational hypertension as documented blood pressure elevation prior to pregnancy or before the 20th week of pregnancy (3). Diagnosis of mild or severe hypertension during pregnancy is based on blood pressures at the initial office visit regardless of anti-hypertensive treatment (2).

When performing pre-pregnancy evaluations in women with hypertension, it is important to keep in mind that organ damage can progress during pregnancy; therefore, maternal assessment for renal disease, retinopathy, or ventricular hypertrophy should be noted in the context of pre-pregnancy counseling (3). During pregnancy, women with chronic hypertension should be monitored for IUGR or superimposed preeclampsia (3). Baseline studies include hemoglobin, hematocrit, platelet count, serum creatinine, serum uric acid, 24-hour urine protein, as well as gestational age by ultrasound as early as possible in pregnancy (3). In addition to the baseline studies, ultrasound should also be performed in the setting of mild chronic hypertension at 16–20 weeks of gestation, at 30–32 weeks, and then monthly to monitor fetal growth. In the setting of severe hypertension, ultrasounds should be performed at 16–20 weeks, 28 weeks, and then weekly until delivery (2). Additional monitoring in the setting of severe chronic hypertension includes a fetal non-stress test or biophysical profile at 28 weeks and then weekly until delivery. In mild chronic hypertension, a fetal non-stress test or biophysical profile is indicated only if growth restriction is documented or suspected (2,3). The development of uncontrolled severe hypertension, preeclampsia, or fetal growth restriction at or beyond 34 weeks of gestation is an indication for delivery (2).

There is a lack of good evidence to guide clinicians regarding the threshold blood pressures at which to initiate therapy, the optimal blood pressures to achieve, and which anti-hypertensive medications to use. In general, oral medications commonly used for the treatment of hypertension during pregnancy are methyldopa, labetalol, nifedipine, and thiazide diuretics. Medications that are used for acute treatment of severe hypertension include hydralazine (IV), labetalol (IV), and nifedipine (PO). No adverse maternal or fetal effects are seen with the use of labetalol, methyldopa, or nifedipine. Thiazide diuretics are not associated with increased risk of fetal-neonatal events. However, these medications are associated with decreased plasma volume expansion in the mother and should be discontinued in the setting of fetal growth restriction (2). Atenolol is associated with reduced fetal and placental growth and weight, effects not seen with the use of other beta-blockers (2). Angiotensin-converting enzyme inhibitors and angiotensin receptor blockers should not be used during pregnancy because of the increased risk of oligohydramnios and fetal-neonatal renal failure (2,3).

Asthma in Pregnancy

Epidemiology

Asthma complicates 4–8% of pregnancies (4). Results regarding the effects of asthma on maternal and perinatal outcomes are inconsistent. Nearly every possible pregnancy complication has been reported to be both associated with and not associated with asthma. Methodological inadequacies may have contributed to these confusing results. Overall, women with asthma experience more exacerbations during pregnancy, and suboptimal control of asthma during pregnancy results in an increased risk to the mother and fetus (4). Forced expiratory volume in 1 second (FEV1) <80% of predicted is associated with increased preterm delivery and birth weights <2500 g (4).

Clinical Features or Presentation

Physiologic dyspnea of pregnancy is common with intermittent symptoms of shortness of breath in the setting of mild exertion. Asthma is characterized by persistent symptoms and abnormal spirometry results. It is important to differentiate between physiologic dyspnea of pregnancy and asthma.

Diagnosis and Differential Diagnosis

Diagnosis of asthma relies on symptom history as well as spirometry results. During pregnancy, the uterus elevates the diaphragm about 4 cm, resulting in a decreased functional residual capacity. Pregnancy does not alter the forced vital capacity (FVC), peak expiratory flow rate (PEFR), or FEV1. Therefore, these measurements should be used when evaluating pregnant patients with asthma (4). Women with symptoms less than twice a week and PEFR or FEV1 of at least 80% of predicted are classified as having mild intermittent asthma; if the symptoms are more often than twice a week but not daily then they have mild persistent asthma. Women with moderate persistent asthma have daily symptoms and PEFR or FEV1 60–80% of predicted, and women with severe asthma have continuous symptoms with PEFR or FEV1 <60% of predicted (4).

Prevention and Clinical Care

Asthma has been associated with IUGR; therefore, an ultrasound during the first trimester for accurate dating may be useful (4). In women with asthma, the effect of pregnancy on their asthma is unpredictable. It is recommended to monitor pregnant asthmatic patients with spirometry measurements of PEFR and FEV1. The goal for these measurements is to maintain them at 70% of predicted or greater (4). One advantage of using the PEFR is that a simple peak flow meter can be used for this measurement, permitting patient self-monitoring. The goal of asthma treatment is prevention of hypoxic episodes in the mother in order to maintain adequate oxygenation of the fetus. The medications used are the same as those used in non-pregnant patients. Inhaled beta 2-agonists are recommended for all degrees of asthma during pregnancy (4). Inhaled corticosteroids are recommended for the management of all levels of persistent asthma during pregnancy. Budesonide is labeled pregnancy class B by the Food and Drug Administration; all other corticosteroids are class C (4). Asthma is usually quiescent during labor;

despite this, asthma medications should not be discontinued during labor. It is also important in the setting of postpartum hemorrhage to remember that carboprost, ergonovine, and methylergonovine can cause bronchospasm.

Chronic Thyroid Disease inPregnancy

Epidemiology

The presence of overt thyroid disease in the pregnant population is approximately 1% (5).

Hyperthyroidism occurs in 0.2% of all pregnancies, of which 85% are due to Graves' disease. Thyroid storm affects 1% of pregnant women with hyperthyroidism and is a medical emergency (5,6).

The prevalence of hypothyroidism in pregnant women is approximately 0.3–0.5%. Hypothyroidism is usually caused by a primary thyroid abnormality. Worldwide, iodine deficiency is the most common cause of hypothyroidism. Maternal hypothyroidism caused by iodine deficiency is associated with congenital cretinism. In industrialized nations, Hashimoto's disease (chronic autoimmune thyroiditis) is the most common cause of hypothyroidism (5,6).

Clinical Features and Diagnosis

During pregnancy, thyroid function test results are affected by the serum thyroid binding hormone level. It is recommended that thyroid stimulating hormone (TSH) and free thyroxine (FT4) or free thyroxine index (FTI) testing be performed in pregnant women with suspected thyroid disease. Symptoms associated with hyperthyroidism include nervousness, tremors, insomnia, excessive sweating, heat intolerance, tachycardia, hypertension, or goiter. Diagnosis is based on an elevated FT4 level or FTI with a decreased TSH level. Symptoms associated with hypothyroidism include fatigue, constipation, cold intolerance, muscle cramps, or hair loss. Diagnosis is based on a decreased FT4 level or FTI with an increased TSH level.

Prevention and Clinical Care

Propylthiouracil (PTU) is used at the lowest dose that maintains the FT4 or FTI at the high end of normal to treat hyperthyroidism in pregnant women. PTU is safe to continue during breast-feeding (5,6). When using PTU to treat hyperthyroidism, the FT4 or FTI should be monitored every 2–4 weeks. Beta-blockers also can be used for short-term symptom management if necessary. Methimazole may be associated with congenital anomalies and should not be used during the first trimester (5). Iodine 131 is contraindicated in pregnancy. In hyperthyroidism caused by Graves' disease, antibodies cross the placenta, and there is the possibility of neonatal hypo- or hyperthyroidism (6). Fetal ultrasound should be performed to evaluate for growth restriction, hydrops, goiter, or cardiac failure in the setting of maternal Graves' disease (5). Newborns of mothers with Graves' disease should be screened for thyroid dysfunction (5).

Levothyroxine is used to treat hypothyroidism in pregnancy. The goal of therapy is to maintain the TSH within the normal range. The TSH level should be monitored during each trimester. The levothyroxine dose usually needs to be increased at 4 to 6 weeks gestation (5,6).

Pregestational Diabetes and Pregnancy

Epidemiology

Pregestational diabetes is observed in 1% of all pregnancies. The most common type of pregestational diabetes is type 2 diabetes mellitus (7).

Diabetic ketoacidosis is observed in 5–10% of pregnancies complicated by pregestational diabetes mellitus (most commonly type 1) and is a life-threatening emergency (7).

Clinical Care

In the setting of pregestational diabetes, perinatal outcomes are best when glucose control is achieved prior to conception and in the absence of maternal vascular disease (7). Poor preconception glucose control is linked to an increased rate of congenital malformations and spontaneous abortion. Major congenital anomalies occur in 6–12% of infants born to women with pregestational diabetes (7). The focus of management during pregnancy is on excellent glucose control. The goals are as follows: fasting blood glucose ≤95 mg/dL, preprandial ≤100 mg/dL, 1 hour postprandial ≤140 mg/dL, 2 hours postprandial ≤120 mg/dL, and glycosylated hemoglobin A1c no higher than 6% (7). Frequent self-monitoring to achieve euglycemia is essential. During pregnancy, there is increased insulin resistance and reduced sensitivity to insulin. It is important to keep this in mind when considering treatment of diabetes during pregnancy.

The medication most commonly used for treatment of pregestational diabetes is biosynthetic human insulin. Oral medications are widely used in the treatment of non-pregnant patients with type 2 diabetes, but many of these have not been well studied in pregnancy. The oral agent, glyburide, does not cross the placenta and has been used during pregnancy. Metformin has been used during pregnancy, but its long-term effects are not well studied. In general, when treating type 2 diabetes during pregnancy the use of oral medications should be limited until more safety information is available.

Antiepileptic Medications and Pregnancy

Epidemiology

Seizure disorders are present in over 1 million women of childbearing age in the U.S. and are the most frequent neurologic disorder in pregnancy, affecting 0.4–0.8% of pregnancies (8).

Clinical Care

There is agreement that all women capable of becoming pregnant in the U.S. should consume 0.4 mg/day of folic acid. However, there is no agreement about whether women with epilepsy should take a higher dose of folic acid. The Centers for Disease Control and Prevention (CDC) suggests a dosage of 4 mg/day of folic acid for women on anti-epileptic drugs. Pregnancy can have variable effects on seizure frequency, and the literature evaluating the effects of epilepsy on pregnancy is conflicting (9). Anti-epileptic drugs have been associated with an increased risk of fetal malformations. If possible, therapy with one anti-epileptic drug is recommended in women of childbearing age (8,9). If drug withdrawal is planned, it should be completed at least 6 months prior to conception (8).

In women who remain on anti-epileptic medications during pregnancy, the use of divided doses of medication or the use of sustained release medication results in lower peak drug levels and has been shown to reduce the risk of malformations (8). Women treated with anti-epileptic drugs during pregnancy should be offered testing with alpha-fetoprotein levels at 16 weeks of gestation, and level II ultrasound, including fetal echocardiography, at 16–20 weeks gestation, and, if needed, amniocentesis should be offered (8).

References

1. **Sibai BM.** Caring for women with hypertension in pregnancy. JAMA. 2007;298:1566–8.
2. **Sibai BM.** Chronic hypertension in pregnancy. Obstet Gynecol. 2002; 100:369–77.
3. **Zamorski MA, Green LA.** NHBPEP report on high blood pressure in pregnancy: a summary for family physicians. Am Family Physician. 2001;64:263–70, 273–4.
4. **Dombrowski MP.** Asthma and pregnancy. Obstet Gynecol. 2006; 108:667–81.
5. **Abalovich M, Amino N, Barbour LA, et al.** Management of thyroid dysfunction during pregnancy and postpartum: an endocrine society clinical practice guideline. J Clin Endocrinol Metab. 2007;92:S1–47.
6. **Schroeder BM.** Practice guidelines: ACOG practice bulletin on thyroid disease in pregnancy. Am Family Physician. 2002;65:2158, 2161–2.
7. Pregestational Diabetes Mellitus. ACOG Practice Bulletin No. 60. American College of Obstetricians and Gynecologists. Obstet Gyn ecol. 2005;105:675–85.
8. **Rose VL.** Special medical reports: new guidelines offer recommendations for women with epilepsy. Am Family Physician. 1999;59:1681–3.
9. **Eller DP, Patterson CA, Webb GW.** Maternal and fetal implications of anticonvulsive therapy during pregnancy. Obstetrics and Gynecol Clinics. 1997;24:523–34.

B. Rashes in Pregnancy

Michael A. Umland and Helen Luce

KEY POINTS

- Rashes are common in pregnancy.
- Many normal skin changes occur in pregnancy and are due to multiple hormonal changes.
- Pruritic urticarial papules and plaques of pregnancy (PUPPP) is the most common rash seen uniquely in pregnancy and is not associated with any harmful fetal outcomes.
- Pemphigoid gestationis is associated with prematurity and low-birth-weight babies.
- Impetigo herpetiformis (also called pustular psoriasis of pregnancy) is an autoimmune disease and should be treated early with steroids to prevent maternal or fetal death.
- Intrahepatic cholestasis of pregnancy causes intense itching and is associated with preterm labor, stillbirth, and fetal distress.
- Oral therapy should be avoided if possible to limit potential fetal toxicity.

Epidemiology

Rashes are common in pregnancy and may be harmful to mother and fetus. Rashes can be caused by allergies, medication, viruses, insect bites, and infection. The most common rashes exclusive to pregnancy include: PUPPP, prurigo gestationis, pemphigoid gestationalis, pruritic folliculitis of pregnancy, and impetigo herpetiformis (1). In pregnancy, skin changes are common; some are normal and should not be mistaken for a skin disorder.

Clinical Considerations

Normal skin changes during pregnancy include linea nigra (vertical dark line on the abdomen from the umbilicus downward), darkening of the nipples and genitals, and striae gravidarum (stretch marks). Striae gravidarum are red lines on the abdomen and/or breasts. In the postpartum period, these will turn into flat, white, shiny bands, and are often smooth to the touch (1). Another normal skin variant in pregnancy is melasma, which are blotchy brown hyperpigmented areas on the face and body, particularly on the cheeks, forehead, and areolae. Darkening of preexisting moles also may occur. Other normal skin changes in pregnancy include spider angiomas (which are small dilated blood vessels on the skin, usually above the waist), varicose veins on the legs, worsening acne, and increase in skin tag number and/or size (1).

Most normal skin changes are due to increasing levels of estrogen and melanocyte stimulating hormone, which derive from the placenta (1). Melanocytes are cells found deep within the skin that are responsible for the pigmentation of the skin. Elastin, a mucoprotein in skin, is stretched in pregnancy with rapid growth of the uterus which causes a loss of elasticity leading to the formation of striae gravidarum. None of these normal variants are harmful to the mother or baby. Most of these changes will resolve within a few weeks or months postpartum, but they can recur in future pregnancies.

The most common skin condition of pregnancy is PUPPP, also referred to as polymorphic eruption of pregnancy (PEP) (Figure 15-1/Plate 1) (4).

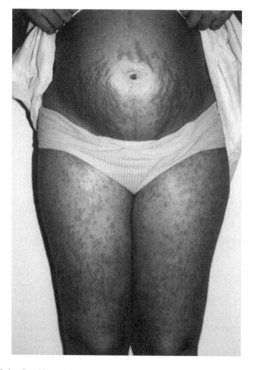

Figure 15-1   Pruritic urticarial papules and plaques of pregnancy (PUPPP). (Reprinted from Medscape General Medicine 1(2), 1999. http://www.medscape. com/viewarticle/408878 ©1999 Medscape; with permission.)

This condition typically resolves spontaneously within a week of parturition (2). There is no mortality associated with PUPPP. It usually occurs in first pregnancies during the third trimester. Women develop an itchy, raised rash, beginning in the striae of the abdomen. These small, red wheals merge into larger wheals and may spread to the trunk, thighs, and extremities (2). They usually do not affect the face, palms, or soles (2). The duration of the eruption is approximately 6 weeks, with associated intense itching usually lasting only 1 week. The cause of PUPPP is unknown and it is not associated with any other pregnancy condition or abnormality of the fetus. PUPPP tends to be more common when the fetus is male (3). There are no diagnostic laboratory studies; the diagnosis is made clinically, and rarely biopsy is needed. Treatment tends to be conservative, with wet soaks, cool baths, and light clothing. Topical corticosteroids help with skin eruptions and pruritis. Systemic corticosteroids and anti-histamines have produced some relief of itching. PUPPP usually does not recur in subsequent pregnancies (2).

Prurigo gestationis (Figure 15-2/Plate 2) (3) is another pregnancy-associated rash. It appears as tiny bumps that look like insect bites (red raised spots), usually on the extensor surface of the extremities (4). The abdomen and buttocks are commonly spared. Lesions are grouped and may be crusted or appear eczematous, closely resembling scabies (4). This can occur anytime in pregnancy and is linked to abnormal hormone levels, especially elevated gonadotropins and low estrogen and cortisol levels. This rash is common in the second half of pregnancy but has been reported in each trimester and is not linked to maternal or fetal morbidity (2). Treatment is conservative with topical corticosteroids and oral anti-histamines in the third trimester (2). Rash is limited and often resolves shortly after childbirth.

Pemphigoid gestationis (Figure 15-3/Plate 3) (4) is rare and not related to the viral infection, Herpes simplex (1). It usually begins in the second

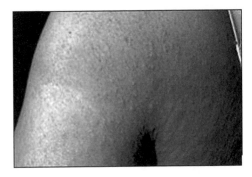

Figure 15-2   Prurigo gestationis. (Image reprinted from eMedicine.com, 2008; with permission.)

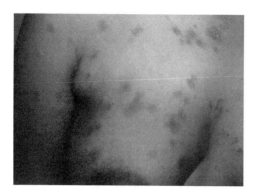

Figure 15-3   Pemphigoid gestationis. (Reprinted from Medscape General Medicine 1(2), 1999. http://www.medscape.com/viewarticle/408878 ©1999 Medscape; with permission.)

or third trimester. The etiology of this rash is unclear, but it is similar in immunologic mechanism to bullous pemphigoid, which is an antibody-mediated, organ-specific, autoimmune disorder (4). Pemphigoid gestationis presents with an eruption of vesicles and bullous lesions that start around the umbilicus and spread to other parts of the body. Lesions may be seen on the palms and soles but rarely on the face or mucous membranes. The skin eruption is similar to hives and may also resemble chicken pox, erythema multiforme, and contact dermatitis (4). The lesions are red, swollen, and fluid-filled. Erosions and crusts are often found because of the pruritic nature of this condition. There is an association with prematurity and low-birthweight, consistent with mild placental insufficiency (2,5). Biopsy can confirm the diagnosis, showing antibodies against the basement membrane. Treatment does not appear to affect the fetal outcome (5,6). The condition can be treated with systemic steroids, which can be used in all trimesters. Antibiotics are recommended to prevent secondary infection. The condition may resolve late in pregnancy, but it usually flares up again at delivery, with oral contraceptive use, and with menses (7). Pemphigoid gestationis usually recurs in subsequent pregnancies, when it tends to be more severe. It also increases the lifetime risk of Graves' disease due to maternal antibodies found in the placenta (7,8).

Pruritic folliculitis of pregnancy, which is very similar to what was previously known as prurigo gestationis, occurs in the second and third trimesters. This rash is often mistaken for acne or microbial folliculitis (9,10). It is characterized by an acneiform eruption consisting of multiple, pruritic, 2–4 mm, follicular papules or pustules, typically on the shoulders, upper back, arms, chest, and abdomen (11). Skin biopsy shows follicular involvement. The diagnosis is made clinically after ruling out other more

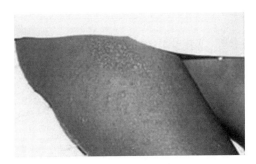

Figure 15-4   Impetigo herpetiformis. (From Tunzi M, Gray G. Common Skin
Conditions During Pregnancy. Am Fam Physician. 2007;75:211–8; with permission.)

common rashes. The etiology is unknown. There is no associated maternal
or fetal morbidity. The rash usually resolves spontaneously 1–2 months
postpartum. In severe cases, topical benzoyl peroxide, oral antihistamines,
and topical hydrocortisone may be used for relief of pruritis (11).

Impetigo herpetiformis or pustular psoriasis of pregnancy (Figure
15-4/Plate 4) (13) can occur during any trimester. The lesions start as small
rings of pustules. The pustules then scab, and the rash dries up, but new
blisters may appear at the edge of the dried rash (1). The lesions are
often found in the groin, axillae, and folds of the knees and elbows (1).
The hands, feet, and face are spared. The rash, unlike the others presented, has no associated pruritis. Chills, fever, vomiting, diarrhea, and
malaise often accompany it (1). This condition remits postpartum but
may flare after delivery and recur with subsequent deliveries, menses, and
oral contraceptive use. It tends to have a more severe and earlier onset
with subsequent pregnancies. The etiology is unclear, but it is likely associated with hormonal changes of pregnancy. Laboratory examination of
patients may reveal elevated sedimentation rate, leukocytosis, hypocal-
cemia, albuminuria, pyuria, and hematuria. Maternal and fetal death
rate is high if the rash is not treated promptly (1). Treatment begins with
adrenocorticotropic hormone and steroids (1).

Intrahepatic cholestasis of pregnancy is a skin reaction on the palms
of the hands and soles of the feet. It usually begins in the second or third
trimester. The skin itself appears normal. Increased serum bile acids cause
pruritis. Mild jaundice can occur. The symptoms arise because the liver
becomes less efficient in removing bile. As the bile backs up, bile acids
increase in the bloodstream and are eventually deposited in the skin which
causes the itching. If a woman scratches, she may develop a secondary
neurodermatitis. The diagnosis is based on clinical findings and laboratory
data. Liver function tests (bilirubin, ALT/AST) can confirm the diagnosis.
This condition is harmful to the fetus and may cause fetal demise, preterm
labor, or fetal distress. It is very important to make an early diagnosis.
Table 15-1 summarizes the various pregnancy-related dermatoses.

Table 15-1 Pregnancy-Specific Dermatologic Disorders

Condition	Rash Presentation	Pregnancy Risk	Treatment
Pruritic urticarial papules and plaques of pregnancy (14)	Intensely pruritic urticarial plaques and papules with or without erythematous patches of papules and vesicles; rash first appears on abdomen, often along striae and occasionally involves extremities; face usually is not affected	No identified adverse effects	Oral antihistamines and topical corticosteroids for pruritus; systemic corticosteroids for extreme symptoms
Prurigo of pregnancy (5)	Erythematous papules and nodules on the extensor surfaces of the extremities	No identified adverse effects	Mid-potency topical corticosteroids and oral anti-histamines
Intrahepatic cholestasis of pregnancy (5,15,16)	Excoriations from scratching; distribution is nonspecific	Risk of premature delivery, meconium-stained amniotic fluid, intrauterine fetal demise	Oral anti-histamines for mild pruritus; ursodeoxycholic acid (ursodiol [Actigall]) for more severe cases
Pemphigoid gestationis (6,17)	Pruritic papules, plaques, and vesicles evolving into generalized vesicles or bullae; initial periumbilical lesions may generalize, although the face, scalp, and mucous membranes usually are not affected	Newborns may have urticarial, vesicular, or bullous lesions; risk of premature deliveries and newborns who are small for gestational age	Oral anti-histamines and topical corticosteroids for mild cases; systemic oral corticosteroids for severe cases
Impetigo herpetiformis (18,19)	Round, arched, or polycyclic patches covered with small painful pustules in a herpetiform pattern; most commonly appears on thighs and groin, but rash may coalesce and spread to trunk and extremities; face, hands, and feet are not affected; mucous membranes may be involved	Reports of increased fetal morbidity	Systemic corticosteroids; antibiotics for secondarily infected lesions
Pruritic folliculitis of pregnancy (5)	Erythematous follicular papules and sterile pustules on the abdomen, arms, chest, and back	No identified adverse effects	Topical corticosteroids, topical benzoyl peroxide (Benzac), or ultraviolet B light therapy

Information from references 5, 6, 14 through 19.
From Tunzi M, Gray G. Common skin conditions during pregnancy. Am Fam Physician. 2007 Jan. 15;75:211–8; with permission.

Any rash developing during pregnancy should be examined by a clinician. The success of dermatologic therapy is based on: the correct diagnosis, the timing of the diagnosis, the type of lesion, the medication, the vehicle (base in which the medicine is delivered), and the method used to apply the medication. Vehicle selection includes powders, oils, and liquids. Powders absorb moisture; oils act as emollients and keep the area moist; liquids evaporate quickly and cool the area. Systemic drugs provide the greatest risk during pregnancy, because of the adverse effects on the fetus and outcome of pregnancy (4). Fortunately, many dermatologic disorders allow alternate treatment methods (topical) during pregnancy (12).

To make the most appropriate treatment decision, a medical provider who treats pregnant and lactating women must be familiar with the potential adverse effects of various pharmacologic agents on the fetus and breast-fed baby (4). Physicians should refer to pharmacologic literature regarding potential risks to the mother and fetus. The following drugs used in dermatology need to be avoided in pregnancy: isotretinoin, methotrexate, trimeprazine, doxepin, hydroxyzine, tetracycline, ciprofloxacin, indomethacin, povidone-iodine, and podophyllin (4). Acetaminophen and topical corticosteroids present a low risk to the fetus.

In conclusion, it is important for health professionals to recognize and treat cutaneous disorders in pregnant and non-pregnant women of child-bearing age. The risks and benefits of medications need to be weighed when prescribing them. Drugs that cross the placenta and have a teratogenic effect on the fetus should be avoided (4).

References

1. http://www2.netdoctor.co.uk/health_advice/facts/skinrashespregnancy.htm
2. **Vaughan Jones SA, Black MM.** Pregnancy dermatoses. J Am Acad Dermatol. 1999;40(2 pt 1):233–41.
3. http://www.emedicine.com/derm/topic351.htm
4. http://www.medscape.com/viewarticle/408878_print
5. **Kroumpouzos G, Cohen LM.** Dermatoses of pregnancy. J Am Acad Dermatol. 2001;45:1–19.
6. **Engineer L, Bhol K, Ahmed AR.** Pemphigoid gestationis: a review. Am J Obstet Gynecol. 2000;183:483–91.
7. **Shornick JK.** Dermatoses of pregnancy. Semin Cutan Med Surg. 1998;17:172.
8. **Jenkins RE, Hern S, Black MM.** Clinical features and management of 87 patients with pemphigoid gestationis. Clin Exp Dermatol. 1999;24:255.
9. **Kroumpouzos G, Cohen LM.** Pruritic folliculitis of pregnancy. J Am Acad Dermatol. 2000;43:132–4.
10. **Fox GN.** Pruritic folliculitis of pregnancy. Am Fam Physician. 1989;39:189–93.
11. http://www.aafp.org/afp/20050401/photo.html
12. **Reed BR.** Pregnancy, drugs, and the dermatologist. Curr Probl Dermatol. 1994;6:33–72.

13. **Tunzi M, Gray G.** Common skin conditions during pregnancy. Am Fam Physician. 2007;75:211–8.

14. **Aronson IK, Bond S, Fiedler VC, et al.** Pruritic urticarial papules and plaques of pregnancy: clinical and immunopathologic observations in 57 patients [Published correction appears in J Am Acad Dermatol 1999; 40:611]. J Am Acad Dermatol. 1998;39:933–9.

15. **Kroumpouzos G, Cohen LM.** Specific dermatoses of pregnancy: an evidenced-based systematic review. Am J Obstet Gynecol. 2003; 188:1083–92.

16. **Riely CA, Bacq Y.** Intrahepatic cholestasis of pregnancy. Clin Liver Dis. 2004;8:167–76.

17. **Shornick JK, Bangert JL, Freeman RG, et al.** Herpes gestationis: clinical and histologic features of twenty-eight cases. J Am Acad Dermatol. 1983;8:214–24.

18. **Stambuk R, Colven R.** Dermatologic disorders. In: Gabbe SG, Niebyl JR, Simpson JL, eds. Obstetrics: Normal and Problem Pregnancies, 4th ed. New York: Churchill Livingstone; 2002. pp. 1283–302.

19. **Lotem M, Katzenelson V, Rotem A, et al.** Impetigo herpetiformis: a variant of pustular psoriasis or a separate entity? J Am Acad Dermatol. 1989;20:338–41.

C. Office Management of Miscarriage

Honor MacNaughton and Linda W. Prine

KEY POINTS

* Early pregnancy loss is common and can be managed in the primary care setting.
* The diagnosis of miscarriage is confirmed by characteristic ultrasound findings or by measurement of serial serum ßhCG levels.
* There are three options for treatment of miscarriage: expectant management, use of medication, or suction aspiration.
* Misoprostol can be used for medical management, with varying success rates depending on whether the miscarriage is incomplete, a missed abortion, or an anembryonic gestation.
* Vacuum aspiration in the outpatient setting is as safe and acceptable as, and more cost-effective than, dilatation and curettage in the operating room.
* No interventions are proven to prevent early pregnancy loss.
* Counseling should address concerns about future fertility and reassurance that the miscarriage was not the woman's fault.

Epidemiology

Miscarriage of pregnancy, or early pregnancy loss, is very common and largely occurs in the first trimester, with a peak incidence around 6 weeks of gestation and a second, smaller peak around 10 weeks. One in four women will have a miscarriage during their lifetimes. It is estimated that 15–20% of diagnosed pregnancies miscarry in the first trimester (1).

Clinical Features or Presentation

There are three common clinical scenarios in which women present with a miscarriage. The first presentation is that of a woman who has had a positive pregnancy test and presents with vaginal bleeding. She may have bleeding alone or bleeding with concomitant cramping, signifying a more likely diagnosis of miscarriage. Alternatively, a woman may be in the office for a routine early prenatal visit at about 10–12 weeks, when the fetal heart tones are not audible by Doppler. In this scenario, a subsequent ultrasound will diagnose a miscarriage. Finally, a miscarriage may present to the primary care physician as a report from a radiologist reading an early obstetric ultrasound or during an in-office dating ultrasound.

Diagnosis and Differential Diagnosis

The diagnosis of early pregnancy loss is made by a combination of historical, physical exam, laboratory, and ultrasound findings. Based on these characteristics, early pregnancy loss can be distinguished from continuing viable pregnancy, subchorionic bleed, ectopic pregnancy, and non-uterine sources of bleeding. Additionally, these findings help to define the subtypes of spontaneous abortion (Table 15-2).

In the scenario in which a woman presents with vaginal bleeding, a careful speculum exam may be diagnostic. The exam should include inspection for sources of non-uterine bleeding, including vulvar, vaginal, and cervical etiologies. An open cervical os with pregnancy tissue in the vaginal vault or coming from the os confirms an incomplete abortion. If the os is closed,

Table 15-2   Definitions of Subclasses of Early Pregnancy Loss

Threatened abortion	Bleeding with a closed cervix and no passage of tissue; pregnancy may or may not be viable
Incomplete abortion	Bleeding with passage of some, but not all, of the gestational tissue
Complete abortion	Bleeding with completed passage of the gestational tissue
Inevitable abortion	Cervix dilated; gestational tissue not yet passed
Missed abortion	Cervix closed; nonviable embryo not yet passed
Anembryonic gestation	Gestational sac without embryonic development; diagnosed by ultrasound; also referred to as "blighted ovum"
Embryonic/fetal demise	Embryonic disc developed or fetus >5 mm, with loss of viability diagnosed by lack of cardiac activity

however, additional testing is needed to distinguish between ongoing pregnancy, miscarriage, and ectopic pregnancy. If a sonogram machine is readily available, an ultrasound exam with the vaginal probe can often make the diagnosis quickly and is most welcome by the worried patient.

An ultrasound revealing an embryo with a crown–rump length of 5 mm or greater, without visible cardiac activity, is consistent with embryonic or fetal demise. Alternatively, the finding of a gestational sac >18 mm without a yolk sac or a fetal pole defines an anembryonic gestation. If the sonogram does not meet either of these criteria, or if the measurements are just on the border of 5 mm or 18 mm, a repeat sonogram 1 week later that shows no interval growth is also diagnostic of a nonviable pregnancy.

In the absence of ultrasound, serial measurement of quantitative ßhCG levels can help to differentiate between a viable and nonviable pregnancy. During the first 10 weeks of gestation, the quantitative ßhCG should rise by at least 66% over a period of 48 hours. A suboptimal rise, plateau, or decrease in ßhCG levels points to a nonviable gestation. In this scenario, if ultrasound has not previously documented an intrauterine gestation, care should be taken to rule out ectopic pregnancy.

Prevention and Counseling

Miscarriage can be a difficult time for a woman. Sometimes, however, if the pregnancy was unintended a miscarriage can be a relief, so it is important not to make assumptions about the woman's attitude toward the pregnancy until exploring her feelings. Most important in counseling is to explicitly address any feelings of guilt and to reassure the woman that she did not do anything to cause the miscarriage. It can be helpful to explain that, while we do not know exactly what causes early pregnancy loss, it is often nature's way of avoiding abnormal gestations. Women with three or more miscarriages should undergo a work up for recurrent pregnancy loss. Women with a history of one or two miscarriages should be educated that they are not at increased risk of future pregnancy problems and that there are no interventions which have been shown to prevent early pregnancy loss. If the physician senses that a woman or her partner are having difficulty accepting the randomness of miscarriage, or there is an undercurrent of self-blame or partner-blame, more discussion or a referral for counseling may be needed.

Clinical Care

Historically, women diagnosed with first trimester miscarriage were referred for dilatation and curettage (D&C) in the operating room. Recent research, however, supporting a variety of outpatient treatments, now allows physicians to offer women a broader range of options. Current management strategies for early pregnancy loss include expectant management, medical management using misoprostol, and outpatient uterine aspiration. These methods all have well established efficacy and safety profiles, and are now favored over the traditional method of dilatation and curettage under general anesthesia, which carries with it increased risk and higher costs. Coupled with clinical considerations, the woman's preference should be primary in guiding the ultimate choice of method.

Expectant Management

Expectant management, or watchful waiting, as the miscarriage process proceeds spontaneously, may be a preferred option for some women. Women who opt for expectant care may do so for a variety of reasons, including the perception that it is a less invasive, more natural, or more private option. Additional benefits include the avoidance of surgical and anesthetic risk and decreased cost.

Contraindications to safely offering expectant care are uncommon, but include suspicion of ectopic pregnancy, excessive bleeding or hemodynamic instability, evidence of uterine infection, and lack of access to emergent uterine aspiration if heavy bleeding or infection should ensue. Similarly, infection, excessive bleeding, and the need for emergent aspiration are rare complications of watchful waiting. It is important to explain to patients that these same risks exist for all management strategies, however, with no overall difference in complication rates among the three methods (2). Physicians should, therefore, feel comfortable in assuring their patients that all options are equally safe.

Potential drawbacks to expectant care include its unpredictable timing, the longer average time to completion, and the lower rate of successfully completed miscarriage, as compared to medical management or immediate aspiration. The success rates for expectant management, as defined by completed abortion without the need for surgical intervention, are shown in Table 15-3 (3). Success rates increase over time and vary significantly depending on the type of spontaneous abortion (*i.e.*, incomplete miscarriage, missed abortion, or anembryonic pregnancy). It is important to note that studies comparing success rates have a fixed time from diagnosis after which the expectant management is considered a "failure." In real clinical settings, however, women can be safely followed indefinitely, allowing for potentially higher success rates (2).

Table 15-3   Types of Miscarriage and Outcomes in Patients who Chose Expectant Management

Category of Early Pregnancy Loss	Completed Miscarriage with Expectant Management		
	by Day 7	by Day 14	by Day 46
Incomplete abortion	53%	84%	91%
Missed abortion	30%	59%	76%
Anembryonic gestation	25%	52%	66%
Total	**40%**	**70%**	**81%**

Adapted from Luise et al. BMJ. 2002;324:873–5. From the BMJ Publishing Group; with permission.

When considering expectant care, women are often anxious about what to expect. Providing detailed anticipatory guidance can help to alleviate this anxiety. Women should be counseled that during the miscarriage process they will have cramping, heavy bleeding, and passage of blood clots. Patients should be offered an advance prescription for NSAIDs and a low dose narcotic in case of severe cramping. Women may or may not notice passage of the gestational sac, appearing as fluffy white tissue the size of a dime at 6 weeks of gestation or a quarter at 9 weeks. Beyond 9 weeks of gestation, patients may rarely note fetal tissue, but they should be told that there is no need to bring any products of conception back to the provider.

It is essential that women know how and when to contact the on-call physician. Women should be instructed to call with signs or symptoms of infection or hemorrhage and, in particular, with fever, heavy bleeding, or pelvic pain not relieved by pain medications. Heavy bleeding should be quantified as bleeding that saturates two or more thick maxi-pads per hour for two consecutive hours, or bleeding associated with hypovolemic symptoms. An example of a downloadable take-home patient instruction sheet is available at: www.reproductiveaccess.org/m_m/menu.htm.

Regardless of management strategy, Rh status should be determined for all patients and all Rh-negative women should be treated with Rhogam. A follow-up visit should be arranged within 1 to 2 weeks to ensure completed miscarriage, address any emotional concerns, and assess the need for future contraception or preconception counseling. A combination of history and either a transvaginal ultrasound or serial quantitative ßhCG levels can assess completion of miscarriage. The traditional criterion used to assess completion with serial ßhCG levels is a decrease of at least 50% within 48 to 72 hours of the passage of tissue (2). Once completed miscarriage has been established, there is no need to follow further ßhCG levels.

If an initial ultrasound documented the presence of a gestational sac, completed miscarriage can be confirmed with a subsequent ultrasound demonstrating absence of the sac. Thickened endometrium or heterogeneous, echogenic material also may be seen on ultrasound following completed spontaneous abortion and is normal rather than an indicator of incomplete miscarriage. If the miscarriage has not completed spontaneously by the initial follow-up visit, choices include continued watchful waiting or switching to medical or surgical management. In the absence of contraindications, expectant observation may be offered for as long as the woman prefers to wait.

Medical Management

Medical management of spontaneous abortion uses misoprostol, a prostaglandin E1 analogue, to stimulate uterine contractions and promote uterine evacuation within a more predictable time-frame. For women facing the process of miscarriage, this increased predictability and the subsequent shorter interval to the miscarriage's resolution may be attractive advantages over expectant management. When compared to aspiration, benefits of medical treatment are similar to those of watchful waiting, including the lack of instrumentation and decreased cost. Contraindications to misoprostol use are the same as those outlined previously for expectant management, with the addition of allergy to prostaglandins. Risks also are the same, and, as with watchful waiting, are rare, occurring at a rate of <1%. (2) As with expectant care, access to emergent uterine aspiration is necessary in cases of heavy bleeding, infection, or failure to expel the gestational sac.

Numerous small studies have looked at varying doses and routes of administration of misoprostol, including oral, buccal, sublingual, and vaginal. (2) Though no one protocol has yet to be codified as standard-of-care, the use of 800 mcg vaginally is common and has been shown to be safe, effective, and acceptable to women. Using this protocol, the woman is dispensed misoprostol for home use and instructed to insert the medication vaginally at a time that is convenient to her. If this dose does not initiate bleeding, a second dose may be administered 24 to 48 hours after the first. The rates of successfully completed miscarriage using this protocol vary between 81% and 93%, depending on presentation, as shown in Table 15-4 (7). Of note, these rates are higher than those with expectant care, especially for missed abortions and anembryonic gestations. Again, studies define treatment "failures" as those in which the miscarriage process does not complete within a fixed number of days or weeks. In real clinical settings, however, the process may be given more time and may thus have a higher success rate (5)

Desired effects of misoprostol are cramping and bleeding, which typically begin within 6 hours of administration and last for several hours. Lighter bleeding or spotting persists for up to 2 weeks and, occasionally, longer. Other transient side effects of misoprostol include flu-like symptoms, such as low-grade fever, chills, and headache, and gastrointestinal symptoms, such as nausea, vomiting, and diarrhea. Women should be counseled that these side effects are short-lived and will resolve within 24 hours. Patient instructions are the same as those with expectant care, but women should additionally be instructed to call if they have no bleeding within the first 24 hours of taking misoprostol as a second dose may be used. For a sample downloadable instruction sheet for patients see:www.reproductiveaccess.org/m_m/MiscarriageUsingMeds.htm.

Table 15-4   Types of Miscarriage and Rates of Successfully Completed Miscarriage in Patients using 800 mg Misoprostol Vaginally

Category of Early Pregnancy Loss	Completed Miscarriage using Misoprostol by Day 8
Incomplete abortion	93%
Embryonic/fetal death	88%
Anembryonic gestation	81%
Total	84%

Adapted from Zhang et al. NEJM. 2005;353:761; with permission.

Follow-up care and assessment for completion of miscarriage are the same as that described for expectant management. The patient should be seen in 1 to 2 weeks to allow adequate time for the miscarriage to take place before assessing completion. If medical management has initially failed, and the patient remains clinically stable, subsequent options include expectant management, a repeat dose of misoprostol, or vacuum aspiration.

Vacuum Aspiration

Surgical management is the most immediate and effective treatment for miscarriage, with success rates of over 98%. While surgical management traditionally entailed D&C under general anesthesia in the operating room, newer outpatient vacuum aspiration techniques have largely replaced D&C due to a number of advantages. The aspiration procedure uses suction to evacuate the uterus, as opposed to sharp curettage, and is associated with less pain, shorter procedure time, and less blood loss (2). Additionally, vacuum aspiration performed in the outpatient setting has been shown to be as acceptable to women as treatment in the operating room and is associated with lower cost (2). From the patient's perspective, perceived benefits of aspiration include its immediacy, predictability, and high efficacy.

Indications for initial management with outpatient vacuum aspiration, as opposed to expectant or medical management, include patient preference, evidence of infection, and excessive blood loss. Immediate aspiration also may be prudent for patients who will not have future access to aspiration should complications arise. Fetal demise beyond 10 or 12 weeks, depending upon physician comfort level, is a contraindication to outpatient office management. Serious complications are rare but include uterine perforation, cervical trauma, infection, and bleeding. Additional anesthetic risk depends on whether a local paracervical block, IV sedation, or general anesthesia is used. Informed consent should include an explanation of the procedure, as well as a discussion of the above alternatives and risks.

When performed in the outpatient setting, using local anesthesia, the procedure takes approximately 10 minutes. For the basic steps of manual vacuum aspiration see Box 15-1. Provided that completion of miscarriage is confirmed by tissue examination, there is no need for repeat ultrasound or ßhCG levels following the aspiration. Women should rest in the office for a while until residual cramping from the procedure resolves, and they then can be safely discharged home, without any restrictions on activity. Patients should be counseled that bleeding following aspiration is typically less than that with expectant or medical management, but that it may be sporadic until the next menses. Though there is little evidence to support the recommendation, common practice is to counsel against the use of anything per vagina for a week following surgical management to decrease the risk of infection. Women should be provided with provider contact information and educated about the

Box 15-1   Technique for Manual Vacuum Aspiration

1. Bimanual exam to determine uterine position and size
2. Insertion of speculum and preparation with antiseptic solution
3. Administration of paracervical block using local anesthetic
4. Application of tenaculum to cervix
5. Dilation of the cervix
6. Insertion of cannula into uterine fundus
7. Application of suction via hand-held syringe
8. Aspiration of the uterine contents
9. Tissue examination of aspirate to identify gestational sac and, if beyond 10 wks, fetal parts

signs of infection and hemorrhage. Though a follow-up appointment is not medically necessary after the procedure, one should be offered to discuss contraceptive management, preconception counseling, and the patient's adjustment to the miscarriage.

References

1. **Wilcox AJ, Weinberg CR, O'Connor JF, et al.** Incidence of early loss of pregnancy. N Engl J Med. 1988;319:189–94.
2. **Joffe C.** Abortion in historical perspective. In Paul M, Lichtenberg SE, Borgatta L, Grimes DA, Stubblefield PG (eds): A clinician's guide to medical and surgical abortion. Philadelphia: Churchill Livingstone; 1999. pp. 3–10.
3. **Sotiriadis A, Makrydimas G, Papatheodorou S, et al.** Expectant, medical, or surgical management of first-trimester miscarriage: a meta-analysis. Obstet Gynecol. 2005;105:1104–13.
4. **Luise C, Jermy K, May C, et al.** Outcome of expectant management of spontaneous first trimester miscarriage: observational study. BMJ. 2002;324:873–5.
5. **Chen BA, Creinin MD.** Contemporary management of early pregnancy failure. Clinical Obstetrics and Gynecology. 2007;50:67–88.
6. **Barnhart K et al.** Decline of serum ßhCG and spontaneous complete abortion: defining the normal curve. Obstet Gynecol. 2004;104:975–81.
7. **Zhang J, Gilles JM, Barnhart K, et al.** A comparison of medical management with misoprostol and surgical management for early pregnancy failure. N Engl J Med. 2005;353:761–9.
8. **Neilson JP, Hickey M, Vazquez J, et al.** Medical treatment for early fetal death (less than 24 weeks) (Cochrane Review) In: The Cochrane Library 2007.
9. **Forna F, Gülmezoglu AM, Forna Fatu.** Surgical procedures to evacuate incomplete abortion (Cochrane Review). In: The Cochrane Library 2007.
10. **Dalton VK, Harris L, Weisman CS, et al.** Patient preferences, satisfaction, and resource use in office evacuation of early pregnancy failure. Obstet Gynecol. 2006;108:103–10.

16

Perimenopausal Women

A. Menstrual Disorders in Perimenopausal Women
Beverly VonDerPool, MD

B. Management of Menopausal Symptoms
Katherine L. Margo, MD

A. Menstrual Disorders in Perimenopausal Women

Beverly VonDerPool

KEY POINTS

◆ Perimenopausal bleeding is a normal variation in a woman's reproductive life.

◆ Menopause is usually reached after 12 months of amenorrhea, reflecting the cessation or almost complete cessation of ovarian estrogen secretion.

◆ In the early menopausal transition stage, the irregularity in the menstrual cycle is due to a declining number of ovarian follicles and declining inhibin B levels.

◆ The distinction between variations of normal bleeding in the perimenopausal stage versus abnormal bleeding is based on the clinical evaluation.

◆ The most common causes of abnormal perimenopausal bleeding are anovulation, fibroids, and bleeding disorders.

◆ Either endometrial biopsy (EMB) or transvaginal ultrasound (TVUS) can be used as the initial endometrial evaluation of the postmenopausal or anovulatory perimenopausal woman.

During the past decade, clinicians and scientists have made substantial progress toward unraveling the mystery of the perimenopausal period. The perimenopause is the period of biologic changes and menstrual irregularities that precede a woman's final menstruation. This chapter will define the stages leading to menopause, the epidemiology, clinical manifestations, and treatment options for menstrual irregularities.

Epidemiology

In the U.S., most women experience menopause between 40 and 58 years of age. The median age of menopause is 51 years (1). Premature ovarian failure is defined as menopause occurring earlier than age 40 (Table 16-1).

Reproductive Stages

The stages of reproductive senescence last from months to years and include the reproductive phase, menopausal transition, perimenopause, final menstrual period, menopause, and postmenopause, as defined by the consensus panel, entitled "The 2001 Stages of Reproduction Aging

Table 16-1   Factors Associated with Age at Menopause

Earlier Menopause	Later Menopause
Lower body weight	Multiparity
Smoking	Prior use of oral contraceptives
Shorter cycle length	Japanese race/ethnicity
Family history of early menopause	Higher body weight
Nulliparity	
Lower socioeconomic status	

From Gold EB, Bromberger J, Crawford S, et al. Factors associated with age at natural menopause in a multiethnic sample of midlife women. Am J Epidemiol. 2001;153:865–74; with permission

Workshop (STRAW)" (Figure 16-1) (2). This staging system is clinically useful, although considerable variation characterizes a woman's movement through the STRAW Staging System (3).

Definitions

The **reproductive** stage is divided into 3 parts: an early (Stage −5), a peak (Stage −4), and a late (Stage −3). In the early reproductive years, the menstrual cycle may be regular or variable. During the peak and late reproductive stages, menstrual cycles are regular and normal. For a menstrual cycle to be normal, the interval between the first day of one menstrual period to the first day of the next menstrual period is no longer

						Final menstrual period		
Stages:	−5	−4	−3	−2	−1	0	+1	+2
Terminology:	Reproductive			Menopausal transition			Postmenopause	
	Early	Peak	Late	Early	Late*		Early*	Late
				Perimenopause				
Duration of stage:	Variable			Variable		(a) 1 y	(b) 4 y	Until demise
Menstrual cycles:	Variable to regular	Regular		Variable cycle length (>7 d different from normal)	≥2 skipped cycles and an interval of amenorrhea (≥60 d)	Amen × 12 months	None	
Endocrine:	Normal FSH		↑ FSH	↑ FSH			↑ FSH	

*Stages most likely to be characterized by vasomotor symptoms
↑:elevated.

Figure 16-1   STRAW Staging System. (Adapted from Soules MR, Sherman S, Parrot E, Rebar. Executive Summary: Stages of Reproductive Aging Workshop (STRAW). Fertility and Sterility, 2001;76:874–878; with permission from Elsevier.)

than 35 days and no shorter than 21 days. The menstrual blood flow does not exceed 80 ml during the cycle (2).

The **menopausal transition** stage has 2 stages: the early (Stage −2) and the late (Stage −1) and extends to the final menstrual period. The menopausal transition stage initiates variability in the menstrual cycle length. In the early stage of the menopausal transition, the menstrual cycle length varies >7 days from the woman's normal cycle. In the late stage of the menopausal transition, a woman typically has skipped at least 2 cycles and has an interval without menstruation for >60 days (2).

The **final menstrual period**, a period identified only in retrospect, is Stage 0 in the STRAW Staging System.

The **perimenopausal** time period includes the menopausal transition stage, the final menstrual period, and the 12 months after the final menstrual period. During the time preceding menopause, neuroendocrine changes (4), vasomotor symptoms, as well as a marked decline in ovarian follicles and estrogen secretion lead to amenorrhea.

Menopause occurs after 12 months of amenorrhea, reflecting the cessation, or almost complete cessation, of ovarian estrogen secretion.

The **postmenopause** stage includes an early (Stage +1) and late (Stage +2) stage. The early postmenopause stage begins at the final menstrual period and ends after 5 years. The late postmenopause stage begins 5 years after the final menstrual period and ends at death.

Physiology

The average woman is born with approximately 2 million primordial follicles in her ovaries, ovulates <500 times in a lifetime, and has follicles that will undergo atresia, resulting ultimately in menopause. The hypothalamic–pituitary–ovarian axis controls the reproductive process by a feedback system (5).

In the late reproductive stage, menstrual cycles remain regular, but the follicular phase shortens. As a woman enters the early menopausal transition stage, the irregularity in the menstrual cycle is due to declining follicles and declining inhibin B, with the subsequent lack of negative feedback causing an increase in FSH (4). With the rise in FSH, a gradual rise in estradiol occurs without a change in LH. During the late menopausal stage, FSH levels inconsistently rise and fall until about 10 months prior to the final menstrual period. Subsequently, a rapid elevation of FSH occurs, reaching a plateau 2 years after the final menstrual period. The estradiol level initially rises, and then follows a reciprocal pattern to FSH, gradually declining for 2 years prior to the final menstrual period with an abrupt drop at menopause (4).

Clinical Presentation

Women can have variable symptoms at each stage of the menopausal transition. These symptoms may continue for years into the postmenopause stage. The symptoms associated with the menopausal transition include uterine bleeding, hot flashes (a sudden sensation of intense heat with sweating and flushing), night sweats, vaginal dryness, and sleep disturbance. The vasomotor symptoms of hot flashes and night sweats are reported most commonly and with high frequency in the perimenopausal stage.

Since menopause is preceded by menstrual variation, the clinician must determine whether a woman is experiencing a normal bleeding variation or abnormal bleeding. In the early menopause transition stage, a woman's menstrual cycle shows a variation of over 7 days from the normal cycle length (21–35 days). Most women have shorter cycles and a shorter follicular stage with increasing age (6). Women with longer cycles tend to have anovulatory cycles (6). In the late menopausal transition, a tendency to skip at least 2 cycles is common (1). However, when bleeding lasts >10 days or occurs between menstrual cycles, the bleeding is abnormal and deserves an evaluation.

Differential Diagnosis of Abnormal Uterine Bleeding

The differential diagnosis of abnormal perimenopausal bleeding is extensive. The most common causes are uterine anovulation (6), fibroids (7), and bleeding disorders (8). One must keep in mind that the risk of endometrial cancer increases in women over 45; postmenopausal bleeding is associated with a 10% prevalence of endometrial cancer (9). Endometrial hyperplasia is also more common in women in this age group and can be a precursor of cancer (9). The women with the highest risk for endometrial cancer are nulliparous, obese, and diabetic, with endogenous or exogenous exposure to estrogen. Exogenous exposure to estrogenic influences includes estrogen replacement therapy and tamoxifen, while endogenous exposure may result from obesity, anovulatory cycles, or estrogen-secreting tumors. Also, when a perimenopausal woman has menorrhagia, she has the same likelihood as an adolescent of having a bleeding disorder (8).

Diagnostic Evaluation

The distinction between variations of normal bleeding in the perimenopausal stage versus abnormal bleeding is based on clinical evaluation. Evaluation begins with a history consistent with the definition of perimenopause. The factors that may indicate a cancer or other problems should be critically assessed.

The history should include information listed in Box 16-1.

The gynecologic exam may facilitate identification of the bleeding site, an infection, trauma, or tumor. A general examination focusing on particular body systems should be performed if indicated by the history.

The initial laboratory studies can be limited to urine (beta-human chorionic gonadotropin B-HCG) to evaluate for pregnancy and a CBC when menorrhagia and anemia are suspected. Because of the fluctuating

---

Box 16-1   Important history in perimenopausal bleeding

- The quality, quantity, and timing of the bleeding (intermenstrual bleeding and menorrhagia are more worrisome for pathology)
- Documentation of the associated symptoms including hot flashes, night sweats, vaginal dryness, and sleep disturbance
- Documentation of specific risk factors associated with endometrial cancer such as unopposed estrogen, late menopause, a history of diabetes, nulliparity, polycystic ovary disease (chronic anovulation), obesity, hereditary nonpolyposis colorectal cancer or tamoxifen therapy
- Obstetrical history (Nulliparous women are at higher risk for endometrial cancer.)
- Past history of medical problems, uterine pathology, or medications that can affect the menstrual cycle
- Family history of gynecologic cancers, benign tumors, or bleeding disorder
- Social history, since lower socioeconomic level and smoking are associated with earlier menopause

---

values of FSH and estradiol during the perimenopause, tests for these hormones are not diagnostically useful unless repeated over time. Other laboratory tests are tailored to the clinical findings. Because the incidence of endometrial cancer in women from the age of 35 to 44 years is almost three times higher than those between 20 and 34 years (10), the American College of Obstetrics and Gynecology (ACOG) has recommended an endometrial evaluation in women 35 years or older with abnormal bleeding (11).

Either endometrial biopsy (EMB) or transvaginal ultrasound (TVUS) can be used as the initial endometrial evaluation of the postmenopausal or anovulatory perimenopausal woman. In ovulating perimeopausal women, an EMB is the best first evaluation because an ultrasound may not be able to exclude endometrial cancer. Each has its advantages and disadvantages in achieving the goals of excluding endometrial cancer and identifying the source of the bleeding. The choice of EMB or TVUS depends upon the physician's assessment of the woman's risk, the patient population, the availability of high-quality sonography, and patient preference. Both diagnostic modalities have similar sensitivity for the detection of endometrial carcinoma in postmenopausal women. However, some clinicians prefer endometrial biopsy as the initial diagnostic test for women with abnormal uterine bleeding due to its high sensitivity, low complication rate, availability, and low cost (11).

When compared to the historic "gold standard" of dilation and curettage, the EMB is an office-based, simple, cost-effective procedure that has high diagnostic accuracy. In the evaluation of abnormal bleeding, studies (11) show the sensitivity for EMB ranges from 90% to 98% when compared with dilation and curettage. A meta-analysis (11) showed that the detection rate for endometrial cancer utilizing EMB in perimenopausal women is less than the rate using EMB in postmenopausal women, with a sensitivity of 91% versus 99.6%, respectively. Endometrial biopsy also has been reported to miss up to 18% of focal endometrial lesions. Overall, EMB utilizing the Pipelle procedure was superior in detection rates of cancer compared to other devices. Transvaginal ultrasound also can be used to evaluate the endometrial layer and measure the thickness of the endometrial "stripe" (the thickness of the endometrium). The sensitivity of TVUS endometrial stripe evaluation for detection of endometrial cancer is reportedly 91–96%, but the specificity is as low as 58% (11). An endometrial biopsy or other evaluation modality is required if the endometrial lining is >4–5 mm in thickness, the endometrial stripe is not well visualized, the endometrial lining is diffusely or focally irregular, or the woman has persistent bleeding.

In the setting of persistent menstrual bleeding with a negative or benign biopsy, further diagnostic evaluation is indicated. Endometrial cancer and atypical hyperplasia have been diagnosed in up to 20% of women studied with an initially negative biopsy (11). Depending upon prior evaluation, a combination of repeat endometrial biopsy or hysteroscopy/dilation and curettage with transvaginal sonohysterography (saline-infused imaging) or ultrasonography should be pursued (12).

Management of Cycle Irregularity and Menorrhagia

Once the perimenopausal bleeding evaluation reveals no cancerous or precancerous lesions, educating and monitoring a patient may be sufficient. Women may not appreciate the lifestyle effects of irregular and unpredictable menstrual cycles bring. After assessing the woman's risks, exogenous hormones are commonly used to regulate menstrual bleeding. Low-dose combined estrogen and progesterone oral contraceptive pills (OCPs) containing 20 µg of ethinyl estradiol have been shown to be effective in reducing blood loss, improving menstrual cycle regularity, diminishing hot flashes, providing contraception, and improving overall quality of life (11). As a woman reaches the average menopause age of 50–51 years, some clinicians discontinue OCPs completely because of the increased risks of breast cancer, blood clots, stoke, and heart disease described in the Women's Health Initiative (WHI) Study (13). To diminish the return of hot flashes, the clinician can taper the OCPs over 6 weeks.

Contraception can be continued until menopause, at which time hormone replacement therapy (HRT) can be instituted, following recommended guidelines to treat vasomotor symptoms, if necessary. Due to the risks described in the WHI, however, many clinicians are cautious about starting HRT and will encourage women to try all other available options first. Although there are no definitive markers of menopause, repeated levels of FSH of 20 mg/dl or higher in combination with vasomotor systems are suggestive of the late menopausal transition. If FSH and estadiol levels are used as markers in women taking OCPs, the levels may be checked on day 5–6 of the placebo pills. After 2 weeks off OCPs, FSH and estradiol levels can be rechecked. An increase in FSH levels and no change in basal estradiol levels indicates menopause. Then, if the woman has moderate to severe vasomotor symptoms and understands her risks and benefits regarding HRT, the lowest dose of HRT can be started. The goal is to taper the patient off HRT after about 3 years and no later than 5 years. A slow taper over a 3-6 month period may decrease rebound vasomotor symptoms (13).

When estrogen is contraindicated (i.e. in smokers, or women with a history of blood clots or breast cancer), progesterone hormonal therapy may be an option. Depot medroxyprogesterone acetate (MPA) may be effective, but women can experience spotting or amenorrhea. Given the high frequency of anovulatory cycles in the perimenopausal stage, some clinicians advocate cyclic progestins for 10–14 days each month, especially in women with infrequent periods (11).

Management of menorrhagia includes many of the same hormonal treatments used to control cycle irregularity but with mixed results. OCPs can significantly diminish menstrual cycle flow. Nonsteroidal anti-inflammatory drugs (NSAIDs) can decrease menstrual cramping and blood loss by up to 40%. Cyclic and depot progestins have not been effective for long-term treatment of menorrhagia (11). The progestin-releasing intrauterine device (IUD) is approved by the US Food and Drug Administration for contraception only, but it is also an effective treatment for menorrhagia (14). The IUD releases levonorgestrel 20 µg/day for 5 years. The levonorgestrel IUD reduces menstrual blood loss more effectively than OCPs or oral progestins, often inducing amenorrhea (14).

When medical therapy is unsuccessful, several effective surgical options are available, including endometrial ablation and hysterectomy. Endometrial ablation is a clinically effective, low morbidity, cost-effective procedure in the short-term, but up to 40% of women will require a repeat procedure or hysterectomy with 4 years of the procedure. Hysterectomy is the definitive therapy for menorrhagia (15).

Summary

Perimenopausal bleeding is a normal variation in a woman's reproductive life. The clinician can determine when such bleeding is abnormal by understanding the normal reproductive physiology and evaluating the patient with a thorough history and physical exam. Only if indicated, other diagnostic tools may be implemented. For the majority of women, the treatment of perimenopausal bleeding is reassurance and observation.

References

1. **Gold EB, Bromberger J, Crawford S, et al.** Factors associated with age at natural menopause in a multiethnic sample of midlife women. Am J Epidemiol. 2001;153:865–74.
2. **Soules MR, Sherman S, Parrot E.** Rebar. Executive summary: stages of reproductive aging workshop (STRAW). Fertility and Sterility. 2001;76:874–8.

3. **Mansfield PK, Carey M, Anderson A, et al.** Staging the menopausal transition: data from the Tremin Research Program on Women's Health Issues. 2004;14:220-6.
4. **Hall JE.** Neuroendocrine physiology of the early and late menopause. Semin Reprod Med. 2007;25:344-51.
5. **HaleGE, BurgerHG.** Perimenopausal reproductive endocrinology. Endocrinology and Metabolism Clinics. 2005;34:907-22.
6. **Jain A, Santoro N.** Endocrine mechanisms and management for abnormal bleeding due to perimenopausal changes. Clin Obstet Gyn. 2005;48: 295-311.
7. **Farquhar CM, Steiner CA.** Hysterectomy rates in the United States 1990-1997, Obstet Gynecol. 2002;99:229-34.
8. **Philipp CS, Faiz A, Dowling N, et al.** Age and the prevalence of bleeding disorders in women with menorrhagia. Obstet Gynecol. 2005;105:61-6.
9. **Albers JR, Hull SK, Wesley RM.** Abnormal uterine bleeding, American Family Physician. 2004;69:1915-26.
10. SEER cancer statistics review, 1975-2004 (serial on line). Available at: http://seer.cancer.gov/csr/1975_2004/.
11. **Espindola D, Kennedy KA, Fischer EG.** Management of abnormal uterine bleeding and the pathology of endometrial hyperplasia. Obstet Gynecol Clin North Am. 2007;34: 717-37.
12. **Goldstein SR.** Abnormal uterine bleeding: the role of ultrasound, Radiologic Clinics of North America. 2006;44:901-10.
13. **Reed SD, Newton KM, LaCroix AZ.** Indications for hormone therapy: the post-Women's HealthInitiative era. Endocrinol Metab Clin North Am 2004;33:691-715.
14. **Sitruk-Ware R.** The levonorgestrel intrauterine system for use in peri- and postmenopausal women. Contraception. 2007;75:155-60.
15. **Van Voorhis BJ.** Genitourinary symptoms in the menopausal transition. Am J Med. 2005;118:47-53.

B. Management of Menopausal Symptoms

Katherine L. Margo

KEY POINTS

◆ Vasomotor symptoms are the most common symptoms related to menopause and can last for years.

◆ Estrogen is the most effective treatment for hot flashes, but other medications such as selective serotonin reuptake inhibitors (SSRIs), selective norepinephrine reuptake inhibitors (SNRIs), clonidine, and gabapentin have also been shown to be effective.

◆ Most alternative treatments are not effective for hot flashes, though soy and black cohosh have some weak evidence of effectiveness.

> ◆ Vaginal symptoms, which can be problematic for years, are best treated by topical estrogen.
> ◆ Insomnia and some sexual disorders can be related to menopause, but the possibility of underlying depression must be considered.

Menopause is defined as the cessation of menstruation. It can be diagnosed after a woman has no menses for a year. The average age of menopause is 51, but symptoms can start years before and extend for years after (1). Smokers, on average, have an earlier menopause. There are a multitude of symptoms that relate to menopause. Some symptoms are limited to the perimenopausal period (typically the 3–5 years surrounding the menopause), but some, particularly the urogenital symptoms, can continue for many years after menopause occurs. The psychological symptoms, too, may be ongoing, depending on a woman's psychological state predating the menopausal period (2).

Treatment of Vasomotor Symptoms/Hot Flashes

Vasomotor symptoms (hot flashes or night sweats) are the most common symptoms related to menopause. Most women (85%) have hot flashes, but only half are disturbed by them (1). Fifty percent of women have hot flashes for 5 or more years. Women who have a surgical menopause have the most severe symptoms. The cause of vasomotor symptoms is not completely understood. These symptoms appear to be related to falling levels of estrogen that trigger a dysfunction in the thermoregulatory system. Not all women get vasomotor symptoms. Levels of estrogen cannot predict who will have the most severe symptoms. While not all women need to be treated, for some women hot flashes are intolerable and interfere with daily activities and sleep. Although the duration of vasomotor symptoms can be years, most women are relieved to know that the symptoms will resolve eventually.

Lifestyle Treatments

Several lifestyle changes have been studied in relation to the severity and number of hot flashes (3). Exercise has been shown in observational studies to reduce the frequency of hot flashes, but the evidence is not strong (3). Exercise does, however, improve the quality of life in the menopausal period. Dietary changes, especially increase in soy and flaxseed, have been recommended but have not been shown to be effective in rigorous studies. Smoking is associated with earlier, more frequent, and more intense hot flashes, so smoking cessation may benefit women with vasomotor symptoms (3). Similarly, a BMI >30 is associated with more hot flashes making weight loss beneficial (3).

Hormonal Treatment

Hormone treatment (HT), either with estrogen alone or in combination with progesterone in either a cyclic or continuous manner, is the most effective treatment to decrease the frequency and severity of hot flashes (4). Because of the association of HT with increased cardiovascular disease and breast cancer in the Women's Health Initiative (WHI) study, many women and their healthcare providers are reluctant to use HT, or, if they do, limit its use to a short duration (5). However, many physicians and their patients feel that the benefits can outweigh the risks, especially in women in the perimenopausal and immediate postmenopausal periods when the symptoms are the worst and the risks the least. In general, the lowest dose of estrogen that is possible is used for as short a time as possible (3). Estrogen can be given orally or by patch and has been found to work in low doses. Progesterone in combination with estrogen is used for women who have a uterus in order to prevent the development of endometrial cancer.

Synthetic progesterone alone also can decrease vasomotor symptoms, but its use is limited because of side effects. Plant-derived micronized progesterone cream was shown in one small study to decrease hot flashes with minimal side effects (6).

Non-Hormonal Treatments

Several other classes of medications have shown some effect compared to placebo in treating hot flashes. Antidepressants of the SSRI or SNRI type, such as venlafaxine, paroxetine, and fluoxetine, have the most evidence. In addition, clonidine and gabapentin also have some effect in reducing hot flashes (5). The side effects of these medications may limit their use.

Herbal Treatments

Many herbal treatments have been tried for treating hot flashes. The use of botanicals can be problematic because they are not regulated by the FDA. Some women have good results with herbal treatments despite the lack of evidence supporting their use. Red clover isoflavone extracts did not reduce frequency of hot flashes, and there were mixed results for soy isoflavone extracts in several studies (7). Black cohosh may be somewhat effective; dong quai (used alone) and evening primrose have not been shown to be effective. Acupuncture has not been shown to be effective (8).

Vaginal Symptoms

Vaginal symptoms can be the most troublesome of all menopausal symptoms, since they do not get better over time. The main symptoms of atrophic vaginitis are vaginal irritation, dryness, and pain with intercourse. In contrast to vasomotor symptoms, which usually develop in the perimenopausal time frame, vaginal atrophy does not occur until a woman's estrogen levels have been low for some time. Vaginal lubrication provides some relief, especially before intercourse. Women can use vaginal moisturizers to keep the tissue from cracking. Estrogen is the most effective treatment and can be given systemically and locally. Local treatment is first line, since it does not have the side effects of systemic estrogen administration (9). Local treatment with estrogen cream or an estrogen-containing vaginal ring can be used long-term without the complications of oral estrogen. Women who use vaginal estrogen cream do not need concomitant progesterone administration because the risk of endometrial proliferation from low-dose local estrogen is very low (9).

Insomnia

Insomnia is often related to hot flashes at night (nightsweats) that can be treated as above. The cause of insomnia is often multifactorial, including medications, depression, anxiety, and other chronic medical problems. In addition to treatment to reduce nightsweats, eszopiclone (brand name Lunesta) has been shown to decrease insomnia in the setting of menopause (10).

Sexual Symptoms

As women age, many experience variable changes in their sexuality. Responsiveness to sexual stimuli for menopausal women and their partners tends to decrease with age, and libido can be significantly decreased in some women. Many menopausal women have pain with intercourse from vaginal atrophy. Sexual issues may also be related to whatever psychological or relationship issues that are present. Treatment of the vaginal symptoms can be very helpful. Testosterone treatment may be helpful for decreased libido, based on a few small studies (11). The only readily available testosterone treatment for postmenopausal women in the U.S. is a combination of testosterone and estrogen.

Psychological Symptoms

Menopause represents a significant transition in a woman's life. It reflects not only the loss of fertility but is also an unavoidable sign of aging. Some women find it a difficult time for these reasons, but some enjoy the fact that they no longer have periods and do not have to worry about contraception. A number of psychological symptoms, such as irritability, depression, and anxiety, have been associated with menopause, and women with preexisting anxiety have more menopausal symptoms (12). The healthcare provider is challenged to determine whether a woman's symptoms reflect a psychological or psychiatric disorder versus normal changes related to menopause. Psychotherapy and appropriate psychiatric medication should be considered for any troublesome psychological symptoms. Estrogen has been shown to increase the overall quality of life and decrease depression, though it should not be relied upon for women with moderate to severe depression or anxiety (13).

Conclusion

Menopause is a normal transition in a woman's life. Most of the symptoms can be treated with multi-dimensional therapies. HT continues to be the most effective treatment for many menopausal symptoms, but side effects and long-term health risks limit its usefulness and it is therefore used infrequently.

References

1. **Mitchell ES, Woods NF, Mariella A.** Three stages of the menopausal transition from the Seattle Midlife Women's Health Study: toward a more precise definition. Menopause. 2000;7:334–49.
2. Our Bodies, Ourselves: Menopause. The Boston Women's Health Book Collective. Touchstone. New York 2006.
3. **Santoro NF, Clarkson TB, Freedman RR, et al.** Treatment of menopause-associated vasomotor symptoms: position statement of the North American Menopause Society. Menopause. 2204;11:11–33.
4. **MacLennan AH, Broadbent JL, Lester S, et al.** Oral oestrogen and combined oestrogen/progestogen therapy versus placebo for hot flushes. Cochrane Database Syst Rev. 2004;(4):CD002978.
5. **Rossouw JE, Anderson GI, Prentice RI, et al.** Risks and benefits of estrogen plus progestin in healthy postmenopausal women: principal results from the Women's Health Initiative randomized controlled trial. JAMA. 2002;288:321–33.
6. **Leonetti HB, Longo S, Anasti JN.** Trandermal progesterone cream for vasomotor symptoms and postmenopausal bone loss. Obstet Gynecol. 1999;94:225–8.
7. **Nelson HD, et al.** Nonhormonal therapies for menopausal hot flashes: systematic review and meta-analysis. JAMA. 2006;295:2057–71.
8. **Morelli V, Naquin C.** Alternative therapies for traditional disease states: menopause. Amer Fam Phys. 2002;66:129–33.
9. The role of local vaginal estrogen for treatment of vaginal atrophy in post-menopausal women: 2007 position statement of the North American Menopause Society. Menopause. 2007;14:357–69
10. **Soares CN, Joffe H, Rubens R, et al.** Eszopiclone in patients with insomnia during perimenopause and early postmenopause: a randomized controlled trial. Obstet Gynecol. 2006;108:1402–10.
11. **Margo KL, Winn R.** Testosterone treatments: when, why and how? AFP. 2006;73:1591–8.
12. **Freeman EW, Samuel MD, Lin H, et al.** The role of anxiety and hormonal changes in menopausal hot flashes. Menopause. 2005;12:258–66.
13. **Hlatky MA, Boothroyd D, Vittinghoff E, et al.** Quality-of-life and depressive symptoms in postmenopausal women after receiving hormone therapy. Results from the Heart and Estrogen/Progestin Replacement Study (HERS) trial. JAMA. 2002;287:591–7.

17

Postmenopausal Women

A. Postmenopausal Bleeding

Judith A. Gravdal

KEY POINTS

- Postmenopausal bleeding (PMB) is a common symptom encountered in the primary care setting.
- Malignancy is identified in 10–20% of patients with PMB.
- An evaluation to rule out malignancy is mandatory.
- Many tests and diagnostic approaches are available; tissue sampling for pathologic evaluation is generally recommended.
- Recurrent or persistent bleeding must be reevaluated.
- Obesity prevention and treatment may decrease the risk of malignancy.

Epidemiology

Postmenopausal bleeding (PMB) is defined as bleeding that occurs >12 months after the last menstrual period (1). The incidence of PMB varies with the time lapsed since the last menstrual period. An overall incidence of 10.7% was found in one Danish study (2). During the first 1–2 years of menopause, the rate was higher, 409/1000 person-years. In later menopause (>3 years since the last period), the rate dropped to 42/1000 person-years. Although a minority of women who experience PMB are found to have endometrial carcinoma, this diagnosis must be excluded (3). Recommendations for evaluation are guided by the risk of malignancy and the sensitivity and specificity of the available diagnostic tests.

Clinical Presentation

The climacteric or perimenopausal period may be marked by either regular periods that suddenly cease or by increasingly irregular periods with ultimate cessation of bleeding. Postmenopausal bleeding most commonly presents with spotting or light flow. Heavy flow with clotting is uncommon in the postmenopausal woman. Associated symptoms are infrequent. Hale and Fraser (3) report that 4.5% of all postmenopausal women have at least one episode of bleeding that occurs more than a year after the last menstrual period and that 10–20% of these will be due to genital tract malignancies.

Bleeding can be the presenting symptom of many conditions. The postmenopausal endometrium is atrophic and, thus, very thin, usually

≤3 mm. Although a benign etiology is found in the vast majority of women experiencing postmenopausal bleeding, premalignant and malignant causes are the underlying consideration of the physician evaluating a woman who presents with bleeding after menopause.

Diagnosis and Differential Diagnosis

The most frequent causes of PMB are atrophic endometrium, neoplasm, and hormone replacement therapy. With the declining use of hormone replacement therapy, this will become a less frequent factor in PMB. Box 17-1 outlines the differential diagnosis of PMB.

Benign, premalignant, and malignant neoplasms can present with postmenopausal bleeding. Neoplasms may be focal, that is, localized to a specific site in the endometrium. Endometrial polyps are common

---

Box 17-1   Causes of Postmenopausal Bleeding

- Atrophic endometrium
- Neoplasia
  - Benign
  - Premalignant
  - Simple hyperplasia
  - Hyperplasia with atypia
  - Complex hyperplasia
  - Malignant
  - Metastatic
  - Breast, gallbladder, bladder, and sarcoma
- Medications
  - Estrogen
  - Tamoxifen
  - Anticoagulants
- Genetic
  - Hereditary nonpolyposis colorectal cancer
- Coagulopathies
  - Thrombocytopenia
  - Acute leukemia
  - Liver disease
- Mechanical
  - Trauma to external genitalia
  - Advanced pelvic prolapse with irritation to vagina and/or cervix
  - Foreign body
- Infectious
  - Tuberculosis
- Vascular
  - Arteriovenous malformation
- Trophoblastic disease—hydatidiform mole

focal lesions and carry an increased risk of malignancy in the postmenopausal woman (4). Common among diffuse or non-focal lesions that result in PMB is hyperplasia, which may be simple, atypical, or complex. The most frequent malignant cause of PMB is adenocarcinoma of the endometrium, although it is important to recognize that not all endometrial cancers present with bleeding.

Well-established risk factors for uterine malignancy include nulliparity, obesity, unopposed estrogen use, and tamoxifen. A family history of hereditary non-polyposis colorectal cancer increases the risk of endometrial cancer (1). Evidence also suggests that diabetes, alcohol intake, and high fat diet confer higher risk. Patients with one or more risk factors require a more urgent and thorough evaluation. Rarely, postmenopausal bleeding is caused by metastatic cancer from remote sites, such as breast, gall bladder, sarcoma, or bladder.

Medications such as estrogen, tamoxifen, and anticoagulants uncommonly cause postmenopausal bleeding. The patient taking tamoxifen, especially after longer duration of therapy, is at higher risk for developing uterine malignancy. Some herbal medications, such as garlic, gingko biloba, and ginseng, interfere with coagulation and may result in PMB.

Underlying coagulopathies, which increase the risk of bleeding in general, may lead to postmenopausal bleeding. Thrombocytopenia, acute leukemia, and severe liver disease are examples. Mechanical causes of non-uterine bleeding include trauma to the external genitalia, irritation to the vagina and/or cervix due to advanced pelvic prolapse, and the presence of a foreign body. Very rare causes include uterine infections (of which tuberculosis is probably the most common), arteriovenous malformations, and trophoblastic disease (hydatidiform mole).

Diagnostic Evaluation

Diagnostic evaluation always begins with a thorough history. Box 17-2 outlines important areas to be covered. The pertinent examination begins with the pelvic exam. A thorough pelvic exam can assist in the identification of non-uterine causes of PMB, such as vaginal atrophy, foreign bodies in the vagina, urethral, vaginal, or vulvar lesions, or trauma. The history may suggest the need for examination of other body areas.

A Pap smear should be performed, if not done recently. The Pap smear is necessary to evaluate the cervix but does little to aid in the investigation of PMB. Blood tests are of little value in the evaluation of PMB. If the patient is hemodynamically unstable, a hemoglobin is warranted. If the history and physical examination suggest coagulopathy, liver disease, or other non-uterine cause, then appropriate studies are indicated.

The evaluation of the endometrial lining is the key aspect of the diagnostic work-up of any woman who experiences PMB. Many options are available. The work-up for a patient with PMB is in evolution. Both imaging and tissue sampling are warranted. Factors that influence the choice of test include availability of procedures, convenience, patient acceptability, and cost. As the available technology evolves, recommen-

---

Box 17-2   Important Elements in the History of Postmenopausal Bleeding

- Nature of bleeding
  - Quantity
  - Frequency
  - Duration
- Prior history of bleeding or bruising problems
- Trauma history
- Associated symptoms
  - Pelvic discomfort
  - Vaginal discharge
- Medical history
  - Diabetes mellitus
  - Obesity
  - History of malignancy
- Drugs
  - Prescription
  - Over-the-counter
  - Herbal supplements
  - Alcohol use
- Pregnancy history
- Menopause history
- Family history
  - Hereditary cancers
  - Bleeding disorders

---

dations for the work-up will change. Figure 17-1 summarized current recommendations.

Endometrial biopsy — Obtaining tissue for pathological evaluation is crucial to the assessment of PMB. The development of devices such as the Pipelle™ has made uterine sampling safe and easy in the office setting. This procedure is well within the scope of most primary care clinicians. The procedure may even be performed during the presenting visit.

Because this procedure samples the uterus in a limited and non-directed way, lesions can be missed. Haung (5) reported a sensitivity of 93.8% for low-grade cancer and 99.2% for high-grade cancer. Unsuccessful attempts may result from patient intolerance of the procedure, cervical stenosis, or other reasons, and in those situations, referral for further testing is needed. A non-diagnostic sample also requires further evaluation.

Ultrasound — As the technology of ultrasound evolves, its use permits one to distinguish with acceptable reliability the thickness of the uterine lining. The lining of the atrophic endometrium is about 3 mm. Ultrasound can generally provide accuracy within 2 mm. The most widely accepted cut-off for a normal postmenopausal endometrial lining (stripe) is 4 mm. Heterogeneity of the endometrial stripe is of concern. Ultrasound can often delineate fibroids and polyps. The correlation of

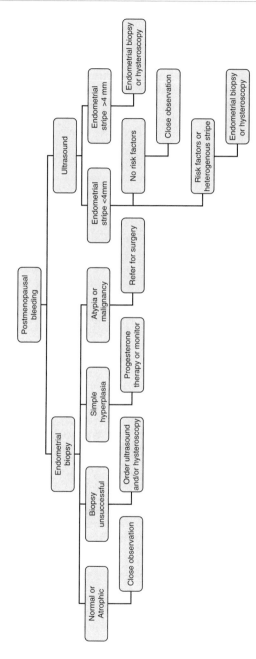

Figure 17-1   Algorithm for the evaluation of postmenopausal bleeding.

uterine lining thickness and malignant or premalignant conditions has been described by Opmeer (6).

Ultrasound alone cannot provide tissue for evaluation. Transvaginal ultrasound, which is relatively low in cost and high in safety and reliability, can guide the clinician in determining the appropriate next step. Watchful waiting may be acceptable in patients who have been on hormone replacement therapy for <12 months or in patients who have an endometrial stripe of 4 mm or less.

Transvaginal power Doppler sonography provides blood flow mapping and can suggest neovascular causes of bleeding, but it is still under investigation (7). In the future, this technology may play a role in the evaluation of PMB.

Hydrosonogram (or Sonohysterography)

The injection of 10 cc of saline into the uterine cavity in conjunction with ultrasonography permits more accurate depiction of the surface of the endometrial lining. Focal lesions, such as polyps or submucosal fibroids, may be identified (8). Like ultrasound, this test does not allow for tissue sampling.

Dilation and Curettage

Although dilation and curettage can be both diagnostic and therapeutic, it is no longer recommended in the evaluation of postmenopausal bleeding. The risk-benefit ratio is not acceptable when the risk of anesthesia, the risk of missing focal abnormalities, and the availability of alternative approaches are considered.

Hysteroscopy

This procedure permits diagnostic evaluation of both focal and diffuse disease (9). The limits of hysteroscopy are primarily availability and cost. It is an excellent secondary test in the evaluation of PMB.

Hysterectomy

Hysterectomy provides definitive evaluation and treatment for PMB. This major surgery is associated with significant morbidity, mortality, and cost. In selected patients, it may be the approach of choice.

Prevention and Clinical Care

The multiple causes of PMB preclude any one method for preventing bleeding after menopause in all women. The risk factors for malignancy in PMB have been outlined by the American Cancer Society and include nulliparity, obesity, diabetes, and years since menopause (10). Although there are no studies providing evidence that weight reduction can prevent or reduce the risk of either PMB or endometrial cancer, the prevention and treatment of obesity is warranted.

The clinician trained to perform office endometrial biopsy may offer this as initial evaluation. A biopsy result of either normal endometrium or endometrial atrophy can be followed by watchful waiting. Hyperplasia without atypia can be managed by evaluating hormonal status and a consideration of progesterone cycling (daily for 2 weeks, followed by 2 weeks off, for 3–6 months). If biopsy is unsuccessful or if the pathology shows atypia or malignancy, referral for further evaluation and treatment is warranted. Persistent bleeding after a negative work-up always warrants further or repeat evaluation. Close follow-up of women experiencing recurrent or persistent bleeding should be ensured.

References

1. Postmenopausal uterine bleeding. Available at www.guideline.gov December 31, 2007.
2. **Astrup K.** Frequency of spontaneously occurring postmenopausal bleeding in the general population. Acta Obstst Gynecol Scand. 2004;83:203–7.
3. **Hale Georgina E, Fraser Ian S.** Changes in the Menstrual Pattern During the Menopause Transition. In Lobo, Rogerio A (ed): Treatment of the Postmenopausal Woman: Basic and Clinical Aspects. 3rd Edition. Burlington, MA: Elsevier; 2007. p. 152.
4. **Ben-Arie A.** The malignant potential of endometrial polyps. Eur J Obstet Gynecol Reprod Biol. 2004;115:206–10.
5. **Huang GS, Gebb JS, Einstein MH, et al.** Accuracy of preoperative endometrial sampling for the detection of high-grade endometrial tumors. Am J Obstet Gynecol. 2008;196:243:e1–243, e5.
6. **Opmeer BC.** Improving the existing diagnostic strategy by accounting for characteristics of the women in the diagnostic work up for postmenopausal bleeding. BJOG. 2007;114:51–8.
7. **AlcAjzar JL.** Reproducibility of endometrial vascular patterns in endometrial disease as assessed by transvaginal power Doppler sonography in women with postmenopausal bleeding. J Ultrasound Med. 2006;25:159–63.
8. **Meng K.** The short-term clinical outcomes after saline infusion sonohysterography in women with postmenopausal bleeding. Acad Radiol. 2005;12:136–41.
9. **Litta P.** Role of hysteroscopy with endometrial biopsy to rule out endometrial cancer in postmenopausal women with abnormal uterine bleeding. Matuitas. 2005;50:117–23.
10. What Are the Risk Factors for Endometrial Cancer? Revised November 27, 2006. Available at www.cancer.org. December 31, 2007.

B. Falls Assessment

Melissa M. Stiles and Kathleen E. Walsh

KEY POINTS

- Thirty percent of people over the age of 65 fall annually.
- Falls result in significant morbidity and mortality.
- Postfall anxiety syndrome can lead to self-imposed functional limitations.
- Multifactorial interventions can reduce the rate of falls up to 30–40%.

Epidemiology of Falls

Falls result in significant morbidity, mortality, decreased function, and an increased rate of nursing home placement. Yearly, approximately 30% of persons over the age of 65 fall at least once and the incidence increases with age. Up to 10% of falls result in serious injury such as hip fracture, other fracture, or head injury including subdural hematomas. In the U.S., hip fractures currently account for more than 300 000 hospitalizations with a 1-year mortality rate of up to 33% (1,2). By 2050, it is estimated that the worldwide number of hip fractures will rise to 6.26 million. Falls also cause functional limitations by both direct injury and indirect psychological consequences. Loss of self-confidence in ambulation can lead to postfall anxiety syndrome and self-imposed limitations in activity. Postfall anxiety syndrome can also result in depression and social isolation. The cause of falls is often multifactorial and so the assessment and intervention targets a number of areas (3).

Risk Factors

The following risks factors for falling have been identified in at least 2 observational studies:

- Arthritis
- Depression
- Decreased muscle strength
- Age
- Past history of a fall
- Impairment in cognition
- Four or more prescription drugs

- Visual impairment
- Gait disturbance
- Impairment in balance

The risk of falling increases significantly in people with multiple risk factors. Taking 4 or more prescription drugs is in itself a risk factor for falling. Also, several medication classes have a higher potential to cause falls, including tricyclic antidepressants, neuroleptic agents, serotonin-reuptake inhibitors, benzodiazepines, and class 1A antiarrhythmic medications (4).

Screening

The US Preventive Services Task Force (USPSTF) recommends that all persons older than 75, as well as those 70–74 with known risk factors be counseled on measures to reduce falls (5). "Have you had any falls in the past year?" is a simple screening question that can be answered by the patient or caregiver in a previsit questionnaire. For those patients who have not fallen, the pretest probability of a fall in the upcoming year ranges from 19% to 36%. In these patients, assessment of gait and balance offers the highest potential yield from screening. Gait and balance risk factors have been found to more frequently predict future falls compared to other domains. Asking the patient, "Have you noticed any problems with gait, balance or mobility?" is another easy screening question. Answering "yes" to either screening questions warrants further assessment (Figure 17-2) (6,7).

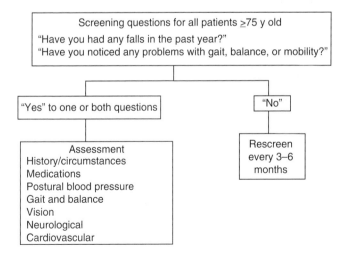

Figure 17-2   Clinical approach to falls assessment.

Assessment

The assessment should begin with a multifactorial evaluation followed by interventions targeting the identified risk factors (Table 17-1). A history of previous falls and the circumstances surrounding the fall(s) can help pinpoint which of the risk factors are involved. One of the most prominent modifiable risk factor is medication use. Central nervous system (CNS)

Table 17-1   Assessment and Management of Community-Dwelling Older Persons at Risk of Falling

Risk Factor	Management/Intervention
Circumstances surrounding fall (e.g., location, activity)	Changes in environment and behavior
Medications High risk: benzodiazepines, neuroleptics, antidepressants, anticonvulsants, class IA antiarrythmics) 4 or more medications	Review, change, or eliminate medications
Postural Hypotension ≥20 mm Hg (or ≥20%) drop in systolic pressure with or without symptoms, either immediately or within 2 min or standing	Diagnosis and treatment of underlying cause. Change or eliminate medications; adequate hydration; adjustment of salt intake; compensatory strategies
Gait and Balance Self report or observation Impairment on brief assessment (e.g. Get-Up and Go test*)	Diagnosis and treatment of underlying cause. Environmental interventions; physical therapy; assistive devices
Vision Acuity <20/60; decreased depth perception decreased contrast sensitivity; cataracts; glaucoma; macular degeneration	Appropriate lighting without glare; avoid multifocal glasses when walking; ophthalmologist evaluation
Neurological Impaired cognition Decreased proprioception Diminished muscle strength	Diagnosis and treatment of underlying cause; assistive devices; appropriate footwear Change in medications; caregivers awareness of impaired cognition
Cardiovascular Syncope Arrhythmia	Cardiology referral; medication adjustments
Home Hazard Evaluation	Remove loose rugs; use of nightlights; nonslip bathmats; bath and stair rails

*Get-Up and Go Test: The patient gets up out of a standard armless chair, walks 10 feet, turns and walks back to chair and sits down. <10 seconds: freely mobile; <20 seconds: mostly independent; <30 seconds: variable mobility; >30 seconds: impaired mobility. From Podsiadlo D, Richardson S. The timed "Up & Go": a test of basic functional mobility for frail elderly persons. J Am Geriatr Soc. 1991 Feb;39:142–8; with permission.

medications, such as benzodiazepines, antidepressants and neuroleptics have been linked to the occurrence of falls. Use of 4 or more medications, frequent medication changes and increased dosages are also risk factors (8). Dizziness or lightheadedness, which can be associated with postural hypotension, can affect up to 30% of elderly patients. Disturbances in gait and balance can be identified either through the patient or caregiver's direct report or a simple office-based assessment such as the "Get-Up and Go test" (9). Impaired vision resulting from decrease in visual acuity, depth perception, contrast sensitivity and dark adaptation has been associated with both falls and hip fractures. Decreased proprioception, impaired cognition and decreased muscle strength are important risk factors that need to be assessed during the neurological exam. Targeted cardiovascular conditions associated with increased fall risk include history of syncope and/or arrhythmia. Finally, home-hazard evaluation and intervention is an essential component in the assessment of falls in the elderly (10,11).

Summary

Falls are one of the most common and treatable geriatric syndromes. Approximately 30–40% of community-dwelling patients older than 65 years fall each year. All patients 75 years and older (or younger patients known to be at risk) should be screened for falls every 6–12 months. Evidence has demonstrated that a multifactorial approach and intervention strategy is needed to effectively reduce the rate of falling in older patients.

References

1. **Sattin RW.** Falls among older persons: a public health perspective. Annu Rev Public Health. 1992;13:489–508.
2. **Tinetti ME, Speechley M, Ginter SF.** Risk factors for falls among elderly persons living in the community. N Engl J Med. 1988;319:1701–7.
3. **Nevitt MC, Cummings SR, Kidd S, et al.** Risk factors for recurrent nonsyncopal falls. A prospective study. JAMA. 1989;261:2663–8.
4. **Rubenstein LZ, Josephson KR.** The epidemiology of falls and syncope. Clin Geriatr Med. 2002;18:141–58.
5. U.S. Preventive Services Task Force. Guide to clinical preventive services: report of the U.S. Preventive Services Task Force. 2d ed. Baltimore: Williams & Williams, 1996.
6. **Tinetti ME.** Clinical practice. Preventing falls in elderly persons. N Engl J Med. 2003;348:42–9.
7. UCLA Medical Center Geriatrics. Pre-visit questionnaire: initial visit. http://www.geronet.ucla.edu/centers/acove/office_forms/Pre-Visit_Questionnaire.doc. Accessed January 5, 2006.
8. **Hanlon JT, Schmader KE, Koronkowski MJ, et al.** Adverse drug events in high risk older outpatients. J Am Geriatr Soc. 1997;45:945–8.
9. **Podsiadlo D, Richardson S.** The timed "Up & Go": a test of basic functional mobility for frail elderly persons. J Am Geriatr Soc. 1991;39:142–8.

10. **Gillespie LD, Gillespie WJ, Robertson MC, et al.** Interventions for preventing falls in elderly people. Cochrane Database Syst Rev. 2001;(3): CD000340.
11. **Stevens M, Holman CD, Bennett N.** Preventing falls in older people: impact of an intervention to reduce environmental hazards in the home. J Am Geriatr Soc. 2001;49:1442–7.

C. Geriatric Assessment

Melissa M. Stiles

KEY POINTS

- The goals of the geriatric assessment are to maintain function and preserve quality of life.
- The geriatric assessment domains are medical, functional, psychological and social.
- A medication review is an essential component of a geriatric assessment.
- A multidisciplinary approach is used to identify intervention and management strategies.

Background

According to the U.S. Census Bureau predictions, the percentage of people over the age of 65 will almost double by the year 2020 (1). The purpose of a geriatric assessment is to identify conditions which lead to significant morbidity in the elderly. Elders identified at risk in the initial assessment are then targeted for further evaluation and interventions to modify risk. The emphasis of the assessment is to preserve function and quality of life. Key components include medical, functional, psychological, and social assessments (2,3).

Medical Assessment

The components of the medical assessment include a review of the medical record, medication overview, and a nutritional assessment. The medical review focuses on conditions which are more common in the elderly (geriatric syndromes) and have significant comorbidities. Review of systems should be complete with special emphasis on sensory impairment, dentition, mood, memory, urinary symptoms, history of falls, nutrition, and pain. The US Preventive Task Force recommends routine screening for visual and hearing impairment (4). Adverse drug reactions (ADRs) are a significant public health issue, especially in the elderly (5). Polypharmacy (>4 medications) is an independent risk factor for both delirium and falls (6,7). Review of the current medication list including over the counter medications is an essential component of the assessment. Malnutrition and undernutrition can lead to significant problems including delayed healing and longer hospital stays. A good marker of nutritional problems is weight loss; >5% in the past month and a 10% or greater weight loss in the last 6 months (8).

Functional Assessment

One of the primary goals of the geriatric assessment is to identify interventions to maintain function and thus lengthen duration of staying at home in independent living situations. The functional assessment focuses on activities of daily living (ADLs) and falls risk screening. The basic ADLs include eating, dressing, bathing, transferring, and toileting. The instrumental ADLs (IADLs) are shopping, managing money, driving, using the telephone, housekeeping, laundry, food preparation, and managing medications (9). Home health and/or social services referral should be considered for patients who have difficulty with the ADLs. The patient should also be screened for gait and mobility problems by first asking: "Have you fallen all the way to the ground in the past 12 months?" A positive screen should lead to a more thorough evaluation and consideration of a physical therapy referral (see Section B).

Psychological Assessment

The psychological assessment screens for cognitive impairment and depression, 2 conditions which significantly impact both the patient and their families. The most studied test to screen for cognition is the mini-mental state examination which is best for identifying patients with moderate or severe dementia (see Chapter 7D). Depression can be readily screened with shorter versions of the original 30 item Yesavage geriatric depression scale (GDS) (10). The 5 item version of the GDS involves asking the following:

1. Are you basically satisfied with you life?
2. Do you often feel bored?
3. Do you often feel helpless?
4. Do you prefer to stay home rather than going out and doing new things?
5. Do you feel pretty worthless the way you are now?

A score of greater than two positive answers is positive (Sensitivity 97%, Specificity 85%) (11). The Yale Depression Screen ("Do you often feel sad or depressed?") is a validated one-item GDS screening tool (12).

Social Assessment

It is important to assess the patient's living situation and social support when performing a geriatric assessment. The living situation should be evaluated for potential hazards especially if the patient is identified as a fall risk. The social assessment also includes questions about financial stressors and caregiver concerns. Advance planning is a key component of the assessment and includes clarifying the patient's values, setting goals for care in case of future incapacity, including identifying the patient's power of attorney for health care.

Summary

A geriatric assessment can identify frequent problems, thus leading to earlier interventions for the common medical and social concerns of the elderly. The keys to an effective assessment are to have a questionnaire targeted to the geriatric assessment domains completed ahead of time and to utilize a multidisciplinary approach to interventions and management. Preserving function and maintaining quality of life are the primary goals of the assessment.

References

1. U.S. Census Bureau, 2004, U.S. Interim Projections by Age, Sex, Race, and Hispanic Origin.
2. **Miller K, Zylstra R, Standridge J.** The geriatric patient: a systematic approach to maintaining health. American Family Physician. 2000;61;1089–104.
3. **Wiland D, Hirth V.** Comprehensive geriatric assessment. Cancer Control. 2006;10:454–62.
4. U.S. Preventive Services Task Force. Guide to clinical preventive services: report of the U.S Preventive Services Task Force. 2d ed. Baltimore: Williams & Williams, 1996.
5. **Thomsen LA, Winterstein A, Sondergaard B, et al.** Systematic review of the incidence and characteristics of preventable adverse drug events in ambulatory care. The Annals of Pharmacotherapy. 2007;41:1411–26.
6. **Moylan K, Binder E.** Falls in older adults: risk assessment, management and prevention. The American Journal of Medicine. 2007;120:49e1–493e6.
7. **Inoye S.** Prevention of delerium in hospitalized older patients: risk factors and targeted intervention strategies. Ann Med. 2000;32:257–63.
8. **Huffman G.** Evaluating and treating unintentional weight loss in the elderly. American Family Physician. 2002;65:640–50.
9. **Katz S.** Assessing self-maintenance: activities of daily living, mobility, and instrumental activities of daily living. Journal of the American Geriatrics Society. 1983;31:721–7.
10. **Yesavage JA, Brink RL, Rose TL, et al.** Development and validation of a geriatric depression screening scale: A preliminary report. Journal of Psychiatric Research. 1983;17:37–49.
11. **Rinalde P, Mecocci P, Benedetti C, et al.** Validation of the five-item geriatric depression scale in elderly subjects in three different settings. Journal of the American Geriatric Society. 2003;51:694–8.
12. **Mahoney J, Drinka TJ, Abler R, et al.** Screening for depression: single item GDS. Journal of the American Geriatrics Society. 1994;42:1006–8.

D. Urinary Incontinence

John W. Stutsman and Paul G. Schoon

KEY POINTS

- Incontinence is a very common medical problem, affecting up to 30% of the adult female population.
- It is far more common in young and middle-aged women than in men, and the incidence increases as people age.
- Most cases can be evaluated and treated by a primary care provider.
- Based on the working diagnosis, many treatment options exist, including behavior modification, pelvic exercises, pharmacologic agents, vaginal pessary, and surgical procedures.
- Stress incontinence is the most common type of incontinence, followed by urge incontinence.

Epidemiology and Economic Impact

The involuntary loss of urine affects approximately 20–30% of women >18 years, with the incidence 2–3 times greater for women than men (1,2). No more than a third of incontinent women will present with this complaint unless specifically screened during an office visit (3). Economic impact of routine care for each incontinent woman ranges from $50 to 700 each year. In 1995, estimates of annual direct costs in the U.S. were >$16 billion (4).

Anatomy and Physiology

The bladder and the proximal urethra are intraperitoneal organs that rest on the pelvic diaphragm; this allows increased intra-abdominal pressure transferred to the bladder to be transferred to the proximal urethra to aid in urethral closure and thus continence. The sympathetic innervation originates from the thoracolumbar spinal cord (T11 through L2-L3). Beta receptors are primarily located in the bladder and alpha receptors in the bladder neck and urethra. Stimulation of the beta receptors promotes relaxation, while stimulation of the alpha receptors promotes increased tone, thus assisting urethral closure. The parasympathetic innervation originates in the sacral spinal cord (S2-S4). The postganglionic transmitter is acetylcholine, and it acts on muscarinic receptors (M2 and M3). Stimulation of these receptors (mainly M3) causes detrussor contraction and relaxation of the urethra, promoting micturition.

Continence can be affected at many levels: at the cerebral cortex, affecting conscious control of micturition (e.g., central nervous system trauma or tumors, dementia, cerebrovascular accident); at the spinal level by demyelinating diseases (e.g., multiple sclerosis); damage at the peripheral nerve level (e.g., diabetes and other vascular diseases, obstetric trauma); and pelvic support damage (e.g., obesity, chronic obstructive pulmonary disease, obstetric trauma, connective tissue disorder).

Categories of Urinary Incontinence

1. *Stress incontinence*—This is the most common type of incontinence, in which detrussor (bladder) pressure exceeds urethral pressure, thus allowing loss of urine. History includes urine loss with coughing, sneezing, heavy lifting, laughing, and/or exercise. Conditions that cause increase intra-abdominal pressure, such as chronic obstructive pulmonary disease (COPD) or chronic cough, can increase the risk of stress incontinence. An episode of incontinence coincides with the moment of increased intra-abdominal pressure. The loss is usually a small volume, not the entire bladder content. A good history and Urolog (see below) are quite sensitive for the diagnosis of stress urinary incontinence (5). Medication ingestion should be reviewed, including angiotensin-converting enzyme (ACE) inhibitors (iatrogenic cough), alpha adrenergic antagonists (urethral relaxation), and narcotics (constipation).

2. *Urge incontinence*—Leakage occurs due to uncontrolled contraction of the detrussor muscle, causing urine leakage (one can have urinary urge symptoms without loss of urine in the case of overactive bladder [OAB]). This type of incontinence increases as women age. Patients give a history of losing urine because of a strong urge and are unable to get to toilet in time. They are more likely to report loss of the entire content of the bladder, loss of urine during intercourse, nocturia, or enuresis, as opposed to what occurs in stress incontinence. The hallmark symptom is urinary frequency (voiding more than every 2 hours and >8 times a day). A good history and Urolog are quite sensitive and specific for the diagnosis (5).

3. *Mixed incontinence*—Urinary loss with symptoms of both stress and urge incontinence. This is the second most common type of urinary incontinence in women.

4. *Overflow incontinence*—Incomplete emptying of bladder, allowing an excessive amount of urine to fill the bladder, leading to urinary leakage. This inability to completely void bladder contents is usually due to outflow obstruction (e.g., tumor, urolithiasis) or neurogenic disease (e.g., multiple sclerosis, diabetes mellitus). It is far less common in women than in men. The diagnosis is confirmed by a small, slow void and a post-void residual volume of >100 ml (usually >200 ml) on

more than one occasion. Many medications can cause or worsen the symptoms, including sedating antipsychotic medications with their anticholinergic side effects, narcotics, alpha-adrenergic agonists, beta-adrenergic agonists, or calcium channel blockers.

5. *Bypass incontinence*—Constant loss of urine due to communication of the urinary tract with the outside (usually the vagina). Certain congenital abnormalities (e.g., ectopic bladder, ectopic ureter inserting into the vagina or distal to the external sphincter into the urethra) are major causes of this type of incontinence, but they are typically diagnosed during early childhood. Fistulae (vesicovaginal, ureterovaginal, vesicouterine) due to obstetric trauma, prior pelvic surgery, and/or pelvic radiotherapy are the most likely etiologies of bypass incontinence presenting in the adult.

Evaluation

Evaluation of a woman with incontinence begins with a thorough history and physical examination. The history should begin with review of any event(s) preceding the incontinence episodes, such as coughing, sneezing, laughing, exercise, urge, or intercourse. Other important elements in the history include the duration of symptoms and the presence or absence of nocturia (number of voids/night), enuresis (loss of urine during sleep), dysuria, or pain associated with a full bladder (or relieved with micturition). A full evaluation of current medications, including over-the-counter and herbal preparations, that may affect bladder functioning is also important.

The physical exam of the incontinent patient should include a neurological exam to assess motor strength and reflexes. A thorough pelvic exam should assess pelvic organ prolapse (e.g., cystocele, rectocele, uterine prolapse, etc.) and the presence of an estrogenic effect (e.g., pink vaginal mucosa, normal vaginal ruggae). A stress test should be preformed; this is a Valsalva maneuver (such as a cough) with a full bladder (about 250 cc) to check for demonstrable urinary leakage. If the test is negative when the patient is supine, it should be repeated while standing over a large pad. A Q-tip test can be done by placing a lubricated swab into the urethra to the urethrovesical junction and asking the patient to perform a Valsalva maneuver while supine; a change of >35 degrees is suggestive of poor urethrovesical support (urethral hypermotility). The urethra should be palpated to examine for tenderness and/or urethral diverticulum. With the latter, one may be able to milk purulent material from the urethral meatus by palpating under the vaginal mass.

A Urolog or voiding diary is a chart sent home with the patient to evaluate for excessive fluid intake or for bladder irritants (e.g., caffeinated or carbonated beverages, alcohol), timing of and symptoms associated with episodes of incontinence, and frequency of micturition. It should be measured over the course of 2–7 days (a thorough 24–48-hour diary is better than a poorly recorded week's worth of data). The patient will need an accurate means to measure urinary output. An example is located in Table 17-2 (6).

Table 17-2

Patient name:

INTAKE AND VOIDING DIARY

INSTRUCTIONS:
1. Begin recording upon rising in the morning—continue for a full 24 hours.
2. Record separate times for voids, leaks, and fluid intake.
3. Measure voids in "cc's" using the hat.
4. Measure fluid intake in ounces.
5. When recording a leak, please indicate the volume ("1,2, or 3"), your activity during the leak, and if you had an urge ("yes" or "no").

This chart is a record of your fluid intake, voiding and urine leakage.

Choose 4 days (entire 24 hours) to complete this record—they DO NOT have to be in a row.

Pick days in which it will be convenient for you to measure EVERY void.

Please bring this diary to your next visit.

Examples of entries

DATE:

TIME	Amount voided (in cc's)	LEAK Volume 1 = drops/damp 2 = wet-soaked 3 = bladder emptied	Activity during leak	Was there an urge?	Fluid intake (Amount in ounces/type)
7:00a	240 cc	2	Running	Yes	
7:30a					8 oz. Herbal tea

DATE:

TIME	Amount voided (in cc's)	LEAK Volume 1 = drops/damp 2 = wet-soaked 3 = bladder emptied	Activity during leak	Was there an urge?	Fluid intake (Amount in ounces/type)

DATE:

TIME	Amount voided (in cc's)	LEAK Volume 1 = drops/damp 2 = wet-soaked 3 = bladder emptied	Activity during leak	Was there an urge?	Fluid intake (Amount in ounces/type)

DATE:

TIME	Amount voided (in cc's)	LEAK Volume 1 = drops/damp 2 = wet-soaked 3 = bladder emptied	Activity during leak	Was there an urge?	Fluid intake (Amount in ounces/type)

All women with incontinence should have a urinalysis and urine culture to identify urinary tract infections (UTIs) which can cause acute incontinence. Often, after antibiotic treatment for the UTI, the incontinence will resolve. Persistent glucosuria and hematuria require further evaluation.

A post-void residual (PVR) measures the amount of urine left in the bladder after a routine void. It can be performed by sterile in-and-out catheterization or by transabdominal ultrasound immediately following voiding (7). If the PVR is >100 ml on two occasions, it can signify overflow incontinence (neurogenic or outflow obstruction).

Urodynamic testing includes a cystometrogram to determine bladder capacity and the presence of bladder spasms (detrussor instability, consistent with urge incontinence).

A cystoscopy can be done in the urologist's office with CO2 or saline as a distension medium to assess urethra and bladder mucosa for abnormalities (e.g., urethral diverticulum, bladder mucosal glomerulations of chronic interstitial cystitis, and/or neoplasm).

Intravenous pyelogram (IVP) is used to assess renal function and ureteral integrity (e.g., obstructing urolithiasis). CT or MRI of abdomen/pelvis also provide images of the urinary system with greater definition but at a greater expense. A voiding cystourethrogram (VCU) assesses bladder integrity and helps identify urethral diverticuli. Ultrasound can image the kidneys and bladder, as well as assess urethral motility in real time. It is relatively inexpensive and carries no risk of dye exposure.

Most diagnoses can be made with the urinalysis with culture and sensitivity history, physical, and Urolog, after which the appropriate treatment(s) may be started. If additional testing is required that is unavailable or unfamiliar to the primary care provider, the patient should be referred to a gynecologist, urologist, or urogynecologist, who can perform the additional testing and offer therapies, including surgical options (Table 17-3).

Pharmacotherapy

The mainstay of treatment for urge incontinence is anticholinergic medications (antimuscarinics) (11,12). Many patients (10–25%) abort this therapy because of side effects (e.g., xerostomia [dry mouth], constipation, blurry vision, elevated intraocular pressure, gastroesophageal reflux, urinary retention, cognitive impairment, delirium) or lack of adequate effect. Cessations of treatment rates are even higher (up to 80%) when looking over a year or more of therapy (14,15). The major complaint is xerostomia, which can be minimized by having water available to sip and/or sucking on hard candy (Table 17-4).

As in the case with stress urinary incontinence, large trials have *not* shown estrogen replacement to be beneficial in the treatment of urge urinary incontinence (16,17) (Table 17-5).

Table 17-3 Therapeutic Options

Stress Urinary Incontinence—Nonsurgical Treatment		
Treatment	**Comments**	**Side Effects/Risks**
Behavioral modifications	• Adequate hydration (>1 L but <3 L) Document on Urolog • Smoking cessation (to minimize chronic cough) • Scheduled voiding every 3–6 h • Avoid and/or treat constipation	Minimal to none
Weight reduction	BMI <30 kg/m² (may resolve symptoms or improve outcomes of other therapy) (8,9,10)	None, plus added health benefits
Pelvic floor (Kegel) exercises	See Figure 17-3	• Minimal to none • Requires self-motivation
Pessary	Fit appropriate pessary (i.e. incontinence ring) to aid in urethral closure pressure	• Vaginal irritation or erosion fistula (rare). • Minimize risks with daily cleansing and removal and replacement the next day
Estrogen	• Does not improve incontinence by itself (11,12) • May use topical therapy to treat vaginal atrophy so menopausal patient may better tolerate pessary (13)	Uterine bleeding, endometrial cancer, nausea, local irritation, thromboembolic events, CVA, MI
Absorbent Hygienic Pads	• The major contributor to money spent on incontinence in the U.S. (4) • Change often to avoid breakdown of skin and/or infection from prolonged exposure to moisture	• Expensive over the long term • Skin breakdown and ulcer formation
Stress Urinary Incontinence—Surgical Treatment		
Procedure	**Comments**	**Side Effects/Risks**
Retropubic colposuspension (Burch; Marshall–Marchetti–Kranz)	• Gold standard for SUI w/urethral hypermotility • Open or laparoscopic • Excellent long term results (≥85% 5-year cure rates) (1)	Anesthesia, infection, bleeding, bladder or ureteral damage, new onset or worsening of urinary urgency, urinary retention

cont'd

Table 17-3   Therapeutic Options (cont'd)

Stress Urinary Incontinence—Surgical Treatment		
Procedure	Comments	Side Effects/Risks
Suburethral sling (tension-free vaginal tape)	• Synthetic mesh placed beneath proximal urethra via suprapubic, transvaginal, or transobturator approach • Can be done under local or regional anesthesia • Limited long term data show cure rates comparable to Burch procedure	Anesthesia; infection; bleeding or hematoma formation; bladder, bowel, or major vascular damage; urinary urgency/retention; erosion of mesh into urethra, bladder, or vagina
Periurethral infection of bulking agents	• Done via cystoscope in outpatient surgery or office setting • Bovine collagen, carbon-coated beads, silicone particles	Anesthesia, infection, hematoma, urinary retention (rare), short-lived results (~12 months)

Urge Incontinence—Nonsurgical/Nonpharmalogic Treatments		
Therapy	Comments	Side Effects/Risks
Behavioral modifications	• Avoid possible bladder irritants (i.e., caffeine, carbonated beverages, alcohol, spicy foods) • Adequate fluid intake (>1L/day)	None
Bladder training	• Increase the time patient holds urine before voiding—increase time by 30 min between each void every 1–2 wk until able to limit to 8 voids or less daily • Requires keeping urolog	None (requires self-motivation)
Pelvic floor exercises	See Figure 17-3 (combine w/bladder training)	None
Absorbent hygienic pads	Expensive over the long term (4)	• Minimal • Skin ulcers if changed infrequently

Mixed Incontinence Treatments

The first-line of therapy is a combination of pelvic floor exercises (Figure 17-3a,b) plus bladder training and/or anticholinergics. Weight loss should be encouraged in obese patients. Pessary placement should be considered if there is accompanying pelvic organ prolapse and/or a stress

Table 17-4

Urge Incontinence—Pharmacotherapy		
Drug	**Dosage**	**Comments**
Oxybutynin	• IR—2.5–5.0 mg po TID • ER—5–15 mg po every day • Transdermal 3.9 mg/day patch—apply every 4 d	• ER & transdermal formulations have less anticholinergic side effects (18) • Local skin irritation seen w/patch
Tolterodine	• IR—1–2 mg po BID • ER—2–4 mg po every day	ER appears to be better tolerated than IR formulation
Solifenacin	5–10 mg po every day	In clinical trials, discontinuation rates were similar to placebo
Darifenacin	7.5–15 mg po every day	Less xerostomia but increased constipation
Trospium chloride	20 mg po BID	It is hydrophilic thus should have less CNS effects in the elderly

IR = immediate release.
ER = extended release.

Table 17-5

Urge Incontinence—Surgical Therapy		
Procedure	**Comments**	**Side Effects/Risks**
Sacral neuromodulation	• Mild electrical stimulation of sacral nerve by implanted device (this interrupts reflex detrussor contractions) • FDA approved in 1997	General anesthesia, infection, bleeding, need to redo procedure in up to 1/3 of cases (19)
Cystectomy with urinary diversion or neo-bladder construction	Limited to only the most severe cases that are refractory to all other treatments	General anesthesia, infection, bleeding, damage to bowel (especially if portion harvested for neo-bladder), chronic post-op pain, need for chronic catheterization
Botulinum toxin injections (20)	• Injected into bladder mucosa at 15–30 separate sites via cystoscopy • Off label use, thus some payors may not cover this expensive medication	Anesthesia (can be done under local or regional), urinary retention, short-lived results (6 months)

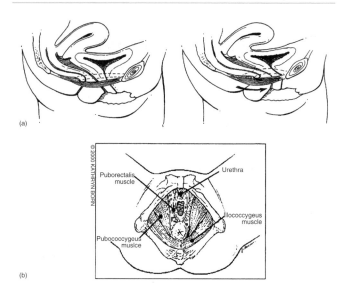

Figure 17-3   Pelvic muscle (Kegel) exercises. (a) Pelvic diaphragm with pubococcygeus at rest and contracting to aid in continence. (From Wall LL. Novak's Gynecology (12th Ed) 1996:621; with permission.) (b) Muscles of levator ani; palpate these during a pelvic exam to help patient isolate for proper pelvic floor exercises. (From Culligan PJ, Heit M. AFP 2000;62:2247; with permission.)

This can be taught at any female health visit (prenatal visit, routine exam) or with any patient suffering from incontinence to increase or maintain health and tone of pelvic floor musculature. During a vaginal exam palpate the pubococcygeus (Figure 17-3b) and have the patient contract her pelvic floor muscles (levator ani which includes pubococcygeus). Assure that she is *not* contracting her abdominal *nor* gluteal muscles; this will only be counterproductive. When the patient is at home, she may isolate these muscles by stopping her stream of urine during micturition. Have her do this only the first few times, as this may cause an unhealthy reflex if done repetitively. The patient should hold the contraction for 10 seconds and do a set of 10, resting 10 seconds between contractions. She should do 3 sets a day each day for ***at least 6–8 weeks***, and then do 3 sets of 10, 3–4 times a week to maintain the strength and hypertrophy of her pelvic floor musculature. One can further this by teaching her to coordinate pelvic floor contractions with inciting events (i.e. lifting, sneezing, coughing).

If one does not have the time or training to instruct patients in your office, some physical therapy groups offer pelvic floor rehabilitation. Biofeedback techniques (electronic or weighted vaginal cones) can be used to augment pelvic muscle exercises, though randomized control trials are mixed as to whether they improve outcome (22,23). These may be considered in patients having difficulty isolating the correct muscles with simple office training and follow-up.

component. The practitioner should allow at least 6–8 weeks of therapy before considering the treatment a failure; such patients, and those desiring surgical options, will need urodynamic testing by a specialist.

Overflow Incontinence Treatment

The etiology should be identified and eliminated if possible. Intermittent self-catheterization approximately every 4–6 hours is the preferred route over a chronic indwelling catheter with its high risk of bacterial colonization and infection. Neurosacral modulation, as with urge incontinence, appears to be of benefit for these patients as well (21).

Women with fistulae generally require surgical repair of the defect and, thus, will need the attention of a specialist. A bladder fistula may be temporized by placing an indwelling urinary catheter (Figure 17-4).

Refer to specialist if:
- recurrent or persistent UTI
- persistent hematuria despite UTI treatment
- patient desires surgical management
- prior urinary incontinence surgery within the past 6 months
- treatment failure after at least 6–8 weeks
- overflow incontinence is suspected (particularly newly diagnosed and/ or in the young patient)
- bypass incontinence is suspected

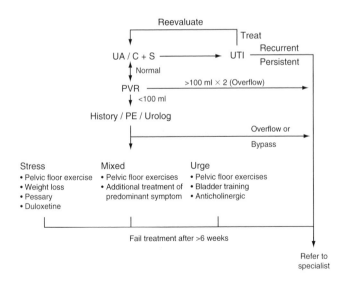

Figure 17-4   Algorithm for assessment/treatment of urinary incontinence.

References

1. **Stenchever MA.** Urogynecology, Comprehensive Gynecology, 4th ed., 2001:607–40
2. **Gibbs CF et al.** Office management of geriatric urinary incontinence. Am J Med. 2007;120:211–20.
3. **Vigod SN, Stewart DE.** Treatment patterns of Canadian women with urinary incontinence: a need to improve case identification. Journal of Women's Health. 2007;16:707–12.
4. **Subak L, Van Den Eeden S, Thom D, et al.** Urinary incontinence in women: direct costs of routine care. AJOG. 2007;197:596–8.
5. **Martin JL et al.** Systemic review and meta-analysis of methods of diagnostic assessment for urinary incontinence. Nerourology and Urodynamics. 2006;25:674–83.
6. **Cholhan HJ.** Female urinary incontinence, www.augs.org
7. **Lertbunnaphong T et al.** Transabdominal ultrasound in the assessment of postvoid residual urine volume in patients after hysterectomy. Journal of the Medical Association of Thailand. 2006;89:152–7.
8. **Lawrence JM, Lukacz ES, Liu ILA, et al.** Pelvic floor disorders, diabetes, and obesity in women: findings from the Kaiser-Permanente continence associated risk epidemiology study. Diabetes Care. 2007;30:2536–41.
9. **Vikrup L, Yalcin I.** Duloxetine treatment of stress urinary incontinence in women: Effects of demographics, obesity, chronic lung disease, hypoestrogenism, diabetes mellitus, and depression on efficacy. Ejogrb. 2007;133:105–13.
10. **Townsend MK et al.** Body mass index, weight gain, and incident urinary incontinence in middle-aged women. Obstetrics and Gynecology. 2007;110: 346–53.
11. **Hashim H, Abrams P.** Overactive bladder: an update. CurrOpin Urol. 2007;17:231–6.
12. **Wagg AS et al.** Overactive bladder syndrome in older people. BJU International. 2007;99:502–9.
13. **Hanson LAM, Schulz JA, Flood CG, et al.** Vaginal pessaries in managing women with pelvic organ prolapse and urinary incontinence: patient characteristics and factors contributing to success. Int Urogynecol J. 2006;17:155–9.
14. **Hashim H, Abrams P.** Drug treatment of overactive bladder: efficacy, cost, and quality-of-life considerations. Drug. 2004;64:1643–56.
15. **Kelleher CJ, Cardozo LD, Khullar V, et al.** A medium-term analysis of the subjective efficacy of treatment for women with detrussor instability and low bladder compliance. Br J Obstet Gynaecol. 1997;104:988–93.
16. **Waetjen EL, Duyer PL.** Estrogen therapy and urinary incontinence: what is the evidence and what do we tell our patients? Int Urogynecol J. 2006;17:541–5.
17. **Palmer MH, Newman DK.** Urinary incontinence and estrogen: is hormone replacement therapy an effective treatment? AJN. 2007;107:35–7.
18. **Curtwright R, Cardozo L.** Transdermal oxybutynin: sticking to the facts. Eururo. 2007;51:907–14.
19. **Elliott DS, Boone TB.** Neuromodulation for idiopathic detrussor instability and urge incontinence, Female Pelvic Reconstructive Surgery 2003 (eds. Stanton SL, Zimmern P):315–20.

20. **Casanova N et al.** Botulinum toxin: a potential alternative to current treatment of neurogenic and idiopathic urinary incontinence due to detrussor overactivity. Int Journal of Gyn and OB. 2006;95:305–11.
21. **Hussain Z, Harrison SCW.** Neuromodulation for lower urinary tract dysfunction – an update. TSWJ. 2007;7:1036–45.
22. **Gray M, David DJ.** Does biofeedback improve the efficacy of pelvic floor muscle rehabilitation for urinary incontinence or overactive bladder dysfunction in women? JWOCN. 2005;July/August:222–5.
23. **Choi H, Palmer MH, Park J.** Meta-analysis of pelvic floor muscle training. Nursing Research. 2007;56:226–34.

E. Caring for the Dying Woman

Rose M. Guilbe and Janet M. Townsend

KEY POINTS

- Healthcare providers can have a profound impact on the experience of a dying woman by careful listening and partnering with her and her loved ones to maximize the quality of her life as she approaches death.
- Women's experience of and response to a terminal illness are influenced by social roles and responsibilities.
- Symptoms at the end of life are very distressing and can be managed by attentive and expert care.
- Mobilizing the support of family, friends and an interdisciplinary team enhances the care of women who are dying.
- Attending to spiritual and religious concerns is important to women at the end of life.

Primary care providers will ultimately care for women who are dying. Though the care of all dying patients is challenging, caring for women in such circumstances poses issues particular to women's multiple social and family roles. This chapter aims to provide a framework for addressing the specific needs of women at the end of life. It is essential to approach each patient's needs systematically, addressing specific goals of care along with the meaning of an incurable illness to the patient, her family, and her loved ones. Achieving relief of important medical symptoms while addressing the patient's (and often the family's) emotional, spiritual, and social distress is the ultimate goal. This frequently involves an interdisciplinary approach and partnership with the patient, her family, and pastoral counselors. Our conversations with dying women must allow us to listen to the their needs, recognize their suffering, validate their experience, communicate hope, negotiate treatment and palliative care options, and support them throughout the trajectory of the illness.

Causes of Death in Women

Women in the U.S. die most frequently from cardiovascular disease and cancer. HIV infection is the third leading cause of death among all U.S. women aged 25–44 years and the leading cause of death among African American women in this age group (1). Cancer, HIV/AIDS, diabetes, violence against women, and mental illness have been identified as the highest priority areas for preventing premature death in minority women. Globally, complications of pregnancy and childbirth are the leading cause of death in women of reproductive age in developing countries, with the greatest burden among young women from 15 to 19 years of age and in Asia and sub-Saharan Africa. HIV/AIDS also has been a major contributor to mortality in women in Africa and Asia in recent decades (2).

The Younger Dying Woman

Younger women's initial responses to a life-threatening or terminal illness are characterized by shock, anger, and fear. A woman in this position experiences: 1) an inability to reconcile the diagnosis and prognosis with her previously healthy and strong self-image; 2) profound fear of the bodily changes that her illness or treatment may cause; and 3) anger at the sudden loss of her life, dreams, and plans. Denial and fear can lead to delays in evaluation and treatment, possibly resulting in a longer and more serious illness course. The effects of the underlying illness and aggressive treatment regimens, such as chemotherapy, can affect her self-image and sense of beauty, due to hair loss, pallor, weight loss, and diminished physical level of function.

Once a young woman has faced her diagnosis, she may still find it very difficult to mobilize the support she needs and to reassess her responsibilities in view of the demands of treatment or the progression of her illness. Disclosure of the diagnosis of a life-threatening illness or, especially, a poor prognosis, to her spouse, partner, family, friends, and children is extraordinarily difficult. Thus, patients frequently benefit from assistance in planning or rehearsing such disclosure. As her illness progresses, she is likely to struggle to maintain the level of multi-tasking and caretaking that typically characterize women's lives. The younger dying woman tends to continue with child-rearing, household, and work obligations as long as she can handle them.

When caring for a woman dealing with conflicts between caretaking responsibilities and her own needs for care and support, healthcare providers can be of great assistance by exploring options for seeking and accepting help from those closest to her. Her loved ones are often

Box 17-3   Healthcare Provider Role: Caring for the Younger Dying Woman

- Support the patient in examining the impact of her terminal illness on her identity, role(s) and aspirations.
- Acknowledge feelings of anger and fear, and support the patient in processing and redirecting these feelings in ways that support her values and beliefs.
- Communicate her clinical status and prepare the spouse/partner and her children according to their level of understanding.
- Discourage isolation and encourage patient to identify a trustworthy friend or relative who can provide comfort and support her in dealing with the fear/pain/conflicts in the dying process.
- Encourage her to connect to and depend upon her support network such as family and friends, pastoral and other community leaders, her children's teachers, and neighbors.

willing to help carry her load but may need coaching on how to proceed. Providers and loved ones need to support a woman's continued participation in roles that are important to her, yet find practical and realistic strategies appropriate for her stage of illness and physical/emotional capabilities. Particularly difficult are decisions about when and how to disclose her terminal condition to her children and how to plan for such issues as custody and their future care. Healthcare providers, family, friends, mental health professionals, and pastoral counselors can all assist in this part of a patient's journey. (Box 17-3)

The Older Dying Woman

The older woman faced with a new diagnosis of a terminal illness or progression of a chronic or previous illness to its terminal phase is likely to understand and accept the diagnosis more readily than does her younger counterpart. She may be better prepared than a younger woman to discuss goals of care and tough decisions with her healthcare provider, especially if the medical, psychosocial, and ethical dilemmas of her terminal illness are dealt with in the context of her individual values and beliefs.

A particular challenge for health professionals assisting an older woman at the end of life is negotiating the involvement of her family in her care and support. The older dying woman may try to protect her spouse, partner, or children, resulting in avoidance of discussion of her diagnosis and condition with them until she is closer to death. This can complicate designation of healthcare proxies or prevent clarity about advance directives and other wishes. Conversely, healthcare providers may face challenges when family members resist informing an elderly woman of her diagnosis and prognosis. Such issues are influenced by cultural norms and need to be addressed respectfully by the healthcare team, while assuring that the older woman does not suffer alone in her knowledge of her impending death (3).

Box 17-4 Healthcare Provider Role: Caring for the Older Dying Woman

---

- Explore the patient's values regarding the care plan and dying process.
- Explore the meaning of the patient's illness and anticipated death in the context of her life history.
- Support the patient in examining her fears about the dying process and provide reassurance about support and medical management.
- Help her to define and communicate values and wishes to family, care providers, and her healthcare proxy regarding goals of care and her specific wishes.
- Encourage her to communicate her needs.
- Assess her level of involvement with clergy or spiritual practices.
- Help her in her transition from caretaker to person in need of help and explore resources for care that are acceptable to her.
- Assess level of responsibilities that she must delegate to others and assist her in asking for help and commitments to carry on key responsibilities.
- Assess financial resources and implication of patient's death on others.

The older woman's role as caretaker also gets in the way of her becoming a patient who needs help. The older woman may in fact be parenting young children (or grandchildren) and feel the need to carry on for their sake. (Box 17-4)

The Influence of Culture on Women and Families at the End of Life

Cultural beliefs, norms and traditions have a tremendous impact on the experience of women and their loved ones as they navigate the final stages of an incurable illness. From the moment of diagnosis through the active dying process and into the mourning period, it is essential to inquire into and assess the relevance of patients' social and cultural context and tailoring plans that meet the particular needs of patient and family members (4). Issues such as disclosure, decision-making, attitudes toward hospice services, and behavior at the time of death are all influenced by cultural beliefs. All of these influences dictate patient and family reactions to their wishes regarding health care (5). Providers should not assume that an individual patient's core health beliefs and current cultural reality necessarily match those of her culture of origin or that of her family. Issues of trust in the healthcare system and in individual providers are especially acute for members of minority communities whose previous encounters with the medical system may have been problematic (6). Health professionals can be instrumental in promoting the integration of healing, family, or mourning rituals and practices into inpatient and outpatient care, and thereby provide tremendous comfort and meaning during difficult times.

Spiritual and Religious Issues

"Regardless of one's particular orientation, every individual has to make a decision as to whether one's life has meaning and value that extends beyond self, life and death" (7). Women often experience profound uncertainty and isolation as they face incurable illness, especially as death approaches. Experiences of "disquieting apprehensiveness" (8) about what the future holds, lack of clarity about what is possible, and a sense of losing control contribute to a woman's uneasiness and discomfort as her illness progresses. Women who have been active in a religious community often draw upon clergy and members of their congregations for support, input regarding treatment decisions, and spiritual guidance. Some women reconnect to the faith in which they were raised. Women who are not involved in organized religion may nonetheless have a meaningful spiritual framework through which they can interpret what is happening to them and the meaning of their death.

Many tools are available to assist providers in exploring the spiritual and religious dimensions of patients' experiences. Collaborating with hospital chaplains or community clergy can support integration of the spiritual and religious dimension of a woman's experience.

Hospice Care

Hospice services, both outpatient and residential, can be a tremendous resource for the patient and her family by providing comfort and support to them when a life-limiting illness no longer responds to cure-oriented treatments. Hospice care aims to improve the quality of a patient's last days by offering comfort and dignity. A team of professionals, volunteers, and family members work together to address all symptoms of a disease, especially pain and discomfort, and to deal with the emotional, social, and spiritual impact of the disease.

Bereavement and counseling services are offered to families before and after a patient's death (9). Primary care and specialist health care providers can offer a great service to dying patients and their families by becoming familiar with local hospice organizations and by making timely referrals.

Strategies to Address Key Issues for Women at the End of Life

Providing exemplary care to women facing incurable disease and approaching death requires a broad repertoire of skills and strategies and, often, a flexible attitude. Access to a trusted healthcare provider over time can help sustain a sense of well-being despite the progression of illness. Family meetings can foster collaboration, clarity about clinical status and expectations, mutual understanding of goals of care, conflict resolution, and shared medical decision-making. Family meetings also offer opportunities to listen to and respond to family member questions or statements, to address emotion through supporting expressions of grief or alleviating feelings of guilt, or to address important aspects of palliative care, including family statements regarding patient preferences or issues related to surrogate decision-making (10). Early and frequent attention to advanced directives, designation of a healthcare proxy, and custody issues is essential to ensuring that patients' wishes are honored.

> Box 17-5   Helpful Questions to Ask Women Who Have a Terminal Illness
>
> ● What do you find hardest about discussing your illness with others?
> ● Who needs to know about your illness (prognosis)?
> ● What are your most important responsibilities? Whom can you trust to carry them on?
> ● What would you most like to accomplish in the next months (weeks)?
> ● Tell me what you think will happen in the next few months.
> ● What role would you like me to play in helping you with your illness?
> ● Tell me (us) something I (we) can do to help you.

Collaboration among diverse members of the healthcare team will result in more appropriate care planning and enhanced services for the patient. Assisting children, other family members, and loved ones through their pain and resulting disorientation are important tasks. Suggesting ways in which family can comfort the dying person is a part of the comfort that the healthcare team can offer. (Box 17-5)

Management of Common Symptoms

Terminally ill women frequently experience troubling symptoms with complicated pathophysiologic mechanisms. Acute pain, shortness of breath, acute delirium, asthenia, anorexia, nausea, and constipation are the more common symptoms presenting challenges to both patient and medical providers. Women may fail to report or minimize symptoms as they struggle to show a good face and continue with "life as usual" for as long as possible. Symptom management at the end of life should not focus on disease management but instead on symptom relief so that women can be comfortable in the presence of loved ones.

Shortness of Breath/Dyspnea

Breathlessness is one of the most frightening and common symptoms for women patients and their families and caregivers. Patients experience a sensation of gasping for air, even when objective measures of respiratory rate, O_2 saturation, or CO_2 retention may not correspond. Air hunger or shortness of breath may result from physical causes, such as pleural effusions, pneumonia, airway obstruction, or pulmonary edema; psychological causes such as anxiety and fear; or religious and spiritual experiences. Approaches to reducing shortness of breath need to be individually tailored and include low doses of opioids or anxiolytics, oxygen and non-pharmacologic modalities such as relaxation techniques, and visual imagery or meditation (11).

Delirium

Delirium and terminal agitation are commonly experienced symptoms during the final stages of life. These potentially reversible changes in cognition are extremely bothersome to both patients and family and should be distinguished from depression/dementia for appropriate treatment. In delirious states, patients exhibit disorientation, perceptual disturbances, fluctuating levels of consciousness, and a decreased ability to focus and sustain attention. The underlying causes include multiple factors, such as infections, metabolic abnormalities, hypoxemia, hypercapnia, tumor burden, renal or hepatic failure, drug interactions, and side effects of patients' medications. A complete review of the patient's physical condition, history, and current medication list is necessary in order to manage the delirium appropriately. Terminal agitation is exhibited by restlessness, a sense of discomfort and inability to cope with their emotional distress caused by physical, psychological, social, or spiritual tensions. Anxiety may contribute to agitation, making assessments very complex, and may require the intervention of an interdisciplinary team of palliative care health providers. Both acute delirium and terminal agitation require pharmacologic and non-pharmacologic management. Medications such as benzodiazepines and narcoleptics (both typical and atypical) and, occasionally, atypical antidepressants can be quite beneficial in managing these symptoms (11).

Pain

Pain is a multi-dimensional experience affecting women approaching the end of life. Effective management must include an effort to identify the underlying cause of the patient's pain and careful assessment of overall pain and sites of pain, with reassessment after initiation or changes of therapy. Analog pain scales, used consistently, provide data that helps with adjustments in management. There are four types of pain, each with different pathophysiologic mechanisms and manifestations: nociceptive pain (somatic/visceral); neuropathic pain; psychogenic pain; and idiopathic pain. Nociceptive pain responds best to NSAIDS and opioids, neuropathic pain to tricyclic antidepressants or anticonvulsants, and psychogenic pain frequently requires a multifaceted approach. The ABCs of pain assessment include **A**. Ask about the pain regularly and assess the pain systematically; **B**. Believe patient and family reports of pain; **C**. Choose a pain control strategy that is appropriate for the specific type of pain the patient is experiencing; **D**. Deliver the intervention in a timely manner; and **E**. Empower and enable the patient to control the management of her pain (12).

Healthcare providers can provide great relief and reassurance to patients by learning effective approaches to managing common symptoms, by consulting palliative care specialists when unsure what to do, and by communicating confidence and commitment to relieving symptoms to both patients and families.

References

1. http://www.cdc.gov/Women/lcod.htm, accessed 4/22/08
2. http://www.populationaction.org/Publications/Reports/Measure_of_
   Survival/sec8.shtml, accessed 4/22/08

3. **Abbott KH et al.** Families looking back: one year after discussion of withdrawal or withholding of life-sustaining support. Crit Care Med. 2001;29;197–201.

4. **Waters CM.** Understanding and supporting African Americans' perspectives of end-of-life care planning and decision making. Qualitative Health Research. 2001;11:385–98.

5. **Trill MD, Holland J.** Cross-cultural differences in the care of patients with cancer: a review. Gen Hosp Psychiatry. 1993;15:21–30.

6. **Hopp FP, Duffy SA.** Racial variations in end-of-life care. J of Amer Ger Soc. 2000;48;658–63.

7. **Okon TR.** Palliative care review: spiritual, religious and existential aspects of palliative care. J of Palliative Med. 2005;8:392–414.

8. **Bunkers SS.** The experience of feeling unsure for women at end-of-life. Nursing Sci Quarterly. 2007;20:56–63.

9. http://www.hospicefoundation.org/hospiceInfo/. Accessed 4/26/08

10. **Curtis JR et al.** Missed opportunities during family conferences about end-of-life care in the intensive care unit. Am J Respir Crit Care Med. 2005;171:844–9.

11. **Ross DD, Alexander CS.** Management of common symptoms in terminally ill patients: Part II: constipation, delirium and dyspnea. Am Fam Physician. 2001;64:1019–26.

12. **Miller KE, Miller MM, Jolley MR.** Challenges in pain management at the end of life. Am Fam Physician. 2001;64:1227–34.

Appendixes

Appendix A. FDA Drugs in Pregnancy Classification

Class A: Adequate, well-controlled studies in pregnant women have not shown an increased risk of fetal abnormalities to the fetus in any trimester of pregnancy.

Class B: Animal studies have revealed no evidence of harm to the fetus; however, there are no adequate and well-controlled studies in pregnant women.

or

Animal studies have shown an adverse effect, but adequate and well-controlled studies in pregnant women have failed to demonstrate a risk to the fetus in any trimester.

Class C: Animal studies have shown an adverse effect and there are no adequate and well-controlled studies in pregnant women.

or

No animal studies have been conducted and there are no adequate and well-controlled studies in pregnant women.

Class D: Adequate, well-controlled, or observational studies in pregnant women have demonstrated a risk to the fetus.

However, the benefits of therapy may outweigh the potential risk. For example, the drug may be acceptable if needed in a life-threatening situation or serious disease for which safer drugs cannot be used or are ineffective.

Class X: Adequate, well-controlled, or observational studies in animals or pregnant women have demonstrated positive evidence of fetal abnormalities or risks.

The use of the product is contraindicated in women who are or may become pregnant.

Available from http://www.fda.gov/fdac/features/2001/301_preg.html#categories

Appendix B.   Levels of Evidence

Level A: Based on multiple high quality randomized controlled trials.

Level B: Evidence from one randomized trial or from other observational studies.

Level C: Based on expert or consensus opinion, case studies, or standard of care.

U.S. Preventive Services Task Force Ratings

Strength of Recommendations

The U.S. Preventive Services Task Force (USPSTF) grades its recommendations according to one of five classifications (A, B, C, D, I) reflecting the strength of evidence and magnitude of net benefit (benefits minus harms).

A.— The USPSTF strongly recommends that clinicians provide [the service] to eligible patients. *The USPSTF found good evidence that [the service] improves important health outcomes and concludes that benefits substantially outweigh harms.*

B.— The USPSTF recommends that clinicians provide [this service] to eligible patients. *The USPSTF found at least fair evidence that [the service] improves important health outcomes and concludes that benefits outweigh harms.*

C.— The USPSTF makes no recommendation for or against routine provision of [the service]. *The USPSTF found at least fair evidence that [service] can improve health outcomes but concludes that the balance of benefits and harms is too close to justify a general recommendation.*

D.— The USPSTF recommends against routinely providing [the service] to asymptomatic patients. *The USPSTF found at least fair evidence that [the service] is ineffective or that harms outweigh benefits.*

I.— The USPSTF concludes that the evidence is insufficient to recommend for or against routinely providing [the service]. *Evidence that the [service] is effective is lacking, of poor quality, or conflicting and the balance of benefits and harms cannot be determined.*

Available from: http:/www.ahrq.gov/clinic/3rduspstf/ratings.htm#irec

Index

Plates

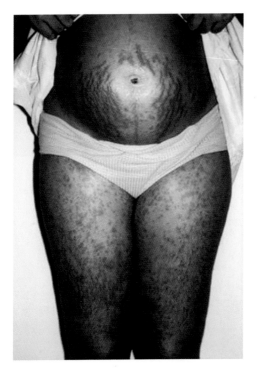

Plate 1   Pruritic urticarial papules and plaques of pregnancy (PUPPP). (Reprinted from Medscape General Medicine 1(2), 1999. http://www.medscape.com/viewarticle/408878 ©1999 Medscape; with permission.)

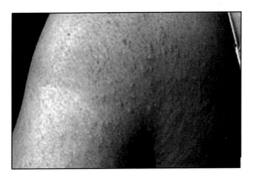

Plate 2   Prurigo gestationis. (Image reprinted from eMedicine.com, 2008; with permission.)

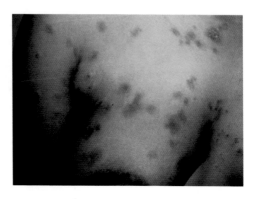

Plate 3   Pemphigoid gestationis. (Reprinted from Medscape General Medicine 1(2), 1999. http://www.medscape.com/viewarticle/408878 ©1999 Medscape; with permission.)

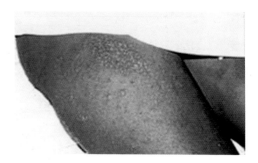

Plate 4   Impetigo herpetiformis. (From Tunzi M, Gray G. Common Skin Conditions During Pregnancy. Am Fam Physician. 2007;75:211–8; with permission.)